Medizinische Informatik und Statistik

Herausgeber: S. Koller, P. L. Reichertz und K. Überla

W0050890

3

Informatics and Medicine

An Advanced Course

Edited by
P. L. Reichertz and G. Goos

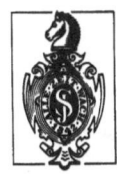

Springer-Verlag
Berlin · Heidelberg · New York 1977

Reihenherausgeber

S. Koller, P. L. Reichertz, K. Überla

Mitherausgeber

J. Anderson, G. Goos, F. Gremy, H.-J. Jesdinsky, H.-J. Lange,
B. Schneider, G. Segmüller, G. Wagner

Bandherausgeber

Prof. Dr. P. L. Reichertz
Abteilung und Lehrstuhl für
Medizinische Informatik
Medizinische Hochschule Hannover
Karl-Wiechert-Allee 9
3000 Hannover 61

Prof. Dr. G. Goos
Universität Karlsruhe
Institut für Informatik II
Postfach 6380
7500 Karlsruhe 1

Library of Congress Cataloging in Publication Data
Main entry under title:

Informatics and medicine.

   (Medizinische Informatik und Statistik ; 3)
   1. Medicine--Data processing--Congresses.
2. Medicine--Documentation--Congresses. I. Reichertz,
P.L, 1930-   II. Goos, Gerhard, 1937-
III. Series.
R858.A1I46   362.1'028'54   77-660

ISBN-13:978-3-540-08120-3   e-ISBN-13:978-3-642-81110-4
DOI: 10.1007/978-3-642-81110-4

Table of Contents

Preface

The modern development of medicine has been characterized by the growing use of new technologies in health care delivery and research. As an empirical science, medicine is based on many types and quantities of information to recognize alterations, explore causes and apply corrective action. Dealing with biological objects, signals have to be collected, processed and interpreted to recognize the state of this object. It is therefore understandable that data processing technology and informatics have been employed to a growing extent in medicine. The increasing economic repercussions of modern medicine lead also to the demand of ways and means to assess the system as such and to develop means for evaluation and regulation.

However, the application of data processing to the medical field has very often grown in parallel to and remote from the development of informatics and data processing in general. Furthermore, difficulties have occurred resulting from the differing concepts of reasoning, decision making and methodology. We therefore decided to start a series of seminars with the attempt to bring scientists from both medicine and informatics together to discuss basic principles of informatics and medicine and to attempt a synthesis between the problems in medicine and health care delivery and methods in informatics to approach a solution of these problems. This volume contains the lecture notes of the first seminar of this type. The goals of this advanced course were:

- to convey knowledge about general and specific problems in theoretical medicine and health care delivery which are suitable for or subject to the application of methods and technology of informatics and data processing,

- to identify and teach systematized concepts and methodology in informatics which relate to the problems and the application of which may open more efficient ways for the solution of these problems in particular and broaden and solidify the knowledge of those who work in leading positions in medical informatics in general.

It is unnecessary to mention that neither the broad field of medicine nor all developments in informatics could be treated during this seminar. Therefore, this volume is a selection of topics presented in a way which still show the inhomogeneity of approaches. The editors hope that this publication will serve as a basis for further seminars of the same type and as a condensation point furthering the development of an adequate methodology to solve specific and general problems in theoretical medicine and health care delivery with its many ramifications.

We are greatly indebted to Mrs. U. Piccolo for her help in preparing this publication and to Drs. Engelbrecht and Wolters who organized the course.

P.L. Reichertz/ G. Goos

Contributors:

ALBER, K., Prof. Dr.
Lehrstuhl A für Informatik
Universität Braunschweig
Gaußstr. 12
D-3300 Braunschweig
Fed. Rep. Germany

ANDERSON, J., M.D.
Professor of Medicine
King's College Hospital Medical School
Denmark Hill
London SE5 8RX
Great Britain

GOLDBERG, M., Dr.
Département de Biophysique
et de Biomathématiques
Faculté de Médecine Pitie-Salpetrière
Boulevard de l'Hôpital
F-75634 Paris Cedex 13
France

GOOS, G., Prof. Dr.
Institut für Informatik
Universität Karlsruhe
Zirkel 2
D-7500 Karlsruhe
Fed. Rep. Germany

GREMY, F. Prof. Dr.
Département de Biophysique
et de Biomathématiques
Faculté de Medecine Pitie-Salpetrière
Boulevard de l'Hôpital
F-75634 Paris Cedex 13
France

GRIFFITHS, M., Prof. Dr.
Departement d'Informatique
I.U.T. de Nancy
2 bis Boulevard Charlemagne
F-5400 Nancy
France

HARTMANN, F., Prof. Dr.
Department Innere Medizin
Medizinische Hochschule Hannover
Karl-Wiechert-Allee 9
D-3000 Hannover 61
Fed. Rep. Germany

LEILICH, H.-O., Prof. Dr.
Institut für Mathematik
Universität Braunschweig
Gaußstr. 28
D-3300 Braunschweig
Fed. Rep. Germany

LOCKEMANN, P.C., Prof. Dr.
Institut für Informatik
Universität Karlsruhe
Zirkel 2
D-7500 Karlsruhe

LODWICK, G.S., M.D.
Professor and Chairman
Department of Radiology
University of Missouri Medical Center
Columbia, Mo 65201
USA

MÖHR, J.R., Priv. Doz. Dr.
Institut für Med. Informatik
Medizinische Hochschule Hannover
Karl-Wiechert-Allee 9
D-3000 Hannover 61
Fed. Rep. Germany

REICHERTZ, P.L., Prof. Dr.
Institut für Med. Informatik
Medizinische Hochschule Hannover
Karl-Wiechert-Allee 9
D-3000 Hannover 61
Fed. Rep. Germany

SCHNEIDER, W., Prof. Dr.
Uppsala Datacentral
Box 2103
S-75002 Uppsala
Sweden

VALLBONA, C., M.D.
Professor and Chairman
Department of Community Medicine
Baylor College of Medicine
Texas Medical Center
Houston, Texas 77025
U.S.A.

WINGERT, F., Prof. Dr.
Institut für Med. Informatik
und Biomathematik
Hüfferstr. 75
D-4400 Münster
Fed. Rep. Germany

BASIC NOTIONS OF INFORMATICS

Gerhard Goos, Karlsruhe

0.Introduction

Informatics is concerned with information processing as supported by technical tools. Today's major technical tool for processing information is the computer. Hence, to a large extent informatics is concerned with computers, their construction and their applications. In the latter area informatics is mainly interested in extracting the common underlying principles of different fields of application and in generalizing those principles to apply them to other fields. This interest is justified by our experience that many applications which, at first sight, seem to not have anything in common, rely on the same methods and can take over many principles from each other.

Historically, informatics arose as an independent science when the growing significance of computers required a deeper understanding of technical information processing. Many insights, however, which were gained in the last decade have a much wider range of applicability than that indicated by computers.

The first part of this lecture discusses the notion of information and its technical representation as data, the notion of algorithm as the fundamental means for describing information processing, and the relationship between algorithms and data. The second part is concerned with how to present algorithms and data to computers and with the development of algorithms for computers.

1. Information and its technical representation by messages

The English word "morning" and the German word "Morgen" represent to those who understand these languages the same information. Without knowledge of these languages this information cannot be derived. We learn from such examples that information is an abstract entity which may be given in various ways by concrete encodings which we call messages. The relationship between a message and its information cannot be deduced; it is a convention which must be learned.

The example further shows that there may be many representations of the same information by distinct messages. Conversely there may be distinct informations which are represented by the same message. Which information is deduced may depend on the context or on the people, or the message is just ambiguous. Whether the sign $\times$ denotes the letter x or a multiplication sign in a mathematical formula depends on the rest of the formula. The letter ε has a very distinguished meaning in mathematics which is usually not deduced by a non-mathematician; the broadcast announcement of a traffic jam carries completely different information for those who are on the road in question than for others. Examples of ambiguities are such well-known sentences as

they are flying planes

or

fruit flies like a banana.

To give a more technical example: 11110000 may be the binary encoding of the digit zero in EBCDI-Code or it may be the binary encoding of the number 240. Also we note that a given message-information relation may hold with a certain probability. Examples are the informations about illnesses deduced from certain chemical determinations in the clinical laboratory.

In conclusion we see that the relationship between messages and informations is a many-to-many relation. An actual relationship is selected by giving an <u>interpretation rule</u> α which states the information $I = \alpha(N)$ for each message N of a class of messages:

$$\alpha : \mathbb{N} \to \mathbb{I}.$$

The interpretation rule is usually given informally, e.g., if somebody understands medical terminology then this means that he knows the interpretation rule for a set of specific medical terms. The interpretation rule could also be stated formally or even by the hardware or software of a computer. For example, a computer in doing floating-point arithmetic shows that it knows how to interpret a bit pattern as a floating-point number.

As the outcome of this discussion, however, we must realize that information processing with technical tools always means message processing with technical tools. If we send informations to a system for automatic information processing e.g., to a computer, then in fact we present messages to the computer which we believe can be interpreted as the required information. If we take results from a computer then we have to interpret them to deriving the information which we require. Also by reasoning about the possible operations which a computer can perform, we easily see that it can only handle messages and can never handle information on the user level.

This insight is important because it shows that in addition to the automatic processing device, we need interpretation rules for how to encode information as input to this device and how to decode the informations from the result messages. A computer never processes medical data but at best bit patterns which might be interpreted as medical data. All too often the computer is blamed for mistakes which result from a lack of knowledge and imprecision in applying the interpretation rules for input or output data.

The interpretation of messages may consist of several hierarchically ordered steps. For example, if we interpret 11 as the binary equivalent of the number 3 then in turn we might see that this is the number of unknowns in a set of mathematical equations, and this value might be implied by the number of dimensions in physical space. In fact, a computer does not work with bits or numbers or strings of characters, for all of these are informations which occur by interpreting certain physical processes, impulses, magnetic states etc. in a suitable manner. We see therefore that whatever we consider as the underlying message M of an information, appears, from another point of view, to be itself an information. Hence, when we say, M is a message, we characterize a certain level of abstraction by showing that it is presently of no concern to us that M itself might be the interpretation of a more elementary message.

2. The Notion of Algorithm

We know now that every information which we wish to process automatically must be encoded as a message and that the result is another message. The word data is commonly used for messages which are the subject or result of such processes. Our next question is: "What are the characteristic properties of processes which can be done automatically, e.g. by a computer?" We restrict ourselves to considering digital computers for which every message is finally coded by a finite sequence of bits. In practice this is no restriction at all, since other types of processing devices, e.g. analog computers, can be simulated easily by digital computers.

For a digital computer every message appears as a sequence of characters or other symbols. This statement is true as well for the input as for the output data. Hence the most general process which we have to consider is the transformation of strings of characters. All such transformations can be composed of elementary replacements of the form

(*) If a substring $a_1 \ldots a_{k-1} \, a_k \, a_{k+1} \ldots a_n$ occurs in the given string then it should be replaced by $a_1 \ldots a_{k-1} \, b \, a_{k+1} \ldots a_n$. If there are more such substrings then replace the leftmost one.

(The string b may be empty, i.e. a_k is deleted). In order to build constructively from such elementary replacements a procedure describing arbitrary processes, we must specify also the order of execution of these replacements and state when the processing ends. Since every replacement (*) requires a certain execution time we cannot execute infinitely replacements if the process is to end at a certain time. Hence, all processes must consist of a finite number of steps: The description of such a process is called an <u>algorithm</u> (from the name of AL KHWARIZMI who lived in the 9th century. In fact the geometric constructions of EUCLID and his method for getting the greatest common divisor were already algorithms). If the algorithm is presented in a form suitable for execution by a computer we call it a <u>program</u>.

There are many distinct ways for describing algorithms. The use of replacements is only one of them. Already in the early days of computers it was recognized that not every algorithm needed to be decomposed into elementary replacements. It is sufficient to start from operations for which how to decompose them further is already known. For example, if one has shown that the usual addition and the other arithmetic operations may be done using elementary replacements, then one can use these operations in formulating algorithms; the operands of these operations are interpreted as numbers and not considered only as sequences of binary characters. These operations correspond to a higher level of abstraction in our hierarchy of interpretations as introduced in section 1.

Algorithms can also be constructed on a higher level of abstraction which is specifically developed for this purpose. The level is determined by first asking: "What are the basic operations and operands most suited to the problem to be solved? Once the algorithm is described in terms of these operations, one has the (simpler) problem of describing these operations and the data in terms of simpler operations and their data. This method is called construction of algorithms by <u>step-wise refinement</u> (cf.[Wirth 1971])

Algorithmic processes are not the only ways of deriving new informations, but they are the only ones which are constructive and lead effectively to the desired result after a finite amount of time. Examples of nonalgorithmic processes are all mathematical constructions which do not end after a finite number of steps, e.g., the computation of the decimal representation of π or other decimal fractions with infinitely many digits. Other examples include reasoning by analogy or by intuition. Even if it can be shown that some intuitive reasoning has an algorithmic basis complexity and the time required by such algorithms would mostly be so high that it is prohibitive for practical use.

Information processing by means of algorithms is thus restricted compared with information processing by human beings. Not all information processing by human beings can be taken over by computers. Expecially in medicine the class of algorithmically solvable problems seems at present to be rather small.

3. The relation of data and algorithms

Up to now we have looked at information processing systems from the point of view of a designer. It is this view which puts the main accent on algorithms and programs. From the point of view of the user of such a system we see mainly the data which we input or receive as results. The transformations which lead to these results remain mostly invisible. Nevertheless it is the algorithm to be performed which determines the amount of input data required, and the form and the order of these data. On the other hand we must not be satisfied by any coding, amount and order in which the resulting data are presented; it is usually not too difficult to modify an algorithm in such a way that it presents its results in an understandable form (e.g. as character strings or decimal numbers instead of sedecimal numbers), orders them in a proper fashion and, most importantly, delivers only those results which we are interested in.

These considerations lead to the conclusion that the order in which we design the input and output data and the algorithms is of some importance. It is necessary that we define first the required results, then outline the algorithms which lead to these results and finally determine the required input data. If we wish to use the input data for several applications, ideally we should proceed in this way for all applications. If this is impossible because some of these applications will be designed much later in time, we must still determine carefully what requirements may be imposed on the input data by these as yet unknown applications. All too often we see that the design is started first by outlining the input data, but the question should be: "What data do we need to derive these results?", not "What results can be derived from this data?". To think first of results and algorithms and only then of input data is of particular importance when we build information systems. An omission in entering patient histories into a computer probably can never corrected; even if we know the missing information the large number of records which must be corrected guarantees that the correction will never be done.

Also the form in which we store the data internally may be important. If we want to sort records in a file in order of increasing dates it is useful to have stored the dates in the format YY.MM.DD and not as they are usually written with the month or day first.

4. The external representation of programs and data

From now on we devote our discussion entirely to information processing using computers. One of the basic concerns is how to present algorithms (i. e. programs) and data in a way suited to both the human writers (and readers) and to the computer.

It should be clear from our remarks on how to present results that the form as bits, or a binary number, which is used inside a computer is not a suitable representation outside the computer. Instead we use representations which are more suited to human beings and which can be converted to the internal form for a computer by special programs in the computer itself. In the case of programs we call the set of rules which determine such an external representation a <u>programming language</u>. The converting program is called a <u>compiler</u>. In many cases the compiled program can be executed directly because it consists of instructions which are basic operations of the computer. If this is not the case (the compiled program is still on a higher level of abstraction) we need in addition an <u>interpreter</u>, a program which simulates the instructions in the compiled program with the help of the instruction set of the computer.

We distinguish three classes of programming languages:

- <u>machine-oriented languages</u>, in particular assembly languages. The basic operations of these languages coincide with the instructions (e.g. the use of mnmonics to denote operations or operands). There is usually one such language for each particular computer type.

- <u>high level languages</u> (also problem-oriented or procedure oriented languages). These languages allow, as far as numeric calculations are concerned, for a notation similar to standard mathematical notation. They furthermore contain means for expressing the structure of an algorithm and the flow of control in a neat and lucid way. Most well-known languages like FORTRAN, ALGOL 60, ALGOL 68, PL/I or PASCAL but also special language like' SNOBOL 4, a language particulary suited to text processing, belong to this class.

- <u>declarative languages</u> (very high-level or problem-defining languages). High-level languages serve for formulating algorithms to solve a given problem. Declarative languages describe the problem; it is assumed that from this description one can automatically derive an algorithmic solution by selecting amongst well-known algorithms. Hence, a declarative language requires a good overall view of all important algorithms in a field of application, and a library of such algorithms ready for automatic adaption to a given problem. Declarative languages can thus be defined for relatively narrow fields of application only. They are the most convenient tool for users which one could think about. But practically speaking they are still of minor importance since the costs for developing and implementing such languages are still too high.

It is not our concern here to teach any of these languages. But in view of their importance we give a classifying overview of the characteristic properties which one can find in most high-level languages. We take our examples from ALGOL 68 [Wijngaarden 69].

A program is a collection of statements describing actions to be executed on certain data. As the basis for structuring programs one finds in most newer languages blocks and procedures (fig. 1). A block is a parenthesized sequence of statements which if seen from the outside form a new (composite) statement. A procedure denotes a statement, or more generally, an algorithm which can be invoked at arbitrary points during program execution by just quoting its name.

The sequence of execution (flow of control) of such statements is controlled by a set of special statement types which we describe in figure 2.

For manipulating data one must know how these data are coded and how they are to be interpreted. This knowledge determines what operations are admissible We characterize this knowledge by the type or mode of the data (figure 3). Whenever we introduce a named data object we indicate its type. Besides the simple types we have type constructors for describing groups of data (arrays, records). Pointers serve to show the (dynamically changing) relations between objects. The most important operation which is explained for objects of all types is the assignment:

$$a:=formula$$

It allows for assigning the result of the formula to the variable a. By using the name a later on, this result may be retrieved (cf. [Goos 75] for a broader discussion of language properties).

There is a well-known relationship between a natural language and the thinking habits of the people using this language. The language mirrors the thinking habits of the people creating it. At the same time it forces people to think and to express themselves in the frame of this language. Ideas which cannot be expressed by simple means are likely not to be thought. Conversely ideas which can be expressed by simple means are considered to be simple even if they are of great complexity. The same arguments apply to programming languages, which in addition reflect, the structure of present-day computers and our understanding of what computers should do. Hence, the programming language influences at least the following:

- The conceptual understanding of how a problem can be solved by computers.
- The range of problems which can be attacked by programming.
- The set of basic notions available in programming.
- The style of programming (clarity, readability, modularity etc.).
- The reliability and correctness of a program.
- The meaning of efficiency.

Thus, the proper choice of a programming language may influence considerably the solution of a problem, the amount of time spent for design, coding, testing and maintenance and the overall costs of the project. This influence and its economic consequences are usually very difficult to estimate since rarely does one guide the same project twice just to obtain comparable figures (see [Goos 73] for a continuation of this discussion).

In an analogous fashion the proper design of input data for a program may influence considerably the reliability in use of this program. The very simple method of not coding everything numerically but having the computer look up the coding internally (e.g., that "wednesday" is coded by 3) avoids a lot of mistakes. An additional degree of reliability can be obtained easily by giving not only the values of the input data but also their meaning. The input line

$$age=43$$

is much preferable to simply giving the value 43, as far as convenience and reliability of usage are concerned.

5. The program development process

The development of a program may be subdivided into several steps (cf. [Metzger 73] for a similar scheme):

- system analysis and problem definition
- program design
- implementation
- system integration
- acceptance test and installation
- maintenance.

This section tries to characterize each such step by a few sentences. Each step forms a distinguishable phase of program development. They are not usually executed sequentially but can overlap partially in time. An important aspect of the development process is iteration: the return to an earlier phase, in particular the design phase, for improving and correcting shortcomings which are detected only in a later phase, or for adapting the program to changing requirements.

System analysis and problem definition

The goal of this step is the development of a model of the solution of the given problem, and the writing of a plan of how this solution

can be achieved. The model shows the feasibility of the proposed
solution; if defines the problem in technical terms; it characterizes
the necessary input data and the results to be obtained. Except that
it proposes a certain decomposition of the problem into subtasks which
are believed to be solvable, all specific decisions about algorithms
etc. are deferred to the design phase.

A main concern of the problem definition must be to establish the
criteria to be met by the solution, e.g., the class of computer
configurations on which the program should run, whether the program
should be portable, what are the trade- offs between reliability, date
of delivery, efficiency etc. We discuss some of these criteria in more
detail in the next section.

Program design

The goal of the design phase is a specification of the solution,
its algorithms and data structures. For a large project the design is
divided into a gross design specifying the subtasks which must be
solved by some modules and the relationship between these modules, and
the module design specifying the inner working of the modules. This
subdivision corresponds to the principle of stepwise refinement
mentioned earlier.

Design decisions are very often risky: they are based on incomplete
information about their consequences. Whether the decision was good or
not is seen sometimes only years later. Although the design itself may
constitute only a small percentage of the overall costs of a project
the costs of all later phases and the overall costs are implicitly
determinded by the design. From an economics point of view the best
people should therefore work on the design.

Whenever possible the design should include a rational - not an
intuitive - reasoning about the correctness of the solution. It is
much simpler and cheaper to correct mistakes and omissions now then in
later phases.

Implementation

This phase codes and tests the solution developed in the design
phase. It constitutes the last step in the refinement

gross design -> module desgin -> coding.

While creativity is a virtue of a designer the required property in
implementation is utmost accuracy in all activities. Ideally, testing

is required only for removing the clerical errors introduced during the implementaion itself. One should always keep in mind Dijkstra's famous statement: "Program testing can be used to show the presence of bugs, but never to show their absence."

System integration

This step is done successively after the programmers deliver their tested modules. It is the attempt to put these modules together and to test the program as a whole. Usually this attempt fails in the beginning due to bad documentation of interfaces, misunderstandings, lack of communication about changes etc. At latest in this phase, the need to prepare from the beginning against misunderstandings, imprecision and other human inadequacies has been learnt.

Acceptance Test and Installation

This phase includes the thorough testing of the whole program by a group of people distinct from those who wrote the program. This acceptance test must show the functional correctness, the robustness and the performance of the program. It is a prerequisite to the installation of the program for practical use. At the same time it has to clarify whether the other prerequisites for installation, e.g., a user guide, program documentation etc. are in a satisfactory state. The group performing the acceptance test should design sets of test data with which the program has performed well and which can be used by customers to check that the program as installed performs well, at least in its main parts.

Maintenance

This phase consists of correcting detected errors, adapting to new environments (new hardware, new problem specification), and improving the performance of the program. It lasts for the whole life-time of the program. There are numerous examples that maintenance may incur more than half of the total costs of a project. It is therefore important to check again and again how long the maintenance should be extended and when it should be stopped in favour of a newly developed program which takes into account the lessons learnt from the last development.

6. Qualitative properties of programs

What constitutes a "good" program? We have mentioned a few properties of programs which are relevant in this context. This section is devoted to defining some of these properties and to discussing why they are relevant. We are not concerned about how to achieve these properties.

Functional Correctness (A)

The main requirement of a program is that, given an admissible set of input data, it precisely does what it is supposed to do. No other property of the program is of any concern if the program does not solve the specified problem. This requirement may be difficult to meet if the problem was not specified precisely enough and a proof that the progam is solving the problem is impossible. The situation should be carefully avoided by precise specification of the problem. Otherwise the result may surprise greatly both the programmer and his customer.

Being in Time (B)

This is another requirement which must be met if the problem is to be solved at all. It is not unusual for the programmers to exceed the date of delivery by continuously improving the performance of their program. Meanwhile the customer loses orders of much greater value than can ever be saved by the improvements.

Modularity (C)

A program is called modular [Dennis 73] if it consists of pieces, the program modules, such that

(a) the correctness of a program module can be demonstrated regardless of the context of its use in building larger units of software;

(b) program modules written under different authorities can be conveniently put together without knowledge of their inner working.

To be more precise this definition defines functional modularity. Other definitions, e.g., separate compilability are of minor significance. A sufficient modularization is a prerequisite for most of the program properties which follow.

Adaptability (D)

A program is adaptable to a new or changed problem specification if it can easily be modified to conform to the new requirements. An increase in efficiency usually diminishes the adaptability of a program.

Portability (D)

A program is portable if it can be easily transferred to a new base system, e.g., another type of computer, or another computer configuration with new peripheral devices. Hence, portability and adaptability are like the two sides of a coin. Portability is a prime requirement for all software house products. It should be a requirement of all adacemic software developments. For obvious reasons computer manufacturers have a minor interest in portability. Programs are claimed to be portable much more often than it is actually the case.

Compatibility (D)

Compatibility is the harmonious coexistence of several programs. It exists if we can use programs in combination (e.g., the use of FORTRAN subprograms in an ALGOL main program), or if two programs show similar behavior to the user and can be used alternatively. Compatibility is a primary requirement whenever one develops an existing system further or replaces it by a new one. Very often, however, the pursuit of compatibility leads to stagnation and prohibits the use of newer scientific insights.

Reliability (E)

Reliability comprises all properties which guarantee that the program is working properly. It thus includes <u>functional correctness</u>, i.e. safety against internal faults of the program, and <u>fault tolerance</u>, i.e. safety against faults in the base system, such a faults at the cpu, the main store, parity errors, faults of peripheral devices or break-down of electrical current. Ideally such faults should lead only to a drecrease in program performance and never to a complete break-down. Finally reliability includes <u>robustness</u>, i.e. safety against erroneous input data and wrong operating. Robustness requires that such errors should be detected at the earliest possible time and that recovery is made so that the program can continue, e.g., by requesting new input data.

Absolute reliability can never be achieved. In particular fault tolerance and also robustness may have a very high price. We can only achieve a certain <u>degree</u> <u>of</u> <u>reliability</u>. It is an important engineering decision to determine this degree such that the price is worth the profit.

Availability (E)

This property is not always required, but for important base systems and for process control it is often necessary that the system should never stop. An extreme example is the requirement of telephone companies: They tolerate a failure of the total system for at most one hour in forty years. Available is helped by the same methods which support fault tolerance.

Efficiency (F)

Efficiency is the optimal use of all available resources in order to fulfill the given tasks. In programming one usually concentrates on the best possible use of cpu time and storage. This technological efficiency may often lead to inefficient solutions because the cost of programmer- and testing time, the cost of inconvenience to the user and the cost of maintenance may outweigh the benefits. Another common mistake is to avoid simple solutions because a more complicated one seems to be more efficient. It should be stressed that simplicity and clarity of a design which may be necessary for correctness can never be added later, whereas efficiency can be improved later.

Conclusions

Not all of the properties which we have discussed can be achieved together. In particular efficiency conflicts with nearly everything else. It is therefore necessary to discuss in an early stage of program development the trade-offs between the relevant properties. The letters attached to the properties in the above discussion may serve as an indication of priorities.

Literature

[1]   Dennis, J.B.:
      Modularity,
      Lecture Notes in Economics and Mathematical Systems,
      vol. 81, pp. 128-182, (1973)

[2]   Goos, G.:
      Language Characteristics,
      Lecture Notes in Economics and Mathematical Systems,
      vol. 81, pp. 47-69 (1973)

[3]   Goos, G.:
      Systemprogrammiersprachen und strukturiertes Programmieren,
      Lecture Notes in Computer Science,
      vol. 23, pp. 203-224 (1975)

[4]   Metzger, P.W.:
      Managing a Programming Project. Prentice Hall:
      Englewood Cliffs, N.J.. 1973

[5]   van Wijngaarden, A., ed.:
      Report on the Algorithmic Language ALGOL 68,
      Numer. Math. 14, pp.79-218, (1969)

[6]   Wirth, N.:
      Program Development by stepwise refinement,
      Comm. ACM 14, pp.221-227, (1971)

Block Structure

begin statement; ....; statement end

composite statement

Procedures

PROC name of procedure =
        (formal parameters) type of result, if any:
        statement

PROC arithmetic mean = (REAL a, b) REAL : (a + b)/2

PROC Check input   = (INT mother age, child age):
                      IF mother age - child age ≤ 10 OR
                         mother age - child age ≥ 50
                      THEN print ("input data not plausible")
                      FI

Figure 1   Program Structure

16

Sequence: S_1 ; S_2

Collaterality: S_1 ; S_2

Selection: IF condition THEN S_1 ELSE S_2 FI

                   CASE formula IN S_1
                                  S_2
                                  ...
                                  S_n
                            OUT S_{n+1} ESAC

Enumeration: FOR counter FROM start BY step TO end
                   DO S

Iteration: WHILE condition DO S

Procedure call: P
                   P (actual Parameters)

Exit: BEGIN statements ...; EXIT; statements END

JUMP: GOTO labelled statement

                   Figure 2 Flow of control
                   (S denotes a arbitrary statement)

Simple data types	Characteristic operations
INT(integral number)	$+,-,*,DIV,MOD,<,\leq,>,\geq,=,\neq$
REAL(floating-point number)	$+,-,*,/,<,\leq,>,\geq,=,\neq$
BOOL(character)	$=,\neq$

Type constructors:

Arrays: [1:n] REAL vector   vector[i]

        [1:n,1:n] REAL matrix   matrix[i,j]
        STRING character sequence   character sequence[i]

Records: MODE person = STRUCT (STRING name, INT age);
        person richard := ("richard", 46)

Records including pointers:
        MODE person = STRUCT (STRING name,
                        REF person father, mother)

      person richard, henry, maria;
      father OF richard := henry;
      mother OF richard := maria

Figure 3   Data types

Hardware

by H.-O. Leilich

1. Introduction

Computer hardware is often considered by computer users as
   a mysterious link between electronics and those black (or blue)
   boxes, which understand computer languages and data and perform all
   kind of computations and storage actions at a phantastic speed. They
   are supposed to work with binary signals and consist of an ever-
   growing number of AND- and OR-circuits. These black boxes are prai-
   sed by salesmen as ultimate and finalized - at every instance of
   time - , designed by producers and configured by computer specialists
   only, so that a user must not worry with any internals nor interfere
   with his ideas relating to system design.

One should not join this tune, that computer hardware is a finished task
which merely yields faster, smaller, cheaper and more reliable circuits.
One the contrary: modern technology and design techniques introduced
a new phase of dynamic architectural development - as well as and in
conjunction with software efforts - and are therefore pacing the way to
new applications and system concepts. Computer have been and are being
developed to serve the user and everybody concerned with the application
of automatic data handling - esspecially in new fields like medical informatics - should have some insight in the internal concepts and the
potential of future equipment including the possibilities of development
of special hardware for certain applications.

The next three sections are therefore intended to convey some basic
understanding of internal hardware organisation - three brief textbook-
like chapters, which link the AND-OR-circuit level to the level of
functional units and explain the basic operation of a program-controlled
computer. Section 5 analyses the general charcteristics and trends in
computer hardware. Section 6 emphazises the hierarchical design of
building blocks and gives raw ranges of speed and memory capacity and
their relations to the interface to the technical and human world . It
stresses the possibilities of adapting devices and system organizations
to the user need.

2. Combinational Networks

Fig. 1 a is the general representation of a combinational network with
yields for each element X_i of the finite set X one (and only one) element Y_j of the finite set Y.

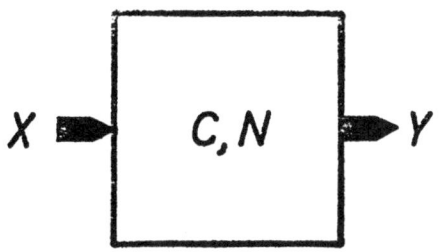

(a) Combinational Network

Input X	Output Y
X_1	Y_8
X_2	Y_5
...	...

(b) Transformation Table

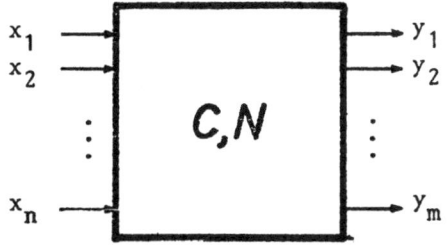

Input x_1 x_2	Output y_1 y_2 y_3
0 0	0 0 0
0, 1	0 1 1
1 0	0 1 0
1 1	1 0 1

(c) Variables X,Y presented by binary components   (d) Example

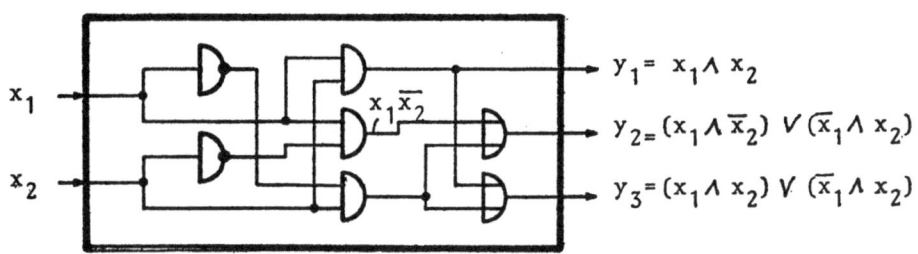

$$y_1 = x_1 \wedge x_2$$

$$y_2 = (x_1 \wedge \bar{x}_2) \vee (\bar{x}_1 \wedge x_2)$$

$$y_3 = (x_1 \wedge x_2) \vee (\bar{x}_1 \wedge x_2)$$

(e) Switching Network   (f) Boolean Functions

FIG 1   COMBINATIONAL NETWORKS

If X is represented by binary components x_1, x_2, ... x_n (Fig. 1c), there are 2^n combinations, i.e. 2^n elements of X can be distingnished and for each one, one combination of the y's is produced (where m may be smaller or larger than n). The full description of this basic transformation of X to Y can be thought of as a table (Fig. 1 b in general form, Fig.1 d is a specific example).

A combinational network may perform an arithmetic function (here X and Y are binarys numbers and the function may be $Y = X^2$). It also can be viewed as a static code translater or as a read-only-memory, where X means the address and Y the contents of the cell number X.

Any combinational network can be realized by AND,- OR- and NOT-switching elements, which should be obvious from the following verbal description of the table in Fig. 1 d:

"if (x_1 is 1 AND x_2 is 1) y_1 becomes 1, else 0,

if (x_1 is 1 AND x_2 is NOT 1) OR

if (x_1 is not 1 AND x_2 is 1) y_2 becomes 1, else 0,

if (x_1 is NOT 1 AND x_2 is 1) OR

if (x_1 is 1 AND x_2 is 1) y_3 becomes 1, else 0".

or in brief Boolean notation as shown in Fig. 1 f.

It is well known, that the basic logical functions (AND, OR, NOT) can be performed by mechanical, electrical or electronic arrangements (for instance two contacts (a, b) in parallel let a bell ring if a OR b are closed.). Electronic elements are much faster and smaller and are designed such, that the output ("bell rings") can be used as input to other logical elements (compatibility).

3. Sequential networks

If one feeds back (part of) the output (Y') of a combinational network to (part of) its input, one creates the structure of a sequential network (Fig. 2 a).

Imagine what may happen if a certain combination X_i is assumed to exist at a given time at the input of the combinational network, depending on the specific transfer function:

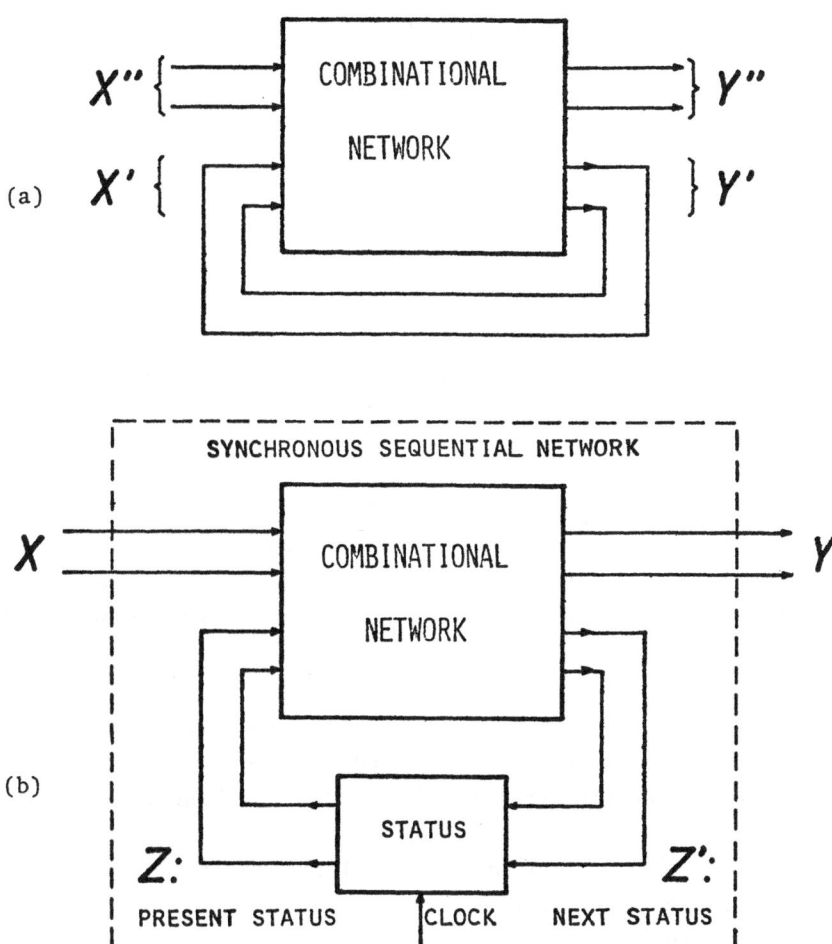

FIG. 2   ASYNCHRONOUS AND SYNCHRONOUS SEQUENTIAL NETWORKS

a)   if the fed back output part (Y_j') is different   from the original
     input part (X_i'), the C.N. transformes this new input to a new
     output Y_k $(X' = Y_j')$

b)   if Y_j' is the same as X_i' nothing else happens, the process is
     finished, the circuit is "stable" ("dead"!)

In the first case the newly generated output Y_k' may be identical with
the input Y_j', then the circuit becomes stable. It may recycle several
times and become stable. Yet it may also generate one of the previous
instable states and run in circles forever unless the steady part (X_i'')
is changed.

If one eliminates wild races by unifing all delays (clocking the feedback - Fig. 2 b), one gets an orderly time-sequentially working circuit,
which, once started at a given input state, generates a sequence of
states and outputs exactly "programmed" by the transfer-function of
the combinational network.

Mathematicians call this structure a "finite, deterministic automaton"
and computer scientists recognize the prototype of a program controlled
computer, as basic and universal as the "Turing machine".

Since a sequential network may have several stable states, it is also
the logical prototype of a memory. The structure of a "flip-flops, me-
a special case of such a network. Registers consist of flip-flops, memories of registers with a certain access-structure (decoders, transfer
circuits).

All futher computer structure concepts are based on these nets, motivated
by technical-economical reasons. One of these reasons is that of rational
design, which leads to the definition of different hierarchical levels
 - as it is very common in all technical fields as well as in public,
economic and daily life.

We have moved from the AND-OR-level to the network-level. The next level,
consisting of certain network configurations is called the "functional
unit"-level, examples are arithmetic units, memories, communication and
control units.

4. Central Computer

Fig. 3 shows the main functional units of the classical general purpose computer structure, still hinting their composition of networks
(the previous level!).

The arithmetic unit - often considered as the "working horse" - where
"the real computing" is finally done - is a combination of number registers, combinational networks (adders, shifters, communication circuits)
and a sequential control network for the detailed stepping through multiplication etc. algorithms. It needs data and a command what to do, for
instance "multiply!", similar to a pocket calculator. Other working
horses may be apt to perform operations like "Check for correctness!"
or "Fourier transform!".

The main memory in a classical computer stores all types of data and
programs, usually in form of fixed portions (words), appropriate for
interpretation in the other functional units. Programs are mostly stored
in "machine oriented" format, instruction by instruction, each consisting
of a data address and an operation code. (Programs may also be stored
symbol by symbol according to a user language before they are translated
to machine format).These memory words are picked or loaded, one at a
time, via an address decoder and a transport network.

The internal bus-system connects the memory and the other functional
units (including I/O-channels and control). Its functions became very
important in more recent computer structures with sophisticated parallel
operations and I/O-organizations.

The control unit steers the transfers of data and instructions, inter-
pretes the instructions and is responsible for the right sequence of
commands to the other units. It containes a sequential network (micro-
program control) and the important program status register, which at
any instance of time points to the "current" instruction in the program,
stored in memory, i.e. it knows at which address the next instruction
can be found. In a linear sequence of instructions the "program status
register" is just stepped by a counting network. In case of a branch
instruction, the control network inquires the branching condition (e.g.
the sign of the previous result in the accumulator) and either steps
the program status by one or resets this registers according to the jump
address contained in the branch instruction.

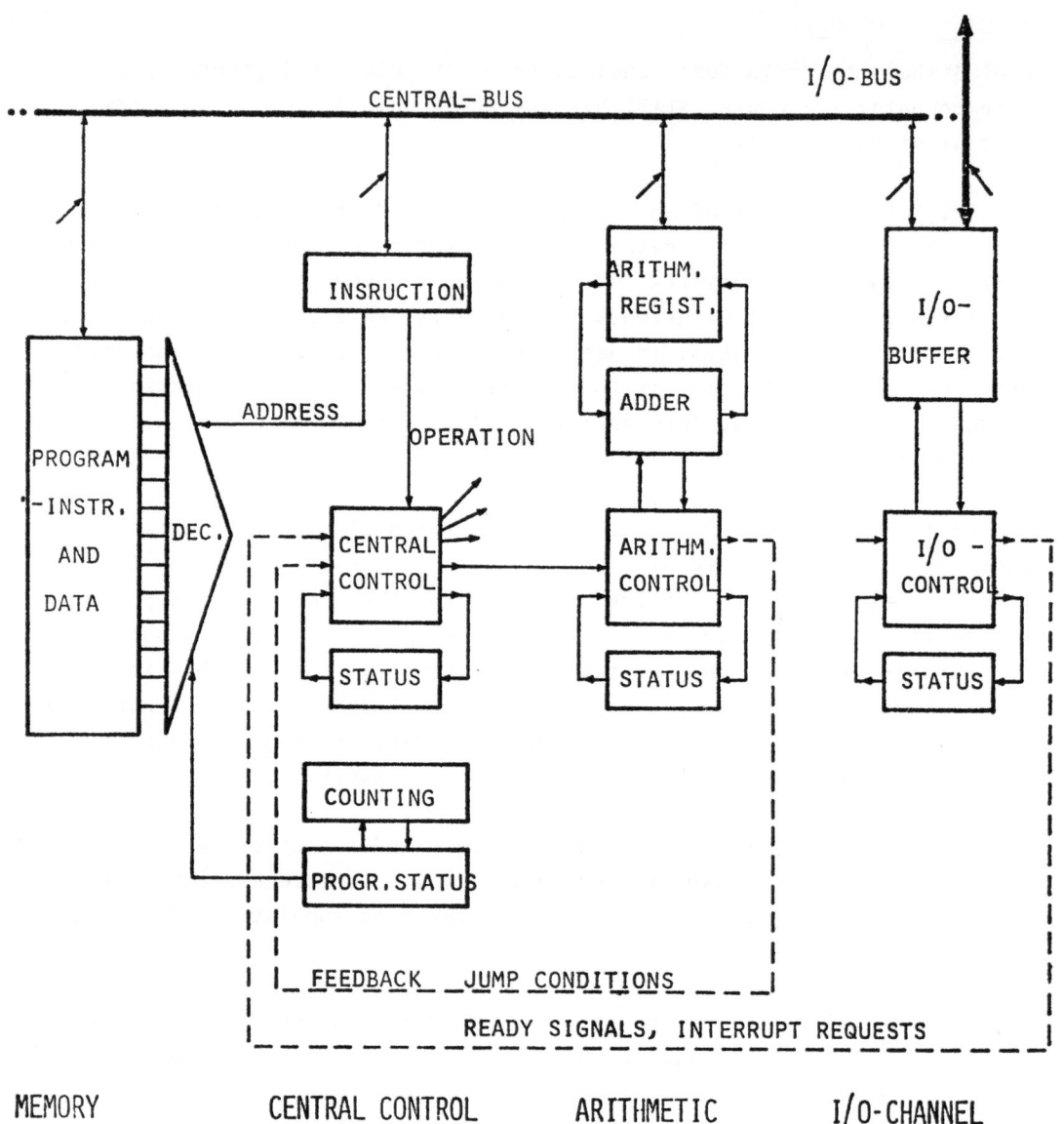

FIG 3 CENTRAL COMPUTER COMPONENTS AND INTERRELATIONS

The conditional jump causes the computer to react on results of calculations or counting or interrupts from the periphery etc. rather than
merely executing a preprogrammed string of orders. During the first years
of the computer age this ability of responsiveness was enthusiastically
phrased as "thinking", "decision making" of an "electronic brain" -
although the computer is just a mechanism, which executes in a predetermined way a programmed algorithm.

5. Characteristies and trends of computers

There is not the space to explain any details of machine codes, address
manipulation systems, subcontrollers and microprograms generated and
modified for efficiency and economies in building and operation of
computers. The important points for a general overview are the following:

Computer hardware provides means of data transformation, storage and
communication, to implement - within economical limits - the execution
of all programming structures which may be conceived.

Due to the advances made in electronics, these universal-purpose information handling machines are today capable of performing several thousands to millions of basic instructions per second and of storing thousands to billions of words of data and/or program instructions. Costs
and prices per intruction performed and per memory word decreased due
to technical progress and competition and they are still expected to
decrease in the years to come. Compactness and costs allow constructions
of very powerful large machines and multiprocessors als well as "minicomputers","microprocessors" and pocket calculators. It became also
economically feasible to distribute "intelligence" to the places were
it is needed, thus avoiding excessive communication problems and indi-
gestion of central computer installations with simple small jobs.

Since computer hardware is no longer the main and most costly part in
computer systems, it is icreasingly used to facilitate its use, i.e.
its programming and operation. The user-oriented presentation of programs
and data is converted to the required internal codes by the computer
itself executing a translation program - a "compiler". So the actual
operation sequences and numbers in the computer differ drastically from
the program viewed by the user (e.g. "do procedure X" may be performed
in thousands of machine steps). Due to the compiler action the programmer
has, generally speaking, not even to know which computer will execute

his program. Virtual memories are implemented by hardware and software
means, so that the user "sees" a memory of a size, speed and structure
which can never be ralized by a single hardware device (e.g. a 16-M-Byte
random access memory with 100 nanoseconds access time). Also virtual
structures and complete machines are implemented by internal automatic
simulation techniques.

Operating systems - again programs executed by the computer itself -
have been developed to unburden the user from internally necessary
management tasks like availling the necessary memory space for a certain job or waiting for certain peripheral actions or other programs
to be finished.

The multi-purpose - <u>universal</u> - computer has the ability to serve many
(all) purposes and yields a broad spectrum of users - resulting in an
economic mass production and reasonable development and maintenance
efforts. For each specific purpose - say for one program (e.g. converting measurement data in a space vehicle) - a special, <u>dedicated</u>
<u>computer</u> can be conceived, which performs this job with much lesser
hardware.

The decision for a systems engineer to use a general purpose or a special
piece of equipment is an economical one, for computers as in all other
technical fields. These decisions should be done in a rational rather
than in an emotional - ideological - way. And the ability to judge what
instruments to use for a job requires a knowledge of those instruments
as well as of the job, i.e. a physician designing a medical system with
automatic data handling got to know something of computer hardware in
addition to the art of its application (programming at any level).

With falling prices for electronics and with automatic (computer-aided)
design tools already in use, the trend leads to diversification although
a rational management fosters general-purpose devices or a least standard
building blocks at a certain level. "Microprocessors" (small, slow, cheap
but rather flexibel programmable electronic building blocks) seem to be
optimal compromises. They are presently attached to many measurement
devices, enhancing their performance and easing their operation.

6. Computer speed and the human interface

One can easily impress a layman with numbers concerning speed and capacity

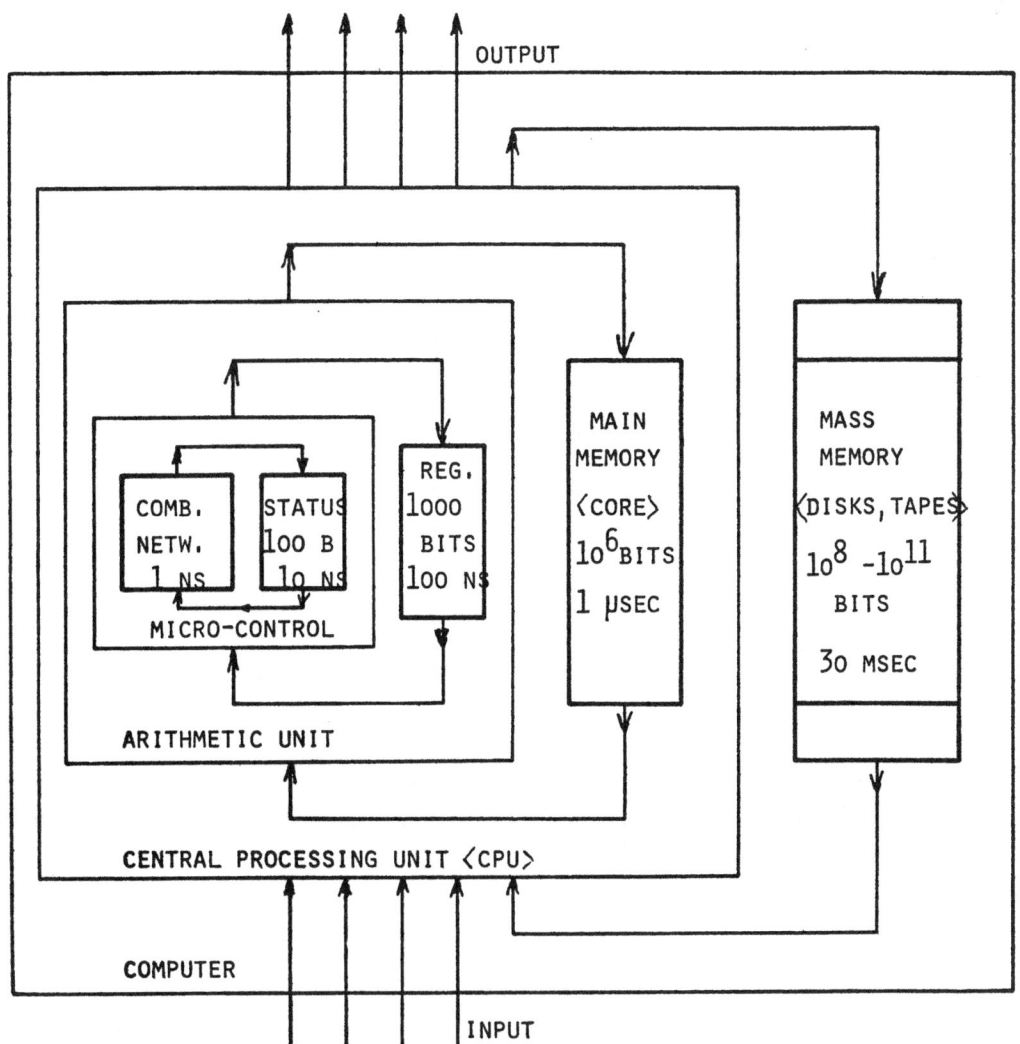

OUTPUT

MAIN MEMORY
⟨CORE⟩
10^6 BITS
1 μSEC

MASS MEMORY
⟨DISKS, TAPES⟩
$10^8 - 10^{11}$ BITS
30 MSEC

REG.
1000 BITS
100 NS

COMB. NETW.
1 NS

STATUS
100 B
10 NS

MICRO-CONTROL

ARITHMETIC UNIT

CENTRAL PROCESSING UNIT ⟨CPU⟩

COMPUTER

INPUT

FIG 4   HIERARCHICAL COMPUTER HARDWARE STRUCTURE

Device	Information Unit Size $\lfloor$bits$\rfloor$	Parallelism	Processing Time	Transfer-Speed $\lfloor$bits/sec$\rfloor$
log. elements	1	100 ÷ 1000	1 ÷ 10 ns	1,000,000,000,000 ÷ 10,000,000,000
registers, microprogram	100	1 ÷ 10	0.1 ÷ 1 µs	10,000,000,000 ÷ 100,000,000
main memory machine progr.	32	1 ÷ 8	0.2 ÷ 1 µs	1,280,000,000 ÷ 32,000,000
mass memory (disc. tape)	32000	1 ÷ 8	25 ms	50,000,000 ÷ 2,000,000
Card Reader Mech. Printer	1000	1	20 ms	50,000
Telefon line	1	1	0.2 ms 0.4 ms	4,800 2,400
Teletype (human reading and writing rate)	5	1	140 ms	35

Fig. 5:   Processing and Transfer Speeds
of Computer Levels and Periphery

of computer components: "A fast elementary electronic switch with 1
nanosecond reaction time can perform 10^9 operations per second, as
many as there are heart beats in one human generation". Or: "One magnetic disc memory ($\approx 10^9$ bits) stores the contents of several hundred
books and requires 100 hours for its complete transmission over a
telephone channel (2400 baud)", "Large-scale integrated semiconductor
elements comprise a complete microprocessor or thousands of memory bits
on a simple silicon chip of a few square millimeters".

On the other hand: "an educated human being can recognice a contour
of an organ in a (X-ray-)picture much faster than a computer". The
reasons are probably, that the human brain works with a huge number of
(slow) "microprocessors" and it is developed and trained to perform
certain programs very efficiently. Even more impressive than technical
data are storage capacities and densities in biological cells (e.g.
in the DSN-molecule, Lit. $\sqrt{37}$).

Rather than wondering one should face the numbers and try to put them
in proper relations. Fig. 4 and 5 should convey two essentials:

a) Attached to the structural levels of the hardware hierarchy (AND-OR-
circuit, networks, working horses etc.) are speed and capacity levels:
with higher structural levels capacity increases and speed decreases.

b) The communication activity, measured in raw transfer speed (bits/sec),
decreases from level to level.

One can explain both facts partially by physical limitations: smaller
units have shorter wires and operate faster due to the finite speed of
light and electrical signals. There is also the structural trend: each
level has more internal activity than external communication (data
shuffling and control activity).

Realizing these ranges of numbers, one notices the need of adapting
equipment to the human interface and organizing the total structure
such, that unnecessary information shuffling is avoided. Fig. 6 extends
the onion-model of the computer (Fig. 5) to the human interface, showing
some of the well-known peripheral devices. Each of the devices has already some logical capability, often realized with a special internal
processor (e.g. picture memory and manipulation facilities in a visual
display). In respect to data transportation and organizational overhead
one may conjecture, that it makes no sense to funnel a simple sensor

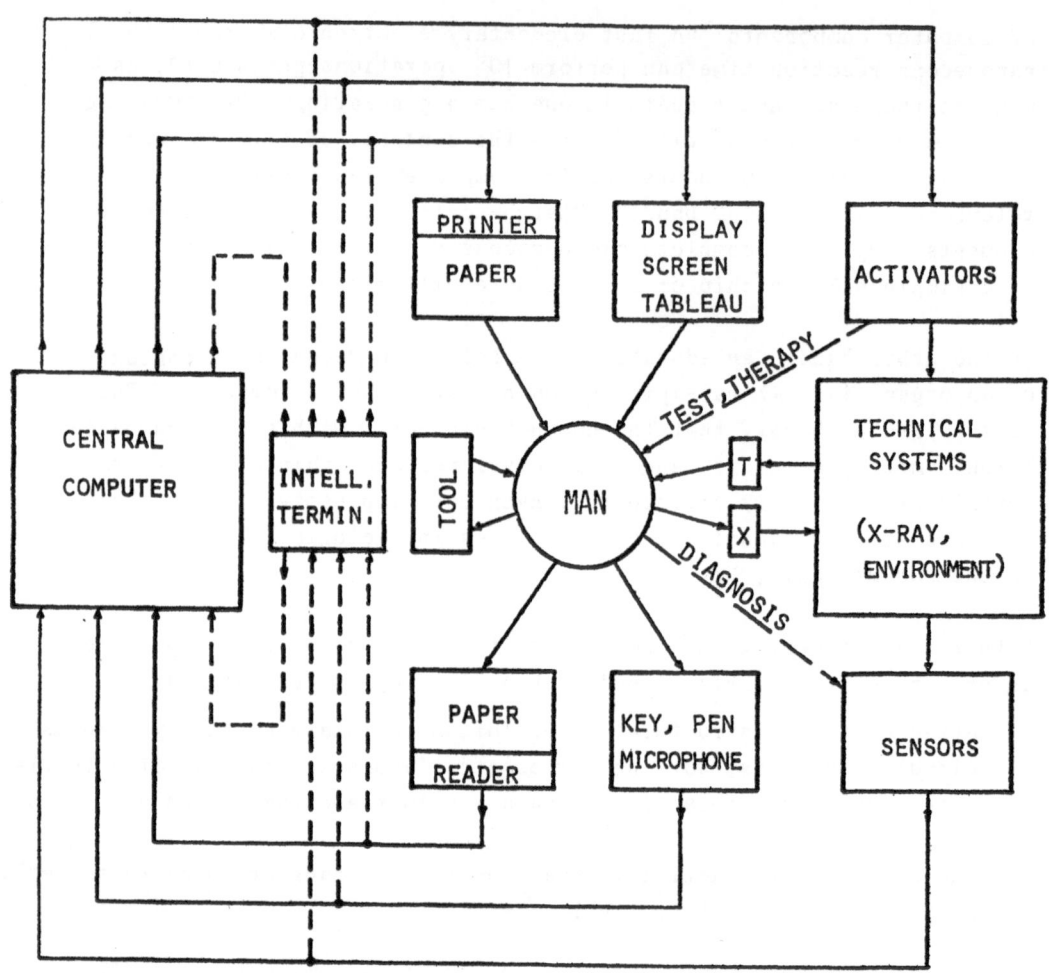

FIG. 6: MAN-COMPUTER INTERFACES

output (e.g. heart beat sensor) through the arithmetic unit of the
central clinic processor in oder to ring an alarm in case of emergency.
This certainly can be done locally or with a small miniprocessor in
a proper position, called an "intelligent terminal".

In conclusion, the application of informatics to medicine requires understanding of medical systems and methology as well as priciples of
informatics, including those of hardware - its principles, its state
of the art and its trends. Present technology and design techniques
not only offer a rich palette of ready-to-use devices and systems, they
also have the potential for dedicated hardware and specialized systems
similar to the application of computers for physics research in space experiments.

Lit.:

/1/ I. Flores: Computer Organization
                                            Prentice Hall, 1969
/2/ H.W. Gschwind, E.J. Mc Cluskey: Design of Digital Computers
                                            Springer 1975
/3/ H. Kaufmann (Ed.):   Daten-Speicher
                                            (German) Oldenburg, 1973

Health Care Delivery as a System

Peter L. Reichertz

Department of Biometrics and Medical Informatics
Medical School Hannover
Hannover, Fed. Rep. of Germany

1. Introduction and definition of goals

The life of an individual is limited by principal and accidental factors. Furthermore, his physical and mental well-being may be influenced in many ways during the course of his life.
It seems therefore logical to desire to

-maintain or restore physical and/or mental well-being in case of impairment and to
-attempt to influence those factors which limit the life span.

When a system is defined as a conceptual set of interdependent units, as health care delivery all systematized efforts can be defined that attempt to achieve these goals.

The development of social structures has to be added to the goal of health care delivery, which above has only been defined in regard to the individual. These structures depend on productivity of their members. Well-being of an optimal number of its productive members is therefore essential. Furthermore, these structures have to meet generally recognized objectives as is the individuals' wish to be healthy. Since members want to participate in resulting benefits, this might restrict the individual's share. Attempts to achieve the greatest amount of collective health may conflict with requirements for greatest individual health, e.g. expensive programs directed towards seldom, but for the individual lethal or seriously imparing diseases might need more resources than general programs that attempt to improve the conditions of a larger population.

Thus the main goals of health care delivery may be formulated as to

-provide individual health
-provide for collective health
 and
-avoid impairment of health

at, it may be added,

-reasonable cost.

Skills to perform the desired services depend upon knowledge and training. The development of medical science has therefore become a necessity, as well as the efforts to teach and develop skills. This sub-objective may partially be combined with the other goals already described, but may compete with these for existing resources.

During the history of mankind, these efforts, which require certain skills, have been more and more provided by individuals or groups of people as a service to others. The recompensation for this service, either material or immaterial, has subsequently become an additional

objective for the delivery of these services, though naturally not
being a goal of the system itself. This certainly may lead to
conflicts.

Attempts to generalize procedures and concepts in health care delivery
and to describe them in a formal way in order to instrument changes and
improvements have to recognize the possible conflicts between its goals
and means for this achievement. Health care delivery shares this fact
with other real systems in the sociological environment.

The various elements in this system, institutions and individuals, are
neither centrally directed nor do their goals coincide. This seems
natural for a real system. Nonetheless, when the necessity is
recognized to improve the quality of health care delivery or to
optimize its cost, it is a precondition to control and supervise its
information flow.

Since human beings are both objects and subjects in these systems,
psychological and sociological factors have to be taken into
consideration when analyzing the system. It does not suffice to base
conclusions on objective output alone. Ways and means have to be
developed to measure, monitor and motivate psychological involvement
and concern. Subjective value scales have to be studied for assessment.

There may, however, be trade-offs between the competing goals. The
reduction of risk within a population , may decrease the need for
individual health care and research efforts may make substantial
contributions to the methodology to deliver care. Educational training
can be combined with actual care delivery. Some of these trades-offs,
however, occur on a deferred time scale and within different sectors of
the real world.

The applications of methods of informatics in medicine or, as some call
it, medical information science, are addressed to the problem of

-documentation
-analysis
-guidance
-control and
-synthesis

of information processes within the health care delivery system,
especially in the classical environment of hospitals and medical
practices.

In this context, documentation is used in the broader sense of the
medical connotation which includes the levels of

-recording of cognitive processes,
-abstraction and condensation of information and
-the classification of processes (diseases) and elements of
 processes.

Often medical practice is used synonymously with health care delivery
as pars pro toto. It should be clearly understood that not only
physicians are involved in the process, that they even constitute a
minor part of the various professionals involved, though the ones with
the greatest weight in the decision making process. It should be
recognized that health care delivery reaches beyond the practice of
physicians and that this part will become more and more important in
the future. The position of the physician, however, is characterized by
an important particularity. Not only is he the main source of often far

reaching decisions, but often he is also at the operational level of
care delivery. This creates requirements for information flow different
from the usual industrial environment, which is mainly characterized by
a condensation towards the higher levels of management. Certainly, this
hierarchical condensation also occurs in the management of health care
delivery or in health care planning, but a direction of the information
flow towards the operational level is typical for delivery of
individual health care.

In Russian literature (1,2), systems have been described as to be
defined by their output. Health care delivery, in a strict sense, does
not produce output in terms of a measurable good. It attempts to
interfere with biological processes in order to

    -restore or preserve functions or
    -reduce or reverse trends.

Diseases do not exist as such. What is called an illness is the
reaction of a biological systems.

Health care delivery interacts with its objects. The information coming
from the patient is perceived, interpreted and leads to actions, which
attempt to evoke a desired change in the objects (10,11). This
interaction occurs with biological and psychological systems, namely
the patients.

Health care delivery is organized in various structures. Information
processing is a major part both in the overall management of health
care delivery as well as in the management of the patient with his
specific diseases and problems. Good design of information processing
and its structuring according to recognized requirements opposed to
historical development may have an important influence on the future
structure of health care systems. The quality of such an improvement
will depend on a thorough analysis of the goals of health care
delivery, the possible conflicts between various objectives and an
understanding how the system works today. Also no change will be
accepted by those who deliver health care unless they are properly
motivated. This implies also the understanding of the psychological and
sociological components of the system.

2. The overall system of health care delivery
==

When analyzing the system of health care delivery, one first is
impressed by the great variety and complexity of appearances as is
typical for an empirical and applied science. This is reflected also in
the teaching and research techniques of medicine, where abstraction and
generalization only gradually penetrate into the scientific concept.
This is caused not only by tradition, but also by the fact that the
dynamic evolution of patho-physiological concepts and understanding
encompasses various stages of description of phenomena, classification
of observations, and causal relations. As will be shown by various
contributions of other authors in this volume, general abstraction is
not always possible and the stage has to be set for further
investigations by description of observations and relationships, before
they can be formalized. The difficulty does not lie in the depth of the
logical process, but in the complexity of the interconnections and the
amount of facts. It is therefore understandable that first approaches
of data processing techniques in medicine were based on ad hoc concepts
serving a finite and limited application rather than attempting to set
up general procedures.

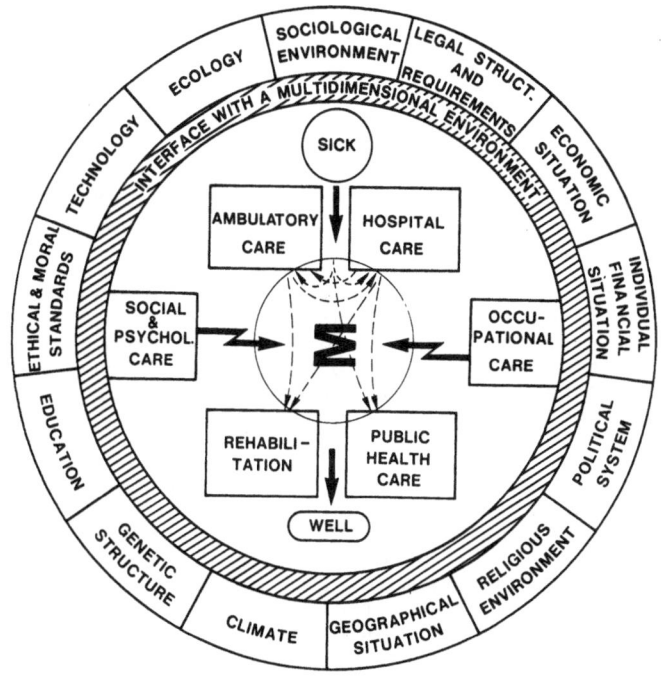

Fig. 1:
      Generalized and simplified model of the environment of health
      care delivery. The basic institutional components are
      ambulatory care, hospital care, rehabilitation and public
      health care. The patient flow between institutions is indicated
      to be not optimally controlled (if controlled at all). Social
      and psychological care as well as occupational care gain
      increasing importance (From 13).

Certainly medicine encompasses characteristics of a natural science.
This is especially true for academic medicine. However, the involvement
of psychological factors both from the side of the physician and the
patient introduces other elements of decision making than a purely
scientific thought process. It also has to be recognized that the
decision making process is very often under time constraints and cannot
wait, until all possible relevant information has been obtained. This,
however, implies the possibility to improve this process by providing
relevant information by information processing techniques. Nonetheless
it has to be accepted, that probably not every decision in medicine can
be completely rationalized.

2.1 Environment

Fig.1 (13) attempts to give an impression of the complex environment,
into which health care delivery systems are placed. They interface with
the sociological groupings and ramifications into which they are

placed, are dependent upon ecology, technology, and technological development, have to meet legal requirements and, at their turn, influence legal structures. The economic situation is of relevance both for the system and the consumer of the system. The political system sets priorities of developments, religious convictions interfere with human behavior and decision making, the geographical situation is of importance both for the occurrence of diseases and the delivery of health care as is climate. The genetic structure of the population has influence on disease incidences and, last but not least, the education and ethical and moral standards are of great importance for behavioral patterns of people in the system.

One of the particularities of health care delivery is the fact that the consumption is not directly controlled by the consumer. It has been found that the number of procedures ordered or performed in the health care system is directly proportional to the number of physicians in the area and that the consumption of health care procedures does mainly depend on the distribution of those delivering health care. (Further reference see 13,4). This is partly caused by the fact that there is only a restricted access limitation of the consumer to the elements of health care delivery. The more advanced the insurance system is, the less financial aspects of the instigated procedure are of noticeable influence on the consumption. The effect is not directly measurable and the benefit of health care procedures is highly dependent upon individual value scales. Furthermore, the decision making process is subjected to many influences without direct feedback from the outcome of the action taken as a result of the great number of interfaces with other systems. Since medicine is an empirical science, standardization of procedures is only very limited and constant changes in the state of knowledge certainly are not facilitating validation and standardization of procedures.

2.2 Structures

The main structures of health care delivery systems are shown in Fig.1. Various institutions may provide

    -ambulatory
    -hospital
    -rehabilitative and
    -public health care.

This enumeration does not yet show institutions of preventive care. This function is mainly provided, at the moment, by all the above mentioned institutions to a varying degree. But health care screening centers come into being as special features as well as other institutions dedicated to preventive medicine, which is gaining an increasing importance in modern medicine.

Fig.2 illustrates that the main functions are provided by all institutions and are financed from various sources. In modern industrialized society, occupational care (as in industrial medicine) becomes increasingly important as well as social and psychological care which addresses itself to those ailments which are directly or indirectly caused by the psychological and societal situation of individuals resulting in various complaints and phenomena of not well-being.

As already indicated in Fig.1, the flow of patients between the various structures of the system is ill-defined and very often determined at random. This is partly because most subsystems have grown independently from each other. Access time to the system varies and the elapsed time to arrive at the optimal place for treatment. This is not necessarily in the institution most advanced in technology.

2.3 Functions

The traditional functions (see Fig.2) of health care systems are

-diagnosis
-prognosis
-therapy
-rehabilitation
-prevention.

In general terms, diagnosis is the recognition of the state and hopefully cause of the deviation from normality, prognosis is the attempt to describe the time vector and direction of the process, therapy is the action taken to exercise an influence on the course, rehabilitation are measures to reintegrate individuals after events and prevention are means and measures to avoid the incidence of a possible event.

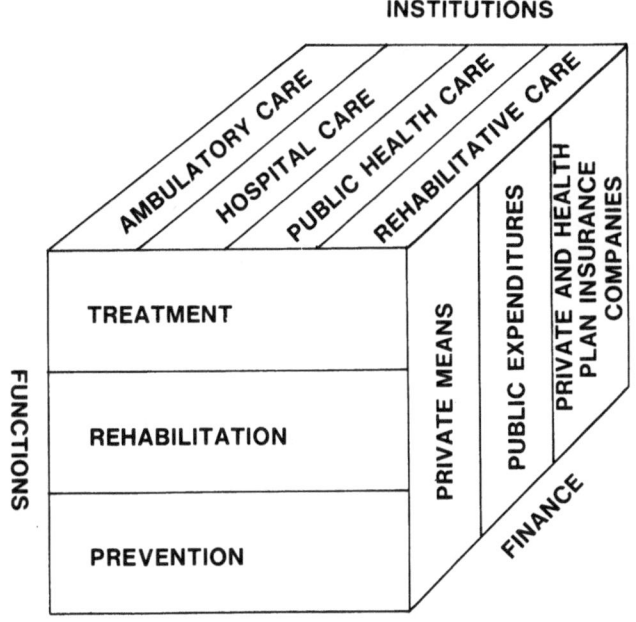

Fig. 2:
        Functions, institutions and major sources of finance in health
        care delivery (According to BESKE, personal communication).

All these functions are not by necessity provided by the medical profession alone, but more and more by other health care providers, mostly under the direction of physicians as the managers of a health care providing team. Besides looking at the institutions and medical functions the following groups may be distinguished:

- care providers (i.e. medical and paramedical professions)
- carriers (i.e. those institutions financing care delivery like insurance companies), and
- consumers (i.e. those who enter the process of care delivery).

Also between these groups conflicting interest may arise, definitely their criteria and aims are not necessarily concordant.

2.4 Evaluation criteria

Since the health care delivery system has so many interfaces with various environments, it is difficult, if not impossible, to evaluate all the various outcomes in their ramifications. However, it is possible to assess the cost of at least conventional health care delivery. Most evaluations therefore address themselves to the process of delivery, not to its product.

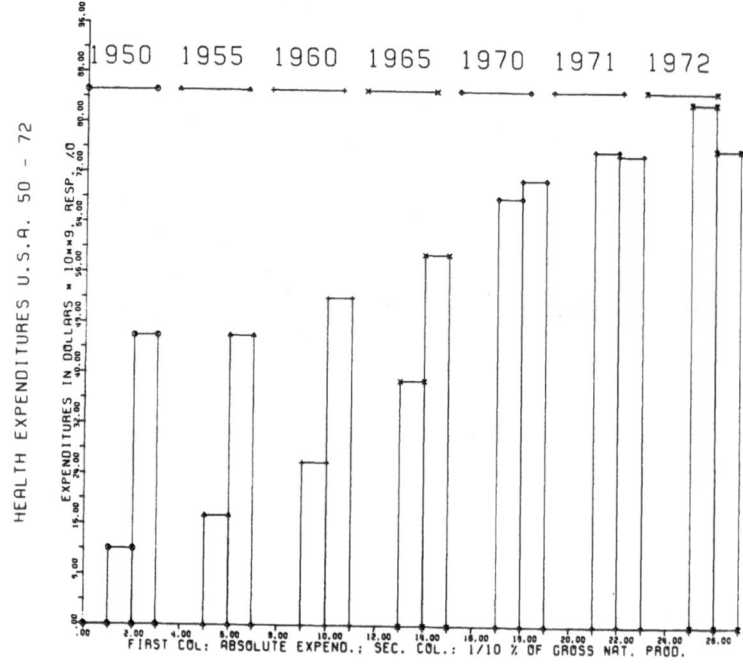

Fig. 3:
        Development of gross national product and cost for health care in % of the GNP, United States 1950-72. (18, see also 13)

During the last decades, in all industrialized countries a continuous increase of the cost of health care delivery has been observed. The roots of this increase go back to the introduction of technological

procedures into medicine. This started at the turn of this century,
reaching an almost exponential growth during the last two decades.
Fig.3 describes the development of cost compared with the gross
national product in the U.S.A. during the years 1950 to 1972. Though
the social and insurance system is different in the Federal Republic of
Germany, the trend is quite similar (12).

A breakdown of the various expenditures shows hospitals as the major
part of these expenses being followed by fees for physicians and
general procedures like private care, rehabilitation and other support.
The fourth largest item are expenditures for drugs. Within hospital
personnel expenses account for roughly 55% (Fig.4).

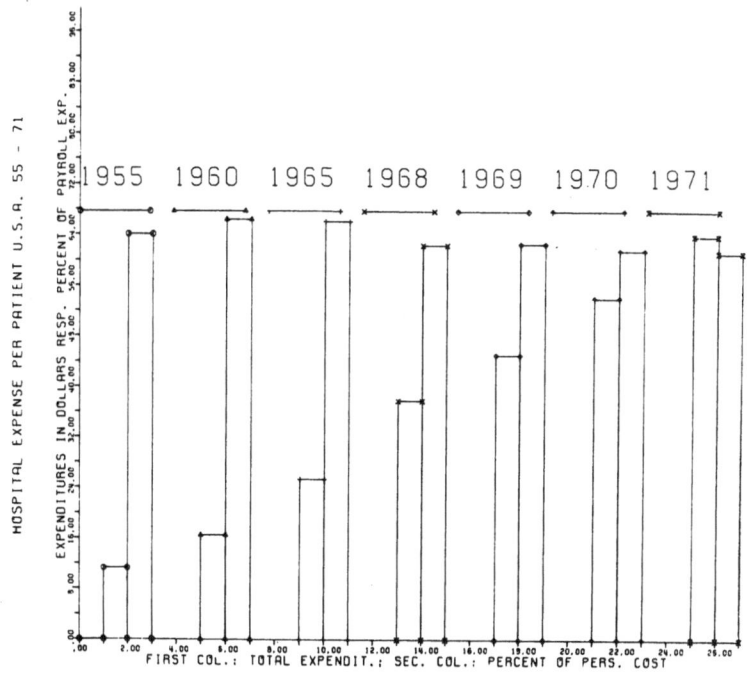

Fig. 4:
    Increasing hospital expenditures and percentage of personnel
    cost (material from 18).

This development of cost naturally indicates hospital care as the
primary target for investigations and attempts to improve the
situation. It has to be pointed out, however, that cost in this
subsystems may accrue due to the fact that longterm control mechanisms
or lack of control mechanisms may have occurred prior to the entrance
of the individual into the system, already determining his course or a
sequence of actions following their own intrinsic rules.

In analyzing the rate of increase of the various items, nursing home
care and research show the greatest ratio. Hospital cost rank third;
however, they have the greatest absolute value anyhow, and so the
absolute increase is also the greatest.

The raising hospital costs show a fairly constant percentage of personnel cost in this increase (Fig.4). Physicians' income, in the United States at least, shows a steady increase since '59 for the various disciplines, the general price increase, however, has a steeper gradient. The greatest ratio of increase can be seen in the discipline of internists, general practitioners, and obstetricians/ gynecologists in this order.

In addition to the increased prices for health care provided, the number of health care personnel has been increased with the greatest ratio for physicians and nurses. Also here the trends in the United States are almost identical with those in the Federal Republic of Germany. Incidences of health care encounters show a clear relationship to economical development (Fig.5), as do incidences of retirement.

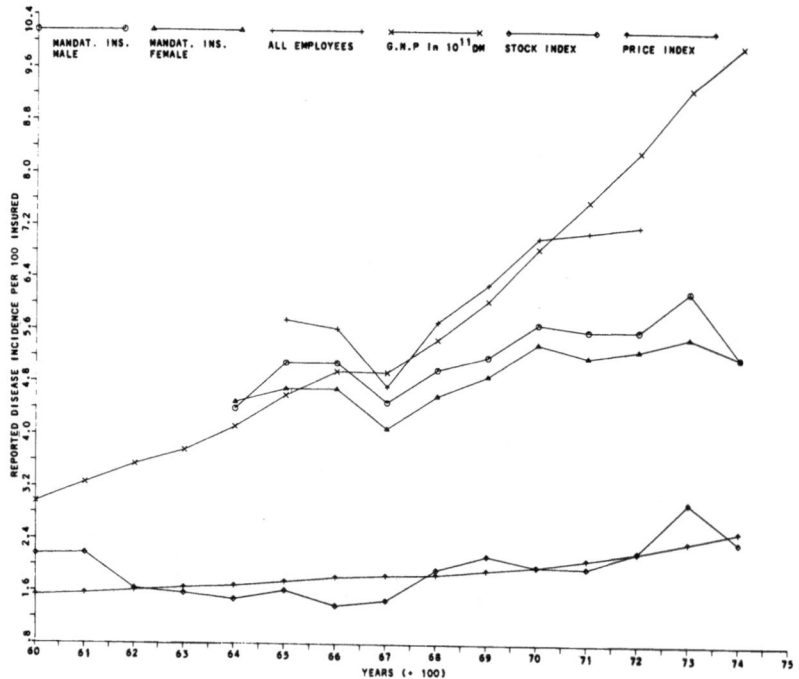

Fig. 5:

      Relations between economical indices and health care encounters. Significant decrease during the recession period 1966-68. Members of the mandatory and optional health insurance (approximately 35-90% of all patients) in Germany.

The increasing cost naturally are of concern to economists and politicians. Furthermore, high cost may, in some incidences, reflect optimal scheduling and treatment, as e.g. when the cost per day is calculated in a hospital where diagnostic and therapeutical actions follow each other in close sequence. Effective and expensive treatment may carry on into the other environmental systems and reduce obligations and support of society for an individual that can be rehabilitated and re-integrated into the working process. At the moment, however, there is very little or no cross-accounting. On the other side, it has to be mentioned that intensive care may save lives of people, but may make it necessary to provide continuous support.

The high cost therefore could be tolerated if the increasing input would result in an appropriate output, i.e. a measurable increase in individual and collective health. The contemplation of cost would have to take cross benefits into consideration such as occurring in the social section. To do this, indicators to describe the health status of a population would be necessary as well as models to assess consequences of disease categories.

It therefore seems necessary to look for indicators to describe the systems' output. Performance figures for institutions of the system only indicate the amount of services rendered, not the effectiveness of these services. Furthermore, these performance indicators, as e.g. for hospitals, do not necessarily show an increase beyond the proportion of services per capita, as shown for hospital utilization data (13).

Much of the cost is generated by the application of technological procedures. It has been said that the increased costs are not reflected in those indicator variables that traditionally have been used in the attempt to describe the quality state of health care delivery. These indicators have been used in health statistics:

    -life expectancy
        . male
        . female
    -infant mortality
    -mother mortality
    -death rate
    -birth rate
    -average hospital stay
    -disease
        . morbidity
        . mortality
        . hospitalization
        . stay per hospitalization
    -days away from work and
    -access time to system.

For some of these indicators, there exist biological differences between sexes as e.g. for female and life expectancy, which show a significant difference (73.99 versus 68.1 years) in 28 countries of the European WHO region;13).

Health care planning tries to improve indicators by factors, which subsequently will be called extrinsic. The main extrinsic factors are

    -expenditures
        . per capita
        . per hospital stay
        . per visit
    -numbers (per capita) of
        . physicians
        . nurses
        . other health personnel
        . encounters
        . hospitals and
        . beds.

It is rather disappointing, how little influence these extrinsic
factors seem to have on the indicators described above. It has to be
taken into consideration, however, that most of these indicators are
indicators of collective health and that individual events are not
reflected in their values. For instance, it can be found that adequate
treatment of ten thousand people out of a city like Hannover with the
result of gaining 20 years of life span of the individual increases
the overall life expectancy of this population only by half a percent.
If this type of treatment is projected on a larger population, the
increase naturally becomes smaller and negligible. For the individual
involved, however, special value scales apply which vary according to
character, environment and many other factors.

INDICATOR: INFANT MORTALITY

CONSTANT OF EQUATION: 53,67

VARIABLE	FACTOR	RANK
POLITICAL SYSTEM	+7,024	2
NURSES	-0,38	5
NUMBER OF HOSPITALS/10,000	-10,07	6
HEALTH EXPENDITURE PER CAP.	-0,054	3
MIDWIVES PER 10,000	+2,064	4
DENTISTS PER 10,000	+1,85	7
PHYSICIANS PER 10,000	-2,168	1
BEDS PER 1,000	+0,26	9
POPULATION DENSITY	-0,007	8
TOTAL POPULATION	-	-

Fig. 6:
      Regression analysis of the relation between the indicator
      infant mortality and extrinsic health factors, 33 countries of
      the European WHO region, including the U.S.A. and Japan.

A regression analysis of data from 34 nations in WHO statistics (3)
only indicates a weak relationship between the extrinsic factors and
the listed health indicators. For instance, life expectancy of females
varies between countries with different political systems and seems to
be dependent upon the number of nurses, shows a positive relationship
to the number of hospitals and health care expenditures, just to name a
few. Some of these relationships definitely may not be considered to be
causal but to be caused by third factors, which cannot yet be described
properly. This becomes evident when the indicator male life expectancy,
e.g. shows a primary correlation to dentists per 100 population. Even a
negative correlation seems to exist in regard to physicians, while
nurses rank in the third place. However, on the other side, infant

mortality is negatively correlated to the number of physicians per ten thousand and to health care expenditures per capita (Fig.6). All this indicates a complex interrelationship and gives little clues as to what input increases the expected benefit. This question can only be answered when the benefits are clearly defined, known in their ramification and examined from a certain value scale or reference context, as, e.g., the incidences of certain infectious diseases like poliomyelitis, malaria, smallpox, etc.

In exploratory factor analytical techniques, the described indicators and input variables form various groups which sometimes seem to describe a logical relationship and common trend and in other incidences do not give further clues. For example, the variables birth rate, growth rate, death rate, and infant mortality seem to be projected on one factor as well as number of physicians, number of nurses, and number of dentists into an opposite direction. Number of beds per capita, hospitals per capita and male life expectancy as well as female life expectancy seem to form another factor on which the very crude variable of political classification in East- or West-block-countries seems to have a negative loading. As always, factor analytical techniques may not be used to give causal explanations, but just describe variances of data collectives. Other factors in the same material show similar, mostly confusing, pictures.

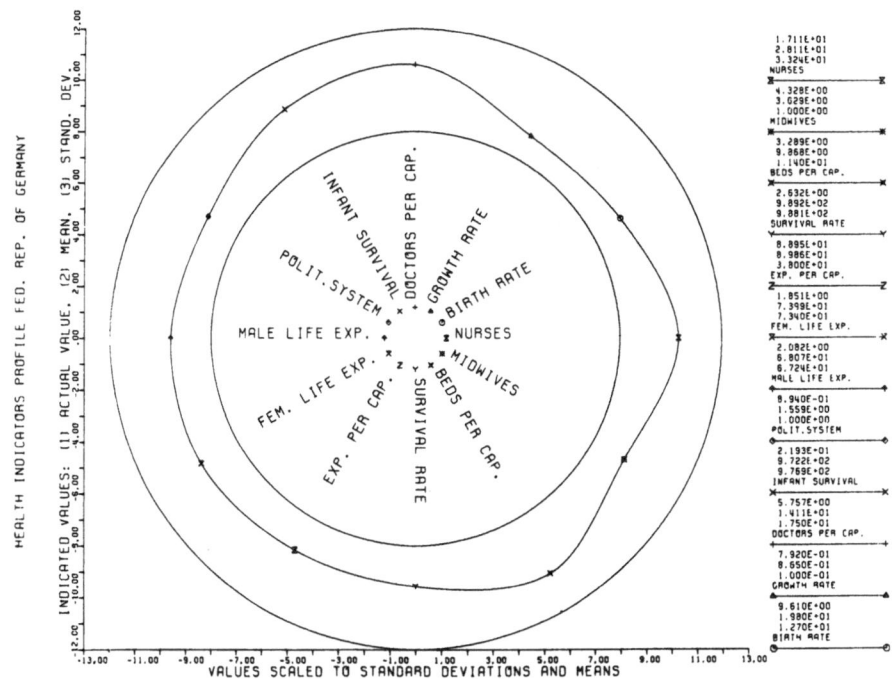

Fig. 7:
Profile of health indicators of the Fed. Rep. of Germany in comparison with the mean values and (+2) standard deviation of the other countries in the European WHO region including Japan and the U.S.A. (33 countries).

Further investigations indicate that other factors than those described
as extrinsic may have equal or even greater influence (e.g. 7). These
factors, which may be called intrinsic, are
     -nutrition
     -hygiene
     -alcohol
     -accidents and
     -education.

Especially education seems to have a very strong influence on the
general incidence of diseases and life expectancy. Probably, collective
health seems to be stronger influenced by these mostly longterm factors
which affect a great number of people and constitute risks for chronic
disease and ailment.

2.5 Summary of system aspects

The functions treatment, rehabilitation and prevention are expected to
be performed by health care delivery systems through institutions of
hospital care, ambulatory care, public health care and rehabilitation
care. These gross classifications of institutions encompass various
elements which are to be basically described when discussing these
subsystems, which will be done in other contributions of this volume.

Financing, which so far has only been regarded from a global
standpoint, is provided by
     -private means
     -public expenditures and
     -private and health plan insurance companies

according to the various health care plans of the countries which may
vary from predominantly basing the health care system on private means
to comprehensive state health careplans. In between are those
countries basing their health care system on semi-state insurance
systems with comprehensive legislature regulating access and payment
structure.

The discussed functions can be abstracted as functions of recognition,
evaluation and action (productions):
          -recognition
              . diagnosis
              . analysis
                    i.e. functions of pragmatic or systematized
                    semantic classification
                        = cognitive function
          -evaluation
              . prognosis
              . (therapy) planning
          -action
           (productive or prohibitive)
              . therapy
                    . . drugs
                    . . operation
                    . . diet
                    . . nursing
                    . . etc.
              . rehabilitation
              . prevention
                    i.e. interference with the **objects** system
                        = active (productive) function

In describing the health indicators in polar coordinates, profiles can
be created which allow for a certain comparison of data (Fig.7)
However, it has to be borne in mind that many statistical data of this
kind have a uncertainty factor lying in the various methods of
compiling statistics and even defining the criteria for the elements
of the statistics.

When the described variables are examined with discriminant function
analytical techniques, female life expectancy can be predicted
correctly in approximately 60% of the cases using the variables
political systems, growth rate, physicians per capita, and number of
nurses. Infant mortality when grouped into 4 classes, can be predicted
correctly in approximately 80% using the variables expenditures per
capita, doctors per capita, political system, dentists per capita and
beds per capita; thus it seems to be roughly determined by the
"traditional" extrinsic factors. Even the political system can be
grossly classified using health indicators like birth rate, infant
mortality, female life expectancy, expenditures per capita and
physicians per capita. These last results, however, should be regarded
with greatest caution. Environmental factors may influence variables
into the same direction which then not necessarily have the casual
interrelationship.

TABLE 1:   DISCRIMINANT ANALYSIS (8) PREDICTION RESULTS
           FOR INFANT MORTALITY, SAME MATERIAL (3) AS
           USED FOR FIG.7. FOR THE PREDICTION THE VARIABLES:
           EXPENDITURES PER CAPITA, M.D.'S PER CAPITA,
           POLITICAL SYSTEM, DENTISTS PER CAPITA, BEDS PER CAPITA
           WERE USED.

ACTUAL GROUP	NO. OF COUNTRIES	PREDICTED GROUP MEMBERSHIP			
		GR. 1	GR. 2	GR. 3	GR. 4
GROUP 1 10 - 15 PER 1000	9.	7. 77.8%	1. 11.1%	1. 11.1%	0. 0.0%
GROUP 2 16 - 20	6.	1. 16.7%	4. 66.7%	1. 16.7%	0. 0.0%
GROUP 3 21 - 30 - 40	13.	0. 0.0%	2. 15.4%	11. 84.6%	0. 0.0%
GROUP 4 41 AND ABOVE UP	5.	0. 0.0%	1. 20.0%	0. 0.0%	4. 80.0%
UNGROUPED CASES	1.	0. 0.0%	0. 0.0%	0. 0.0%	1. 100.0%

PERCENT OF 'GROUPED' CASES CORRECTLY CLASSIFIED: 78.79%

Briefly, it can be stated that so far the traditional indicators have
failed to give reliable measurements for the general health status and
its relation to input into the system (called extrinsic factors).
However, greater statistical material and methodological research may
yield more results in the future. Further work is necessary. The
discussed grouping techniques and results of analyses are unreliable so
far but may point into a possible direction.

Despite of sporadic and partial results attempts have failed so far
to produce reliable evaluation means to determine the result of these
functions, especially in their relation to the input. Further research
is necessary and probably the variables included in this research must
not be restricted to the traditional medical indicators.

The complexity of the overall system calls for defined approaches in
limited areas as well as modelling and analytical techniques to study
the interrelationship between the various inputs and the system
functions. There simply cannot be easy or global solutions. It has to
be distinguished between the optimization of the process of care
delivery and the optimization of the input-output relationship. Also
process optimization may have its value, but must be recognized or
intended as such.

3. Subsystems
=============

As a consequence of this complexity, the traditional global approach in
medicine enters into competition with the engineering techniques to
form successively conceptual subdivisions and to look for solutions in
well defined areas. Certainly, 'suboptimized' subsystems may resist
integration which has to be borne in mind. But the understanding of
subdivisions makes it possible to treat them as single variables and/or
modules in more complex arrangements. A system which cannot be
understood cannot be controlled, and its information flow cannot be
modelled.

Subsystems may be identified as structures, that is subsets of elements
of a system, with a high degree of communality in communication
channels and procedures and less intense interaction with other
elements. In health care, the most distinct subsystems are institutions
for ambulatory care and even more, hospitals. Subsystems in the public
health sector are institutions for chronic care, institutions for local
public health administration and operations including vaccination and
epidemy control.

In this context, subsystems in ambulatory care hospitals and public
health will be briefly described in their main system aspects.

3.1 Ambulatory care

Institutions in ambulatory care may be
     -private practices
            . general practitioners
            . specialists
            . group practices of either combinations or single
              specialties
     -ambulatories
     -hospital outpatient departments
            . clinics
            . dispensaries

or combinations of these, either as private institutions or maintained
by other structures in the national or local system.

The units comprise a varying number of members of the health care
delivering team, i.e.

-doctors
-nurses
-aids
-technicians
-secretaries.

These units are mostly characterized by a closed loop of communication, mostly involving only a small number of people. Own investigations within general practices have shown, that only 10 percent of all communications in these units go outside, the rest includes the stages
-physician
-patient
-aid, technician or nurse.

Fig. 8 describes this situation and gives examples of means of communication.

The documentation (definition see above) is done for purposes of
-treatment
   . recollection of own cognitive processes
   . justification (medical and forensic)
   . communication
-billing and administration
-planning of therapy and operations of the unit.

AMBULATORY CARE

STAGES OF COMMUNICATION

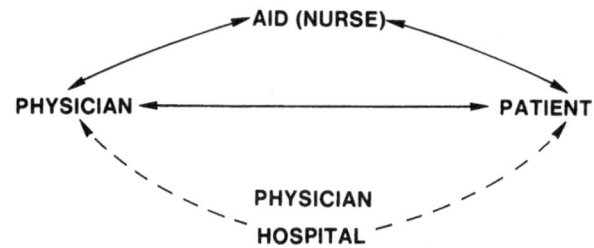

CHANNELS OF COMMUNICATION

— PATIENT

— VOICE

   — DIRECT

   — TELEPHONE

— WRITTEN MATERIAL

   — RECORD

   — NOTES

   — FORMS

   — PRESCRIPTIONS

   — REPORTS

   — BILLING/ACCOUNTING

   — SYMBOLS

Fig. 8:

Communication in ambulatory care.

The principle event in ambulatory care is the encounter. Most
documentation is related to this encounter.

The elements recorded are:
    -location or type of encounter
        . office
        . patient's home
        . dispensaries
        . nursing homes or similar institutions
        . by telephone
        . through third persons
    -findings
        . history
        . examinations and observations
        . laboratory examinations
    -procedures
        . diagnostic
        . therapeutic
    -prescriptions
    -planned actions.

Legal and administrative requirements dictate parts of the information
flow. Medical requirements are satisfied mostly in an individual manner
and with great variance (17).

3.2 Hospitals

The main functional areas within hospitals have been described (11,6,9)
as
    -hospital management
    -patient management
    -medical tasks and science
    -public health tasks.

Hospital management in this context includes also technical and
supportive functions. Patient management encompasses auxiliary services
and laboratories. The operations of the hospital are directed towards
the goals (13):
    -individual health
    -collective health
    -hospital economy
    -employees' satisfaction
    -professional recognition as basis for professional and financial
     support.

The main benefits of hospital operations group around the two main
objectives - system patient and system hospital -
    -through patient
        . improvement of patient health
        . decrease of disability payment or supportive actions
        . increase of gross national product
    -through hospital operations
        . employment of personnel
        . local economic factor
        . education of health personnel
        . contribution to general knowledge.

Attempts to optimize the system 'patient' and the system 'hospital'
certainly may and do conflict. Scheduling problems involve
consideration for both types of systems. Planning for the system
'patient' has to take also into consideration psychological limitations

besides limitations by sequences of procedures dictated by their specific characteristics, besides the possible physical stress.

The main control functions for the system 'patient' originate in the treatment units
    -wards
    -outpatient departments,

from where the patients are dispatched to the various diagnostic and treatment units (see 14,16). Consequently, these treatment units are the main target for the patient optimization of related information flow, both in terms of administrative as well as medical procedures.

The subsystems, to which the patients are dispatched for diagnostic or therapeutic services have their own communication and information systems. It has always been assumed, that many detail information in these subsystems is necessary for the decision making in other units, investigations, however, seem to indicate, that communication mostly occurs in an abstracted or condensed form, so that closed information systems with definded interfaces may be used. The experiences with existing hospital systems gradually yield the material to analyze the actual information flow and subsequently requirement between the various units. This experience is necessary, it does not suffice to know the conventional information exchange. The behavior influenced by the new tools of information exchange has to be analyzed in terms of their repercussion on the set of information actually used.

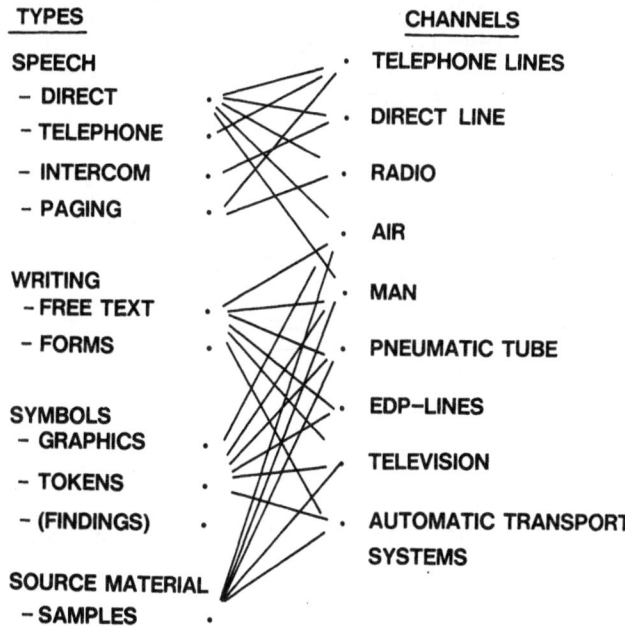

COMMUNICATION

Fig. 9:
    Classes and channels of communication on a ward in a tertiary care hospital.

The main forms of communication within a hospital, as related to the patient, are given in Fig.9 (15) for a ward in a tertiary care hospital as a result of an analysis in the Medical School Hannover.

The main vehicle for documentation is the medical record. Here systematic and chronological data are recorded and collected. Information generated in ancillary departments (radiology, laboratories, etc.) and related to the patient are also made part of this record.

3.3 Public Health

The functional areas in the public health subsystems are basically the same as in the other parts:

- administration
- care (and 'health') delivery
- research
- general services and planning.

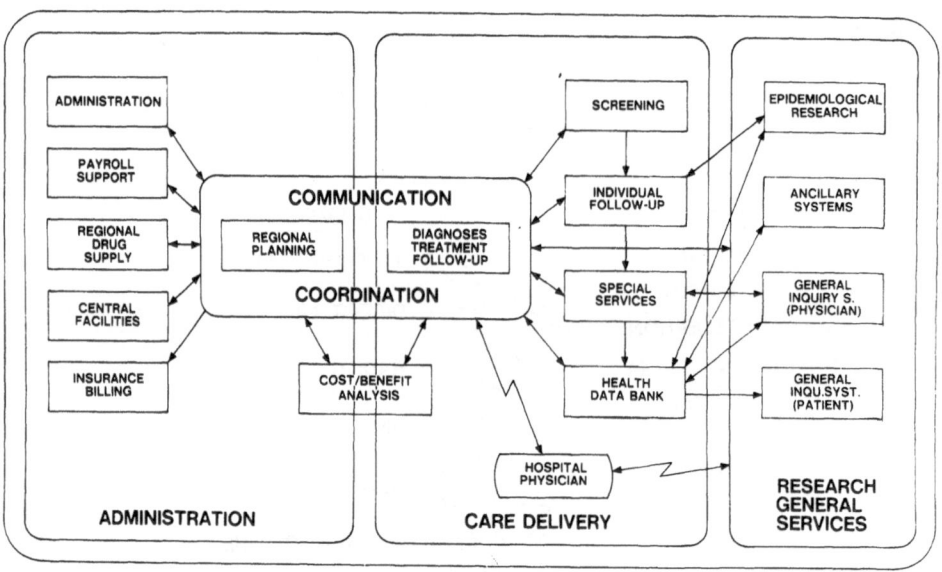

Fig. 10:
        Principle of functions and of information control in public health

Fig.10 gives an exemplary concept of information flow.
The institutions in this sector vary between countries and the borders between the subsystems described in this chapter wander in respect to

the national health and political concept of a region and/or country.
The chapter on information system in public health in this book will
deal with some details of system aspects in this subsystem.

4. Communication between subsystems
=======================================

The communication between the various health care delivery subsystems
is mainly

    -through the patient and
    -in written form.

Since most information is pertaining to the disease process, being
derived in several hierarchies of message processing, this disease
process being dynamic and the physician having the responsibility for
his diagnostic and therapeutic action, it is probably an illusion to
reduce duplication of diagnostic procedures more than only to a minor
degree by increasing the very limited amount of communication between
systems, which in most cases is monodirectional from the institutions
of higher specialization of care to referring systems and 'source
carried' (by the patient) into the other direction.

It is generally felt, that improvement of communications between
subsystems will

    -improve the quality of health care delivery and
    -reduce cost.

Both assumptions seem to be logical but have not been proven so far.

5. Dynamic of systems
============================

The dynamics of the health care delivery system(s) are determined by
    -the functional requirements and operational dynamics of the care
     providing institutions
    -the environmental and personal requirements of the patient and
    -the dynamics of the disease processes.

The statistics of hospital admisssion for example reflect primarily the
first two elements. The typical weekly ondulations in statistics of bed
occupancy (5) reflect the working habits in the hospital as well as the
preference of the patient population. The superimposed pattern of
reduction during holidays and general vacation periods reflect the
general environment. The functional requirements and dynamics of wards
can be recognized by further analysis in regard to the services
performed on these wards.

The increasing amount of data in hospital information systems provides
the material to investigate seasonable fluctuations of occurences of
diseases and disease categories (6,5). We know too little yet about
these factors, but they may be of certain importance for both teaching
and planning.

Certainly, the diagnostic mix of the catchment population is of
importance both for the hospital operations as well as for the analysis
of the accruing costs. Information has to be broken down to disease

groups or actions performed in order to be able to make comparisons and
adjustments. It is, however, a problem, that the most common disease
groups or diagnoses occur in combinations.

Functional characteristics and medical practice of an institution are
also reflected in the profile of main activities, as e.g. medication.
It is surprising to see, that in the own institution e.g. 40% of
expenditures are caused by less than ten different kinds of drugs.

Hospital information systems gradually yield information about the
system aspects of the delivery of health care. Research is only
gradually progressing in the field of system analysis of the system
patient. Modelling of pharmcocinetic activities is one of the areas of
interest, as well as chronic diseases and management of chronic
diseases. Here certainly is an area of interesting work in the future.

6. Problems and goals of information treatment in health care systems.
===

This basic description of the system aspects of health care delivery is
intended to set the stage for further discussion of the various
subsystems and their aspects. Only after the clear perception of the
various environmental and output aspects it is possible to derive the
criteria for an overall evaluation. It is necessary to study subsystems
of limited abilities. When they are sufficiently known, complexer
problems may be attacked.

In discussing the various aspects, general problems in regard to
information processing could be observed. They may be summarized as
follows and may require further attention in regard to possible methods
and techniques to cope with these problems. Furthermore, these problem
areas constitute weak parts in the traditional systems and give targets
for a system analytical approach which may impact on the overall
system.

(1) A major problem is the complexity of output and input in context
with the great variety of interfacing systems of the real world. This
leads to conflicts of goals and creates fuzziness and varying bases for
value scales and evaluation.

(2) Very often the elements to the process of information treatment are
     -ill defined, both as elements and as
      ordered groups or tuples of elements
     -and serve as input to non-standardized and
      varying rules for processing.

Very often items are treated as elements and described as elements,
when they are in reality n-tuples, where the other elements are
substituted from other sources of information in associative or
subconscious processes. The complementary elements are provided from
the whole set of pragmatic data generated by the patient contact and
the multiple interfaces.

The recognition of theses facts has generated many efforts to collect
elements in terminologies and to define their semantic content in
nomenclatures. This is the basis for effective information systems, but
has already as such improved communication and systematic research.

(3) Most decision making (information treatment) process consists of a
long and often recursively processed chain of message - information

hierarchies. This is the problem of prevailing secondary information,
i.e. the primary process cannot be measured and peripheral variables
are collected respectively multiple steps of deduction occur. Very
often then the final step of transformation is taken or described as
being representative for the whole process, while in reality this step
has been already been pretty much determined by previous steps.

Work in this area contibutes to the systematic approach to causal
relationship in a quantitative way, thus slowly providing the input to
the systematization of the medical decision making process.

(4) There is no formal theory in medicine. Information processing
efforts generate systems analytical approaches which may introduce the
system concept into this field. Gradual expression of medical findings
and reasoning in a formal way will enable further quantitative analysis
and will allow for the formulation of hypotheses and their testing in a
more abstract and generalized way.

(5) There exists a high degree of network structures between subsystems
without clear definition of interfaces.

Health care delivery consists of a number of elements, which have
historically grown and have, by experience, developed a modus vivendi
which is far away from a planned system construction. Such a system
construction will provide the basis for the elimination of unnecessary
and costly redundancy and loss of time.

Given this situation, the consequences have to be determined, both from
the standpoint of medicine with all the various aspects as they have
been described as well as using the experience and methodology of
informatics. The following articles will give some of these aspects and
will continue to analyze the situation. Several attempts have
originated in the immediate past to design new types of delivery
systems. Some will be discussed in this context.

LITERATURE
==========

1 ANOKHIN, P.K.: Fortschritt der biologischen und medizinischen Kybernetik. Moskau (1974), 52-110.
2 ANOKHIN, P.K.: Biology and Neurophysiology of the Conditioned Reflex
  and its Role in Adaptive Behavior. Pergamon Press, Oxford (1974).
3 ANONIMOUS: Les Services de Santé en Europe. Organisation Mondiale de
  la Santé, Bureau Regional de l'Europe. Copenhague (1974).
4 BAILEY, N.T.J., THOMPSON, M.: Systems Aspects of Health Planning.
  North Holland Pub. Co., Amsterdam (1975).
5 ENGELBRECHT, R., SCHMEETZ, D., LAUDE, G., V. GAERTNER, H.-O.,
  REICHERTZ, P.L.: Patients' Dynamics and Functional Administrative
  Behavior of a Multi-Disciplinary Medical Center. MEDIS'75, Tokyo,
  (Oct. 7-9, 1975), 144-155.
6 HILL, R.D., SAUTER, K., REICHERTZ, P.L.: Data Bank Concept of the
  Medical System Hannover and the Analysis of Patient Data. In:
  ANDERSON, J. and FORSYTHE, J.M.: MEDINFO 74, (Amsterdam 1974),
  399-406.
7 LETOURMY, A.: Some Aspects of the Relationship between Mortality,
  Environmental Conditions and Medical Care. IIASA - Conference
  'Systems Aspects of Health Planning'. Schloss Laxenburg/Oesterreich,
  (Aug. 20-22, 1974), in: BAILEY, N.J., THOMPSON, M.: Systems Aspects
  of Health Planning. North Holland Pub. Co., Amsterdam (1975),
  267-278.

8 NIE, N., BENT, D.H., HULL, C.H.: SPSS - Statistical Package for the Social Sciences. McGraw-Hill, New York (1970).

9 REICHERTZ, P.L.: Medizinische Informatik - Aufgaben, Wege und Bedeutung. Verhandlung der Ges. Deutscher Naturforscher u. Aerzte 1972, 107 (1973), 106-120.

10 REICHERTZ, P.L.: The Medical System Hannover (MSH). In: COLLEN, M.: Hospital Computer Systems, Wiley & Son, New York, (1974), 598-661.

11 REICHERTZ, P.L.: Hospital Information Systems, Concept and Implementation of the Medical System Hannover (MSH). In: MAROIS, M. (Edit.): Man and Computer. North Holland Pub. Co., Amsterdam (1975), 153-186.

12 REICHERTZ, P.L.: Computer im Dienste der Medizin - Aufgaben, Wege und Bedeutung -. IBM-Seminar 'Datenverarbeitung und Wissenschaft in Verwaltung: Einsatz im Krankenhaus'. (Maerz 20-22, 1973), Bad Liebenzell, IBM-Form: GE 12-1275-0.

13 REICHERTZ, P.L.: Hospitals and Health Care. IFAC75, 6th Triennial World Congress of the International Federation of Automatic Control. Boston/Mass./USA, (Aug. 20-30, 1975), P.7.1-P.7.23.

14 REICHERTZ, P.L.: Informationssysteme in der Medizin. IBM-Verlag, Bonn-Bad Godesberg (1975).

15 REICHERTZ, P.L.: Strategy Considerations for Hospital Information Systems. MEDIS '75, Tokyo, (Oct. 7-9, 1975), 11-18.

16 REICHERTZ, P.L.: Datenbanken/Informationssysteme. In: KOLLER, F., WAGNER, G., (Edit.): Medizinische Dokumentation. Handbuch der Datenverarbeitung in der Medizin. Schattauer-Verlag, Stuttgart (1975).

17 REICHERTZ, P.L., MOEHR, J.R., HOLTHOFF, G., FILSINGER, E.: Struktur und Funktion der allgemeinmedizinischen Praxis. Bericht einer Projektstudie an das Zentralinstitut fuer die kassenaerztliche Versorgung in der Bundesrepublik Deutschland (1975).

18 U.S. DEPARTMENT OF COMMERCE, BUREAU OF THE CENSUS. The American Almanac. Grosset and Dunlap, New York (1974).

J. R. MOEHR, HANNOVER

1. Introduction

It has repeatedly been pointed out that information processing, generally speaking, constitutes an important activity of our medical care systems. It absorbs a substantial fraction of available manpower. Demands concerning information processing have considerably increased in recent decades. This is due in part to recent advances in medical technology which entailed a pressure towards subspecialization in medicine with consequent increase of the number of spezialists involved in treating a particular case. This in turn increased the need for documentation of the information gathered by a given subspecialty and the need for communication of this information. Another cause can be seen in the fact that modern techniques for automated data generation are widely employed in many laboratory procedures. Another feature of modern technology is the increased use of reproduction techniques such as photography or radiography which contribute considerably to the massproduction and dispersion of data with an ensueing increase in the demand for availability, correctness and intelligibility of the data. Modern medical technology also influenced the demand for medical care. More derangements have become distinguishable and amenable to various kinds of treatment. Disease in general has become detectable at earlier stages. Cure, however, is not always attainable, with the consequence that more patients have to be treated chronically. Early detection and the need for protracted care both increase the fraction of people demanding medical attention in a given population. The continuous trend towards socialization of medical care has the effect that the subjective need for medical care results in actual requests for it. So far this request for medical care is in most countries controlled only by the patient, who sometimes adopts the attitude of a consumer. Efforts to control the consumption of health resources by some kind of objective measure are yet scarce.

The described situation creates a need to react by adapting means for information processing to the altered situation. Automation of information processing is one way to meet this demand. This, however, requires understanding of the role of information processing in medical care systems and of the related medical concepts. The goal of the following discussion is to contribute to a clarification in this respect.

2. Basic Concepts

The medical care system, health and disease.

As a basis for the following discussion, let us first examine a few basic notions.

A 'system' has been defined as a set of a mutually interrelated elements (29). In medical care systems, two principal components may be differentiated: the provider of medical care and the consumer of medical care. Since the provider may not only be an individual physician, but a hospital or even a public health system, just as the consumer may not only be a single patient, but e.g. a whole population, it seems more appropriate to distinguish a subject system and an object system. The subject system corresponds to the provider, the object system to the consumer of medical care. The subject system acts upon an object system with the purpose of influencing its behaviour, for instance by converting a state of disease into a state of health. The subject system also collects information about the object system with the aim of assessing the object system's behaviour, in order to select appropriate actions.

The subject system is then what is frequently called 'medicine' - the materialized, personified or institutionalized effect of an attempt to provide professional help on the basis of a scientific approach where health is impaired or endangered (11). It is important to note that medicine has in the past directed its attention almost exclusively at the analysis of its object systems. As a result we dispose of a great number of techniques for the analysis and description of the behaviour of entire populations, of physical or psychical reactions of individuals as well as for analysis of structure and function of single organs or their components down to the submicroscopic and molecular level. Consideration of the subject system has virtually been ignored. Neither do we have sufficient knowledge of the various subject systems' requirements and constraints, nor is an instrumentarium of methods available to diminish this ignorance. Least of all seems to be known about the manner in which the knowledge gained as a result of the analysis of the object systems is used in the process of medical care.

Clarity about this issue, however, is crucial if automated means of data processing are to be successfully incorporated into medical care systems, in which case they become part of a subject system. In this respect computer based information systems have much in common with a graft which is implanted into an organism. One of the important effects of the past successes and failures of computer based medical information systems was that they pointed out the need for more knowledge about the subject system and for better methods for the advancement of this knowledge. Apart from the immediate benefit that such information systems may have, they contribute in this fashion to our understanding of medicine which has broad implications not only for medical care but also for medical didactics and professional politics.

If the goal of medicine has been described above as providing help where health is endangered, the definition of health becomes a crucial issue. Health has been defined by the World Health Organization as a status of 'complete physical, psychical and social well-being' (12). Despite of the wide acceptance of this definition it suffers the disadvantage that its strict application makes it hard to consider anybody healthy. This has lead to attempts to arrive at better definitions. Most appropriate seem definitions which view the state of health as that of a stable equilibrium of an object system and its environment. Thus 'health' has been defined as a 'state of complete and persistent adaptation of an individual or collective to its environment' (41) or as a state where an individual is able to maintain 'its psychical integrity and physical and social identity' (11).

These definitions do not state a distinct or absolute goal of medicine, which would be desirable as a measure of effectiveness and achievement.

Neither do they serve to define the requirements for attainment of such a goal. Instead they make clear that the goals of medicine are relative to environmental circumstances. Health is a desirable state and disease a perceived objective or subjective difference between an actual state and this desired state.

The given definitions also emphasize the cybernetic nature of modern disease concepts (27, 39). The object system may be viewed as a complex system of mutually interrelated and superimposed control circles. What we perceive as disease are the expressions of the derangement of such control circles. Different kinds of derangements may have the same effects. Single causes may have different effects depending on the state of the object system under consideration. This state of the object system and consequently the appearence of disease varies with time and location. The perceived effects are further more dependent upon the means applied for observation.

Different medical specialties employing different means of observation will arrive at different results regarding a diseased system. Also, as the means for observation evolve historically, the picture of disease does change.

An important consequence of these concepts is that we are not dealing with 'diseases' corresponding to distinguishable natural entities. Disease is but an expression of the derangement of complex systems, and does not exist independently of the afflicted object system (14,15).

Medicine did since the times of Hippocrates strive to derive its conclusions from patterns of observed findings. Until the late middle ages these conclusions were predominantly of the prognostic type, i.e. the physicians attempted to forecast the outcome of a given course of disease. Since this type of reasoning was based on the interpretation of signs, the process was called 'semiology'. Under the influence of the developing natural sciences in the 17th and 18th century the emphasis shifted to a diagnostic classification of disease. An ontologic disease concept evolved which assumed that disease has its own natural history independently of the afflicted organism (14,15).

If a disease is a natural entity, it deserves its propper designation, - a diagnostic label -, requires a defined set of actions and, most important, is essentially unchangeable. Recognition of the fact that disease is only what we are able to perceive of the derangements affecting a patient, and that a diagnostic term assigned to a set of such perceivable derangements of a patient is influenced by the means with which, the situation in which, and the goals for which such derangements are assessed , should make the physician aware of the fact that the terms he uses are relative to the circumstances of their use. As will be demonstrated in greater detail below, this has decisive implications for what we may expect from automatic processing of such terms.

Distinctions between different states of the object system have the nature of model concepts and are due to artificial delimitations. A model is a simplifying representation of a complex system which serves the purpose of facilitating understanding of the latter (31). The systems, which are the objects of medical science, have many features in common with objects of other empirical sciences. They are an integral part of nature, which has to be artificially delimited, in order to become suitable for scientific understanding. In order to serve its purpose, the model has to be consistent within itself, and behave similarly to the natural system it is supposed to represent. Truths of empirical sciences are truths only within the scope of such a model. If differences in behaviour are observed that are not attributable to errors of observation, the model has to be corrrected. The continuous refinement of model concepts is therefore a primary objective of empirical sciences. In this respect medicine is not different from other empirical sciences.

The objects of medicine, at which the caring physician directs his attention, differ, however, in one important aspect from object systems of nonhumanitarian empirical sciences: in the subjective and active role that they assume in any transactions directed at them. They react physically, intellectually, emotionally and socially to medical actions.

This subjectivity on the part of the object system has various consequences, which cannot be reviewed here comprehensively.

One of these consequences is an impact on medical models. Unlike in other fields of science, these cannot be defined completely according to principles of scientific esthetics. They are actively shaped by influences from the object system. Medical science is furthermore only to a limited extent able to define its goals - much more than in nonhumanitarian sciences, these are imposed by the object system, by society, social subsystems or individuals. The ultimate criterion of the value of medical model concepts - the effectiveness in preservation or restoration of what is perceived as 'health' - is extraneous to the model and itself subject to changes due to the evolution of ideological concepts, environmental conditions, and progress of science - just to name a few. Every failure concerning this fuzzy criterion - 'health' - constitutes an incentive to reconsider the model and to change it.

An example is the continuous refinements of concepts of pathology, which in the past has led to a continuous resolution of the organism into organsystems, these into cells, these into organelles. Since all the physical substructures do not suffice, however, to explain the phenomena observed in medicine, contemporary models tend to comprise elements of the environment, such as social environment, climate, geographic characteristics, but also the microbial flora of the body, food, ethnic background, etc. Further extensions are brought about by inclusion of the emotional and psychic dimensions. These facts account for the great variety of medical model concepts which represent the rules and guide lines for medical action.

There is no hope to arrive at a perfect model which is completely identical with the natural system or which encompasses the complete chain from cause to effect. The chain of cause - effect reactions may be endless. To give a popular example: A coronary infarction is an effect of a discrepancy between blood supply and demand in the heart; the insufficient supply may be caused by coronary artery sclerosis, this by diabetes due to a hereditary disposition; an increased demand may be determined by emotional stress with its variety of possible causes, by physical exertion etc. Unfortunately we are lacking a criterion upon which to decide that a cause - effect relationship is complete in that it permits to establish the true cause (29). For the model one therefore has to create an artificial limit. Within these limits only one may argue.

This means that we have to deal with models that are effective with respect to a predetermined objective, and we have to be ready to change the model if it proves insufficient. The rules determining the behaviour of such a model are therefore provisional rules - in medicine even more than in other empirical sciences. In many instances, the situation is furthermore characterized by the fact that we do not have the means or the time to construct valid models. An example for the former are disease models in psychological medicine, examples of the latter abund in emergency situations. This creates a situation where the goal that is to be achieved is dominant, the means by which it is achieved, its style or elegance are secondary.

3. Types of Data in Medicine

Information processing, as defined in informatics, is achieved at the level of the processing of data or messages under the assumption that procedures exist by which messages of a set $\mathcal{M}$ are converted to messages of a set $\mathcal{M}'$ in a manner corresponding to the conversion of a set of informations $\mathcal{J}$ derived from $\mathcal{M}$ to a set of informations $\mathcal{J}'$ derived from $\mathcal{M}'$. It is assumed, that messages of the type $\mathcal{M}'$ have lower information content than messages of the type $\mathcal{M}$, and that the effort to arrive at informations of the type $\mathcal{J}'$ is smaller on the basis of messages $\mathcal{M}'$ than on the basis of messages $\mathcal{M}$ and informations $\mathcal{J}$. (1).

Automatic data processing then consists in application of a processing procedure to messages of the type $\mathcal{M}$ resulting in the production of messages of type $\mathcal{M}'$, i.e. in the application of a processing procedure to produce a defined output from defined input. Such data processing steps may correspond to a section of a sequence of information processing steps which one might consider discrete in this context.

Essentially then, we need a

- defined input
- defined output and
- processing procedure,
  algorithm or program

for automated data processing. These elements of automated data processing seem to correspond closely to some medical concepts of information. The following discussion is intended to examine this analogy more closely and to show that inconsiderate reliance on such analogies may lead to a wrong emphasis in the automation of medical data processing.

In an attempt to rationalize and discipline medical reasoning and thought processes, it became customary to differentiate at least two classes of medical informations which for this discussion will be referred to as primary and secondary data:

- primary data,
  i.e. symptoms, signs, findings
- secondary data,
  i.e. diagnoses, prognoses, retrognoses.

This differentiation seems to correspond to the technical differentiation between input data and output data.

Symptoms, for instance, used as input to a medical reasoning process are considered to yield diagnoses as output. In line with this concept is an assumption of a fundamental difference between the two classes of medical items of information which is rather widespread in the medical community. Based on this assumption it seemed logical to construct algorithms which e.g. would automatically convert data of the symptom type to data of the diagnosis type. For instance, there exists some controversy in the literature whether one should proceed from diagnosis to symptoms in the way most textbooks are organized or from symptoms to a diagnosis in the way which is required in most practical situations.

However, the attempts of automation of the diagnostic process by providing algorithms which achieve a conversion of symptoms to diagnoses usually fell short of expectations. Their results rarely became widely applied despite of considerable effort directed at their development. It seems necessary therefore to reconsider the basis of these attempts. The following discussion is structured according to the distinction between primary data and secondary data given above. This is used to outline the medical aspects of these concepts. It should be kept in mind that this differentiation applies only to an artificially delimited segment of a sequence of information processing steps. The consequences of this restriction will come out in the discussion of the medical basis for processing procedures termed 'reference data, rules'.

3.1 PRIMARY DATA

Primary data in medicine are of a great variety. They may be broadly distinguished in:

- measurement data and
- observational data.

Measurements are proliferating especially in clinical medicine through increasingly widespread application of laboratory procedures. Commonly supplied as numbers, they have a magic that is often hard to resist.

Observational data may be subdivided into those based on

- direct observation and
- observations related by others.

Observational data are the traditional type of data that physicians had to rely on to arrive at their conclusions. They still constitute the type of data that the majority of conclusions are derived from (13). Typical examples of direct observational data are those of physical examination, or those pertaining to the interpretation of roentgenographic or histologic images.

Related observational data are those related by the patient or by persons from his environment. But they also comprise data related by physicians or other medical personnel.

Unfortunately it has become rather common use to differentiate between 'hard' and 'soft' data. Numbers are usually referred to as hard and related observations as soft data, with direct observations ranking in between. This has resulted in attempts to improve the quality of data by converting them into numbers - in oblivion of the fact that data are only as valid as they are reliable and as valid as the criteria they are compaired against. Since the employed criteria are usually defined by the disease concepts, they are characterized by the fuzziness which is typical for these. This fuzziness is in this way inherited by the data and decreases their validity.

The entire class of primary data is in German referred to as 'symptoms'. This use of the word has a number of advantages, because it denotes a use of a datum as input for some kind of reasoning or processing in the outlined manner. Its quality may be discerned in different ways.

For the purpose of clarity, it should be pointed out that in other languages the word 'symptom' is used in a more restricted sense. Symptoms may be differentiated as to whether they are

```
      - objective or
      - subjective
      and
      - spontaneous or
      - evoked.
```

```
SYMPTOMS
                    I subjective I objective  I
                    I            I            I
                    --------------------------------
                    I            I            I
                    I            I            I
                    I            I            I
   spontaneous      I     a      I     b      I
                    I            I            I
                    I            I            I
                    I            I            I
                    --------------------------------
                    I            I            I
                    I            I            I
                    I            I            I
   evoked           I     c      I     d      I
                    I            I            I
                    I            I            I
                    I            I            I
                    --------------------------------
                    I            I            I
```

```
Engl. : symptom    : a or c
        sign       : b or d

French: symptome   : a or b
        signe      : c or d
```

In medical usage, the English word 'symptom' refers to the subjective variety while the word 'sign' is used for the objective one. In French, 'symptome' refers to the spontaneous, 'signe' to the evoked variety (26). The differentiation was meant to distinguish different classes of quality - analogous to the hard-soft scale. Spontaneous and subjective symptoms such as a headache are difficult to verify. Often this is only possible by inference from other objective data. Evoked spontaneous symptoms may at least be reproduced, which increases their reliability. Objective symptoms, on the other hand, but also e.g. laboratory data are generally most reliable. Their validity depends on the mechanisms used for their detection and the rigor of the criterion that they are measured against. Examples of objective symptoms would be a rash or a tendon reflex.

Still the schemes are not all inclusive and complete. The distinctions were coined by 19th century's medical science, which was predominantly somatically oriented. Today one might include other kinds of symptoms which simply constitute facts pertaining to a given diseased person or group. The fact that a mother has six children, the fact that the male population of a settlement earns its living in an asbestos factory, are examples which have the same characteristic as other primary data for deriving secondary data in medicine. In the following, the word 'symptom' will be used in this encompassing manner to denote primary data.

Examples of different classes of primary data:
subjective:
- sensations
- judgements
- attitudes
- emotions
- motives

objective:
- related observations
- related facts
- direct observation
  = physical examination
  = preparations
- images
- measurements.

3.2 SECONDARY DATA

The most frequently cited example of a class of secondary data in medicine is denoted as

- diagnosis or
- syndrome.

Both terms are conceptually closely related. According to popular understanding as well as to common interpretation by medical professionals these classes comprise terms that denote 'diseases'. They constitute codes or shorthand symbols for an affection that a patient suffers from. This is particularly true for diagnoses, some of which are an expression of rather ancient disease concepts. One frequently cited example is 'malaria' which is derived from an ancient term denoting 'bad air', to which the disease was attributed before the nature of the causative agent of the disease, a microorganism, became known. Another example of similar type is the term 'pernicious anemia', which was coined for a type of disease which is manifested by a lack of red blood cells which inevitably lead to death before the disease could be traced to the lack of a vitamin, and before cure became available through substitution of this vitamin. Pernicious anemia is a good example for the change of the picture that a disease may undergo as a consequence of medical progress. Vitamin B12, one of the vitamins, the lack of which produces what is called pernicious anemia, is readily available today and constituent of many multivitamin preparations, sometimes even an additive to certain food stuffs. Therefore, the full blown picture of perniciuos anemia is rarely seen today. If it appears, it is frequently a consequence of certain types of bowel disease which prevent the vitamin from being made available to the organism even if the food contains sufficient quantities. This means that pernicious anemia has become a symptom of these types of bowel disease. The underlying vitamin deficiency, however, does not only manifest itself in disturbance of the blood production but also in disturbance of nervous function. The nervous system is even more sensitive than the blood system, which has the effect that the disease called 'pernicious anemia' is today often of greater concern for the neurologist (medical subspecialty for nervous diseases) than for the hematologist (medical subspecialty for blood diseases).

The concept of a 'syndrome' differs only slightly from that of a diagnosis. Syndromes are complexes or patterns of symptoms which are observed to occur together and which are distinguished from accidental concurrence by a common underlying pathophysiology or etiology, common means for treatment or common prognosis. The syndrome concept therefore is a step towards the cybernetic disease concept outlined above in that it constitutes less a label for a more or less accidental disease concept, than a term for an expression of a diseased organism which may be observed at a particular stage using certain types of equipment. Syndromes are most frequently named after their discoverer, (e.g. FANCONI syndrome for a certain type of anemia, a blood disease) after a predominant site of manifestation (e. g. lumbar vertebral syndrome), after primary manifestation (e. g. Globus syndrome for a feeling of a lump in the throat), as well as after the major underlying cause (e. g. malabsorption syndrome), a time or place of discovery or even the name of the patient in whom it was discovered.

Besides diagnoses or syndromes there are other classes of secondary or derived data such as

- prognoses
- retrognoses

which may result from processes of medical reasoning. The prognostic conclusion was the dominant goal of medical art and science from the times of the classical Greek medicine until the late middle ages. The goal was to forecast the fate of the diseased for himself or for the people of his surroundings, since means of cure were vastly less powerful, and the need to adapt to fate was dominant (14,15). Retrognosis is a rarely used term for a type of conclusion which is complementary to the attempt to predict subsequent events as a prognosis. Retrognosis tries to guess past events from current evidence. As such it is an element of the anamnestic and diagnostic process. By eleciting possible past events and verifying their occurence, for instance by interviewing the patient or his relatives, assumptions concerning the current affliction may be corroborated or ruled out. These latter classes of secondary data do then point out the close association between the use of terms like diagnosis and prognosis for secondary data and their use for the processes by which these data are arrived at. Although usually terms like 'prognostics' or 'diagnostics' may be used to distinguish the processes from the data they result in, this differentiated use is not strictly observed. In the case of 'anamnesis' for instance the same term is always used for the process as well as its result.

It should be mentioned that the therapeutic conclusion is another type of conclusion which should be counted as one of the secondary data. In this instance one is less used to strict categorization in the many disciplines where therapy consists in behavioral changes, diets and drugs that accompany a continuing disease process. In surgical disciplines, where alternative operative procedures are employed at defined stages of disease, categorization is easier and more readily apparent. Typically, therapeutic classification schemes were first developed and are most widely employed by surgical disciplines.

The purpose of the preceding two paragraphs was to discuss some aspects of common medical understanding of classes of terms distinguished here as primary and secondary data of medical reasoning process. The following paragraph on the concepts corresponding to processing procedures in medicine will bring up some additional aspects of controversy concerning these concepts.

Examples of different classes of secondary data:

- diagnoses
- syndromes
- prognoses
- retrognoses
- therapies.

3.3 REFERENCE DATA, RULES

Medical professionals frequently allude to the procedure by which secondary data are derived from primary data as a reference to some kind of data determining guide lines, normative concepts of professional behaviour. This reference knowledge is stored in textbooks and exists for the practicing physician as some kind of condensed abstract from the textbooks and other literature that he was exposed to, as a condensation of the practical part of his training and as a result of his continuing practical experience. We are only at the very beginning of an exploration of means and possibilities for extracting this condensed form of subjective knowledge and making it available for automated data processing (24). So far, the assumption was dominant that the knowledge stored in textbooks and similar media was an adequate representation of the medical rules and reasoning processes and that transfer of it to computers would be possible and constitute an advantage. The experience with computer systems aiming at the support of the medical decision and reasoning processes pointed out some shortcomings, the reasons for which shall be discussed in the following.

The contents of medical textbooks and similar media are a direct consequence of currently prevailing concepts of disease models and designed for didactic purposes. They are designed to teach students, i.e. human beings with a high capacity for adaptation and compensation. They present their contents in a variety of forms, such as narrative, tables, pictures and make explicit use of the complementary role of practical training. It is evident that different means would be necessary to have machines which lack the human properties of compensation, accept and use this knowledge. The question arises therefore, whether other representations of this knowledge are achievable. This question shall be examined in the light of the characteristics of medical model concepts which were outlined above.

The rules according to which medical secondary data are derived from primary data were related by WESTMEYER (37) SADEGH-ZADEH (26) to the logic structure of scientific explanation proposed by HEMPEL and OPPENHEIM (17).

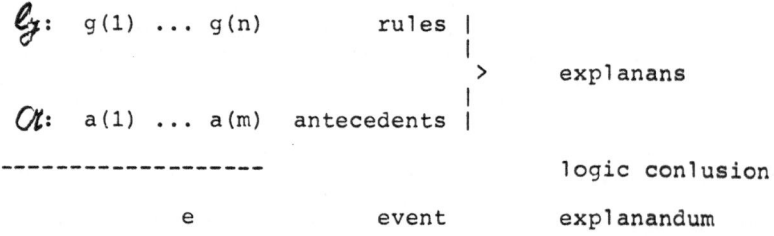

$\mathcal{G}$: g(1) ... g(n)   rules |
                                        |
                                        | >   explanans
                                        |
$\mathcal{A}$: a(1) ... a(m) antecedents |

--------------------   logic conlusion

              e   event   explanandum

H - O Scheme of scientific explanation

also demonstrated by the evolution of medical science, which may be viewed as an account of a continuous reduction of what is considered a 'diagnosis' at one point in the time to a 'symptom' at the next. 'Jaundice' (yellow skin coloration due to bile pigment) and 'dropsy' (swelling of subcutaneous tissue due to fluid) are examples for which the process has been decided. For notions like 'leukemia' (abundance of abnormal white blood cells) and 'diabetes mellitus' (sugar disease), the process of assigning them a place in valid concepts of disease, is still in progress.

The syndrome concept illustrates the relation between diagnostic conclusion and scientific explanation particularly well – the set of symptoms corresponds to a set of antecedents, their common cause or other underlying phenomena to the rules.

Apart from the consequences for the medical concepts of information, the relation between medical conclusions and scientific explanation makes clear that the rules governing medical conclusions are the same as in other empirical sciences. This issue has been elucidated comprehensively by WESTMEYER (37) and SADEGH-ZADEH (28). The latter showed that medical rules are either logical deductions or statistical implications or not scientifically acceptable. SADEGH-ZADEH (28) has also made clear that the essential characteristic of data with respect to their use in scientific explanation is not sufficiently described by such adjectives as 'subjective' or 'objective' , but is essentially a linguistic property which may be decharacterized as the degree of common acceptance of a term. This insight has decisive consequences for what we may expect from automatic processing of medical data, as well as for the choice of techniques employed in such processing, since common agreement is limited for most medical data.

One immediate consequence for medical data is that logical deductions may rarely be based upon strict logical implications of the type

$$\forall X : (x,a) \rightarrow (x,b)$$

(For all x: if x equals a then x equals b).
In an effort to find a rule for which this strict formulation would be acceptable HARTMANN (16) gives as example that all humans must die if exposed to an oxygen free atmosphere. Usually logic deductions will result in a rather lengthy statement about alternatively acceptable propositions. An example would be that humans, if exposed to carbon tetrachloride will either stay healthy or become sick for a certain time or suffer from acute damage of parenchymal organs leading to death. In actual practice the series of conditions connected by 'or' will be much longer. Although it has been attempted to base systems for automated processing of medical data on strict logical deductions (2,3,21,22), the cited example shows that in such a case a probabilistic approach would be preferrable. This might produce the (fictitious) result that the conclusions leading to the three alternatives given in the latter example (if exhaustive and mutually exclusive) have the following probabilities associated to them:

will stay healthy	.6
will become temporarily ill	.1
will die	.3

The initial attempt to approach medical diagnosis as a probabilistic problem by using BAYES' theorem to calculate the conditional probabilities of a set of diagnoses given a set of conditions (symptoms) from the conditional probabilities for these symptoms given each of the diseases and from the a priori probabilities for each diagnosis is due to WARNER (33). It created an uproar in the medical

The H - O scheme of scientific explanation states that scientific explanations consist in explaining an event e by logic conclusion from a set of antecedents $\mathcal{A}$ and a set of rules $\mathcal{L}$. If all rules are logical implications, the logic conclusion is called deductive nomologic. If at least one rule is probabilistic, it is called inductive statistical conclusion. In this latter case, the logic conclusion is assigned a probability, a numerical value which can be calculated according to the axioms and theorems of probability theory. The problems connected with this definition are beyond the scope of this discussion and have been covered extensively in the literature of the theory of science (cf. e.g. 30).

HARTMANN (16) relates medical conclusions to the H - O scheme in distinguishing the diagnostic and prognostic conclusion and the scientific discovery. In the diagnostic conclusion, an event is explained by referring to rules and concluding upon a set of antecedents:

diagnostic conclusion: $e, \mathcal{L} \rightarrow \mathcal{A}$

In prognostic conclusion, a set of antecedents is explained by referring to rules and concluding upon an event:

prognostic conclusion: $\mathcal{A}, \mathcal{L} \rightarrow e$

In scientific discovery, a set of antecedents and an event is used to conclude upon a set of laws:

scientific discovery: $\mathcal{A}, e \rightarrow \mathcal{L}$

It is apparent that there exists no difference between the propositions describing antecedents or events except for the way in which they are used in scientific explanation. One consequence of this relates to the medical distinction between the types of data which have been termed primary and secondary data above. The difference suggested by the medical distinction between symptoms on the one side and diagnoses or prognoses on the other side is not a distinction pertaining to the type of data but a distinction pertaining to the use of the data in medical scientific explanation. Since there is no criterion for completeness of a model used in scientific explanation, there is no way to arrive at a complete diagnosis in the sense of fully understanding the antecedents that explain an event. Failure to realize this relativity of data and laws has been a continuous source of misunderstanding in medicine. Declaring diagnoses derived from morphologic evidence in pathology, or from contemplative research models in clinical medicine, as the only acceptable diagnoses, has led to complete abjection of the term diagnosis in other disciplines (c.f. e.g. 4) which have to rely on different kinds of evidence, have to suit different needs, and hence developed different models.

Another inappropriate effect of a misunderstood distinction between symptom and diagnosis is that frequently 'diagnoses' which are arrived at on the basis of the models of one particular discipline in medicine, - e.g. pathology - are accepted as absolute truths were they should rather constitute a symptom in an ongoing process of medical reasoning. The clinical diagnosis might be a valuable constituent in the pathologist's reasoning, just as the pathologist's diagnosis should be treated as an event to be explained by antecedents available in the process of patient care at the bedside.

The interchangeability of the concepts of 'symptom' and 'diagnosis' is also demonstrated by the evolution of medical science, which may be viewed as an account of a continuous reduction of what is considered a 'diagnosis' at one point in the time to a 'symptom' at the next. 'Jaundice' (yellow skin coloration due to bile pigment) and 'dropsy' (swelling of subcutaneous tissue due to fluid) are examples for which the process has been decided. For notions like 'leukemia' (abundance of abnormal white blood cells) and 'diabetes mellitus' (sugar disease), the process of assigning them a place in valid concepts of disease, is still in progress.

The syndrome concept illustrates the relation between diagnostic conclusion and scientific explanation particularly well - the set of symptoms corresponds to a set of antecedents, their common cause or other underlying phenomena to the rules.

Apart from the consequences for the medical concepts of information, the relation between medical conclusions and scientific explanation makes clear that the rules governing medical conclusions are the same as in other empirical sciences. This issue has been elucidated comprehensively by WESTMEYER (37) and SADEGH-ZADEH (28). The latter showed that medical rules are either logical deductions or statistical implications or not scientifically acceptable. SADEGH-ZADEH (28) has also made clear that the essential characteristic of data with respect to their use in scientific explanation is not sufficiently described by such adjectives as 'subjective' or 'objective' , but is essentially a linguistic property which may be characterized as the degree of common acceptance of a term. This insight has decisive consequences for what we may expect from automatic processing of medical data, as well as for the choice of techniques employed in such processing, since common agreement is limited for most medical data.

One immediate consequence for medical data is that logical deductions may rarely be based upon strict logical implications of the type

$$\forall X : (x,a) \rightarrow (x,b)$$

(For all x: if x equals a then x equals b).
In an effort to find a rule for which this strict formulation would be acceptable HARTMANN (16) gives as example that all humans must die if exposed to an oxygen free atmosphere. Usually logic deductions will result in a rather lengthy statement about alternatively acceptable propositions. An example would be that humans, if exposed to carbon tetrachloride will either stay healthy or become sick for a certain time or suffer from acute damage of parenchymal organs leading to death. In actual practice the series of conditions connected by 'or' will be much longer. Although it has been attempted to base systems for automated processing of medical data on strict logical deductions (2,3,21,22), the cited example shows that in such a case a probabilistic approach would be preferrable. This might produce the (fictitious) result that the conclusions leading to the three alternatives given in the latter example (if exhaustive and mutually exclusive) have the following probabilities associated to them:

will stay healthy	.6
will become temporarily ill	.1
will die	.3

The initial attempt to approach medical diagnosis as a probabilistic problem by using BAYES' theorem to calculate the conditional probabilities of a set of diagnoses given a set of conditions (symptoms) from the conditional probabilities for these symptoms given each of the diseases and from the a priori probabilities for each diagnosis is due to WARNER (33). It created an uproar in the medical likely he is to record the necessary input data unreliably. The efficiency of the system will then largely depend on the quality of the user. This problem has to be investigated for every particular application. Again examples are available which show that this problem can be managed (19).

4. Medical information
and the care process

The process of medical reasoning is still badly understood. In individual care situations the physician is usually consulted because some problem has arisen - the 'chief complaint' or reason for consultation. In the ensuing process of medical care, an attempt is made to explain the problem in the light of an appropriate model and, if possible, to eliminate the problem. The way in which this is done has scarcely been analyzed. So far, some normative models and prescriptions exist. A particularly instructive and clear one has been proposed by WEED (34,37). It advises the medical student to proceed according to four phases of medical action:

1. assemble a defined data base,
2. identify all existing problems,
3. select a course of action,
4. follow up the results and developments

It is the merit of WEED to have furnished a concept that avoids the value judgements that are attached to the symptom diagnosis dichotomy and therefore makes less biased workup in patient care possible.

This is the concept of a 'problem' which is part of the problem oriented approach at patient care and medical record keeping.

WEED is usually asked by those used to the traditional medical terminology to define normatively the nature of a 'problem'. This has never been done. Instead WEED gives examples which include symptoms and diagnoses as described above. In this way it becomes apparent that a problem is in some way a point of origin for a process of medical care and medical reasoning. It eliminates the disadvantages of the traditional concepts such as the fuzzy limits between symptoms and diagnoses. This, however, is not done by substituting a different, encompassing concept but by providing a different model of the medical care process, which does not use the traditional concepts.

According to WEED's suggestion, the first phase of medical action consists in an assembly of a 'defined' data base, the term implying that the data base is different depending on factors such as age and sex of the patient or type of medical specialty.

Even in this more formal approach, the main problem is the lack of a criterion by which to tell whether a defined data base is complete. What is accumulated depends largely on the alternative or concurrent models considered and on the skill with which the symptoms are selected which prove or disprove these hypothetical models. Once selected they may still not be observed if they are present or erroneously assumed to be present by false interpretation of available evidence. The method therefore consists largely in proving and disproving one after the other the elements of a set of hypotheses, until a satisfactory one remains. In this process, each item of information has to be assessed for validity and correctness with respect to

- hypotheses considered so far
- other alternatives, and
- previous information.

Much of this is accomplished subconsciously. An account of something considered to be relevant is passed over, an unfitting lab result is justly discarded without being able sometimes to explain it. In the same fashion, the selection of tests - in the form of a question, posed during an interview, or in the form of an examining view at a hidden area - may be part of subconscious efficient routine. The process, however, desirable it is because of its efficiency, also represents an abundance of excuses, if it fails or is ineffective. Since the process so far eludes definitions and therefore teaching and analysis, it has repeatedly been tried to substitute a consequently scientific approach without being able to achieve the efficiency of this artful kind of medical practice.

Problems analogous to those concerning the establishment of a complete data base exist for the establishment of a complete list of problems. This is usually referred to as a list of 'working diagnoses', reflecting thus the largely hypothetical state of the conditions.

Conscious actions during the second phase of medical action are directed at corroborating the evidence suggested by items of information by more reliable tests, in order to zero in on a fitting pattern of the actual problem constellation. The process also includes:

- disproving wrong hypotheses
- proving correct ones
- distinguishing what appears to belong together
- summing up as an entity what appeared to belong apart.

In the same way, in which diagnoses were dissolved to symptoms of a number of different disease states during the history of medicine, it is frequently encountered in patient care that what is considered various independent diagnoses becomes a syndrome, a pattern of symptoms within a common frame.

The process usually involves two different tactics:

1) Screening for disease
In this approach, a battery of tests of high sensitivity is applied which if positive would suggest a rather broad variety of problems, which then would have to be worked up in the manner which constitutes the second kind of tactics.

2) Single out disease.
In this process a hierarchy of progressively more specific tests is applied, until the appropriate action can be chosen.

The process is complicated, because many actions may conflict with each other. An x-ray investigation of the bowel precludes for a number of days an investigation of the gall bladder. This in turn - like a number of other roentgenologic investigations using iodine compounds as contrast media - precludes an investigation of the thyroid gland for weeks.

Also there may be a conflict between various alternatives at the same time - the choice of further diagnostics as opposed to initiating therapy for instance. Giving an antibiotic will prevent identification of the agent which in turn is sometimes a prerequisite for selecting the most appropriate antibiotic. The decisions concerning the selection

of actions have to consider the urgency of the need for care as well as
the utility and cost of the measures taken. The value judgements are
variable, depending on the setting and the goals pursued. For patient
care purposes, the utility of further diagnostic activity has to be
weighed against the prognosis of therapeutic alternatives. In a
research and teaching environment, the utility of the same measures may
appear different and hence a complete data base will be something
different.

Evidently then, the definition of the problem list, though initially
attempted, is not a one stage procedure but accompanies the treatment
process. 'Treatment' in this respect is not identical with 'therapy'.
Treatment, as should be evident from the discussion so far, involves
simultaneous and consecutive application of diagnostic and therapeutic
measures. Therapeutic measures in themselves have frequently diagnostic
properties, since the response or lack of response to therapy is
crucial evidence for the physician. It appears thus that treatment is a
continuous process, which evolves frequently in highly redundant
fashion. Several tests are frequently applied, one being used to back
up the result of the other. Due to this redundancy the process is
surprisingly successfull, despite of the weakness of the foundations,
on which it is sometimes based.

The third phase of medical action, the definition of a treatment plan
is then obviously done once, at the time of initiation of treatment,
but afterwards continuously repeated. Also, emergency situations, which
call for immediate action provide an example for situations where a
clearcut differentiation of the described phases of medical action is
never possible. Most important is then the fourth phase of medical
action, the phase of follow-up of the ongoing process.

During the fourth phase of medical action according to WEED the concept
of problem oriented practice and documentation seems particularly
promising. If, as advised by WEED, the actions and their results are
indexed during this phase according to the problem which prompted them,
a kind of red thread becomes available, along which the treatment
process may be traced back. This should not only be of value for
different persons involved simultaneously in the treatment process
because it improves communication about a problem constellation and
resultant actions. It should also make the process more intelligible to
the initiating physician himself. Obviously, also, problem oriented
documentation lays the process of medical care open to criticism and
assessment. This property may account for some reluctance in adopting
the process. Also, it is certainly more demanding than less formal
approaches. The concept has led to a kind of crusade, especially among
the young generation of physicians in the United States and gradually
becomes tried out outside the United States. It is, however, too early
to decide definitely upon its value. It has to be stressed at this
point, that the process of medical care evolves overwhelmingly in a far
less formal way. Part of this is due to tradition, most physicians
simply being not used to this kind of procedure. Also WEED's
suggestions may not be universally applicable since they were developed
in the clinical care setting which is different from some other care
settings, such as ambulatory care in physicians' offices and public
health or social medicine.

While in clinical medicine an attempt is made to provide integral care,
general medicine is dominated by special problem management. Clinical
medicine zeroes in on a disease pattern, general medicine tries to sort
out dangerous states. Also general medicine constitutes an environment
of long-term continuing medical care where clinical medicine focusses
on particular episodes in patients that have previously been unknown by
their physicians. For example, the need to assemble a defined data base

exists in general medicine in a sense very different from hospital medicine: A lot is known about the patient from previous encounters. The defined data base is markedly determined by the problem offered by the patient in a particular instance. Still other differences exist in preventive and social medicine. In these settings, highly spezialized problem management is often possible. Attention has mainly to be directed towards arriving at effective and economical solutions in a situation where the incentive for the action taken stems frequently less from the patient himself but where it may be imposed upon him, by legal regulations.

5. Medical information and medical classification schemes

As pointed out above, the nature of medical model concepts results in a multitude of classification schemes. They exist for therapeutic measures, prognostic evaluation schemes and above all for diagnostic classification. The latter shall be examined as an example of the other in the following.

Perhaps the internationally best known diagnostic classification scheme is the International Classification of Diseases and Causes of Death (42). It originated in the late 19th century as a tool of health management and epidemiology and has since been revised 8 times. Items contained in it are arranged monohierarchically and sequentially and identified by a three digit code. Due to the sequential numbering used, it is a rather rigid code, different editions being partly compatible with each other. For clinical purposes it is not detailed enough. This has lead to a number of attempts of adaptions (e. g. in the USA, ICDA,) and Germany (ICDE, 42). Due to its use for epidemiological surveys, it has nevertheless gained widespread acceptance despite of its drawbacks.

In Germany, an index for clinical diagnoses developed by IMMICH is widely applied (20). It is called 'Klinischer Diagnosenschluessel', KDS. It is multidimensionally and hierarchically arranged. Each of the approximately 10,000 entries is identified by a 5 digit number, the first two digits referring to topography, digit 3 and 4 refer to nosology and digit 5 to etiology or other types of modification. The index is used in our institution and is continuously modified. In this way we account for needs of disciplines which were not covered by the original KDS, as well as for needs arising as a consequence of the progress of medical science. Also some disciplines feel that the distinctions provided by KDS are not detailed enough for their needs and therefore ask for subdivision of available terms. In this latter respect however, our experience shows that one has to be very critical in responding to the claims of the physicians. A prominent tendency to be too detailed exists. Frequently it turns out afterwards that a great part of the detailed distinctions are hardly if ever used. In any case, our approach at providing an open, adaptive rigorously controlled and continuously updated coding system has proven to be acceptable and practically used (18).

Another index with predominantly scientific and therapeutic focus of attention developed by LEIBER (23) is on its way towards 30,000 syndromes. This index gives for every syndrome a description of authors, etiology, and the pattern of symptoms defining it, an account of etiology and pathogenesis if available as well as references to relevant literature. Also the use of synonymous designations for given disease conditions are dissolved and crossreferences between symptoms and disease conditions given. This index of syndromes is also continuously updated.

The possibilities of distinction, however, are probably infinite. PAYCHA (26) arrived at some thousand syndromes for the human cornea alone - a part of an organ half an inch in diameter and an eights of an inch thick. Compared with the possibilities of distinction exemplified by these figures, the capacity of the human brain is limited. This limited capacity for conscious reasoning creates part of the urge towards specialization and is an incentive for the call for computer help.

Another diagnostic index, the International Classification of Health Problems in Primary Care (ICHPPC) has been developed for the need of the primary care setting. It contains only 371 entries arranged in 17 chapters and identified by 3 to 4 digit codes (40). A similar code for use in general practice, the Verden Problem List, was developed on the basis of an analysis of the cases encountered in general practice. It contains only 222 positions, (8,9) arranged in 18 chapters using hierarchical code numbers (two digits identifying the chapter, two the problem category within each chapter, with 8,9 and 0 as last digits being reserved for pools of disease categories). All of the cited examples except for the one from PAYCHA aim at encompassing all medical problems - with some emphasis on a somatic orientation. The differences are not only quantitative in that one scheme consists of few hierarchically superimposed items where the other has a greater number of subgroups. Instead they differ in many more respects, based on different principles of classification suiting different needs, and different means of distinction used in actual practice.

The problem lists for general medicine, for example, contain items such as family problems and financial problems which are not covered in the other examples. The differences between e.g. ICD and KDS can also be qualitatively characterized. ICD, being primarily devised for epidemiology and mortality statistics, distinguishes the states of the deceased, while KDS, devised for use in clinical medicine, distinguishes the states of the diseased.

The cited examples may suffice to illustrate the degree of diversity existing in medical classification schemes. A glance at the tables of content of any selection of medical textbooks will serve as further illustrations of the diversity of medical classification schemes.

It should be remarked that the cited examples of diagnostic indices are mainly relevant for a static disease concept and do not make the dynamic relation between different states of health and disease readily apparent. Several different states seem to coexist alternatively and in parallel. Nevertheless, there are alternative attempts to arrive at disease classification. FEINSTEIN (10) has widely employed classification schemes differentiating between different stages of disease complexes. Using this approach he arrived at improved prognostic and therapeutic assessment of the examined conditions.

The described diversity makes the need to arrive at standardization obvious. The attempts of standardization, however, are in themselves problematic. The more a classification scheme strives to be encompassing and usable by multiple disciplines, the greater the tendency to resort to a specialized subset for a given discipline. At our institution, only roughly 1/4 of the diagnostic items offered by the KDS had ever been used by any discipline during a recent survey (36). The spectrum used by Internal Medicine comprised some 1000 items. 520 entries covered 90 percent of diagnostic classifications, only some 100 were sufficient to cover 50 percent. In contrast we found in employing the Verden Problem list that 203 of the 222 available entities had been employed (25). In this case of a highly specialized index with relatively coarse distinctions the rate of utilization of the available entities exceeded 90 percent. Despite of this, individual physicians' offices still had quite disjunct subsets comprising between 38 and 122 different items. Again relatively small subsets were sufficient for most classifications. 114 of the 203 items were sufficient to code 95 percent of diagnoses in all offices. (30 and 70 respectively were sufficient for 95 percent of diagnostic classifications in the 2 extreme offices cited above). It is unlikely that the differences between offices illustrated by these figures are entirely due to differences in the supply and demand situation of different offices since all were offices of general medicine. The differences are then most likely to be explained by differences in the focus of attention and perhaps even in the semantics of the use of various terms - even within this relatively homogeneous group of medical practitioners. It is quite likely then, that the use of medical terminology varies to a considerably greater extent between representatives of different specialities. Terms like 'goiter' or 'psychosis' may mean quite different things, whether employed by an endocrinologist (specialty for hormonal disturbances) or a psychiatrist. These semantic differences are likely to limit the value of automatic textprocessing even if systematized nomenclatures such as SNOP (5, cf. also WINGERT's contribution in this volume) or SNOMED (6) are employed.

The only way out of this dilemma seems to consist in a coordinated effort to arrive at definitions of the employed terms which are acceptable by all concerned with the use of a given terminology, and to enforce adherence to these definitions. If this is not achievable, one has to insure at least that the terminology used by a certain population for a certain purpose is accepted among these. Doing this, one has to weigh the disadvantages of creating specialized terminology in order to improve performance in a comparatively small group or team with the danger of an ensuing babylonian type of confusion against the disadvantages of striving forever to achieve a terminology which is acceptable on a large scale basis. The preceeding discussion should have shown at least that terminology has to be considered carefully in attempts at automation since it may be coined for different types of applications than the ones pursued in a particular application. It should also have shown that a necessity for continuous, however considerate adaption exists, and that adaption is possible and permissable. This should be taken into consideration by physicians in their actions as well as by engineers coming to their help.

Literature

1 BAUER, F.L., GOOS, G.: Informatik, Erster Teil (Berlin, Heidelberg, New York: Springer 1971)
2 BAUER, P. et al.: Ein Computerverfahren zur Unterstuetzung des Arztes bei der Erstellung von Differentialdiagnosen Impuls 10 (1968) 705-712
3 BAUER, P., GANGL, A., GRABNER, G.: Ein Computerverfahren zur Zuordnung eines Krankheitsbildes zu einer Diagnosengruppe Wien.Zeitschr.Inn.Med. 51 (1970) 497-509
4 BRAUN, R.N.: Lehrbuch der aerztlichen Allgemeinpraxis (Muenchen, Berlin, Wien: Urban & Schwarzenberg 1970)
5 COLLEGE OF THE AMERICAN PATHOLOGISTS: Systematized Nomenclature of Pathology (Chicago, 1965)
6 COTE, R.A.: SNOMED - A Tool for the Computerized Management of Medical Data in: Internatl.Symp.Med.Inf.Syst. Proceedings of Medis '75

Tokyo, 1975, p.66-75

7 DE DOMBAL, F.T., GREMY, F. (eds.): Decision Making and Medical Care
Can Computer Science Help? Conference sponsored by I.F.I.P's TC 4
Dijon, May 24-29 (1976) Proceedings in Preparation (Amsterdam: North
Holl.Publ.Comp.)

8   DREIBHOLZ, K.J., ROHDE, P.A.: Die Verdener Diagnosenliste Der
Praktische Arzt 10 (1972) 1824-1838

9 DREIBHOLZ, K.J. et al.: Ergebnisse, Probleme und Konsequenzen einer
vergleichenden Diagnosenstatistik Allg.Med.Int. 1 (1972) 103-110

10 FEINSTEIN, A.R.: Clinical Judgement (Baltimore: Williams & Wilkinson
1967)

11 v. FERBER, C.: Die Rolle des Arztes in der modernen Gesellschaft
Prakt. Arzt 8 (1971) 1146-1163

12 GUENTHER, S.: Die Entwicklung des Krankheitsbegriffes in der
Krankenversicherung Med.Sachverst. 68 (1972) 44-48

13 HAMPTON, J.R. et al: Relative Contributions of History-taking,
Physicial Examination and Laboratory Investigation to Diagnosis and
Management of Medical Outpatients Brit.Med.J. 2 (1975) 486 - 489

14 HARTMANN, F.: Der historische Diagnosebegriff und seine Entwicklung
Muench.Med.Wschr. 114 (1972) 90-96

15 HARTMANN, F.: Begriff und Funktion der Diagnose Muench. Med.Wschr.
114 (1972) 117-126

16 HARTMANN, F.: What Could and what Should Doctors Learn from their
Experience with Computers in Medicine Medinfo '74 Amsterdam:
North.Holl.Publ. Comp. (1974) 1155-1170

17 HEMPEL, C.G., OPPENHEIM, P.: Studies in the Logic of Explanation
Philosoph.Sc. 12 (1948) 98-115

18 HOLTHOFF, G.: Aufbau einer multidisziplinaeren zentralisierten
medizinischen Basisdokumentation Dissertation, Tieraerztliche
Hochschule Hannover, 1976

19 HORROCKS, J.C., DE DOMBAL, F.T.: Diagnosis of Dyspepsia from Data
Collected by a Physician's Assistant Br.Med.J.3(1975),421-423

20 IMMICH, H.: Klinischer Diagnoseschluessel (Stuttgart: Schattauer
1966)

21 LEDLEY, R.S., LUSTED, L.B.: Reasoning Foundations of Medical
Diagnosis Science 130 (1959) 9-21

22 LEDLEY, R.S.: Use of Computers in Biology and Medicine (New York,
McGraw Hill, 1965)

23 LEIBER, B., OLBRICH, G.: Die klinischen Syndrome 5th Edition
(Muenchen, Berlin, Wien: Urban&Schwarzenberg 1972, Urban &
Schwarzenberg)

24 MAI, N.: Bestimmung subjektiver Wahrscheinlichkeiten Training von
Wahrscheinlichkeitsschaetzern in der medizinischen Diagnostik
Dissertation, Universitaet Hamburg (1975)

25 MOEHR, J.R., HAEHN, K.D.(Hrsg.): Verdenstudie Strukturanalyse
Allgemeinmedizinischer Praxen in preparation 1976 (preprints available)

26 PAYCHA, F.: Codification des Connaissances Int. Kongress fuer
Kybernetik/Namur 22.-29.6.56 S. 55-62

27 REICHERTZ, P.L.: Auswirkungen der elektronischen Datenverarbeitung
auf die Struktur der Medizin Vortrag, 4. Deidesheimer Gespraech
25.-26.4.1970

28 SADEGH-ZADEH, K.: Zur Logik und Methodologie der aerztlichen
Urteilsbildung Meth.Inf.Med. 11 (1972) 203-212

29 STEGMUELLER, W.: Das Problem der Kausalitaet in Topitsch, E.,
(Hrsg.): Probleme der Wissenschaftstheorie Festschrift fuer Viktor
Kraft. Wien, 1960, 171-190

30 STEGMUELLER, W.: Probleme und Resultate der Wissenschaftstheorie IV
Personelle und Statistische Wahrscheinlichkeit (Berlin, Heidelberg, New
York: Springer 1973)

31 STEINBUCH, A.: Technische Modelle biologischer Vorgaenge In H.v.
Ditfurth, (Hrsg.): Information ueber Information, Probleme ueber
Kybernetik Hamburg, 1963, 73-104

32 STERLING, T.D., POLLACK, S.V.: Is Medical Diagnosis a General

Computer Problem? JAMA 198 (1966) 191-196

33 WARNER, H.R. et al: A Mathematical Approach to Medical Diagnosis JAMA 177 (1961) 177-183

34 WEED, L.L.: Medical Records that Guide and Teach N.Enq.J.Med. 278 (1958) 593-600, 652-657

35 WEED, L.L.: Medical Records, Medical Education and Patient Care (Cleveland: Press of Case Western Reserve University, 1969)

36 WEINGARTEN, W. et al: The Patient Information System and its User Reactions Journees d'Informatique Medicale Toulouse, 1975

37 WESTMEYER, H.: Logik der Diagnostik (Stuttgart, Berlin, Koeln : Kohlhammer, 1972)

38 WINKLER, C., REICHERTZ, P.L., KLOSS, G.: Computer Diagnosis of Thyroid Diseases Amer.J.Med. Sci 253 (1967) 27-34

39 WIENER, N.: The Concept of Homeostasis in Medicine Trans. Stud. Coll. Physicians Philadelphia 28, (1953) 87-93

40 WORLD ORGANIZATION OF NATIONAL COLLEGES, Academies and Academic Associations of General Practitioners/Family Physicians (WONCA), AMERICAN HOSPITAL ASSOCIATION (AHA): Informational Classification of Health Problems in Primary Care (ICHPPC). Chicago, 1975

41 WYLIE: Public Health Report 85, 100 (1970) Zit. n. (Guenther, S. (12))

42 INTERNATIONALE KLASSIFIKATION DER KRANKHEITEN Stuttgart (1968)

LANGUAGE INTERFACE
==================

K. Alber, Braunschweig

1. *COMMUNICATION MAN - COMPUTER*

Computers are means to assist men in solving information processing
problems. In order to use these means, men have to communicate with
their assistants. They have to tell them what to do and get back answers
what has been done. This communication is an *exchange of information*
in both directions, *from men to computers* and *from computers to men*.

Primarily, the information to be exchanged is *abstract* in nature. E.g.,
it is the idea of an algorithm, how to process certain information; or
it is a certain item of knowledge to be processed, or the knowledge
resulting from such processing. Like communication between men, abstract
information can only be transferred as a message in a certain *concrete
representation*. Both parties, the man and his computer, have to agree
upon certain fixed *coding rules*. By means of these rules the sender
has to represent his abstract information as *coded messages* to be
transferred. Conversely, the receiver has to have the possibility to
decode the transferred messages, i.e. uniquely to recognize the intended
information and to handle it properly.

Generally, the concrete representation of information is a *sequence of
symbols* out of a finite set, the *alphabet*. These symbols may be printed
characters, sequences of electrical signals, positions of holes in
punched cards, intensities of magnetizations, etc. We are not interested
here in these technical details; it is sufficient to know that there are
fixed finite alphabets and that informations can be coded as sequences
(in space or time) of symbols out of these alphabets and transferred
in this form.

As an example, the information in the doctors mind is the temperature
of his patient, say measured as $38,5^{\circ}C$ (or $30,8^{\circ}R$ or $101,3^{\circ}F$ or $311,5^{\circ}K$).
A datum representing this temperature, which can be manipulated by a
program, may be the real number "thirtyeight and a half" (or 77/2 or
385/10), i.e., an abstract mathematical object, which can be added,

subtracted and in particular compared with other real numbers, yielding again real numbers or truth values respectively. A possible "concrete" representation of this datum as a message is the sequence of symbols (digits and decimal point) "3", "8", ".", "5". Each of these symbols can be represented even "more concretely" by a certain sequence of bits. And furthermore a bit may be represented by an intensity of magnetization of a specific position on a magnetic tape. I.e., it is just a question of the level of abstraction what to denote as "abstract" or "concrete", and what to denote as "information" and what as "message".

On the side of the man, the information is some abstract idea in his mind and the coding and decoding (in accordance with the agreed coding rules) is done more or less by human intuition. On the side of the computer, which has no human intuition, the coding and decoding is performed by programmed analysis and synthesis algorithms to or from internal data structures. And the abstract information represented by these data structures is characterized by their behaviour with respect to programmed transformation algorithms, e.g. by the results of arithmetic machine instructions applied to them.

We can say, that each communication between men and computers, like communication between men, is performed *by means of a language*. This language has a *syntax*, specifying *the agreed form* of the messages. It is realized on the computer side by the analysis and synthesis algorithms. And the language has a *semantics*, specifying *the agreed meaning* of the messages, i.e. the represented abstract information. It is realized on the computer side by operations and transformation algorithms defined for the analyzed internal data structures.

Considering the above example, the syntax of the language used specifies that the sequence of symbols "3", "8", ".", "5" is a valid message. This may be verified by a computer by means of a simple analysis algorithm (which checks that it consists only of decimal digits and at most one point). The semantics of the language specifies that this message denotes the real number "thirty eight and a half". This may be verified by a computer by an analysis algorithm transforming the message into a specific internally stored bit pattern, namely that one which is handled by the computers floating point operations as representation of that real number.

All these considerations are valid both for informations being *algorithms* and for *informations processed by algorithms*. The messages representing the former are usually called *programs*, the messages representing the latter are usually called *data*.

But it should be stated that there is *no principal distinction between programs and data,* or between programming languages and data languages. E.g., a program is processed as "data" by a compiler or interpreter, and conversely in a data directed system, "data" may more or less immediately control running algorithms, i.e. be interpreted as "programs"

From a user's point of view, a *pragmatic distinction* between programs and data may be the following: Consider as "programs" those items satisfying the rules of programming languages established in the computer system, i.e., where the analysis and transformation algorithms are built in into the computer system as integrated language processors. Consider as "data" those items corresponding to "languages" provided by the user himself, i.e. where the analysis, synthesis and transformation algorithms have to be programmed by the user according to his own needs, regardless whether they are processed by algorithms or they describe and govern algorithms.

In the following sections of this paper certain linguistic aspects of the communication between men and computers are discussed. In the main part concepts of programming languages are considered. Some thoughts on principles of user defined data languages are added at the end.

2.   *USE OF PROGRAMMING LANGUAGES*

As discussed above, programming languages serve to formulate algorithms and to communicate them to computers. As is well-known, many programming languages exist, i.e. are implemented in computer systems, and many new programming languages are invented by computer scientists every year. Thus, in a particular case, the question arises: Which programming language should I use to communicate my problem to my computer? Or, a bit more general: Which linguistic concepts should a programming language contain to be useful for certain algorithms?

First of all, to destroy possible misunderstandings, we should remark, that the question is not: "Which programming language *can* we use to formulate a certain algorithm?", but rather: "Which programming language *should* we use?" For, apart from questions of availability of a language on a specific computer system and of time and storage capacities, we can state that nearly *every algorithm*, which can be executed by a computer at all, *principally can be formulated nearly in every programming language*. For, each computer finally is based on the ability to store and retrieve bits and manipulate them by logical operations like "and",

"or", "not", etc. This ability can be simulated by any programming
language which can express storing and retrieving integers, adding and
multiplying them and recognizing whether an integer is even or odd.
Of course, this principal consideration is of a very theoretical nature
and will not help very much to answer our questions.

To the use of a particular programming language for communicating an
algorithm to a computer similar considerations apply as to the use of
a natural language in a conversation between men:

- It is necessary that both partners "understand" the
  language.

- Principally nearly everything can be expressed in any
  language (possibly using more or less complicated
  circumscriptions).

- The language used highly influences the thinking habits
  of the speaker.

For our problem of man-computer communication the first of these points
has been discussed in some detail in the first section of this paper.
It means that algorithms processing the programming language to be used
have to be implemented and stored in the computer. The second point
has been scetched shortly above. The last point will be the main topic
of the rest of this paper.

As is well-known, a, say German, learner of a foreign language, say
English, takes the following way to express some thoughts in the foreign
language: He first formulates his thoughts in his mother language and
then translates them. The result is a very bad, though possibly correct,
"German English sentence". The advanced man thinks his thoughts in terms
of English notions from the outset and formulates them directly in
English. The result is a, hopefully, good and understandable English
sentence.

What do these statements say for the use of programming languages? A
programming language is not just a means to formulate predesigned
algorithms. Rather, a programming language in mind highly influences
the programmer's way of thinking, the design of algorithms and the
programming style. I often saw programs, written in a high-level programming language, say ALGOL 60, which looked so terribly complicated
and hard to understand, until I finally found out (from the program
itself) that apparently the programmer used to think in terms of an

assembly language, but had been forced (e.g. by his manager) to program
in ALGOL 60. Of course, this is not the intended style of ALGOL 60 programming, like "German English" is not the style of English speaking.

E.g., consider the problem to program an ALGOL 60 procedure for the
well-known algorithm of Euklid determining the greatest common divisor
of two integers (given a procedure mod(p, q) which yields the remainder
of p modulo q). A typical assembly programmer could have found the
following solution:

```
int proc gcd (m, n); value m, n; int m, n;
begin
  l1: if n = 0 then goto lm;
      m := mod (m, n);
      if m = 0 then goto ln;
      n := mod (n, m);
      goto l1;
  lm: gcd := m;
      goto l2;
  ln: gcd := n;
  l2: end
```

A typical ALGOL 60 programmer could have found the following solution:

```
int proc gcd (m, n); value m, n; int m, n;
  gcd := if n = 0 then m
                  else gcd (n, mod (m, n))
```

An algorithm is not a notion *per se*. It is a function composed as a terminating sequence of elementary steps. Essential properties are not only
the function realized, but equally:

- the *way of composition* of these steps,

- the *basic operations* constituting the steps,

- the data structures handled by these operations.

And just these three points are highly influenced by the choice of the
programming language used to formulate an algorithm.

As the above example demonstrates, the choice of a programming language
(or of certain language concepts) for the solution of a problem is not
just a question of program "efficiency", rather it strongly urges upon
one specific solution and prevents another one. By the way, very often
"efficiency" it thought to be measured in computer time needed for executing a program, while the programmer and computer time needed for

producing and testing a program is neglected. This is not the most economic way to consider efficiency.

Of course, independently from a specific programming language, there are always good programmers applying systematic and disciplined thinking and programming and bad programmers applying unsystematic and tricky thinking and programming. But, if certain desirable concepts are not existent in a programming language, programmers are forced to replace them by other concepts and, as a rule, will come up with worse solutions. In the contrary, if not desirable concepts are existent in a programming language, programmers will use them, even in cases where they are not appropriate.

3.   *CONTROL STRUCTURES IN PROGRAMMING LANGUAGES*

The most important point that influences the programmers thinking, his programming style and the quality of programs is the presence or absence of concepts for control structure in a programming language. That means concepts enabling (and possibly forcing) the programmer to compose the whole algorithm from its single steps in a systematically structured way. Not certain details in a program, but the overall shape and structure of the whole program, its readability and probably its correctness are determined by them.

A programming language should contain few simple general concepts for control structure. In a systematically structured program the same fact should always be expressed in the same way. This could be arrived at by leaving it to the discipline of the programmer. Or, better, the definition of the programming language should follow the goal not to enable to express the same fact in two different ways.

Which control structure concepts are needed in order to overcome the design of programs describing complicated algorithms? A natural way to master this complexity is to apply the following strategy:

- construct the algorithm by stepwise refinement, i.e.
  compose it of a set of simpler actions which themselves
  are described by more detailed algorithms (and may be
  composed of even simpler subactions in the same way again);
- describe all these single subactions by algorithms as
  independent from each other as possible.

Thus, a programming language should provide concepts to support the programmer in applying the two principles of *hierarchy and modularity*

for the structuring of programs. These concepts are discussed in the
next two sections of this paper.

3.1. *HIERARCHY*

The goal of *hierarchically structuring* programs, to be constructed by
step-wise refinement, requires linguistic concepts describing the
composition of actions.

We call the *execution* of an algorithm described by a program an *action*
(which may possibly depend on certain data). An action will generally
be composed of a set of subactions. Each of them will be described by a
specific program part and may itself be composed of a set of subactions,
and so forth. In this way finally all actions are composed step by step
from basic actions which are executions of certain basic operations
provided by the language.

So, what we need in a programming language are concepts describing the
composition of actions to form major actions. Thereby the program part
describing such a composed major action has to express *the way of composition and* to denote *the single subactions*. The latter may be done either
by directly containing the corresponding program parts or by containing
references to them.

E.g., the part

  begin a := 1; p(a); if a>0 then a := 0 else b := 1 end

of an ALGOL 60 program describes an action composed of three subactions
to be performed in the given sequence. The first of them is an assignment
described by the program part a := 1. The second one is an action described
by a certain program part written somewhere else and referred to by the
procedure call p(a). The third one is an action which is itself composed
of two subactions (described by a := 0 and b := 1) to be performed alternatively to each other depending on the selection criterion whether
a>0 or a≤0 holds.

The following composition concepts have proven to be useful and more or
less necessary and sufficient for programming all practical problems:

  - *serial composition* of a sequence of actions,

  - *collateral composition* of a set of parallel actions, combined
    with suitable synchronizing facilities,

  - *conditional selection* of an action out of a set of two or more alternatives,

- *iteration* of an equal action either until a certain
  condition has been satisfied dynamically or until a certain
  set of data to be manipulated has been exhausted.

In higher level programming languages these composition concepts are
available more or less directly (e.g. compound statement, collateral
clause or coroutines, if- or case-statements, while-, repeat-, for-
statements). In lower level programming languages (e.g. assembly
languages) they can be expressed more or less easily using the means of
these languages (e.g. expressing iteration by means of conditional and
unconditional branching in instruction sequences). A programmer forced
to use a programming language, which does not have the above concepts,
should nevertheless conceptually try to design his program using the
above notions. After having this design he has to transcribe them into
standatd instruction sequences (either by means of a macro-generator if
possible, or by hand). Such transcribed algorithms then will result in
clear well-structured programs, making disciplined use of the low
language primitives.

Besides the mentioned four composition concepts a programming language
should provide means to express a *premature termination* of an action
under certain (e.g. exceptional) conditions. E.g. to search a sequence
a[1], ..., a[n] of n variables for the index i of the first one, if any,
having the value c may in an appropriate programming language be expressed
by the following iteration:

    i := 1;

    while i≤n and a[i] ≠ c do i := i + 1

But this solution does not look very natural. What one really wants to
iterate is not the counting i := i + 1 but the check a[i] = c:

    for i from 1 to n do if a[i] = c then "found!"

What has to be expressed by "found!" is this: Terminate the iteration
now, though the sequence i from 1 to n has not yet been exhausted.

Such a possibility of a premature termination of an action is particularly
useful in cases, where a major action or even the complete program
execution shall be terminated when erroneous situations have been recognized. Instead of proper return- or exit-statements to-day's programming
languages provide for this purpose the goto-statement. This statement
however (inherited from the branching concept in machine language
instruction sequences) is a too powerful one and tempts programmers

to misuse this power destroying the logical structure of programs.

3.2. *MODULARITY*

As mentioned above, *modular programming*, besides hierarchical structuring, is the most natural and promising strategy suited to master the design of complicated algorithms. This means that the different subactions, of which the complete action described by the program is composed, are to be programmed as independently from each other as possible. Each of the corresponding program parts has to satisfy these two conditions:

- it can be used externally for composing
  major parts without detailed knowledge of
  its internal structure and behaviour,

- it can be constructed internally without detailed
  knowledge of its external use.

This concept of modularity requires language facilities which allow to express actions by separately written closed program units called *modules*. Such a module consists of its private *local data and algorithms* and has a clearly defined *interface of specified data and control links* to the outside. At best, it could be programmed, compiled and tested separately and lateron incorporated into a larger program.

The possibility to incorporate separately written modules (whether precompiled or in source language text) containing their own local data and algorithms requires a structure of nested levels of nomenclature with locally declared names at each level. This is realized by the well-known *block-structure* concept of higher level languages. When inserting blocks into each other one only has to be careful with global names (which are part of the outside interface) while local names are protected against each other.

E.g. a module designed to calculate the average of n real values a[1], ..., a[n] and to assign it to a variable av can be programmed without further knowlege of its environment:

```
begin real sum := 0;
      for i from 1 to n do
            sum := sum + a[i];
      av := sum/n
end
```

Even if this block is inserted into another one containing the names

sum or i they are protected by scope rules against the local names sum
and i of our block.

Nesting of blocks means incorporation of modules into each other by
literal textual insertion. A better solution is to use the subroutine
or *procedure* concept. Define a module by a separately programmed
procedure definition and use it in the composition of other modules by
procedure calls, i.e. parameterized references to the procedure definition: In each position, where the procedure is to be used, just its name
stands for the complete text of the procedure. Conceptually the notion
of procedure enables the programmer

- to specify once a predefined action, denote it by
  a procedure name and then use it without regard of
  its internal structure,

- to write short comprehensible program units making use
  of such predefined actions,

- to guarantee (by calling the same procedure several
  times) that intended equal actions are really done
  the same way.

The above module calculating an average value may be written as procedure
declaration:

```
proc average = (real[]x, int y, ref real z):
    begin real sum := 0;
        for i from 1 to y do
            sum := sum + x [i];
        z := sum/y
    end
```

and used at different positions by shortly writing, e.g.,

```
average (a, n, av).
```

The mechanism for *passing parameters* to procedures in a programming
language should be so general that any data linkage between the procedure
and its caller can be done via parameters and no other "side effects"
are necessary. In particular, this means that any data structure
available in the language can be passed as a parameter both as a value
and by reference (i.e. by passing a reference for the data structure as
a parameter, to which the procedure may assign a new value to be passed
back). So, in the above example, the values of the array a and of its
upper bound n could be passed as well as the reference av to which the

resulting value is to be assigned.

Here just a remark on *recursive procedures* should be made. One often
hears the opinion that recursive procedures are so complicated that
only mathematicians use them in sophisticated programs. This is not true.
Often it is conceptually the easiest way to express a problem recursively.
It means just: The solution of the problem contains the solution of the
same kind of problem applied to reduced data. E.g., to scan a given
list for an element with a certain property p, one needs just to test
the first element for this property and then, if the list is not yet
exhausted, scan the rest of the list in the same way:

```
proc scan = (list l, ref element el):
       if first elem of l has property p
       then el := first elem of l
       else if l not exhausted
              then scan (remainder of l, el)
```

If a programming language does not allow recursive procedure calls, it
often prevents the programmer from finding the most appropriate solution
for his problem.

A procedure call denotes an action to be performed once, doing its job
and vanishing. In the contrary to this concept, a type of modules is
needed denoting actions which permanently exist collaterally to each
other. For this purpose there are different language concepts:
concurrent processes and *coroutines*.

Concurrent processes are executed conceptually "in parallel", i.e. in
unspecified order relatively to each other, at least in general. Data
communication between such processes is performed by access to common
data. Here one has to prevent unpredictable results yielded by means of
simultaneous access of different processes to the same data. For this
purpose *access to common data* by a process is possible only within a
critical region, which (controlled by means of synchronizing timing
signals exchanged between the processes) cannot be executed at the same
time as critical regions of other processes.

In the contrary to this concept of unspecified order of execution,
coroutines are modules executed in well-determined sequential order.
Each of them consists of a set of data and algorithms. Among the data
there are specified external ones, i.e. such ones accessible also to
the other coroutines, enabling data communication. The algorithms have
specified entry points, enabling control link. At each time one of the

coroutines is active, executing a part of its algorithms, until it transfers the control to another one which then is activated to continue its algorithms at a given entry point.

4. *DATA STRUCTURES*

Another important point that essentially influences programming is the question what kind of data and data structures are expressible in a programming language. In which form can information be represented as data and how can it be processed?

We call *data* the objects which can be manipulated by the algorithms described by programs according to the rules of the programming language. They are considered independently from possible "concrete" representations by messages as parts of programs on the one hand and from possible "abstract" meanings as some information or knowledge in the programmers mind on the other hand. E.g., we consider a real number to be a datum independently from its representation by a sequence of digits on the one hand and from its meaning as, say, a temperature on the other hand.

Data are themselves *abstract* in nature, but they are uniquely *characterized by the operations* applicable to them and the data resulting from these operations. They are classified into *classes of data* of the same *data type* (e.g. integer, logical, array of real). Each type is characterized by the basic operations defined for all data of this type. These operations are the elementary actions from which the actions described by a program are composed as discussed in the previous sections. That means that we cannot consider data and their data types separately from their corresponding basic operations.

Data can be denoted in programs either by *constants* or by *identifiers*. A constant is a message inherently denoting a fixed datum defined by the rules of the language. An identifier is a name defined by the programmer to denote a certain datum inside a certain scope of his program. This definition is introduced either explicitly, by means of a declaration, or implicitly, by standard conventions of the language. E.g., in a program the real number π may either be denoted by the constant 3.14159 or, after having introduced a declaration

<u>real</u> pi = 3.14159,

by the identifier pi. To be general and flexible, a programming language should provide the possibility to denote any data by any freely choosen name within the scope of any module.

Data are either *simple data* or more or less complex *data structures* built up from them.

4.1. *SIMPLE DATA*

Simple data are the elementary objects, characterized by elementary operations, from which all data structures are constructed. The "standard" simple data types needed are the types *integer, real, logical* (Boolean), *character*. The values of type character belong to a (possibly ordered) standard alphabet of symbols of the language (a, ..., z, 0, ..., 9, +, =, ...). The corresponding basic operations are the usual arithmetic, logical and comparison operations and possibly operations transferring data of one type to such of another type (e.g. rounding of real to integer values, or numbering of character values according to the given order of the alphabet).

Besides the "standard" data types the programmer should have means to define his *own simple data types* describing a finite, ordered set of *symbolic values*: E.g.,

  type weekday = (monday, tuesday, wednesday,
                  thursday, friday, saturday, sunday).

Use of such a facility, if present in a language, makes a program more conceivable than e.g. misusing integer values as encoding of such symbols: Then one can write program parts like

  if day = sunday then ...

instead of writing, say,

  if day = 7 then ... .

If a programming language does not contain this concept, one can simulate it by introducing corresponding names for integer values, if this concept is present in the language.

The dynamic property of computers, namely the ability to store and retrieve data is regarded in programming languages by the concept of *reference*. We denote by the term "reference" what in the different programming languages is called a variable, pointer, name or address. We consider references as special simple values having the basic property to refer at each time to a determined datum (either simple datum or data structure). The essential corresponding basic operations are *assigment*,

i.e. changing the value referred to, and *content*, i.e. retrieving the
value currently referred to, which is the last assigned value. Further
operations are *generation* of a new reference, which often is, but need
not necessarily be, combined with a declaration introducing an identifier
naming the newly generated reference, and *deletion* of a reference.

For program security, the programming language should (not all programming
languages do so) fix for each reference the *range of data*, to which it
can refer, to be the class of data of one specific data type. Conversely,
for each data type, including all types of structured data and of references themselves, there should be references available.

One consequence of considering references as data themselves is that a
reference can refer to another reference, i.e. we can construct data
structures which indirectly, by reference chaining, refer to values.
Another consequence is that actions described by program modules can
manipulate both, "usual values" and references, as data. E.g. when
defining and activating procedures we have both possibilities for passing
parameters, and we have carefully to distinguish them: either pass a
value itself or pass a reference referring to it (like a vessel containing this value, into which the procedure may fill in another one to be
returned).

4.2. *STRUCTURED DATA*

In section 3 the possibility to build up hierarchies of actions composed
of simpler ones and finally of basic operations was discussed. Analog-
ously, the programmer needs the possibility to build up hierarchically
structured data composed finally of simple data. What composition
facilities for data are available in programming languages?

Generally, we call a *data structure* a collection of data, *its components*,
which is uniquely characterized by:

> - the components themselves, and
> - the logical way of their composition.

This corresponds to the fact, that a composed action, as explained in
section 3, is described by specifying its single subactions and the way
of their composition (serial, collateral etc.). This definition of the
general notion of a data structure is recursive, since each component
may be a datum of any type,i.e. either a simple datum or a data
structure, which itself is composed of component data.

Examples of such data structures are:

    (a) ordered pairs of real numbers;

    (b) character strings (texts), being ordered sequences
        of characters, i.e., of simple data mentioned above;

    (c) personal records, each consisting of, say,
        a "name"-component which is a character string,
        an "age"-component which is an integer,
        a "sex"-component which is one of the programmer
        defined symbolic values "male" or female", etc.;

    (d) personal files, being either ordered sequences
        or just unstructured collections of components,
        which are such personal records;

    (e) sets of chained elements: each element of the
        set is a data structure consisting, say, of two
        components, namely a "value"-component which is
        a datum of any type and a "next"-component which
        is a reference (see section 4.1) referring to any
        other element of the set.

As the last of these examples shows, the possibility to handle references
as data, and in particular to use them as components of data structures
supplies the means to construct any cross-referenced network of data.

The logical way of composition of a data structure from its components
(ordered sequence, collection of uniquely named components, unordered
set, etc.) has nothing to do with specific concrete representations of
the data structures by written messages. Rather, it describes the abstract structuring of the data structure. It is characterized by two
kinds of basic operations, namely:

        operations applicable ro collections of data
        and producing data structures composed of them,

and conversely and even more important,

        operations applicable to data structures
        giving access to their single components.

Thus, specifying classes of data structures mainly means specifying these
basic operations corresponding to them.

Now, what special cases of this general concept and which linguistic
means to express them in programming languages are the most important
ones? In particular, how can the access to the single components of a

data structure be expressed?

There are two general possibilities of structuring. Either the data structure as such is a completely unordered and *unstructured set of components*. Or it is a *collection of components*, each of which is *uniquely determined by its logical position* within this collection.

In the case of a *set*, access to components is possible in three ways: First, by actions accessing *all* components equally, e.g. by an action composed collaterally of equal subactions, each of which handles one component of the set:

> for all x from s do action(x).

Second, by operations selecting single components uniquely determined by properties to be specified:

> that x from s with prop(x).

Third, indirectly by means of a reference to which a single component to be accessed had been assigned previously. Today's programming languages, however, do not contain general sets as data structures.

In the case of data structures structured by the logical positions of their single components within them, usually each of these logical positions can uniquely be identified by some characteristic datum which we call its *selector*. In this case each single component can be accessed by an operation, called *selection* or *indexing*, which applied to the data structure and the selector immediately yields the identified component. Different kinds of such data structures are to be distinguished by different types of selectors.

If there is a logical *ordering sequence* of the components, natural identifications of them are ordering numbers, i.e. integers to be used as selectors. This is the concept of *arrays* which in all high level programming languages are available in some form or another and in assembly languages can easily be simulated by indexing mechanisms.

The other important kind of such structured data is the case where the logical positions of the single components are uniquely identified by names chosen by the programmer, i.e. identifiers to be used as selectors. This is the concept called *structures* or *records* in different high level programming languages. Nesting of such records, i.e. using records as components of records again, allows to build up data with a static hierarchical structure. E.g.,

```
                  (name: (first: "John", family: "Smith"),
                  sex: male,
                  age: 45)
```

describes such a nested data structure s, where iterated application of
the selection operation, say,

family _of_ name _of_ s

uniquely yields the subcomponent "Smith". In combination with references
used as components (see example (e) above) any dynamically changing
data structure can be expressed. Thus a requirement to a powerful programming language is to provide both records and general references as
data types.

4.3. _USER DEFINED DATA TYPES_

A very useful concept in programming languages is to provide means for
language extension. To satisfy his specific needs, a programmer should
particularly have the possibility to _define his own types_ constructed
from the simple data types mentioned in section 4.1 using the structuring
means explained in section 4.2. As has been stated earlier a data type
determines a class of data and is characterized by a set of operations
applicable to them. So, to define a new data type, a class of data and
a set of operations on these data has to be defined.

To define a _class of data,_ there are two possibilities: _Either_ specify
a set of simple values belonging to this type. This can be done by
explicitly enumerating a finite set of symbolic values, as mentioned
in section 4.1, or by referring to an existing data type and restricting
its range, e.g. the integers out of a specified interval. _Or_ specify a
class of structured data by means of a structure description. This means,
that the class consists of all those data structures satisfying this
structure description.

E.g., assumed lists of data of some given type are needed, whose elements
are chained to each other and where at each time one of its elements
has to be denoted as the current one. For this purpose a data type list
could be defined by structure descriptions of the following kind:

```
        type list = record (first: ref elem,
                            last: ref elem,
                            current: ref elem)
```

```
type elem = record (value: sometype,
                    next: ref elem,
                    prev: ref elem)
```

To define a *set of applicable operations*, the possibilities discussed
in section 3 to define and compose actions can be used. The operations
to be defined may be expressed as procedures with data of the new data
type as parameters. In many cases the composition of such procedures
from subactions corresponds to the composition of the data structures
from the components: The operation applied to the data structure is
built up from operations applied to its components. E.g. a lexical
comparison of two character strings can be defined by comparisons of
corresponding single characters of the two strings.

E.g., assumed that standard actions to be performed with lists of the
type list introduced above are: extracting the value of the current
element, denoting as new current element the first or last element of
the list or the next one before or after the current element, insertion
of a new given element at the end of the list, etc. For these purposes
appropriate operations could be definded by procedure definitions of the
following kind:

```
proc currentval (list l) sometype:
    value of current of l
proc setfirst (list l):
    current of l := first of l
proc setlast (list l):
    current of l := last of l
proc setforw (list l):
    current of l := next of current of l
proc setback (list l):
    current of l := prev of current of l
proc add (list l, sometype v):
    begin elem new = (value: v,
                      next: genref elem,
                      prev: genref elem);
        if last of l ≠ nil
        then begin prev of new := last of l;
                   next of last of l := new;
             end
        else first of l := new;
        last of l := new
    end
```

In fact, principally this concept of data definition does not extend
the power of a programming language. But it increases conceivability of
programs: It allows to *name* classes of data structures and operations on
them. Using these names the programmer can handle the complete data
structures like simple values: He does no more need to consider their
internal structure, when operating them. In particular, by these definitions of data types such data structures and applicable operations
can be defined which are organized appropriately to their use by algorithms. Often used examples of such data structures and operations are:

(a) *queues*, i.e. linearly chained lists of elements, with an
operation adding a new element at the end and an operation
reading and removing the first element.

(b) *stacks*, i.e. linearly chained lists of elements, with an
operation adding a new element at the end and an operation
reading and removing the last element.

(c) *ordered lists*,i.e. lists of elements which are linearly
chained according to an ordering criterion, with an operation
inserting a new element at its right place according to
this criterion and an operations reading or removing the
first or the last element or an element at a specified
position within this order.

(d) *sequential files*, i.e. linearly chained lists with an
accompanying current position pointer, as in the above
example.

(e) *trees*, i.e. structures of elements, each of which may be
chained to two (or more) descendent elements, with
appropriate operations searching through the branches of
the tree and operations adding or removing elements.

5. *CONSIDERATIONS ON DATA LANGUAGES*

So far, we discussed the linguistic aspect of programming languages:
By which means can the programmer communicate algorithms to the
computer? One should not forget that the linguistic aspect of data
languages is not less important: By which means can data processed by
these algorithms be communicated between man and computer?

Each single program defines (at least) two specific languages, its input
data language and its output data language: The input data accepted and
the output data produced are sequences of symbols representing certain

information. Thus, in fact, by producing a program the programmer defines the syntax and semantics of two languages, one by which men can communicate information to the computer and one by which the computer can communicate information to men. When producing a program, the programmer should be aware of this fact and pay special attention to it, especially since in most cases the program will not be used by the programmer himself. It will be used by non-programmers who later will have to write the input messages and to read the output messages by means of these languages.

What does this mean for the programmer? He has to take care of the representation and layout of the input and output of his program, in order to make it writable and readable for others than himself, even for non-programmers.

Of course, to a certain extent the programmer is bound by the input and output facilities of his programming language. For this purpose, a programming language should provide flexible editing facilities and they should be used appropriately. If the language offers only very primitive input and output facilities, the user should not avoid to define his own appropriate input and output procedures based on these primitives.

How should the input and output languages look like? Just in order to initiate thinking about this qestion, some ideas shall be listed below, without going into details or claiming to be complete.

The main demand is this: Make the user's life as easy as possible! For the input language the following points should be obeyed:

- Do not require the user to write too much.

- Allow for a flexible syntax, e.g.:
  - no formatted input,
  - arbitrary order of input items, as far as
    it is uniquely recognizeable.

- Do not force the user to keep hyroglyphs in mind, but
  allow him to use notions of his own language.

- Build all possible consistency checks on the input
  into the program.

For the output language the followin points should be obeyed:

- Make the output self-explaining.

- Write it in a good formatted layout.

- Do not avoid redundancy at any prize.

- Produce readable detailed error messages as
  reply to inconsistent input.

REFERENCES

[1] Rosen, S. (ed.): Programming systems and languages.
              (Mc Graw-Hill, New York 1967).

[2] Sammet, J.E.: Programming languages: History and
              fundamentals. (Prentice-Hall, Engle-
              wood Cliffs N.J. 1969).

[3] Sammet, J.E.: Programming languages: History and
              future. Comm.ACM 15 (1972).

[4] Dahl, O.J., Dijkstra, E.W., Hoare, C.A.R.: Structured programming.
                    (Academic Press, London - New York 1972).

[5] Naur, P. (ed.): Revised report on the algorithmic language
              ALGOL 60. Comm. ACM 6 (1963).

[6] IBM Corporation: PL/I Language specifications,
              IBM Systems Reference library.

[7] Dahl, O.J., Myrhaug, R., Nygaard, K.: SIMULA 67, common base
              language. (Norwegian Computing Center, Oslo 1968).

[8] Wirth, N.: The programming language Pascal. Acta Informatica 1 (1971).

[9] van Wijngaarden, A. (ed.): Report on the algorithmic language
              ALGOL 68. Num. Math. 14 (1969).

FROM PROBLEM TO PROGRAM
========================

K. Alber, Braunschweig

1.   *INTRODUCTION*

"Programming" is commonly understood to be the human activity of
writing computer programs which direct computers to solve information
problems.

What does this mean? If someone wishes to get certain information, does
he just need to hire a programmer and ask him to translate his question
into a language understood by a computer, such that the computer will
yield the required information? Is, thus, programming nothing else but
the mystery of the knowledge and correct use of computer languages, like
professional language translation, e.g. from German to English? Certainly not.

The activities of a programmer may well be compared to those of an
architect: Starting from more or less specific and more or less realistic
wishes of his customer, he has finally to come up with a well formed
and reliable construction. It has to meet the customer's wishes as far
as possible, to be useful even beyond them, if faesible, to provide
means for repairing and possibly extending and, last not least, it has
to satisfy secondary conditions like financial and time limits, available
material and tools and adjustment to its environment.

These activities have the characteristics of a science, engineering and
art as well. They comprise the following points:
- *analysis of the problem* to be solved, to recognize
   not only the wishes, but the underlying needs of the
   user and the requirements necessary for a solution,
- *design of an algorithm* solving the problem, consisting
   of a finite number of steps which are selected out of
   a set of well-defined operations,
- *construction of a program* which realizes this algorithm
   within the environment of the available computing system,
- *verification* of the constructed program, in order to

guarantee that it really solves the stated problem,
- *documentation* of the program to describe the functional
properties for users, and the internal structure for people
who later have to repair, change or extend it.

The following sections of this paper will discuss these different activities of programmers in some detail.

A particular question is the order in time of these five tasks for one
project. Ideally, the first three of them should be performed in the
stated order: First complete the problem analysis before starting the
algorithm design and then complete this before starting program construction. The last two, verification and documentation should be done
simultaneously with all other activities. In practice, the different
tasks will be iterated, and changes in one of them may require reconsideration and changes in earlier ones. One point we have to obey is
the question how to minimize and localize the consequences of such
changes.

2.   PROBLEM ANALYSIS

The first task to be performed in order to solve a given problem by
means of computer programs is the *analysis of the problem* itself. What
are the characteristics of the kind of problems which might be attacked
by computers and what are the points we have to analyse when going to
solve such problems?

First of all, computable problems are concerned with *informations,* i.e.
abstract items of knowledge about the real world. Thus, the first question
to be answered is this: What items of knowledge might be relevant to our
problem? These items of knowledge include in particular:
- Informations we expect to receive from the computer
  as solutions of our problem.

- Informations we have (or can receive from other sources),
  which we can offer to the computer as input for the job.

- Any other possibly relevant information, e.g. information
  which can be deduced from other available information.

We should obey, that at the moment we do nothing else but state as complete as possible which items of knowledge might be related to our problem. Thereby we should state which of these informations are already
available and which can be made available in principle if needed. However, we are not yet concerned with the question which informations are

really needed to be supplied, or even the question how these informations are to be coded and structured as data.

Secondly, computable problems are determined by *interrelationships* existing between the different related informations. Thus, the second question to be answered is this: Which dependencies and relations are known to hold between the informations? These relations between informations constitute the core of any computable problem at all. They have to be analyzed and described completely and exactly in such a way that they can be considered as well-defined for all following activities.

The relations may be of different nature, e.g. the following may hold:

- One information is completely determined by others,
  but not vice versa (e.g. compression of a collection
  of informations, like the sum or average of a set of
  numerical values).

- Different informations determine each other mutually, i.e.
  any of them can be deduced if the others are known.

- The range to which informations belong is restricted
  by conditions determined by other informations (e.g.
  inequalities holding for numerical values).

Now, from these well-defined relations, we have to analyse which informations are *logically deducible* from which ones. By the set of all dependency relations a whole network of deducibilities between the different informations is defined stating which informations, directly or indirectly, are completely determined by each other. From this investigation of deducibilities we can conclude in particular, whether the informations required as answers of our problem can logically be deduced from informations which are available or can be made available. Additionally, this analysis may yield answers to the following questions:

- Which informations are really needed to solve our
  problem, and which can be deduced or are unnecessary anyhow?

- Is our problem possibly only a special case of a more
  general problem which could be solved as well? Could
  we try to modify the solution in such a way that further
  similar problems may be solved using the same method?

3. ALGORITHM DESIGN

The next task to be performed in order to solve a computable problem (if

it is computable at all) is the design of appropriate *algorithms*. The
deductions discussed so far were defined by logical dependency relations
between abstract items of knowledge. An information B deducible from A
was defined by a statement of the form "B is that information for which
the given property P holds with respect to A". No such logical assertions
are of any worth for a solution by means of a computer, unless there are
constructive realizations of the described deductions.

These constructive realizations of the deductions are the algorithms to
be designed. They have to consist of a *finite number of steps*, each of
them being one out of a set of well-defined operations of the computer
system. Thus, the algorithms to be designed essentially depend on two
things:

- the *functions to be realized* by the algorithms,
- the *functions to be used* by the algorithms as their
  single operational steps.

Design of an algorithm is nothing else but composition of a complex
function as a finite sequence of steps out of a set of well-defined simpler functions. In order to do the design we have to know *both* of them,
the function to be composed and the set of functions to be used as its
elementary building stones. And of course one is forced to design very
different algorithms if these sets of building stones differ.

3.1. *FUNCTIONS AND DATA*

What does the notion of *function* mean here? As a function we shall denote a well-defined *transformation mapping data onto data*. In order to
define a function we have to specify

- the *range* of data transformed ("input data")

- the exact *operation* performed on data out of this range,
  in particular, the data resulting from the transformation
  ("output data") in dependency on the input data.

Depending on the level of the functions (whether they are elementary
hardware functions or complex functions realized by sophisticated algorithms), these data can be bits, bytes, words, characters, fixed and
floating numbers, pointers, etc., and data structures built of such elementary data by composition like strings, arrays, lists, trees, networks
etc.

We should emphasize here, that the definition of a function just determines a range of such data and an operation performing a transformation
between such data. Principally, it does not say anything, however, about
the interpretation of such data as encoded representation of abstract
information. (Though, of course, in many cases an anticipated interpretation, e.g. of bit strings as numbers, stood sponsor to the design
of the function.)

One point of our design problem is the question how to represent our
abstract information, as discussed previously, by encoding and structuring them as data to be transformed by the designed algorithms.

Thus, in order to design an algorithm for the solution of a computable
problem we have to perform the following three, *highly interrelated,*
things:

- establish representations of the relevant informations
  by encoding and structuring as data and, vice versa,
  decoding data as informations,

- define functions transforming these data, which realize
  the wanted information deductions,

- design algorithms which realize these functions composed
  of given functions to be used.

It should be emphasized that none of these three problems can be considered isolated from the other two. So the representation and especially the structuring of informations as data has to satisfy the following
conditions:

- The resulting output data have to be easily interpretable.

- The input data have to fit to the data ranges of the elementary
  functions to be used for the algorithm.

- Its structure has to be such that an effective algorithm
  for the problem is possible. (E.g. an alphabetic address
  directory is one possible structured representation of the
  information "addresses of all people in the town", it is
  not well suited, however, for an algorithm to find out, who
  lives in a given house).

- It has to assist easy acquisition, encoding and structuring
  of input information.

As a consequence, when going to solve a certain problem, one should not
start to collect a mass of informations, coming out with large boxes

of punched cards, before having designed the algorithms and knowing
which informations in which representation and structure are appropriate.

3.2. DECOMPOSITION OF FUNCTIONS

As stated above, the design of an algorithm is just composition of a
complex function from simpler functions. Usually the gap between the
complexity of the function to be realized and the simplicity of the
functions to be used as building stones (e.g. the basic computer instructions) is so big, that it is impossible to master at once the
complete problem of designing the algorithm.

In this case the motto "divide et impera" may help. I.e., the whole
function is split up into subfunctions which solve subproblems of the
original problem and which hopefully can be mastered easier. Each of
these functions may again be split up and use other functions which
either again have to be defined in this way or are elementary functions
of our computer system.

For each such splitting up two things have to be done:

- Define exactly each of the single functions by
  specifying their behaviour with respect to the outside,
  i.e. specifying the ranges of data and the operations
  performed on them (without saying at the moment how this
  is achieved).

- Define exactly how the functions are composed in order to
  realize a major function by specifying how they work together,
  i.e. in which order, under which conditions and especially on
  which part of the data of the major function they have to
  operate.

By separating these two aspects, namely the definition of the interface
of each component to the outside and its internal composition from other
functions, we try to come into a position, where it is possible to consider the design of each of these functions separately.

By this process of splitting up the algorithm to be designed we possibly
come up with a large number of functions communicating with each other.
The communication between different functions can take place by mutual
procedure calls with parameter passing, exchange of common data, synchronization signals, etc. These communications will often lead to a
very complex network of mutual dependencies between the different functions of the algorithm to be designed. This complexity may be such

that our aim to separate the design of the single functions and to consider them independently from each other cannot be reached. This will
particularly be true, if two or more functions depend cyclically from
each other.

What we have to do is to try to design the different functions in such
a way, that as much as possible dependencies between them exist only in
one direction and not cyclically. This is the case if one of two functions uses the other as a closed auxiliary subfunction, e.g. by a procedure call, but not vice versa. Following this design strategy we attain
a partially ordered set of classes of functions, where dependency cycles occur only between functions of the same class. Combining these
classes in an appropriate way we finally get a linearly ordered set of
function *layers*.

In this way, we have split up the algorithm to be designed into a *hierarchical structure of functions* belonging to different layers. The functions of one layer work together and communicate mutually with each
other. They use the functions of the next lower layer as more primitive
subfunctions.

3.3. *LEVELS OF ABSTRACTION*

The role of the layers of functions described above is the following.
Each layer L_i comprises the definition of a complete set of functions
and a range of data and data structures on which these functions work.
These functions and data are provided as tools to be used by the functions of the next higher layer L_{i+1}. They are designed as constituted
from the functions and data of the next lower layer L_{i-1}. The solution
of our complete problem will be performed by functions of the highest
layer L_n, while the lowest layer L_o for us consists of the functions
and data structures provided by the computer system, our *host system*.

By the *computer system* here we mean the complete system of hardware and
system software available to us for our problem solution. It appears as
a consistent unit providing us with a set of services, namely functions
and data structures. Its internal structure of different hardware and
software components is of no interest for us and is hidden to us. In
fact it is itself set up as a hierarchy of layers (e.g. hardware, operating system, language processor, etc.).

In the same way as the internal structure of our host system is hidden
to us, the internal composition of the functions and data of layer L_i

from those of L_{i-1} is hidden to layer L_{i+1}. In fact all of layer L_{i-1} and lower layers is hidden to layer L_{i+1}. This means that each layer L_i can be considered as an *abstract machine* and all of layer L_{i+1} is designed only in terms of this abstract machine.

By this concept each layer L_i can be designed as an abstract machine, completely independent from the higher layers (though, of course, their needs have to stand sponsor for its definition) and also completely independent from all layers lower than L_{i-1}.

So each layer consisting of a specific abstract machine allows and forces a specific *level of abstraction*. When using L_i to design L_{i+1} we can abstract from the detailed properties of the lower levels (and forget the specific problems and difficulties concerned with these properties). Conversely, we are not concerned with the complexity to be mastered at higher levels (and can forget the specific problems and difficulties of that). So each problem of the complete design is to be decided and solved at its appropriate level of abstraction and can be separated clearly from problems logically belonging to other levels.

What are the design criteria for each single layer of our system? Every design decision should be measured under the following two criteria:

- good usability for higher levels, this usually includes generality of functions

- clear and efficient implementability from lower levels.

It is a question of experience and personal taste, in which order the design of the complete hierarchy of layers is performed, from top to bottom (i.e. from our original problem down to our host system) or from bottom to top.

When *designing top-down*, we start with a presumably good decomposition of the original problem at the highest level. We continue at each level by anticipating useful definitions of the next lower level and using them for the design. It is up to our intuition, that we finally come down to functions, which easily and efficiently can be composed from the functions of the given host system.

When *designing bottom-up* we start with the given host system. At each level we continue by designing functions which are well composable from those of the next lower level. Now, it is up to our intuition, that we finally come up and provide all functions necessary to solve the original problem.

Certainly, in general the design will be iterated several times top-down and bottom-up. Design decisions made at one level will come out to be inappropriate at later (lower or higher) levels and have to be revised. Additionally questions of efficiency may force us to shift functions between different layers.

4. *PROGRAM CONSTRUCTION*

After having performed the complete design of the algorithms, the final construction of the corresponding program is nothing else but writing down the designed algorithms obeying the rules of given programming languages. Indeed, no definite border line between the design of algorithms and the construction of programs can be drawn. Exactly described algorithms *are* programs. The better and the more exactly the definitions of functions and data structures at each layer and the design of their internal algorithms are described, the less work is left to be done to transscribe these things into running programs. Even, the designed algorithms may be laid down in the final programming languages from the outset, if the design of the function layers is good enough to provide good linguistic tools.

The main difficulty to be mastered when going to write good and correct programs is the problem of complexity. And again we have to master this problem by dividing into manageable parts. For this division into parts there are two main principles:

- *Hierarchy,* i.e. cutting down of the whole into steps of growing refinement. Hierarchical decomposition is mainly realized by the described program layers, but should also be applied within single layers.

- *Modularity,* i.e. cutting down of one hierarchical level into closed parts interacting with each other according to fixed interface rules. Modular decomposition realizes the different functions in the same layer.

4.1. *HIERARCHY OF LAYERS*

As stated in the previous section, in a good hierarchically structured design of an algorithm each layer defines an abstract machine. Each of these abstract machines (as each computing machine) defines an individual programming language as its machine language. This language is given by the data structures and operations on them, defined in that layer. Thus

the hierarchy of layers defines a hierarchy of *linguistic levels* of
programming languages.

Programming with this hierarchy of linguistic levels means nothing else
but implementing each of these abstract machines, i.e. programming its
operations and data structures, as programs in the programming language
of the next lower abstract machine. Hereby a strict programming discipline has to be obeyed: only the language features of that one single
linguistic level of the next lower abstract machine have to be used.
The following are the purposes of this discipline:

- Clarity of programs. Each layer may be described,
  implemented, verified, tested, corrected, changed
  and, last not least, understood completely independently from all other layers, as soon as the linguistic
  levels are exactly defined. No work on other layers,
  as long as it yields a correct implementation of
  the specified abstract machine, will affect this layer.

- Security. Using internals of lower layers is like working
  of a layman on an open electrical socket. It is (or should
  be) by good reasons, that primitive functions of one
  layer are replaced by more comfortable *and* more secure
  ones in higher levels. Any access to internals may
  produce unknown effects in the misusing or misused parts,
  possibly after later program changes which are not aware
  of the misuse.

But how can the programming languages of the different abstract machine
layers in reality look like? How is one such abstract machine implemented
by means of the lower programming language?

The language of the lowest level is the programming language of our host
system. The easiest (though not safest) way for a programmer to implement
one level on top of the previous one is extension by adding new functions
and restriction by discipline. That means, both levels base on the same
host language. They coincide on large parts of it, e.g. its control
structures. The lower level possibly makes use of a larger subset of
the host language than the higher level. Instead of that, the higher
level uses additional functions defined by the lower level within the
frame of the base language. The way of this definition of additional
functions depends on the definitional facilities of the host language.
It may be a set of procedure declarations of high-level programming
languages, a set of macro definitions of assembly languages or PL/I,

type and operator declarations, or use of extension facilities of other languages. More sophisticated ways of implementing a language level by another one are translation and interpretation. In this case also the protection against misuse of lower language features can be built in and does not rely on programming discipline only.

Here again the question arises, in which order, top-down or bottom-up, the single layers should be programmed. After having completely fixed the definitions of the interfaces between all layers, i.e. the definitions of the different languages, the order of *coding* the different layers is, of course, completely irrelevant. For the purpose of *testing*, however, one should *start from the bottom*. Having implemented one level, one is able to run and test the programs running on that level and implementing the next one.

4.2. *STRUCTURED PROGRAMMING*

Also within single layers it is necessary to follow the principle of hierarchical structuring of programs. This principle is mainly a matter of thinking discipline yielding a programming style, which since several years is used to be termed *structured programming*. The essence of this programming style is to reflect clearly in each part of a program the logical structure of the programmed problem. Usually a problem to be programmed can be logically split up into a set of distinct, but somehow interconnected subproblems. Each of them can be split up in the same way, and so forth, into more and more details.

To this corresponds, that each program part implementing one logical problem is composed out of distinct program parts which correspond to the different subproblems. These distinct program parts have to be programmed as much as possible as closed units, modules as to be discussed in the next section. This means a very careful handling of data to the outside and mainly such control flow, that they can be used as building stones with completely predictable behaviour for the composition of the surrounding program part. This behaviour with respect to the control flow means that they act like single machine operations, i.e. have one predictable entry and one predictable exit only (apart from "emergency exits" in exceptional situations).

How are problems composed out of subproblems and thus programs to be composed out of subprograms? There are the following possibilities:

Serial composition. A problem may be completely solved by solving a fixed set of subproblems in a given sequence. Accordingly the program part is composed as a fixed sequence of units. This is the common program structure of combining a sequence of statements or instructions into compound statements, blocks, procedures, modules, macros etc., where each statement or instruction itself may be such a unit.

Parallel or collateral composition. A problem may be completely solved by solving a fixed set of subproblems without any specific order. In this case it may be that the solutions of these subproblems are completely independent or that they influence each other in some wanted or unwanted way. Accordingly the program part is composed as a fixed set of units, which, depending on the programming language and the facilities of the host system, potentially or really can be executed in parallel. This is done by such program structures as collateral clauses, coroutines or parallel programming. Mutual influences have to be directed by appropriate synchronizing facilities of the language.

Alternative composition. A problem may be solved by first testing for a certain condition and depending on the outcome of the test solving a specific one out of a set of alternative subproblems. Accordingly the program part is composed of a test condition and a set of alternative units. This is realized by if- or case-statements or similar constructs.

Iterative composition. A problem may be solved by solving the same kind of subproblem several times, either each time for another one out of a whole set of data items, or each time for new data resulting from the previous solution until these data satisfy a certain given condition. Accordingly the program part is composed of a unit to be executed iteratively and a control part controlling the iteration and in particular its terminating condition. This is realized by the control constructions of so-called program loops as for-, do-, while-, repeat-statements or similar constructs.

In the great majority of all cases these four principles are completely sufficient to build the control structure of programs: serial, parallel, alternative and iterative composition of program units out of smaller ones. Using only these four ones and replacing larger units within them by the substitution mechanism of procedure calls results in a clear, understandable program which by that has a good chance to contain less errors than others.

4.3. *MODULARITY*

The concepts of *hierarchy* discussed in the previous sections were concerned mainly with "horizontal" partitioning of a complex program system
into layers or nested levels of program units. The "vertical" partitioning of one such level into these cooperating program units is the
concept of *modularity*.

The concept of modularity is to compose programs out of preformed building stones with standardized interconnections like the building of pre-
fabricated houses. These building stones are called *program modules*.
They can be composed to form larger modules as described in the previous
section. Program modules are closed program units satisfying the following two conditions:

- The *composition* of modules can be performed *independently*
  from their *internal construction*.

- The *construction* of a module can be performed *independently*
  from its *external composition*.

This means that, once the *interfaces* of all modules to the outside have
been defined completely and exactly, their constructions and uses can
be separated. The programming of a single module can be done "context-
independently", i.e. by a programmer not knowing for which purpose, by
whom, where and how often this module will be used. Conversely, a module
can be used for composition in larger programs by programmers not knowing how and by whom it is programmed.

An important consequence hereof is the fact that single modules can be
exchanged against reprogrammed ones without affecting the programs using
them. Such exchange of single modules may become useful or necessary in
order to correct detected errors, extend (compatibly) the functions,
realize more efficient implementations, or adjust the program to another
host system.

How can the defined interface of a module to the outside look like, and
by which linguistic means can it be realized? In particular, we have to
discuss, by which means data are communicated between a module and the
outside world.

The simplest (and safest) kind of a module is a closed subroutine, i.e.
a *procedure without use of global data*. It has the following behaviour:
Whenever any program part needs the service of this procedure, it pro-

vides a set of input data as actual parameters, activates a new incarnation of the procedure and waits, until this activated procedure incarnation has done its job. The activated procedure takes over the actual
parameters and works. For its own purposes it can create its private
new (*local*) data and use the services of other modules. But the only
interface to the outside, in particular the only knowledge of outside
data (and of the history of the program execution), is via the passed
actual parameters. Also, the only effect of the procedure given to the
outside is via the actual parameters, i.e. there may be passed actual
parameters specifying where to leave results. After the procedure has
done its job, the activated procedure incarnation dies, in particular
its local data are no more available to anybody, and the original program part continues. To sum up:

- The procedure behaves as a closed action used (*"called"*)
  by others.

- The data communication from and to the outside is only via
  actual parameters passed by the calling program part.

- The procedure has no knowledge (except if passed by
  parameters) of the history of the program, even not
  of other calls of itself (other incarnations of the
  same procedure existing or having existed).

A bit more general are procedures which, besides the data traffic by
means of the actual parameters, make *use of global data*. In this case
certain names of outside data are known and used within the procedure.
Then the procedure can use also these global names as communication
links to and from the outside. There is no *principal* difference between
the communication to the outside by means of parameters or by means
of global names. It might be just a question of usefulness which way
to choose: Parameters have to be provided explicitly by the caller,
while by global names those data are made known which are known by
these names anyhow. On the other hand, it is a question of safety:
Calling a procedure, one has to be aware that it does not only use *and*
affect those data explicitly passed to it, but possibly also others
made known to it by global names, whether one wants that or not, even
if one is not aware of this fact. Furthermore, procedures using global
names cannot be used freely, but only within that scope of program,
where the used global names are known. To sum up: For procedures, whose
services are used only within a certain range, use of global names may
be an appropriate way to perform the communication between the procedure
and the outside, but one has to be aware of this fact and explicitly to

specify it as a part ot the interface of this procedure.

For many purposes the procedure concept is not sufficient for what we want from a module. In the contrary to a procedure incarnation, once activated doing its job and dying, it might be necessary that a module be in existence permanently. E.g., it might be necessary that a module, when activated, in order to do its job has to know what it has done at previous activations. This could be realized using the procedure concept in the following way: The procedure creates and uses private data and entrusts them via global names to an outside program part, within the scope of which it always is called, hoping that this program part never will use or indeed affect them. Of course, this solution is very arti-ficial and by no means safe.

Thus, another kind of module has to be programmed as a closed set of routines and private data, which are available to these routines and only to them, with well-defined communication links to the outside. Over these links the module receives input data from other modules and sends transformed output data to other modules. These communication links may be realized, e.g., by global names as described above. Or they can be realized by names provided by one module and accessed by others. These names may refer to places for single data or to queues which are filled by one module and emptied by another one.

A module of this kind is *permanently in existence*, whether currently do-ing something or waiting and offering its services. This concept of module presumes, that different modules work together at the same time. It may be realized by means of programs running really *in parallel*. In order to transfer their data correctly to each other, they have to communi-cate by sending and receiving synchronizing signals. Or it may be realized (e.g. using the programming language SIMULA67) by means of *coroutines*. These are program units ready for action and pushing each other into motion mutually, when their appropriate services are needed, in the manner of a relay race.

5.   *PROGRAM VERIFICATION*

Producing a program as discussed in the previous sections, how can one make sure that it does what it shall, i.e. solve the given problem?

It is a widespread superstition that this can be done by running a suf-ficiently large number of test cases after having produced the program: Try to run the program with input data for which the resulting output

data are known. If in a sufficiently large number of different such
test cases the program runs at all and in addition yields the expected
results then one has convinced oneself sufficiently that the program is
"correct enough". But what to do if such a test case does not run correctly? How to find and correct the error?

The more complex a problem and the produced program are, the more the
only thing, that *is* sure, is that this method will fail. What one really has to do is at each stage of the described way from problem to program carefully to convince oneself that this stage is correct. Not just
test the final product, but verify each step leading to this product.
Again: Partitioning of the complete problem of program verification
into manageable parts.

This means:

- Convince oneself, that the problem description resulting
  from the problem analysis really meets the stated problem.

- Verify, by proving formally if possible or at least by
  making evident, that the designed algorithm really is
  a solution for the problem as analyzed and described.

- Verify, by proving formally or at least by making evident,
  that the produced program really represents the described
  algorithm.

- Supplement this last verification by program testing.

Each of these four steps means verification that the outcome of a single
stage of the complete program development is correct with respect to
the input of this stage. This presumes that the outcome of each stage:
the analyzed problem, the algorithm and the program, are described in
a formal way exactly and completely. And, of course, these four steps
of verification have not to be done after program construction, but
permanently and carefully during the corresponding steps of the complete
development.

In general, each of these four steps is too large to be manageable at
once. But, at least for this purpose we get the pay out for all our
efforts for clean structuring. At each stage we can do the verification
separately for each single subalgorithm, for each single program layer,
for each single hierarchical structure component, for each single program module, etc. This separation means that, once the interfaces between these items have been fixed, we can for each of these single items
separately verify that it meets its required interface. And the better

and cleaner the structuring and cutting down into parts and the fixing
of the interfaces has been done, the easier is the job of verification.
Thus, we have to prove, make evident or test, whatever applies, each
single item in itself and separately its use by other items.

If one finds by this strategy any incorrectness, then this incorrectness
does not mean that the program as a whole has some unknown error to be
sought, but that one specific known limited part is erroneous. I.e.,
the error is located and can be corrected by changing just this part
without affecting all others.

For program construction and testing this means, that one should start
from the bottom layer. Construct and test first those modules which are
the building stones for the other ones. After these have been recognized
as correct each for itself, the higher ones can be constructed from them
and tested, based on the safe grounds of the established correctness of
the parts.

This separation into the verification of the single parts has not only
the effect to ease the verification by splitting up into manageable parts,
but also the effect to complete the verification. Test cases for the
complete program will pass the single parts in a more or less random
manner: one will never be sure that all parts have been tested completely. Testing each small part separately means testing all possible
cases orthogonally with less effort.

REFERENCES

[1] Bauer, F.L. (ed.): Advanced Course on Software Engeneering.
                    (Springer-Verlag, Berlin-Heidelberg-New York 1973).
[2] Brinch-Hansen, P.: Structured Multiprogramming. Comm. ACM 7 (1972).
[3] Buxton, J.M., Randell, B. (ed.): Software Engeneering Techniques,
                    Report on NATO-Conference Rome 1969.
                    (NATO Science Committee Brüssel 1970)
[4] Dahl, O.J., Dijkstra, E.W., Hoare, C.A.R.: Structured Programming.
                    (Academic Press London-New York 1972).
[5] Denning, P.J. (ed.): Programming. Special Issue of:
                    ACM Comp. Surveys 6,4 (1974).
[6] Dennis, J.B.: Segmentation and the Design of Multiprogrammed
                    Computer Systems. Journal ACM 12 (1965).
[7] Dijkstra, E.W.: The Structure of the "THE" Multiprogramming System
                    Comm. ACM 11 (1968).
[8] Dijkstra, E.W.: Cooperating Sequential Processes.
                    In: F. Genuys (ed.): Programming Languages.
                    (Academic Press London-New York 1968)

[9] Hackl, C. (ed.): Programming Methodology, 4th Informatik Symposium
              IBM Germany Wildbad 1974. (Springer-Verlag Berlin-
              Heidelberg-New York 1975)

[10] Naur, R., Randell, B. (ed.): Software Engeneering, Report on
              NATO-Conference Garmisch 1968. (NATO Science Com-
              mittee Brüssel 1969)

[11] Wirth, N.: Program Development by Step-wise Refinement.
              Comm. ACM 14 (1971)

[12] Wirth, N.: Systematic Programming, an Introduction.
                  (Prentice-Hall Englewood Cliffs/N.J. 1973)

INFORMATION SYSTEM IN THE HOSPITAL

by

Professor J. Anderson,

Department of Medicine,

King's College Hospital Medical School,

Denmark Hill, London, S.E.5.

INTRODUCTION

In dealing with information systems in a hospital, let us agree initially
that they are complex at present, untidy and unkempt, largely based on human abilities
to compensate for system deficiencies and difficult to analyse and change. The
concept of a hospital information system is not new but there is a tendency now to
see a system where in fact none exists and functions are carried out with only
co-operation at the interfaces and driven by the fundamental desire to take care of
the patient. Such institutions do not obey standard business and management conventions, there is no profit but only the care motive to exploit. Thus the setting
of objectives for hospital work is fundamental to the whole operation. These
objectives will try to indicate activities that centre around patient care and the
related activities that make it possible.

Objectives for Hospital Work

Objectives for the hospital include the overall objective, namely to offer
care and treatment to patients whose illness cannot be treated by the family doctor
in their home. Thus these patients require institutional rather than family care
for a whole range of illness and also because of emotional and social difficulties.
Thus institutions not only offer acute short term care but also offer their services
to the chronic sick, ranging from the young chronically disabled patient to the
geriatric patient. Hospitals undertake rehabilitation for those whose recovery and
convalescence is slow.

Figure 1.   Hospital Objectives

1. Institutional care and treatment.

2. Reference centre for investigation of illness.

3. Emergency medical care.

4. Casual medical care.

5. Long term services - rehabilitation

- day clinics

- health maintenance

6. Administrative. Health Centre.

7. Education - doctors

- nurses

- patients

Fig. 1. These functions indicate the wide range of activities covered by a modern
hospital for the community it serves.

Secondly hospitals offer to patients a reference centre for consultation and investigation on an outpatient or polyclinic basis. This is to offer a level of investigation of illness to refine diagnosis and treatment that is not available directly through the family doctor. This is because only 3% to 6% of the patients the family doctor sees will require reference to a hospital. Some of these outpatients may be admitted to the hospital for a short stay in order to undertake a complex series of investigations or where special preparation is necessary for an investigation or an anaesthetic is required.

Thirdly most hospitals offer emergency medical care 24 hours a day, seven days a week, based both on a referred consultation by the family doctor and also in response to patient demand either by themselves or through a social agency, including the police. Such medical care may be medical, surgical, psychiatric or social in nature, or probably a mixture of all three. Usually there is no other way for these acutely sick patients to obtain satisfactory care.

Fourthly hospitals exist to give casual medical care, not only to the acutely ill, but for those who have no doctor or who are away from home and have no other doctor to whom they can turn. Social agencies also refer casual patients to the hospital when other arrangements cannot be made with a family doctor.

Fifthly hospitals offer a wide range of services of a long term therapeutic nature including rehabilitation, day clinics for geriatric and psychiatric patients and health maintenance clinics for chronic disorders such as diabetes, hypertension, epilepsy, asthma, arthritis and tuberculosis. The day clinics for geriatric and psychiatric patients are usually held in separate buildings or annexes to main buildings and are special purpose in nature. They are designed to bring together a range of facilities that such patients might require. The care maintenance clinics are often conducted as part of polyclinics and usually do not require anything more than interview and examination facilities. However, if health surveillance and screening is to become a part of this area of hospital activity, then other facilities will be required. In general, hospitals have so far taken few activities which lean towards the preventive side of medicine. Thus health surveillance would be largely preventive in nature and may or may not be carried out in a hospital.

Sixthly hospitals often become the administrative centre for the health care of a district. Thus medical and administrative expertise is available for solving difficult health care problems in a district or region. Often hospitals are closely linked with other local government care facilities. For example, they may have links with special accommodation for the disabled and the aged. Hospitals, themselves, require many administrative functions to be carried out by lay and sometimes medical administrators. Management of hospital personnel is also an essential function and it is usually left to lay administrators. Thus hospitals themselves have to take care of the personnel who are encompassed within the institution.

Seventhly hospitals are responsible for educating the sick and also their own personnel who render care.   Thus they have to act not only as medical schools to train doctors and nursing schools to train nurses, but also must give technicians a practical training.   Administrators also will receive practical experience and training in such institutions.   The educational functions of a hospital are important both to the patient and to all those who serve in it.

Often to-day hospitals become postgraduate medical training centres, both for doctors and senior nurses.   If hospitals are to maintain a part in the care system, then it is important that they must be able to carry on and improve their educational function.   Eventually this must encompass practice on patients and the various degrees of supervision during such training.

2.0 Functional Requirements for Hospital Work

2.1 The Physician

The physician in a hospital may be a general surgeon, a specialist surgeon such as an orthopaedic or ear, nose and throat, or eye surgeon or a general physician or a specialist physician, and his clinical requirements have to be provided.   For example, whether he is a physician or a surgeon he needs facilities to interview and examine patients, both in the outpatient or polyclinic department and also to have facilities to make the appropriate records so that he can both use his records as a continuing aide memoire when he or his deputy next sees that patient, and also to know what tasks he has delegated or ordered.   Most senior doctors are assisted by junior doctors who are being trained for responsibility and work under the supervision of an experienced physician.   Often certain minimal facilities for investigation may be provided in a polyclinic, but usually the patient is referred to other investigative and therapeutic facilities for further investigation and treatment.   The physician will maintain supervision of these activities and the patient will return to him when these delegated functions are completed.

Figure 2.   Physicians Functions

```
            Patient
            Admission
                          Physician

    General Practitioner                 Laboratory Investigation
         Referral
       Clinical Summary      PATIENT      Radiology
                             CARE
                             RECORDS
                                         Surgical Treatment
         Patient
          Discharge                      Drug Treatment


                      Continuing Care
```

Fig.2.   shows the communication and record facilities appropriate to the investigation and treatment of a patient.

All this already implies the need for a series of records, not only to hold observations about symptoms and signs and diagnoses, but also investigation and treatment records which will be complete over a period of time are necessary. As the physician will see several patients each hour, the number of records he will create, up-date and amend will be considerable during the working day. These records will have to be serviced, i.e. brought to clinics, records made, records removed after a clinic and up-dated, records stored and retrieved for the next clinic for each individual patient. It is important to realise that investigative and therapeutic facilities are usually under the charge of a physician, so that the medical interface can be interpreted correctly and appropriate tests and treatment done, usually by para-medical personnel, acting under medical supervision. This type of communication from the doctor at the bedside to the doctor in the laboratory or elsewhere is between professional equals and is subserved by requests for opinions about investigation or treatment rather than by orders for procedures to be carried out. For example, a doctor will request an investigation or test from the laboratory by giving the medical reasons for the request and really asking if this request is appropriate. The report by the doctor in the laboratory will reflect this consultation aspect.

This is not the same as giving an order for a procedure and receiving a result. Thus the doctor doctor interface has been useful to encourage cross fertilisation of ideas. It has been upset recently by the automation revolution, whereby the doctor has tended to become more involved in computing and automation rather than in improving the medical and clinical aspects of the interface. At present is is still left in biochemistry, for example, for the clinical doctor to do his own data processing without much assistance from the laboratory, except in providing normal ranges of data.

Figure 3. Ward Laboratory Communication

WARD	LABORATORY
Request Patient 'X'	**Report** Results of E.E.G. show
Symptoms headache fits.	dysrhythmia but no
Working Diagnosis:- Cerebral Tumour.	localizing signs. Could
Dept. Physiological Measurement	well be epilepsy.
Opinion on E.E.G.	

OR

Order from	**Result** Slow waves in most leads ...
Dept. of Clinical E.E.G.	
Measurement	

Fig.3. shows the difference between a request report system giving clinical data and an opinion or judgement and an order result system. In the latter system the clinician on the ward is left to interpret the result.

It is also important to remember that investigative laboratories are organized by certain functions. To solve most patient problems it is necessary to use several functions, often correlating one with the other. For example, if the patient has an infection one may culture the wound and blood for organisms,

Figure 4.   Laboratory Functions

1. Biochemical pathology	7. Nuclear medicine
2. Pathological anatomy	8. Cardiac Catheterization
3. Physiological Measurement	9. Pulmonary function
4. Microbiology	10. Psychological testing
5. Haematology	11. Social investigation
6. Radiology	12. Stomatology

Fig.4. gives the usual list of laboratory functions available in most large general
hospitals.

i.e. use the microbiology department, send the blood for immunological tests, i.e.
use the department of immunology, send the blood to have the white and red cell
morphology checked in the haematological laboratory to see if there are changes in
white cell morphology and in the different types of white cell counts.   It is also
possible to correlate this information with radiology of either the chest or other
part of the body to show the anatomical changes of inflammation.

It is of interest that no doctor interfaces are used in pharmacy, physiotherapy or social work, but in radiotherapy where the doctor in charge decides the
dosage and treatment of individual patients who are referred for an opinion about
treatment.   So it is that where there is a definite element of medical judgement
involved there tends to be a medical interface.   It will be seen that there are
fewer doctor-doctor interfaces in relation to treatment than with investigated
procedures.   In relation to pharmacy, physiotherapy and social counselling paramedical personnel act on doctors orders and the doctor assumes responsibility
indirectly for the procedures that are carried out.

Figure 5.   Treatment Functions

1. Surgery (M)	6. Physiotherapy
2. Anaesthesia (M)	7. Psychological counselling
3. Radiotherapy (M)	8. Occupational therapy
4. Pharmacy	9. Rehabilitation (M)
5. Dietetics	10. Chiropody

Fig.5. shows some of the major treatment functions available in a large district
general hospital.   Functions with a significant medical component are
labelled (M).

In relation to administration and management there are some doctors who act
as medical managers of institutions such as hospitals.   Often doctors are
responsible for the administrative aspect of medical practice in institutions but
this is largely carried out by means of medical committees.   In the community
general practitioners usually relate to a community physician or to a public health
officer of a local Goverment district.   Usually in the higher echelons of the
health service doctors act as medical advisors and administrators to executive
bodies.

General practitioners usually act as independent contractors, providing
family health care.   In many countries not only do they provide care, the investi-

gation of illness and treatment but they act as certifying agents for different
conditions, assist public services such as the police and are responsible for
industrial medicine as well as for convalescence and rehabilitation. Thus the range
of medical activity of a general practitioner is wide and all embracing in the
physical, emotional and social spheres of his patients lives.

The general practitioner along with his other duties has an educational
function to carry out both in relation to patients, paramedical personnel and to other
doctors in training or other doctors requiring postgraduate training. The educational function of the doctor is usually forgotten, but it is important for
patients, for it helps to control the demand for services and is helpful especially
in chronic illness and preventive care. In large health care systems other
personnel than doctors may have important roles to play in this area to assist the
educational function of the doctor especially in relation to infectious and other
disease. Patients also need education about preventive measures and also on
personal hygiene etc.

2.2 Auxiliary Services.

Nurses are used to give the essential elements of care to patients and in
hospital are responsible for the patient services around the bedside in relation to
feeding, diet, drug treatment and other procedures. Usually they are responsible
for the organisation of the hotel type of arrangements which are an essential part
of care. Nurses also act as organisers of nursing activities and are responsible
for the detailed administration of drugs and also in many hospitals for part of the
medical record function. Indeed about 70% to 80% of the time of senior nursing
personnel may be taken up by recording and administrative functions. Often the
nurse is assisted by a dietitian in the organisation of special diets. They also
have the assistance of physiotherapists in giving the patients special exercises
prescribed by the doctor and also in relation to physical treatment. Professional
nurses often leave it to nursing orderlies to do some of the more elementary caring
duties. Other orderlies in wards are responsible for the usual housekeeping tasks
such as cleaning the wards, sweeping and washing floors etc. Also hospital porters
become responsible for moving patients around hospitals in response to different
investigation or therapeutic orders.

In the community the nurse assistants help with nursing duties in the
terms of seriously ill or disabled patients. They are responsible for doing
dressings and giving injections as well as for general care. Also in some medical
practices nurses also take over the care of minor illness and are responsible for
patient education and for visiting the elderly. They may also give immunisation
injections and carry out vaccination procedures. In this way they can carry out a
number of functions delegated to them by the general practitioner. Other nurses
often look after industrial health and take care of trauma and illness while
patients are at work. The teaching and training functions for nurses are usually

provided in hospitals.   Recently, however, the universities have moved into the
training sphere for senior nursing officers.   As yet there are few training
situations for nurses in the community and most community services are staffed by
nurses who have been trained in hospital.   Usually nurse training is carried out
by specially selected nursing teachers who are themselves nurses.

2.3 Paramedical Personnel.

There are a large number of paramedical personnel including special
scientists such as Physicists, Biochemists, Pharmacists, Psychologists and
Engineers and many other technical personnel working in both the investigative and
therapeutic areas of medical care.   Usually their functions include carrying out

Figure 6.   Types of Paramedical Personnel

1. Physiologist	9. Physiotherapist
2. Biochemist	10. Dietitian
3. Bacteriologist	11. Social worker
4. Physicist	12. Occupational therapist
5. Pharmacist	13. Chiropodist
6. Radiologist	14. Computer scientist
7. Psychologist	15. Documentation officer
8. Bioengineer	16. Technician

Fig.6.   shows some of the various types of paramedical personnel that may be found
in a large general hospital.

the requests or orders of the Physician responsible for the investigation or
technical or therapeutic procedure which may involve the analysis of data, records
of procedures and communication of the results of the request back to the doctor.
In the investigative areas such scientists and technicians assist in the investigation of the morphological aspects of disease both in morbid anatomy, histology,
cytology and haematology.   Others are experts in microbiology, biochemistry
and radiology.   Some work with the physical aspects of investigation and carry out
such recording procedures as the electrocardiogram, the electroencephalogram and
the electromyogram.   Other scientists use isotopes and techniques which are usually
applied in nuclear medicine.

On the therapeutic side pharmacists, physicists and others help in carrying
out various therapeutic procedures on patients and are responsible for seeing that
treatment is given properly to patients.   Usually all such treatment is at the
request of a physician and scientists and technicians carry out the appropriate
procedures, although some are responsible for checking that what they are doing is
in fact within reasonable limits.   Other scientists including psychologists and
social workers carry out patient counselling, rehabilitation, retraining functions
and occupational therapy.

The range of activities covered by paramedical personnel is large but anyone
person carries out a limited function.   Nevertheless all contribute in a major way
to patient care and are responsible for creating records about their activities in

relation to patients.   Some may be responsible for the correctness of their
technical work in relation either to the investigation or treatment of patients.
As they act on the orders of a doctor he assumes responsibility for seeing that
their work is correct on behalf of the patient.

Other paramedical personnel work in the community, for example physiotherapists and social workers.   Here their activities are similar to those that
they would do in a hospital.   They are requested to perform certain procedures by
general practitioners and are responsible to him for the help and the assistance
they give to patients.   Usually they have the same responsibility for recording the
procedure and for reporting the results to the general practitioner.

2.4 Administration

Much of the activity of administration is directed towards the maintenance
of hotel type of services especially food and supplies.   The paramedical and social
services staff are also looked after by administrators.   The services supplied to
patient care not only include the provision of a bed but also the emergency
services such as to maintain heat, light, water and entertainment such as wireless
and television.   It is important to realise that as with medical and surgical staff
the supporting services must also function 24 hours a day seven days a week.   So
it is that hospitals take on the functions of an institution.

Like all institutions hospitals have medical records and important lines
of communication.   The staff that deal with the medical records, their transport
and preservation and with the main lines of communication are usually under the
direction of the administration.   Often there are special records and documentation
officers responsible for technical staff, including librarians and secretaries as
well as record personnel in a large hospital complex.   These medical records are
absolutely essential for day to day patient care and for communication purposes
between the clinical doctors and the investigative and therapeutic areas.   Abstracts
of these records are used by administrators to provide   management data not only
for their own use but to justify the expenditure of resources and funds.   At present hospitals operate with a whole variety of records about patients designed to
yield different types of information for different purposes.

The problem of contracting and paying for services and the general
financial aspects of running an institution are usually under the supervision of
an administrator.   This is necessary if they are to adapt to changing needs and
circumstances.   Thus the use of resources must be reviewed and their cost effectiveness determined in terms of care and not profit.   Usually this is achieved by
declaring certain areas, such as a laboratory, a department, a ward, or a service,
a cost centre.   This cost centre is credited with the services it renders to
patients for a known cost per patient.   Offset against this are the costs in
running the laboratory, service or ward such as the salaries of the personnel
involved, the cost of the space, equipment, less depreciation, and supplies, the

cost of services and cleaning etc. This relates to the investment in the procedure or service and does not reflect the utility or otherwise of the medical aspects of such a service.

Often cost centre procedures enable a comparison of services used over a period of time to be made. In general because of the cost of obtaining data less use is made of available information than would be necessary or desirable in an automated data analysis system. Naturally the payment for services rendered to the institution and the payment of staff for making the institution perform its functions is essential. This is usually carried out by Finance Departments under the direction of an administrator.

In the community doctors often organise themselves into a group practice as well as having single-handed practices. In group practices an administrator is used to provide some supervision of the use of resources and to deal with the functional support and financial aspects of the practice. Often such group practice administrators deal with secretarial records and other staff and are responsible for the accountancy part of the practice. Thus administrators take part in the community as well as institutional services.

A larger amount of administration also takes place in either local or central Government offices who are responsible for the provision of care. The type of organisation depends on the country and district but inevitably there must be some accountancy for the expenditure of tax payers money. Here income has to be obtained from tax payers, who indeed are the potential users of the system and then transferred to the medical care facilities. Accounting for the use of resources and people again takes place.

In view of the information revolution the time for a new look at the whole procedure of accounting for services and resources is now overdue. It already takes place at many levels but its usefulness is rather in doubt. It is now reasonable to ask how cost effective it is in relation to the actual care process carried out by doctors and nurses.

The issue that is being raised here is that some form of accounting process to check the supply and provision of care has been in use. It does not come for nothing and is therefore an added expense to ensure that the care process fulfills its objectives. There are in addition legal means for ensuring adequate standards of competence on the part of health care personnel. In some countries the additional financial burdens of accounting for care and malpractice law suits are adding a significant burden to the cost of patient care. Some better and cost effective compromise in the means of evaluating the delivery of care must be made available and with the automation of medical information this is now possible.

3.0 Structure of Information Systems in Hospital

There are many and different types of information system or sub-systems in a hospital and some of these can be determined from the preceding description

of the functions of different personnel. In the existing system such information
systems have arisen as necessary either for providing patient care or to deal with
the acquisition and accountancy of the expenditure of resources to this end either
directly or indirectly. The natural tendency is to create small information subsystems whenever this need is apparent. In the present system data has often to
be collected about the same function repeatedly and forms have been developed to
help codify the data and enable analysis to be carried out. Thus the logical
links have been forged by the necessity of accountancy and justification of
services. Often medical indicants are not very well adapted to this purpose and
thus formal financial accounting has been adopted to fulfil this function in part.

Another important aspect is that the structure of this sytem is adaptive
in nature. Much of the accountancy and performance data is temporary in nature
and not held once the basic information has been derived. Indeed it is important
to keep control of the allocation of data between temporary and permanent files,
otherwise we could easily be suffocated by an avalanche of permanent records.
So far these problems have received little attention apart from those which arise
in the medical records area about patient care.

Management justifies its information structures by the demands placed on
it to provide varying types of information for accounting for the use of resources.
Usually the accounting system is based on time comparisons of information rather
than on the actual care procedures. Management too is conscious of the fact that
hospitals are run by people for people and that 60% or more of a hospital budget
goes to pay the people who render such services. So it is that the labour aspect
of any budget is important and must relate to functions described by the information
system. Many views of such activities may be important but only one or two have
been considered at present. A new look at this area is long overdue. In the
ensuing discussion we will look at the structure of the information sub-systems
in the wards, the out-patient department, the auxiliary services including laboratory and therapeutic areas and the administration.

3.1 Ward

The information sub-systems in the ward are structured largely to
capture patient orientated data for each patient during the care process and to
provide other data for administration management both of the ward and the hospital
administrative information system.

3.11 Patient Medical Record

The medical record is one of the major information structures in the
ward and reflects the medical view of patient care and its procedures. The
medical record has been developed over two thousand years and has become a more
complex and elaborate with each innovation in medicine. In the conventional
written record usually the initial part of the record, giving data about the

development and state of an illness at a point in time is fairly complete. However,
once the diagnostic and therapeutic procedures are entered it becomes a pure record
of what is ordered or what is done.   In general because all investigative and
therapeutic departments demand forms with specimens of blood or excreta or the
patient himself, there has been a tendency to assume that these forms can be a substitute for an adequate record.   Usually they are not designed from a medical
record point of view, often lacking essential data, but cover mainly the purposes
of the investigative laboratory or the therapeutic area.   Usually such forms are
designed by those involved in the investigative or therapeutic area data records
and these rarely are thought to be important from the medical record point of view,
although they form an essential part of it.   Similarly the situation of the patient
on discharge is rarely stated so that it is often impossible to deduce the outcome
of care.

The following will given an insight into part of the structure of the
medical record.   Initially there are the identification and admission procedures
which allocate a unique identifier to each patient and relate this to a larger
descriptive sub-set of data which can enable each patient to be positively identified.   Usually in this admission data structure is information about the patient's
name, address, the name and address of next of kin and social and religious data
about the patient which is requested by both the doctor and the hospital administrator.   Such admission data may also reflect the credit worthiness of the
patient if he has to pay for his care.   Thus the admission procedures not only deal
with the procedure itself but provide social and financial information often of a
private and confidential nature.   It also attempts to relate the present episode of
illness with previous episodes and to determine if the patient is already known to
the information system so that previous records can be retrieved.   This implies
the existence of a master index of all patients by the hospital.   The patient is
then allocated a bed in a ward.   The type of admission is recorded whether it is
a routine admission from the waiting list, an emergency admission from the general
practitioner or the casualty department, private patient etc.

The medical part of the record is then created by doctors on the ward
as a means of guiding and controlling patient care.   The initial data structure
in the record is the history of the present illness, including the history of
past illness, the family history of illness, the social and environmental history,
the psychological, and the drug history.   In these data structures all the
important variables in each area will be covered.   This data is obtained from
the doctor/patient interview or from interviews with relatives or other persons
connected with the patient.   In some hospitals medical records of this kind may be
obtained from patient questionnaires which cover information from individual
patients.   In a few experimental areas computer generated histories and information
is also used.   One of the problems here is to select the relevant medical data
sub-set from the patient's total life experience.   Much of this condensation of

data and summary procedures depend on medical judgement as well as knowledge. In
any segment further data that may be relevant can be recorded at a later date
amending the existing data.   This may be obtained as the patient's illness itself
unfolds and the doctors become conscious of new information that has become available but not been so far obtained.

The data structure called physical examination deals with the data
derived from the examination on the patient by the doctors.   Usually this is an
area where opinions differ and the final record reflects the judgement of senior
and experienced personnel.   The data is usually recorded in terms of body systems
and there are conventions about what is essential to be done for all patients and
what may be required if this basic examination raises abnormalities.   Thus the
depth of physical examination relates not only to established conventions in this
segment but also to the type of illness the patient has.   Most patients in a
hospital, however, have a physical examination of one kind or another.

While this data collection is in progress the nurses areusually testing
body fluids such as urine for standard abnormalities.   In some hospitals a
general survey of general morphology and biochemistry may be done as part of bedside tests.   The results of the nurses investigations are reported back to the
physician, who may confirm them if necessary and record them in the bedside test
segment of the medical record.

From this data the doctor decides either the differential diagnoses to
be explored or the working diagnoses or the problems that subsequent investigation
and treatment will take into account.   Here the type of diagnosis considered
depends on the policy of the doctor in charge of clinical ward care.

If it is the policy to consider lists of differential diagnoses then
these lists have to be available and known for a wide range of conditions, so that
they can form a working basis for investigation.   On the other hand a working
diagnosis is usually seen as a hypothesis for exploration by investigation and
treatment in relation to a set model.   Weed (1969) introduced the idea of a
problem list linking the doctors view of the patients problems, which he defines
as a definite existing entity, to investigation and treatment.   Others have
stressed the likely hypothesis model for investigation in other types of record.
Naturally different views can be taken of the diagnostic process and different
types of records will be created about orders, procedures and results to reflect
this view.   As yet there have been few successful experiments in this area and
much work remains to be done to establish better types of medical record fulfilling
different objectives than those at present.

The subsequent organisation of the structure of the medical record covers
investigative and treatment plans relating to working diagnoses or to problems.
It involves recording the doctor's orders and reporting the results of investigation
and treatment.   The clinical state of the patient is also noted and the nurses also

make observations. Rarely are such important aspects of patient care noted such as patient education but it is becoming more important to know what has been said to the patient and what has been understood by him. New types of medical record require this to be done. Rarely is the existing record used to determine what has been ordered and if a response has been made. Basic accounting procedures are just being built into new types of medical record such as the Weed record and the decision directed record.

It will be noted that prognosis or the medically predicted outcome of illness is usually not recorded nor is the outcome from the patient's point of view. Discharge records and procedures are often neglected as they seem an unnecessary chore once a patient is well or has died. Yet such evaluations are necessary if we are to know what has been achieved medically by the expenditure of resources and time.

Clinical data is also transferred from the nursing record. Nurses usually record the pulse rate, body temperature, respiratory rate, body weight and other parameters as requested by the doctor. They also have to be involved both in investigative and therapeutic procedures as some nursing care is a necessary part of such activities. Paramedical personnel will also put reports in the medical record and there have to be segments in which these can be recorded as well as being requested.

Clinical data must also be transferred from the medical record to general practitioners and other doctors. The summary structure of the medical record leaves a lot to be desired. Summary procedures are usually left to junior doctors and the basic procedures are often not well understood. It is necessary also to provide different types of summary for different purposes. The six to twelve weeks wait before general practitioners get the clinical summary after the patient is discharged from the hospital bears witness to these problems. Rarely also is an adequate summary available for hospital doctors. Weed in his record has tried to give a summary structure so as to improve its utility and also to declare which problems had been dealt with and which still existed on the patient's discharge. Other types of record offer different types of evaluation.

3.12 Nursing Record

Nursing records can usually be divided into two types of record structure one of which deals with patient care and the other which provides the necessary information for management and administration.

The nursing clinical record begins with the patient's admission and the nurse may be required to admit the patient who arrives after the admission office is closed at night. Thus the nurse must understand admission procedures. As we have already mentioned the nurse makes a variety of clinical observations and also carries out elementary tests on body fluids such as urine. The results of these observations have to be recorded in the nursing record and transferred to the medical record.

Routine clinical observations of body temperature, pulse rate, blood pressure and respiratory rate, body weight are recorded as often as the doctor requires. This information is transferred to the medical record. At present much of it is held in analogue form in the various charts which adorn the patient's bedside.

Nursing orders also reflect many nursing problems as well, for the nurses are responsible often for the patient's diet and for feeding him if necessary. Nursing orders should include all nursing clinical activities and are usually the responsibility of the ward sister or other nursing person in charge of the ward. Usually accounting for such activities is done by a personal report by nurses and also by direct observation by the sister. In some experiments computerised acknowledgement has been tried. Usually ward activities are carried out by nursing teams. They may use either the patient orientated system of working by doing all jobs on a group of patients or organise their work by a function procedure and thus carry out a single job such as bedmaking or bathing or dressing all the patients who need this type of service.

The nursing record must also carry a list of investigation and treatment orders for such medical orders may need special nursing orders and procedures. For example, before a barium meal the patient may need to be fasted from midnight the day before the investigation and to have no breakfast but fluids only before the test. The nurses carry out this preparation. He may also require a sedative drug. When the patient returns to the ward the nursing staff may need to see if the patient has excreted the barium fairly rapidly. For various other investigations the nurses may have to prepare patients and assist the doctor.

The nurses are responsible for carrying out all drug and other treatment ordered by the doctor and for ensuring that the patient goes to other therapeutic areas for special treatment. Checks about treatment orders under execution are carried out by senior nursing personnel all the time. Some computer systems have tried to cover this type of accountancy.

On the discharge of the patient either to home or on death they also carry out set procedures and duties. They are responsible for conveying information and also for educating both the patient and relatives. They also initiate patients into the conventions of the hospital and the ward and are the main communication link with the patient's relatives. To maintain such communication they often use information obtained from the medical record.

The administrative records that senior nursing personnel create cover nurses on-duty and off-duty time. They also deal with leave rosters. Reports are required about nursing care status whether there are too many or too few nurses on a ward. The bed state is usually required at least once a day, sometimes at midnight and sometimes at other times of the day. This includes all patients occupying beds. The nurses are responsible for dietary arrangements with the kitchen as well as for feeding the individual patients who require it. The giving of and supervision of treatment are important aspects of nursing and care and senior nurses are responsible for accounting for the drugs used. They also request the attendance of doctors, physiotherapists and social workers for patients, whenever they are required. They must also decide which patients are confined to bed and who may be ambulant and keep records if necessary of patients' daily activities. They can also order maintenance services as required on the ward and account for these if necessary.

They are responsible for ward equipment and supplies and for domestic staff. They are also responsible for supplies of dressings and drugs which also must be supervised. Emergencies that involve heat, light and water are dealt with at the request of senior nursing personnel by engineering maintenance workers who are on call for such services. Thus the administrative records carried out by nurses are many and varied.

3.13 Physiotherapy

Physiotherapy covers the activities necessary to keep the patients active and healthy and physiotherapists are responsible for carrying out the exercise programmes for different types of patients using a large variety of techniques. Usually they work under medical and nursing supervision. Their work may extend from the care of the seriously ill patient or the post-operative patient who needs special exercises to supervising the progress and rehabilitation of patients who are recovering from their illness. They need to keep records of the patients progress and activity. They are also required to relate to both nursing and medical records and may keep special rehabilitation records as well.

As well as the physiotherapists being active in the ward they also take patients to the gymnasium with special apparatus for further physical treatment as necessary. They are responsible for running such facilities and seeing that the medical orders in relation to them are carried out. Thus they need to keep records of the activities of patients outside the ward.

On the administrative side the physiotherapy records include the work load of individual therapists and the allocation of physiotherapists to different departments in the hospital. Also the usual administrative arrangements for duty rosters and leave are required for their personnel. There is also the problem that they must see to the maintenance of their special equipment and apparatus and thus relate to the engineering department.

3.14 Social Worker

The functions and status of the social worker vary in different hospitals, some are responsible to local goverment authorities, others are responsible to the hospital employer. Nevertheless all will work in relation to patients in the

ward and in out-patients.   They need to keep clinical records about the patients
they investigate and they may interview not only the patient but relatives and the
employer of the patient.   They will also collect data about special and financial
circumstances as required.   After data collection they exercise their judgment in
deciding the most appropriate social actions and advise the doctor and nurses
accordingly.   Many are involved in long term care especially with convalescence
and rehabilitation.   Some social workers not only have hospital but district
responsibilities and may see the patient in his home.   The usual administrative
arrangements are necessary for social workers, they need duty rosters and leave
accordingly.   They will be allocated for special duties to cover emergency work.
Their visits outside the hospital often require transport and the expenditure of
money in order to achieve the objectives and they are required to account for the
use of these services.

3.15 Management Information

Most management information is derived either from the clinical record or
from nursing administrative data.   For example from admissions and bed state it is
possible to determine such parameters as bed occupany and generally the pressure
on medical care services.   It is possible to analyse patients statistics by
diagnosis, grouping patients into categories.   Recent cost centred operations have
begun and it is possible to regard the ward as a cost centre charging its expenditure against the patients it treats.

However, most of the management information comes from medical and nursing
care.   This has priority for this is the objective of the organisation.   Much
effort is directed to the management of the patient's illness.   This could be
improved by more attention to detail, especially ensuring that orders are carried
through and that investigations are completed.

3.2 Out-Patient Clinics

Out-patient clinics to be effective require a high load of patients so
that the maximum amount of consultation can be achieved with the minimum expenditure possible.   The custom has grown up to adjust the out-patient clinic rate
between new patients requiring the initial consultation and old patients coming up
for review of investigations and treatment.   Maintaining the mix is difficult and
different specialists have different types of consultation.   In general 10 to 20
new patients may be seen in a half day session and some follow up patients.
Again the number of patients seen depends on the type of illness and also the
number of doctors available at the out-patient clinic.

Here the medical information record is structured much as for the in-
patient record.   First there is the phase of registration which records much the
same detail as the in-patient had recorded on admission.   This information is
usually not obtained by doctors and nurses but by the admission department of the

out-patients.   The medical record is similar to the medical record on in-patients except that it may not be so extensive.   It also has to explore diagnosis.   Usually at the initial consultation plans are made for both investigation and treatment. The time scale of investigation and treatment will be much longer than that for the in-patient, as the patient has to return either at weekly or greater time intervals for surveyance.   In many cases the initial consultation may be required only for reaching a decision so that investigation and treatment may be carried out by the general practitioner.   When drug treatment is given such drugs may either be dispensed by the hospital pharmacy or by pharmacists outside the hospital.   The main nursing in out-patients is directed towards making the patients comfortable and ensuring that they reach the doctor as promptly and effectively as possible. Nurses are also responsible for seeing the patients are undressed and prepared for the required examination.   In some hospitals nurses are required to take the blood for investigation and to collect specimens.   This varies with the type of institution.

3.3 Auxiliary Services.

All the Auxiliary Services are basic to the fundamental objective of a hospital rendering adequate patient care.   The housekeeping functions are most important and are usually recognised quite quickly when they are not performed. Their main function is to keep the institution tidy and clean and to ensure that rubbish disposal is complete.   Some housekeeping functions deal with the hotel side of care generally.   They are responsible for ensuring that dishes are washed and that steps are taken to see that the patients surroundings are cared for.

Included in this service may be that of bleeding patients.   In modern medicine blood is required for analysis for different parameters not only to obtain diagnoses but also to monitor the course of disease.   One of the auxiliary services provided by some laboratories is that of providing specialist personnel to bleed patients when required.   These are usually part-time nursing staff or others who have had some training in the laboratory.

The record services provided by a hospital are extensive and important. Record staff are responsible for creating the original blank documents in the record and for keeping the written record up to date with the return forms from investigation and therapeutic areas.   It is the record departments function to amalgamate all information into the record in the appropriate place and to keep this as complete as possible.   Once the patient leaves the ward or the out-patient department the record staff are responsible for updating the record with the remainder of the investigations and filing it for subsequent retrieval when the patient either has a new appointment or returns again for care.   Part of the record department is also responsible for secretarial services which communicate with general practitioners and other bodies outside the hospital.   They also make new appointments and arrange for consultations.

An important part of auxiliary services is the provision of supplies which are required by both medical and nursing personnel and for the ordinary maintenance of the hotel services and buildings.   Institutions like hospitals always have considerable number of supplies, including food and it is important that these be checked and handled correctly.   Supplies also relate to the engineering services for they maintain the building and services generally.   They themselves need supplies for the maintenance work and such supplies are also handled usually by the supply department.

In present day hospitals transport services have become important. These may be by human hand, by porters in the case of specimens and records and other services rendered to patients such as the delivery of mail etc.   Other transport services handle patients themselves both inside the hospital and also between the patient's home and the hospital.   There has been a general decline in the use of public transport for many sick patients and most of this present day hospital work is done by ambulances responsible to the hospital or health authority.

One of the auxiliary services that tends to be forgotten is the religious aspect of a patient's life.   Here arrangements are made for the padre or cleric of the appropriate faith to see the patients when they are in hospital.   Usually information is obtained from the admission data if there is a computerised system or from ward sisters records about the location of patients of differing religious faith.   This religious part of hospital life is important for the relatives as well as the patient.   It helps to keep the patient in touch with his local and family interests.

It is important to create the means for relatives of patients to be able to communicate with different levels of hospital personnel about the patient. The patients relatives must be able to contact the doctor who has admitted him. Usually there is some central organisation for answering relatives enquiries about the location of patients and whether they are seriously ill or not.   Thus relations with the outside of the hospital are important.

It is important not to ignore the services to the patient's family of those who die in hospital.   Death certificates have to be completed and relatives seen by doctors and nurses.   Post mortem examinations are to be undertaken when required.   The mortuary personnel have to deal with undertakers,ensuring that bodies are stored on removal from the ward and are ready for removal by the patients family for burial or cremation.

Any errors by ancillary services can cause a great deal of inconvenience and heart searching to patients.   They are just as much a part of the hospital as the clinical services and just as essential.   They are usually administered by the general administration of the hospital.   The co-ordination of their efforts with those in patient care is one of its responsibilities.

3.4 Laboratories.

Under this section are included the information systems which deal not only with the investigative part of laboratory activities but also with therapy generally.   Both are areas where things are done to and for patients, only the outcome is different.   The investigative laboratories will be considered first and then the therapeutic areas.

Biochemical laboratories are designed to analyse the excretions of the body and body fluids generally, including blood for known biochemical parameters which have importance either in the diagnosis of disease or for monitoring the progress of illness.   The present day laboratory has developed many automated procedures to deal with the increasing burden of work.   Such automatic machines for performing a whole variety of analyses are usually computer driven.

The information system begins when the specimen is obtained from the patient following a request by the doctor which is in the medical record.   Usually not only are the tests that are requested specified but also the essential parts of the diagnosis and the diagnostic problem it is hoped to resolve or what part of treatment is being monitored.

This specimen and the information reach the laboratory and are checked to ensure that the specimen is appropriate to the investigation as requested and that the patient's identity is correct.   If this is not the case then the investigation may abort at this stage.   Usually in the present information system there is no feed-back to the doctor at the bedside who may not know that he has to start the whole process again.   Thus the doctor waits for the report.   After a certain period of time he will in fact decide whether a similar request has to be repeated or not.

Once the laboratory has accepted the investigation the specimens are processed and analysed according to the laboratory system.   The results of the analysis are usually checked for errors and compared with standards before being return to the doctor at the bedside.

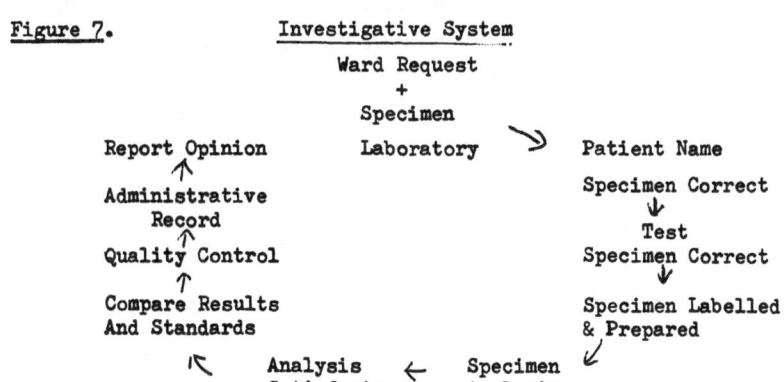

Figure 7.   Investigative System
                          Ward Request
                              +
                          Specimen
Report Opinion   Laboratory   Patient Name
Administrative   Specimen Correct
   Record   Test
Quality Control   Specimen Correct
Compare Results   Specimen Labelled
And Standards   & Prepared
              Analysis ← Specimen
              Satisfactory   Analysis

Fig.7. gives a generalized view of an in-house laboratory sub-system for dealing with an investigation.   Note the many steps where the process can abort and no information goes to the clinician.

The doctor at the bedside then reconciles the information he has with the clinical state of the patient and reaches further clinical decisions. It will be seen that there is a continuing cycle of information both inside and outside the laboratory but that feed-back loops only exist inside the laboratory itself. The link with the clinical area is at the moment rather tenuous because the information system is purely structural.

Similar information systems are created in the morphological laboratories which cover haematology, cytology, pathology of tissues and microbiology. The specimens of tissues, blood or organism are sent to the laboratory and checked for correctness and identification and the purpose of the investigation when they arrive. The investigations are undertaken in the laboratory and then the results are processed and compared with standards and after approval are reported to the doctor who orginated the request.

In all these areas the demand for further investigations due to progress in refining diagnosis, has been increasing in recent years and the information system has had to carry an increasing load. The laboratories themselves have developed their own in-house information systems so that they can document the load and also cost out the resources they consume on behalf of clinicians. In general all laboratories are responsible for their own information and financial and control systems. Usually cost centre practices have been developed in the laboratory to obtain some idea of both their cost and effectiveness.

In the physiological laboratory records are made of electronic functions in the body such as the electrocardiogram, the electroencephalogram and the electromyogram. Some physiological laboratories also undertake pulmonary tests and blood gas analysis. Here again the laboratory acts usually on the provision of the patient or a specimen and the investigation is carried out inside the laboratory itself. The results are then checked for accuracy and in relation to the patient's condition before being reported to the clinician who ordered the investigation.

One of the greatest expansions in laboratories has been in the radiology field. Here more powerful developments have allowed the macro and micro-anatomy of the whole body to be revealed either using radiological techniques or ultra sound. Essentially, radiology reveals structural abnormalities and defects and has enabled this data to be correlated with abnormalities in fuction determined by other investigative laboratories. Recent advances in radiology have also made it possible to administer opaque dyes into the vascular system to determine the circulation of organs and also to allow drugs to be injected into organs. This is an extensive area of investigation and cost centre techniques have been used here to shed light on the utilisation of these resources.

A recent addition to the investigative laboratories has been that of nuclear medicine which uses isotopes to trace metabolic functions in the body and

also to form a dynamic picture of the metabolism of certain organs. In recent
years it has been possible to form images of the uptake and dynamic changes of
isotopes in the body with cameras which detect the radiation emitted by the
isotopes.   This has increased the possibility of further defining diagnosis and
differentiating between different courses of disease.

In both radiology and nuclear medicine there is a need for caution about
the dose of radiation to be administered to the patient.   It is important that
care is taken about the use of ionizing radiation both for patients and for the
personnel who work in such departments.   Thus radiation records are kept of the
amount of radiation received by personnel working in these areas.   It is usually
the responsibility of a physicist acting under medical supervision to supervise
such procedures.   However, few laboratories attempt to keep track of the
accumulative radiation dosage given to patients.   It is not usually documented in
the ordinary medical record.

In the therapeutic area, the first function that is thought about is
that of drug supply whereby doctors, applying pharmacological principles, treat
the disorder of function and structure in the patient with various drugs.
Usually orders and prescriptions for drugs are created by doctors and translated
to the pharmacy through the nursing staff.   The pharmacy then check the dose,
supply the amount of the required drug.   The nursing staff are responsible for
administering this to the patient.

Often in relation to drug routines it is as well to have the patient
know what he is about to receive as well as the nursing staff know what they have
to give.   This acts as a check and can close the difficult loop.   From studies
about the administration of drugs it is apparent that for at least 20% of patients
the right drug may be given at the wrong time or the wrong drug at the right time.
Thus it is important to allow for errors in the system.   Checks must be taken to
keep these to a minimum.   It has to be borne in mind that drugs themselves while
they may cure certain patients may create complications and disorder in another.
Thus some patients may have more trouble from the side effects   of drugs than
the therapeutic action and their administration has to be constantly monitored.
Side effects are evidence that all patients are not the same and we know that
many patients handle drugs differently to others both because of genetic tendencies
and because different illnesses affect them in different ways.

Often treatment may be surgical and this requires both anaesthesia as
well as the provision of operating theatres and surgeons and other ancillary
personnel.   In general surgical intervention is expensive and necessitates a
considerable period of time before full recovery.   The requirement for surgical
intervention has been decreasing in recent years in medicine but is still an
important part of therapeutic endeavour and will remain so.

Other therapeutic systems are physical in nature and much treatment is given to patients with cancer by radiation.   This radiation is generated by a variety of machines designed to produce different types of ionizing radiation.   The most recent additions have been those machines designed to deliver neutron fluxes as well as other particles and radiations to patients.   Treatment in this area is expensive and also requires specialist monitoring.   In general it deals mainly with the group of very seriously ill patients.

On the psychological and social side a considerable amount of behavioural therapy is given either by staff, doctors and psychologists trained in counselling or psychotherapy.   Information structures have to be created about these two activities and the progress of the endeavours monitored and reported back to the doctors who originate the request for therapy.   Other activities may include social support and care of varying kinds.   This support may be personal in nature and involve the adjustment of the patient's environment to his disabilities after an illness.   On the other hand it may involve assistance not only to the patient but his family in a whole variety of ways including financial support.

With modern developments in specialised care, especially in intensive care units and in units taking care of patients with severe renal damage by means of haemodialysis, a large expenditure of resources has become accepted.   These areas of specialist care are both expensive in relation to information handling and demanding on medical and nursing staff.   It is important that they develop their own special information structures.   The development of feed-back systems based on data is important to control the progress of patient care.

3.5 Administration.

The information systems in administration are many and varied and only a few will be discussed here.   One of the important things for an administrator to determine is the resource utilization by patients who are under hospital care. Usually this is done by cost centred information being processed and also by relating this type of information to information about the bed state and the utilization by patients of different diagnostic groups of hospital services.   Inevitably consideration of resource utilization leads to data about other functions.   From data about the supplies coming into the hospital, the upkeep of the building, hotel services and medical and nursing care, the cost of running parts of the institution can be determined.   Already it has been stated that more than half of the budget of the hospital is taken up by salaries of the persons who care for patients.   Thus a major element of the cost is human rather than in machinery, building and plant.

Nevertheless the maintenance of the buildings and the facilities and staff for providing heat, light and water are an important and permanent charge on the hospital system.   They require engineering effort and skills of varying sorts and this has to be supervised.   Hospitals too are changing and growing in various ways and it is important that both financial and engineering functions run hand in hand.

Salaries and pay for all those who work in the hospital create another administrative information system to ensure that all the necessary taxes and regulations at Governmental and other levels are carried out, when the staff receive their reward for the services they have rendered.   It is to be noted that such systems are a charge on the whole hospital system.

The management staff themselves in administration require staff and services to conduct the necessary procedures and committees where decisions are made.   The management of an institution like a hospital requires that doctors, nursing personnel and administrators co-operate in achieving the optimum mix of decisions based on information obtained from the various information systems.   In general the bulk of the decisions are made about occurrences which occur as exceptions during every day practice.   Often much less attention is paid to long term planning, although this in the provision of real facilities may be more important than the short term preservation of existing functions.

Administration has an important function in relation to maintaining the communications throughout the whole organisation and between different groups. This communication function usually requires a great deal of effort on the part of many people but has in the past been largely a human activity.   With the development of automated information systems it is bound to change and therefore its extent and nature must be determined.   The communication systems, as will already be seen from the number of information systems that have been explored, are many and detailed and thus the information load from such systems is not small.   The widespread actions that are required following both clinical and administrative decisions are often quite extensive.   The time scale for appropriate change is usually grossly underestimated.

4.4 Information Flow within Sub-Systems.

4.1 Medical Care.

The information flow within the medical system largely concerns clinical data.   This will be recorded by all doctors contributing to the medical record and understanding its structure and functions.   It is generally left for junior personnel to do most of the recording, while the decision making is the responsibility of the whole team and especially the senior members of the clinical team. Not only is it important to collect a complete initial set of medical information but it is also important to monitor the progress and cause of a disease in response to investigation and treatment.   Thus medical activity is not a once and for all assessment of state but is rather a continuing process of monitoring care and hopefully the patients recovery.   From this it will be seen that, on the whole, clinical data ought to decrease as the patient gets better and investigative results return towards normality.   This tendency is monitored by the clinical team and is the essential part of the information flow in the clinical record system.

Another part of the information flow within the system is the necessity

of keeping track of the investigative and therapeutic plans that are created
around the patient's care.   It is essential to know that investigations have been
ordered and the correct and appropriate specimens dispatched to the laboratory.
It is necessary to follow up the progress of investigations and ensure that they
are completed as soon as possible.   It is important to check that the appropriate
therapy is given to the correct patients and that mistakes are looked for and
errors corrected.   The supervision of both ordering and execution must be
monitored carefully by senior medical personnel.   It is very easy for mistakes
to be made in this area due to the large element of 'noise' in the whole system.
Here, new information systems would in fact be extremely useful in monitoring and
checking the accuracy of the delivery of investigation and care.

It is also necessary to check the functions of auxiliary personnel in
the clinical area such as nurses, physiotherapists, social workers to ensure that
all are generating the appropriate information in relation to their patients
illness and taking the necessary actions where appropriate.   Thus there are
information flows between the different sub-systems inside the ward which lead to
information returning to the medical system.

Information also has to be collected about personnel activity and the
work load.   Provision has to be made for doctors and nurses who have leave of
absence and also for organising the various duty rosters to ensure full clinical
cover 24 hours a day seven days a week.

A great deal of the information that is generated within the ward and
the medical sub-system is important to that system.   Also derivatives of it are
extremely useful in supporting the activities of many other sub-systems and for
checking that the whole system is functioning in an adequate manner.

4.2 The Out-Patient System.

The out-patient system largely consists of diagnostic medical activity
following registration.   The medical data is recorded & diagnostic and therapeutic plans made.   The appropriate investigations and treatment requested and
follow-up occurs later when the patient re-attends.   A monitoring process
usually takes part early after the out-patient clinic when abnormal investigations
are brough to the doctor's notice to see if the patient requires a different plan
of action in relation to the one that was originally given to him in the outpatient department.   A review of the patient's condition as a result of investigation and treatment may change the plan of action.   Much of the activities in
medical out-patients are on a slower time scale than those that take place in
relation to in-patients and involve investigative and therapeutic sub-systems.

4.3 Nursing Sub-System.

The nursing sub-system itself has its own procedures both nursing and
special procedures and is responsible for ensuring that doctor's orders are

carried through.   There is a flow of information from the clinical system by doctors into the nursing system to control nursing activities.   Other activities in relation to patient care are routine and are carried out by the nursing staff themselves. The nursing sister or the person in charge issues the orders and the nursing team carries these out.   It is important that there be information feed-back to those that originate the orders to ensure that these have been carried out.

Nursing information flow may be important when patients are having special care such as barrier nursing or on special diets or requiring special observation after certain procedures.   Here information flows may be more important and it is important that the medical staff obtain quickly and accurately observations made by the nursing personnel.   This is especially important in the post-operative situation and usually close supervision by surgical staff is given during this period.   Thus in the ward system there are close links between various elements of the care system and the nursing sub-system.

4.4 The Laboratory Sub-System.

All types of laboratory act in accordance with a general sub-system set of procedures.   Initially the patient or the specimen has to be identified to the laboratory and correlated with the request for investigation and with an abstract of the appropriate clinical information in order to check that the request is correct.   Thus verification of patient identification and that the appropriate specimen has been received for a procedure are important for the laboratory.

The laboratory must then ensure that the specimen and the patient infor-mation are carried through different channels.   First the specimens are processed and analysed either automatically or serial monitored by certain test routine systems.   As test results are accumulated these are checked against the clinical information provided to ensure that the test result is a likely consequence of the information given.   Test results are also checked to see whether they fall within the normal range or not and are also checked against control specimens which are analysed at the same time.

Thus a considerable number of inter-laboratory data checks are applied before the final results are passed for transmission to the ward.   Results are also held within the laboratory system for varying periods so that reference can be made to these as well as to the clinical record to find out what did happen. Similar procedures and exchange of information within the laboratories sub-systems are used for out-patient orders and requests as well as for in-patient orders. In the therapeutic areas similar types of procedures occur within the system only the checks are different depending on activity that is being carried out.

4.5 Administration and Finance.

The administration is responsible for monitoring the use of resources within its system and also supervising the maintenance both of hotel services and the hospital structure. It also has to try and inform itself about the cost of effectiveness of many of the procedures that are undertaken on behalf of patient care.

The administration exchanges a great deal of information internally in relation to planning and budgeting purposes. In this way it is possible for development and change to be undertaken without throwing the system as a whole out of gear. Part of the administration's function is to ensure that changes ensue as speedily and effectively as possible with the least perturbation of the system. Inevitably this involves a great deal of planning and training and education of different kinds of personnel for change.

4.6 Management.

The management structures for hospitals vary a great deal depending on national situations. Some are managed by a particular individual who heads the administration, others are managed by small groups of people namely doctors, nurses and administrators and others are administered by lay bodies which have overall responsibility for management. The management information system demands that it be cognizant of the parameters which the hospital fulfills in relation to its community. It also has to determine that the system of care for patients is as effective as possible. It has to do this within a budget for resources and finance that is strictly limited. It is also responsible for planning a capital programme as well as for accounting for revenue. Thus managerial functions rely on information systems not only within the administration and management itself but in links with outside sub-systems.

5.0 Information Flow Between Sub-Systems.

5.1 Medical Sub-System.

From what has already been said the medical sub-system relates in the main to the nursing sub-system and to the other record systems rendering services to patient care such as physiotherapy and social work. The medical system also has to relate to the investigative and therapeutic areas of the hospital to ensure that plans are carried through and that information that is generated is received and acted upon. The basic clinical area too has to receive information from the outside, especially from administration and management in relation to the balance of its activities and the control of its endeavours. Usually such relationships outside the sub-system in this area are of a 'stop-go' nature. Rarely has it been proven that regulatory control can be exercised over clinical care with any degree of minor alteration of facilities that are offered.

Indeed this has been one of the major deficiencies of the medical sub-system. Because of the lack of good automatic information systems the doctor has been left to rely only on clinical judgement and to use as much or as little of

the care system as that patient required.   He would therefore only not use
services if they were not supplied.   No element of weighting the cost of care
against its effectiveness has been possible until the development of automated
information systems.

5.2 Medical Out-Patient Sub-System.

Here the information required between other sub-systems is much the
same as in the ward system.   Certainly information about registration from the
administration is continually required.   Also important are investigative and
therapeutic results which have to be reviewed at a later date and on a longer time
scale than usual.   Thus communications with these clinical areas are important.
Also important are communications with the outside especially with the general
practitioner who referred the patient for care so that he can be kept up to date
as to what is being done for the patient whom he has referred to hospital.

Usually information flow is by letters which have to be dictated, typed,
checked and signed by the doctor and posted to the general practitioner.   This
leaves a permanent record of such a communication.   Also telephone calls and
personal visits also assist communication.   The patient too has sometimes been
used to transport information from the hospital doctor to the general practitioner.

5.3 Nursing Sub-System.

The main input to the nursing system is from doctors orders and there is
a considerable flow of information between the medical and the nursing record as
has already been outlined in the information structure.   In the main the nurses
make observations of various variables and parameters that are required from the
patient.   Then the doctors make the plans for treatment and investigation in
response to this data.

The nursing system also has to have information from the investigative
and therapeutic areas in relation to special procedures they might require that
the nurses carry out on patients before they reach the special facility.
Nursing also requires input of information from physiotherapy and social work
areas so that it can be cognizant of these activities and sure that they are
compatible with routine patient care and if necessary communicate these to the
medical record.   Nursing information is useful also to administration.   There
is a considerable flow of basic data about patient care to the administrative
system.

5.4 Administration and Finance.

Administration and Finance require information mainly about clinical
care, although this aspect has not been fully explored yet because of practical
difficulties.   Usually they collect information about clinical care from the
Nursing record and the various other records that are kept on the ward.   Other

information about patient care is obtained from resource utilization whether this
be from the investigative and therapeutical laboratories or from diet kitchens and
those other services that are provided to patients.   They also have to obtain
information about hotel services, engineering as well as from supplies.   From
these inputs the financial situation of the institution can be monitored.   The
most efficient and effective use of resources can then be decided.

5.6 Management.

The input to management system requires information from the clinical
area, the nursing area, investigative and therapeutic services, and from hotel
services, maintenance and other functions such as the administration of hospital
personnel.

From this information it decides about the immediate control of the
institution.   It also makes plans and budgets for the future expenditure of both
capital and revenue.   Thus for management the information flow between subsystems is perhaps more important than the information it generates itself.

6.0 The Organisation of Information.

The organisation of information within the whole hospital system is very
complex and elaborate as the following will show.   Indeed the total volume is
enormous and can be overwhelming unless there are automatic means of dealing with
it.   One of the reasons for lack of progress in medicine has been the difficulty
of dealing with the large information flows and knowing how to use them to the
best advantage.   At present the only solution has been to hire more and more
people to take care of information.   In the end this becomes self-defeating,
because they require administration and management.

6.1 The Medical Record in the Hospital.

The medical record in the hospital requires the services of several
hundred people.   Hundreds of doctors and nurses are involved in its creation.
The data in it involves them as well as many more paramedical and other specialist
personnel.   The organisation of the basic data must be according to data segments
which describe elements of the total information about the patient in a structured
way.   One of the important problems in the medical record has been the lack of
organisation of the information in it.   Given structural data this can be freely
accessible to whoever wants to use such information within the limits of privacy
and confidentiality.   Not only has the medical record to have a structure for the
initial type of data which leads to the diagnoses or problems being formulated but
it also must have a much more elaborate and effective structure, to guide the
execution of plans, to note the results of investigations and treatment.   Such a
structure must promote the development of feed-back loops so that prompt action
can be taken by medical personnel to promote health and treat illness.

Some idea of the numbers of current medical records involved in a hospital are useful to give some idea of the organisation of the information at any one time.   At least 4000 to 5000 medical records will be current in many hospitals including in-patients and out-patients.   Above half a million records are carried by a teaching hospital.   Usually there are legal limits to the medical record.   The minimum legal requirement in some countries is that records will be carried for six years after the patient's last visit, although in many teaching hospitals records are carried for the duration of the patient's life. They are removed only when his death is known to the record system.   At any one time from 1000 to 2000 in-patients in a hospital will be having several parts of the medical record completed each day.   About 100 to 200 out-patients daily are involved in the same procedures.   There will be some 100 to 200 emergency or casualty patients having records created in other departments.   Some of these will be admitted as emergency in-patients.   Thus the flow of information into the hospital medical record system is not small and the data structures must be adequate for its usage.

Different types of medical record will need to be created for different specialties in the hospital.   However, they should still have the same basic structure as all records and only develop new structures when these are required by the specialty.   Obviously surgical records will have more devoted to the treatment segment and there will be a much more extensive record of anaesthesia and the surgical operation than there would be in minor treatment procedures in other records.

It is important that the data structure of the medical record be well defined so that analytical procedures can be applied to the data contained there-in.   One of the major difficulties with the existing written medical record is that it is not possible to analyse in various ways the information that is in the record.   For example, if one wishes to graph the changes in biochemical tests the whole record has to be searched for such information and then the results graphed.   This is largely due to the inadequacy of the existing data structures within the record and the fact that they are seldom complete.   Thus unless a great deal more attention is paid to the organisation of information in the medical record such as in the problem oriented, the decision directed or the newer type of record, then merely recording information is virtually worthless. With the avalanche of present day information the demand for organisation of the information within the medical record is mandatory.

It has already been pointed out that there is considerable exchange of information between different records especially the medical and the nursing record.   Here it is important that these flows be defined and the structures also made compatible so that information can be easily transferred.   Needless to say records must be kept in each record about when and what information has been transferred and to where it has gone.

It is often forgotten that paramedical personnel contribute a great deal of data to the medical record by way of reports in investigative and therapeutic areas.   It is important to see that these reports are incorporated into the structure of the record and not filed in a random fashion as in the present day record.   It is important that investigations and treatment be related to diagnoses or problems so that medical logic can be followed and checked.   Until this can be done it will not be possible to design optimum plans for patient care and the present haphazard system will prevail.

6.2 Volume of Medical Information.

There is a tremendous volume of medical information to be organised every day in the hospital.   At least in each of the eight investigative laboratory areas some 500 to 1000 tests of varying sorts will be completed five days out of every week.   Some of these tests will be emergency investigations, others will be routine.   Even in radiology some 500 to 1000 units of service are processed each day.   Thus the information flow from the investigative laboratories alone is quite large and has to be incorporated carefully into the clinical information structure. In the therapeutic areas as well a similar volume of requests is made each day. For example, in a 2000 bedded hospital there will be some 500 or more prescriptions to be fulfilled by the pharmacy each day and some 50 - 100 or more patients will be seen in the radiotherapy department for treatment.   Thus in the therapeutic area the volume of medical information is not small.

All this flow of data from the investigative and therapeutic areas must be incorporated within the medical record itself as the main permanent record of the patient's illness.   Records are kept in the various therapeutic and investi- gative facilities about what they have done.   Most of these records are temporary in nature and thus there is not such a problem of permanent records as with the medical record system itself.

If in relation to volume of medical information one considers the volume of derived information from laboratories which may be cost centres and from the ward in relation to the facilities used then a considerable larger volume of information flows from the various systems towards administration and management. Unless this is digested and summarized it can rapidly become overwhelming.   This is one of the reasons why to date management has operated largely in an information desert.

6.3 Time Aspects of Information Flow.

There are aspects of medical information flow which are required by the second or minute.   For example, if the patient has a cardiac arrest it is important to know whether the seriousness of his illness does not warrant these procedures being carried out or he has a recoverable condition which requires urgent treatment.   The same problems arise in surgery with shock where what happens in seconds to minutes is vital to the patient's existence.   Thus medical information may be required urgently.   Often blood group information is urgently required for help with cross matching with donor blood.   In these conditions the correct blood may be essential to maintain life by transfusing the severely injured.

Other information may be required within hours especially in investigative procedures and in care.   It is important that plans for investigations be proceeded with as urgently as possible so that the information gets back to the doctor as soon as it can, so that he can take appropriate action.   Here the time scale is in hours.   Most of medical care is conducted in this time scale especially the immediate medical and nursing care of the patient.

In relation to investigations and therapy, results are expected in one or two days especially if the disease is not exceptionally acute.   Here with investigation procedures being on a longer time scale, it is important to know if these have to be repeated quickly if things go wrong as a similar delay cycle will take place when it is known they have not been completed.   Thus the various time aspects of information flow become critical in certain areas.   Unless the patient's clinical condition has changed during one or two days then further investigation and re-thinking of the therapeutic plan becomes necessary.

On the time scale of one week or more, the patient's admission discharge cycle must be considered or at least reviewed.   Thus there are certain essential aspects of the flow of information which relate to time scales.

Because of the tight time scales necessary because of the use of costly resources, it is important that any information processing system be viable and available for most of the time especially if it is taking care of medical information.

In relation to administrative information the time scales are much longer.   Usually action is required about urgent things within a week but otherwise time cycles for information feed-back become months and years.   Thus the information flow in relation to management and administration is not as critical except for emergencies which arise from time to time following major accidents etc.

6.4 Information Archives.

There are problems in relation to archives depending on the volume and flow of information that is required.   Where temporary records are kept either for days, weeks or a month from then archives are not a problem as they are restricted in size and cover a limited time scale.   On the other hand records which are permanent such as the medical record and perhaps part of the nursing record create much more of a problem.   In most hospitals a mass of paper has to be heated, lighted, warmed and serviced at great expense to preserve the permanent records of patient care.

Looking into the medical record problem in a little detail, most archives contain at least 100,000 records in a large district general hospital. Thus the permanent record archive is not small. Usually some 10% to 20% of such records are not in the archives at any one moment in time, being used for a whole variety of purposes either in relation to current patients or patients who are about to arrive or who have just been discharged. The importance of maintaining a master index of the archive cannot be stressed too much for this is the only way in which accurate entry and retrieval of the contents of the archives can be achieved.

As has been stated the archives are dynamic in nature and there is a permanent necessity to update the master index. In relation to the nursing record often certain details are kept on a permanent basis although many of the other observations are temporary in nature, especially those that have been transferred to the medical record. However some parts of the nursing record are kept as a more permanent record , especially that of procedures carried out on the patient. This is largely done for medico-legal reasons to protect the institution.

Laboratory records, both investigative and therapeutic, are kept usually for periods of up to two or four months. This varies greatly with the type of laboratory and the investigations it carries out. Some laboratories which have on-going research programmes may keep records for much longer periods of time. However, if the information has been written to patient records then it should be determined that permanent records should not be kept of laboratory data but they should be purely temporary as a back-up for the patient record for a limited period of time.

Archives for administrative purposes need to be kept for one to five years for the time scales of administrative information and action are much longer than others. The archives here will not be of the basic data but digests, summaries and transformations of such information. Thus the volume of these archives will not be large. It is important to recognised, however, that the information structure and its function has to be described and known before such archives can be created. They are dynamically updated and reflect the on-going nature of the system. Until automated information systems are fully accepted such archives will be very small.

7.0 Concepts of Information Structures.

Information structures can take several basic forms. Most information structures are descriptive in nature and depend on a textual representation of reality. Other information structures are numeric in nature. There are qualifying statements in text to describe the relationships of the numeric variables. Other information structures are logical in nature and this allows for analysis of data by this technique. Other information structures are so designed so that they may have statistical operations applied to them. Other types of information are really structures based on other data of a more fundamental nature.

Much of the medical record has a descriptive information structure and already the elements of such structures have been described. These structures or segments describe the various elements of the medical record and have implications both for the data content and for the functions and procedures so described. Analysis of such structures can be achieved by means of semantic and syntactical analyses. Also a dictionary system will provide the necessary vocabulary on which such descriptions are based.

In the medical record the basic elements of data are known as items. Most items consist of either nouns or noun phrases and may have several qualifiers or descriptors. Those items of data form the basic structure of a segment of the medical record. Such segments together collectively form an individual patient record of the present episode of illness. Other segments will describe past illnesses and other parts of the medical record. A collection of medical records may be described by comparing the elementary data or the data within segments across records. Numeric analysis implies that quantitative data will be stored within the medical record, usually produced as a result of investigative and therapeutic procedures. Some of this data may arise from clinical and medical and nursing observation, others from laboratory data. The importance of numeric data is that it can be manipulated in a different way to descriptive data. Numeric data can also be presented for output in different ways as well. So far in the medical record little analysis of numeric data is conducted in the on-going procedure of care because of the difficulties in handling such data and transforming it appropriately for output.

Logical data structures enable logical manipulations to be carried out on such structures and so create positive states of information. The manipulation of clinical data is often carried out in this fashion. Often feed-back from an information system can be produced from logical as well as numeric data. For example, in the file of input of investigations to a laboratory the logical conclusion may be that this patient has not got a file entry on the entry laboratory file. If the answer is no then the feed-back means there should be another test ordered of a similar kind. Information structures can also be designed so that they can be handled by statistical techniques. Usually aggregations of basic information are transformed and handled in this manner. Some clinical data is of this nature and much administrative and management information is also handled in this way.

Information structures have also to be designed for the other types of record namely the nursing record and the laboratory records. These information structures must not only reflect the on-going process of the laboratory but also must be cognizant of the need to transform that data so that cost and other parameters may be derived from the information structure itself. Now that such

types of transformation can be carried out automatically there is a need for
information structures which can be handled in many ways.

8.0 Concepts of Presentation of Information.

The major type of presentation in the medical record is descriptive in
nature. However, it has to be borne in mind that the total description is generally
required at the basic level of medical activity around the patient's bedside.
Other types of information of a summary nature are also descriptive in kind but
will be presented and used in a different way. Summaries will be required for
different purposes, for example, the summary required for a hospital doctor will be
different from that required by the general practitioner when the patient is discharged from hospital. Thus summary procedures have to be designed to operate on
data. These summaries should then be checked by medical personnel. Thus
appropriate summaries might be composed automatically within an agreed structure
and format. It is important that summaries be structured and the information be
presented in a logical and appropriate fashion.

It is easy to output a great deal of numeric data in tabular form but
much more difficult to comprehend its implications, especially when there is a
large amount of output. Thus numeric presentation should be numeric summaries
of similar kinds of data rather than just print out of figures.

Graphical presentation of changing variables is an extremely useful way
of presenting numeric information to the user. Hospital personnel are already
familiar with graphic output in the shape of temperature, blood pressure and other
charts and are used with handling such information. However, they are not so
familiar with different types of graphical analysis to determine dynamic cycle
times under parameters such as frequency distribution of changing numeric data.
These more sophisticated modes of presentation need further exploration and research
before being generally used.

Much analysis of data is logical in nature and is appropriate for
comparing plans against processes and procedures. Much analysis can be done
logically in the medical record and used to produce adequate feed-back to various
levels of user. It is going to be impossible to design rapidly all the types of
logical analysis required. Most of our present systems tend to leave it to the
user with some formal training in the design of appropriate interpretative systems.
He should be able to write programmes to produce the type of analysis that is
required.

In interpreting the elements of a dynamic system, statistical analysis
can be more appropriate. There are fundamental uncertainties in relation to most
of the data generated in patient care: its uses at management level are perhaps
better presented as statistical digests rather than as absolute collections of
variables. A great deal of information will be transformed and processed to yield

new information to management. As yet little experience has been gained in this type of transform largely because the existing information system has never used this possibility. Thus concepts of scheduling and process control are not able to be carried through unless automatic manipulation of data is possible.

9.0 Possible Ways of Solution.

9.1

It will not be possible to improve the care process in a scientific manner unless adequate systems of information, manipulation and analysis become available. It is quite possible even in the written system to devise new record structures but the time taken to carry these through and analyse them is totally impracticable with the labour force that is available. Until automatic information processing arrives it is not going to be possible to improve the existing utilization of information.

When such automated information handling systems become available the care process in future can be viewed more as a dynamic than a static system and feed-back of information used extensively to control its operation and render it more sensitive to changes.

It will also enable the care process to be monitored more successfully and ensure that effort is not wasted and that results arrive at the appropriate time and not later than expected. Not only have the details of the care process to be monitored in the medical and nursing area but there has to be some monitoring of the overall care rendered by a hospital in relation to the resources expended. Solutions to this problem can only become available if automated data processing is implemented.

9.2 Auxiliary Functions.

It is necessary to have data processing for auxiliary functions as well. It must ensure that communication of their information reaches those clinical staff who require such information. In general it is easy for information from auxiliary functions to get lost or to be overlooked. If appropriate pathways for communications and information processing are created then such information will not be lost and the users of such data can be reminded that it is available. In this way the maximum utility of these functions is realised.

9.3 Administrative Purposes.

In the past administration has found data difficult to collect for its purposes and has had to create separate data collection systems to those used in the clinical care process. Such data collection has been expensive and has restricted the type of purposes for which an administration can use the information. Now that the care process information can be recorded and processed then the types of information that the administration would like to have can now be realised.

Thus various transforms of it are required for administrative purposes at different levels in the management structure. However, the type of information required must be reconciled to the objectives of the administration which even now are not clearly stated. So far administration seems to have got itself locked in job specification rather than in the delineation of appropriate administrative objectives which may be linked to information processing.

9.4 Process Control and Scheduling.

A great deal of administrative effort is directed towards ensuring that processes are controlled and they do not exceed their budgetary limitations. Process control however goes much further and occurs at all levels of the care activity as well as in the administrative situation. Scheduling of activities, investigations and orders is just as important as the scheduling of patients for admission and for investigation. It is important that the concepts of process control are widely applied in the hospital. This has not been possible to date because the lack of adequate information flow with which to institute control procedures. However, with the advent of automatic data processing such objectives are now within sight.

10.0 Case Study Solutions.

It has to be stated at the outset that no total hospital information system exists. This is a theoretical objective or aim towards which most people have been striving. However, a whole variety of solutions have been proposed and implemented at a variety of levels. First many of the basic units or modules of the information system have been created. For example, many projects have registration of patient identity and document the collection of certain basic patient data. Other systems have been designed for scheduling health care intervention, namely those booking systems for hospital admissions and appointments for laboratory tests. Also scheduling is used in the therapeutic area in such departments as the pharmacy and radiotherapy.

Much effort has been expended at hospital and regional and governmental level in the recording of health care statistics about the number of patients seen and the number and kind of health problems that are investigated and treated.

In recent years much automation has been introduced in the various investigative laboratories largely linked with the introduction of machinery to carry out various investigations and tests. Usually computers are used to guide the process, for data analysis and the production of laboratory records. Sub-systems have been implemented in the biochemical laboratory, in haematology and microbiology. Some experiments have also been carried out in recording psychological and pathological data.

Other data processing has gone on in physiological laboratories where automated analyses of the E.C.G. have been made.

Some automation of the results of pulmonary function tests has been investigated. In the radiological field and in nuclear medicine records of the results of investigative procedures have been recorded on a computer and are used to guide clinical procedures. The link between these various sub-systems that have been created and the on-going process of medical care has so far been rather implicit than explicit.

In general medical acts can be divided into two main categories, those of clinical observations and procedures. It is possible to divide observations into symptoms and other data which are recorded in the various histories that can be created about the patient such as the history of the present illness, the family history, occupational and environmental history etc. Doctors also record signs which are obtained according to certain defined minimum standards. A great deal depends on the basic investigation procedures that are particular for that area in medicine. Other data are produced by investigations into body fluids and of the patient himself.

Therapeutic procedures emanate from the various services which the patient may use; these being medical and pharmacological. There may be surgical procedures including anaesthesia, physical procedures instituted for patient care and investigation including the giving of ionizing radiation and the different types of physical treatment. Behavioural procedures may include counselling, psychotherapy and social procedures, including advice to the person and if required family assistance. We have also mentioned the specialised procedures that take place in intensive care and in haemodialysis. There are many common elements to each of these areas and it is possible to generalize about the vast number of test procedures. Such general systems are now being researched.

However, it is much more important to view these acts not only from medical activity point of view but also from the managerial point of view, analysing the actual cost and the benefit obtained from such expenditure of resources. It is the problems of forming basic clinical data for medical, administrative and management purposes that has created problems. Such usages of clinical data have already been considered and ideas of cost of resources and clinical management have not been important parts of medical training as yet.

It is also important to realise that the integration of a sub-system into a larger information system is a much more difficult task than simply designing another sub-system. It requires a new set of knowledge and skills and the recognition that systems integration is a difficult task. To obtain the optimum functioning of a larger system it will often be necessary to drive parts of the existing sub-system at less than optimal level for that part of the system. Most of the mistakes in existing case studies have been due to the lack of recognition of complexity and difficulty of systems integration and of the long time that is required for training and education. So far no ideal solution has emerged but interesting experiments are in progress.

Such difficulties are encouraging a deeper investigation and analysis of the purposes of clinical care. Such an analysis depends on the purpose of care encounters and the state of the patient during the course of his illness. Disability will depend on the changes in the relative signs and symptoms and the manifestations of the illness as it progresses. Thus the expenditure of resources has to be related to patient outcome and the changes brought about by investigation and treatment.

In the preventive care field much has been achieved by maintaining the immunisation and vaccination status of populations of patients who are at risk for various diseases. The comprehensive nature of preventive care has been greatly improved by the introduction of information processing to ensure that a 90-95% of population immunisation has been attained. In this way it has been possible to reduce the incidence of certain diseases, such as diphtheria, virtually to zero.

One of the hopes for the future now that comprehensive care systems exist in most parts of the world is to eradicate the infectious venereal diseases, syphilis and gonorrhea. While case finding takes time comprehensive overall short term treatment could bring eradication about. It cannot happen unless there are adequate information processing facilities, as well as a will on the part of patients to co-operate.

Much work has now been undertaken in the various areas of medicine to form a common data base to ensure that information need only be recorded once and then can be analysed in a variety of ways. Only recently has it been possible to view, not only individual medical care, but the whole medical care system as an entity and institute appropriate information control procedures. It may then become possible for the system to change in a logical and practical fashion using feed-back of information to control its progress.

Such changes as have been achieved have not come about without a great deal of re-education and retraining. Such sub-systems and systems as have been introduced have pointed the way, not only to the training need for those who are implementing such systems, but also to the much wider need to train users and potential users of such systems, on a more extensive scale than has been envisaged so far. Indeed one of the serious factors that has retarded progress has been the lack of education of personnel at all levels.

What is being described now is a total reorientation of hospital information systems and it cannot come about without a total reorientation of those who are going to use and operate them. Such changes cannot be achieved at the instant and take a long time scale. We have already spoken of sub-systems and the modules of such systems being developed. The structures described are not familiar nor are the information transfers and transformations. Thus a great deal more research and education has to be undertaken if we are to ever get the acceptance of such systems and bring about a new information revolution in health care.

REFERENCES

1. Acheson, E.C. (1967) Medical Recording Linkage. Oxford University Press London.

2. Anderson, J. (1970) Definition of Terms Used in Medical Information. P.14. ibid.

3. Anderson, J. (1972) The Medical Student & The Computer. P.151. Pergamon Press.

4. Anderson, J. (1970) Development of Medical Recording. P.3. Information
   Processing of Medical Records ed. Anderson, J., Forsythe, J.M., North Holland
   Press.

5. Anderson, J. (1972) The Evaluation of Technological Practices. P.21.
   Biomedical Technology in Hospital Diagnosis. ed. Elder A.T., Neil W.T.

6. Anderson, J. (1973) Selection Criteria for Health Care Computer Systems.
   Proceedings of International Conference of Health Technology Systems. ORSA. USA.

7. Barnoon S., Wolfe H. (1972) Measuring the Effectiveness of Medical Decisions.
   c.c. Thomas, Illinois, USA.

8. Brolin, I. (1970) Medela - A System for Compiling Radiological Reports.
   P.179. Information Processing of Medical Records. North Holland Press.

9. Coull D.C., Manson A.C., Crooks J., Weir R.D. (1968) Drug Monitoring and
   Health Services. Health Bulletin Scottish Home & Health Dept. 26, 38.

10. Cros R.C. (1970) Free Text Analyses and Coded Information. P.328. Information
    Processing of Medical Records.   North Holland.

11. de Dombal F.T., Hartley J.R., Sleeman D.H. (1969) A Computer Assisted System
    for Learning Clinical Diagnosis.   Lancet $\underline{1}$, 145.

12. de Dombal F.T., Horrocks J.C., Clays, S.E., Store J.E. (1974) Simulation
    Techniques and Computerised Teaching of the Clinical Diagnostic Process.
    Medifo '74, P.274.

13. Feinstein A.R. (1973) The Problems of the 'Problem Orientated Medical Record'.
    Ani. Int. Med. 78, 751.

14. Flynn F.V., Piper K.A., Roberts, P.K. (1966) J. Clin. Path. 19, 633.

15. Flynn F.V. (1969) J. Clin. Path. $\underline{22}$, 62.

16. Flynn, F.V. (1970) Computerised Facilities for Clinical Chemistry Services.
    Information Processing of Medical Records. North Holland.

17. Gledhill V.X., Matthews J.D., MacKay I.R., Strickland R., Stevens, D.P.,
    Thompson, C.D. (1973) The Problem Orientated Medical Synopsis. Ann. Int.
    Med. $\underline{78}$, 685.

18. Gordon B.L. (1966) Current Medical Terminology. Amer. Med. Assoc. Chicago.

19. Gorry, G.A. (1973) Decision Analysis for Computer Aided Management of Acute
    Renal Failure. Amer. J. Med. $\underline{55}$, 473.

20. Hale, P., Mellner, C., Danielson T. (1967) J5 A Data Processing System for
    Medical Information.   Math. Inform. Med. $\underline{6}$, 1.

21. Hallen B. (1973) Computerized Anaesthetic Record Keeping.
    Acta Anaesth. Scand. Suppl. $\underline{52}$, 1.

22. Hedley, A.J., Scott, A.M. (1969) Debenham C.A. Computer Assisted follow-up Register Method. Inform. Med. $\underline{8}$, 67.

23. Henney C.R., Brodie P., Crooks J. (1974) Medinfo 74, P.271.

24. Administration of drugs in a Hospital ed. Anderson J., Forsythe J.M. Hill R.D., Sauter K., Reichertz P.L. (1974) The Data Bank Concept of the Medical System of Hannover andthe Analyses of Patient Data. P.399. Medinfo '74. North Holland.

25. Korein J. (1970) The Computerized Medical Record. The Variable Field Length Format System and its Application. P.259. Information Processing of Medical Records. North Holland.

26. Lindberg D.A.B. (1968) The Computer and Medical Care. C.C. Thomas, Illinois, USA.

27. Lusted L.B. (1968) Introduction to Medical Decision Making. C.C. Thomas, Illinois, USA.

28. Martin J.M., Germain P., Drovin P., Martin J. (1971) Modular Integration of a Coded Record. Journee d'Informatique Medical - IRIA France.

29. Murnagha J.H., White K.L. (1971) Hospital Statistics New Eng. J. Med. $\underline{284}$, 828.

30. Oldham P.D. (1968) Measurement in Medicine. English University Press.

31. Pratt A.N. (1973) Advances in Biomedical Engineering $\underline{3}$, 97.

32. Pratt A.W. (1971) Journee d'Informatique Medical IRIA France. P.595.

33. Pacak M., Pratt A.W. (1971) Symposium on Information Storage & Retrieval. p.5. University of Maryland.

34. Pratt A.W. (1974) Medicine & Linguistics. Medinfo '74 ed. Anderson J., Forsythe J.M., North Holland.

35. Pockington P.R. (1973) A general OMR Form Evaluation Program. Method. Inform. Med. $\underline{12}$, 211.

36. Pockington P.R. (1974) The Necessity for Requirements of a Basic Design of a General Data Interpretation & Evaluation System (DIES) P.411. Medinfo '74, North Holland.

37. Reichertz P.L., Sauter P. (1973) Computer File Structure & Data Presentation in Hannover Medical System: Proc. of International Conference of Health Technology Systems. ORSA. USA.

38 Reichertz P.L., Sauter K., Hill O. (1973) The Data Base Concept of the Medical System Hannover. Medis. $\underline{30}$, 4.

39. Reichertz P.L. (1974) The Medical System Hannover (MSH) ed. Collin. Hospital Computer Systems.

40. Sauter K., Reichertz P.L., Lowe W. (1972) Method Informat. Med. $\underline{11}$, 91.

41. Sauter K., Reichertz P.L. (1972) The Integrated Patient Data Bank of a Hospital Information System. Journee d'Informatique Medicale. P.9. IRIA France.

42. Schwartz W.B. (1970) Medicine and the Computer. New Eng. J. Med. <u>238</u>, 1253.

43. Selander H. (1970) Patient & Resource Allocation. P.149. Information
     Processing of Medical Records.   North Holland.

44. Simmons E.M., Miller O.W. (1970) A New Concept in Automated Patient
     Histories. p.116.   Information Processing of Medical Records. North Holland.

45. Weed L.L. (1969) Medical Records, Medical Education & Patient Care.
     Western Reserve University. USA.

46. Weed L.L. (1968) Medical Records that Guide & Teach. New Eng. J. Med. <u>278</u>,593.

INFORMATION SYSTEMS IN AMBULATORY CARE

Carlos Vallbona, Houston, Texas
Susan Beggs-Baker, Houston, Texas
Robert L. Baker, Houston, Texas

INTRODUCTION

The health care systems of most industrialized nations depend on advanced technology for the delivery of health services to individuals or to community groups.
Technology oriented health systems are complex in their organization, require expensive equipment and supplies, and are heavily dependent on the availability of medical
specialists and highly trained technicians. Consequently, technology oriented health
care systems are very costly. Not surprisingly, the cost of health care in many
countries has increased at a much higher rate than the cost of living. In the
United States, the cost of health care in 1950 was estimated at $12 x 10^9$, which
represented about 4.5% of the gross national product. Ten years later, the cost had
risen to $25.9 x 10^9$, or 5% of the gross national product. During the '60s and the
first half of the '70s there have been staggering increases in total expenditures
and in the proportion of the gross national product spent in health care. Recent
figures compiled by the U.S. Department of Health, Education and Welfare show that
during fiscal year 1975 (from July 1, 1974 through June 30, 1975) the cost of health
care was $118.5 x 10^9$, or 8.3% of the gross national product. This is indeed a high
investment in health care which represents an average annual disbursement of $547.03
per person, the expenses being much higher for the elderly (1).

If we accept the notion that it is not economically sound to sustain a high rate
of inflation in the health field, it is imperative that health planners seek potential solutions to the problem. If the only objective were a decrease in health care
costs, several measures could be considered: put a moratorium on the development of
expensive technology, establish rigid price controls, constrain overall utilization,
and restrict services provided by specialists. However, these measures cannot be
instituted without regard for their impact on the overall state of health of the
population. Thus, health planners face the challenge of seeking strategies which
have a reasonable chance of achieving societal health goals and which are also economically affordable.

The National Center for Health Services Research estimated in 1970 that 55% of
the cost of health services in the U.S. was incurred in ambulatory care and 45% in
hospital or inpatient care. The volume of services rendered, however, was much
greater in ambulatory care settings than in hospitals. One type of system which
emphasizes ambulatory care (referred to as Health Maintenance Organization) seems to
maintain an adequate level of health in the population served at a cost considerably
lower than that of systems which emphasize hospitalization (2). We should point out
that most Health Maintenance Organizations provide care to groups that are not representative of the general population, and because of this, cost extrapolations may be
unwarranted.

A recent study conducted by the National Center for Health Statistics in the
U.S. showed that during the one-year study period (May 1973 - April 1974) there were
$650 x 10^6$ ambulatory visits (a national average of 3.1 visits per person per year).
Of these visits, 80% were of a curative type (i.e. for the purpose of treating a specific medical problem), while only 20% were of a preventive nature (i.e. for services
aimed at avoiding specific health problems). It is well accepted that ambulatory services of a preventive nature are much less expensive than those of a curative nature,
and in turn, ambulatory services are less expensive than hospital services. Therefore,
it would appear highly desirable to change the pattern of utilization of health care
in the U.S. from hospitals to ambulatory settings, and in turn, to change the purpose
of the visits from curative to preventive.

The U.S. health care system's gradual adoption of the alternative of ambulatory care is illustrated by the fact that medical schools are devoting more curriculum time to the teaching of primary care and more and more of the practical training of medical students occurs in ambulatory settings. Having stressed the importance of ambulatory care, we propose in this paper to make a detailed analysis of the organization of ambulatory care systems, to describe the flow of information within those systems, and to point out the significant contributions that information science can make to ambulatory medicine.

GOALS OF AMBULATORY CARE

The goals of an ambulatory care system must, of course, be congruent with those established for the overall health care system of which the ambulatory system is a component. A health care system may be defined as a functional organization that provides special services to individuals or community groups with the purpose of improving and maintaining their state of health.

WORLD HEALTH ORGANIZATION GOAL

In the above definition, the key word is "health". The World Health Organization defines health as "a complete state of physical, mental and social well-being and not merely the absence of disease or infirmity." If the goal of a health care system is to improve and maintain the state of "health", it is clear that the system must provide for all three of the basic components of health and disease implicit in the WHO definition: physiological, psychological, and sociological. Of course, the medical profession has serious reservations about accepting responsibility for effecting changes in the social system which could have a bearing on health and disease. The American Medical Association feels very strongly that the physician should not assume responsibility for solving social problems and that it would be a mistake to train physicians in this difficult field. However, the AMA's position must not be construed to mean that physicians should not be aware of the relationships between the social and the health systems.

SOCIAL GOALS OF HEALTH

Clearly, the overall goal of any health care system which incorporates the definition of health adopted by the WHO is too broad and has implications that transcend the capability of existing health care systems or of health care providers. The U.S. Public Health Service articulated more explicit goals in the decade of the '60s:

1. Every person should have maximum protection against diseases which need not happen and against illness and injury resulting from the hazards of the modern environment.

2. Every person should have ready access to basic medical care, despite social, economic, geographic and other barriers, and should have the assurance of continuity of quality service through diagnosis, treatment and rehabilitation.

3. Over and above these measures of prevention and cure, every person should have maximum opportunity to develop his capabilities, in an environment that is not merely safe but conducive to productive living.

4. All activities conducted in pursuit of health should be carried out with full attention to the dignity and integrity of the individual.

In the early '70s the U.S. Public Health Service formulated a somewhat less ambitious set of goals: a) to improve accessibility to health care for all individuals, b) to provide health services of the highest possible quality, and c) to contain the cost of health care delivery.

Although the above goals are more explicit than the broad statement which embraces the WHO concept of health, it is necessary to express ambulatory care goals in realistic terms according to the needs and available resources of specific communities, and to translate those goals into quantifiable objectives which can serve as the basis for evaluating the system's performance.

SPECIFIC AND QUANTIFIABLE OBJECTIVES FOR AN AMBULATORY CARE SYSTEM

To illustrate this point, we list below the goals established for the ambulatory care system operated by the Harris County Hospital District (Houston, Texas). The system includes a network of seven neighborhood health clinics staffed by physicians on the faculty of Baylor's Department of Community Medicine.

Service Goals

1. To ensure that primary care in all the neighborhood clinics of the HCHD is delivered in a standardized (yet individualized) manner, with full attention to the following components of comprehensive care:

    a. general health education
    b. preventive care (primary and secondary) through:
       - health screening
       - immunizations
       - genetic counselling
       - physical fitness
       - prenatal and postnatal care
       - infant care
       - dental hygiene
       - mental health
       - family planning
    c. episodic care of acute illness or injury
    d. anticipatory and functional management of chronic illness (tertiary prevention)
    e. medical social services
    f. management of disability (through the Rehabilitation Service of the HCHD)

2. To improve the effectiveness of the primary care delivery system in the neighborhood clinics by utilizing health care teams which include:
       - primary physician as the team leader
       - physician extenders
       - community health nurses
       - nutritionists
       - medical social workers
       - pharmacists (within the constraints of existing HCHD policy)

3. To facilitate early implementation of proven new technological developments in the neighborhood clinics of the HCHD.

4. To ensure that the primary care services delivered in the neighborhood clinics are of high quality through development of peer review standards and through participation in the medical audit procedures developed by the Peer Review Committee of the Community Medicine Service.

From these goals we have formulated specific objectives for one of the neighborhood clinics (Sunnyside Clinic), which has a defined enrolled population, a reasonably well documented list of community health problems, and clearly designated resources available to accomplish the objectives.

Service Objectives for the Sunnyside Clinic

1. Extend the ongoing services of the Sunnyside Neighborhood Health Clinic
    to an active enrollee population of 8,000 by the month of June 1975.
    To be considered as an active enrollee, the patient must live in the
    target area and be eligible for services at the Harris County Hospital
    District, have been evaluated at the clinic at least once during the
    period July 1, 1974 - June 30, 1975, and have a complete health-illness
    profile recorded in his chart.

2. Provide complete pediatric care to 1,000 new infants and to 5,000 chil-
    dren of 1 - 19 years of age in order to:

    a. Reduce the infant mortality rate by 25% (25.30/1000 live births
        to 18.98/1000 live births) in the aggregate of census tracts of
        the target area (see objective 3).

    b. Increase the level of complete or up-to-date immunizations in at
        95% of all the children who are active enrollees of the clinic.

    c. Insure that 90% of all pre-school children who are active enrol-
        lees exhibit growth and developmental patterns along an acceptable
        percentile established in three consecutive visits to the clinic.

3. Increase provision of prenatal care to at least 10% (200) of the eli-
    gible pregnant women of the target area from the current 2.5%, in order
    to maintain the incidence of avoidable prenatal complications at a
    level comparable to that of a similar group of pregnant women followed
    regularly in the Maternal and Infant Care Program of the City of Houston.
    Specific efforts will be made to reach mothers of those census tracts
    with the highest infant mortality rates, in order to facilitate the
    achievement of 2.a.

4. Institute a family planning program in cooperation with the City of
    Houston Health Department in order to reach at least 90% of all eligible
    women of child-bearing age who live in census tracts 327, 330, and 343,
    which have exhibited the highest natality rates in 1973. It is antici-
    pated that complete family planning services would be provided at the
    Sunnyside Clinic for at least 1,000 women (25% of the estimated non-
    pregnant population in the child-bearing age group) and that the others
    would be referred through an appropriate mechanism to the neighborhood
    clinics of the City Health Department.

5. Provide health screening (with a minimum set of tests) to all the adult
    new patients who enroll in the Sunnyside Clinic, and to those already
    enrolled who have not had one complete screening within the twelve
    months preceding the visit.

6. Modify the current health service utilization behavior of all active
    enrollees of the Sunnyside Clinic who are known to have diabetes or
    cardiovascular disease (the number is estimated to be about 1,000
    patients) in order to achieve greater utilization of tertiary preven-
    tive services. It is expected that the current average level of less
    than three visits per year for this patient group will increase to at
    least five visits per year with evidence of a greater number of encoun-
    ters for health education, anticipatory and functional management of
    chronic illness, etc. In the case of patients with hypertension, this
    should result in control of blood pressure to systolic levels less than
    140 mm Hg and diastolic levels below 90 mm Hg under 40 years of age and
    95 mm HG for those over 40 years of age in at least 75% of all the
    patients with a diagnosis of hypertension.

7. Provide preventive dental services to all children less than five years of age enrolled in the comprehensive pediatric program listed in objective 2.

8. Provide restorative and prophylactic dental services to all patients with diabetes and/or cardiovascular disease who are enrolled in the comprehensive care program outlined in objective 6.

9. Increase the level of efficiency of physician services to a desired end point of four follow-up visits per hour or two new evaluation visits per hour for primary physicians.

10. Insure continuity of services within the clinic, and between the clinic and the central back-up facilities of Ben Taub and Jefferson Davis Hospitals (both in the outpatient specialty clinics and inpatient services) in order that appropriate and cooperative relationships be established between patient, physician and health teams.

FUNCTIONAL REQUIREMENTS

THE DONABEDIAN MODEL

Donabedian (3) has suggested that a health care system has three basic components which can serve as a suitable framework for assessments of the quality of care provided: structure, process, and outcome. In order to analyze the functional requirements of an ambulatory care system, it is pertinent to examine these components.

The structure refers to the setting in which health services are rendered and the organization which facilitates the provision of such services. Elements within the structure are: facilities, equipment, medical staff, administrative and fiscal personnel, by-laws, policies, etc. Using a human analogy, we could say that the structure of a health care system is its anatomy.

The process is the provision of health services. The following are elements of the process: flow of individuals through the system, volume and types of services rendered to them, flow of information generated in the care process, health manpower inputs, economic inputs, etc. Again using the human analogy, we could consider the process of the health care system as its physiology.

The outcome relates to the impact that the structure and process have on the individuals or community groups who utilize the health system. The outcomes are the results obtained by the health care delivery system. Some outcomes are concrete and may be readily measured (mortality, morbidity). Other outcomes, such as the state of health of individuals, are more difficult to assess because they require complex physiological tests, psychological assessments, and measurements of social performance. A human analog of the outcome is the set of purposeful actions of an individual.

LEVELS OF CARE

If we analyze the health care system from the standpoint of complexity of health problems and facilities, we may distinguish three levels of care: primary, secondary, and tertiary.

Primary care includes a variety of health care services rendered to individuals where and when they encounter the health system on their own initiative. That initiative is usually prompted by the perceived presence of a particular health problem. Less frequently, individuals seek primary care for the purpose of disease prevention. The problems dealt with at the primary care level are rather common and do not require complex facilities beyond those available in ambulatory care settings. The primary care provider is the physician of first contact, usually a family practitioner, a general pediatrician, or a general internist. In the case of women of reproductive age, the primary care provider may be an obstetrician-gynecologist. Typical primary care settings are physicians' offices, group practices, hospital outpatient departments, emergency rooms, and neighborhood health centers.

Secondary care includes the services provided for problems of greater complexity than those handled at the primary care level. Usually, the patient needs to be admitted to a community hospital where his care is provided by a primary care physician or by a specialist to whom the primary physician has delegated the responsibility of treating his patient.

Tertiary care is provided for very unusual or complex problems that cannot be handled adequately in community hospitals. Tertiary care is usually provided by specialists trained in the management of specific diseases or problems. These specialists must have access to sophisticated diagnostic and treatment resources (both equipment and manpower) which are available only at regional medical centers usually connected with a medical school.

Fry (4) has depicted the relationship of these three levels of care in a diagram that clearly shows the decreasing volume of services rendered as their complexity increases. Fry's diagram indicates, in point of fact, that the majority of health problems are self-limited in nature and are handled by the patient and/or his family at what may be termed the self care level. In Figure 1, we present a modification of Fry's diagram which relates the severity of the health problems to the levels of care.

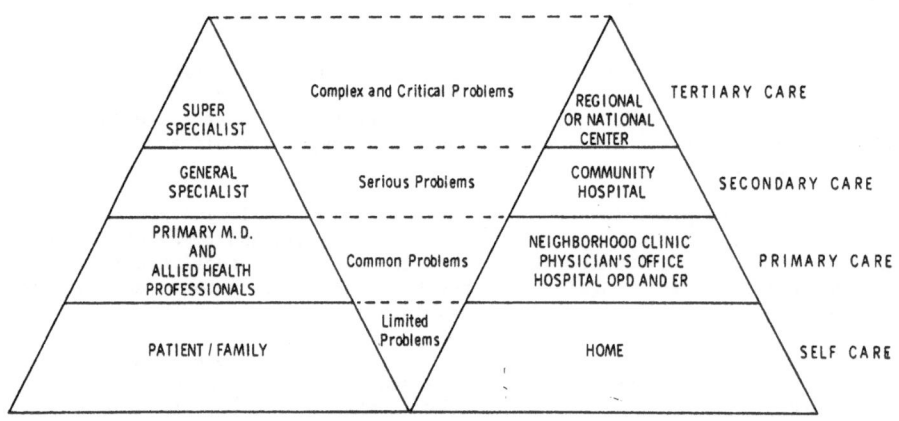

Figure 1. Levels of Care, Complexity of Problems, and Complexity of Facilities (modified from Fry). Reproduced from (8)

PERSONNEL REQUIREMENTS

An ambulatory care system which provides preventive and curative comprehensive services must rely not only on physicians, but on allied health professionals. These health care providers can work more effectively if they are organized into health care teams in which each member has specific responsibilities in the ambulatory management of patients.

A typical health team is composed of: a primary care physician (a family practitioner, a general internist, or a general pediatrician), physician extenders (nurse clinicians or physician assistants), nursing staff, other allied health professionals (nutritionist, social worker, clinical pharmacist, and health educator), and community health workers (also referred to as health advocate). The physician is the leader of the health team and assumes full responsibility for all aspects of the management of the patient, but he delegates various tasks to other members of the team taking into consideration the competence of each team member and the institutional policies under which the ambulatory care system operates.

The dynamics of primary health care teams have been studied by Parker (5). We believe that a harmonious relationship among team members can be achieved if the following principles of team work are kept in mind: a) understanding and sharing of philosophical and operational goals of the program; b) acceptance of specific responsibilities by each member of the team; c) mutual respect for the competency of the team members; d) constant communication among team members and with the patient and/or the patient's family; e) joint periodic review of each patient's progress and problems; f) joint establishment of specific long-term and immediate objectives of each patient's treatment; g) revision and adjustment of objectives of specific programs in light of information provided by other members of the team or the patient's family; h) coordination of team efforts with those of community agencies involved in specific aspects of management.

Adequate support personnel (clerical and administrative staff) is essential, of course, to guarantee the smooth operation of an ambulatory care system. Figure 2 is an example of the organization of personnel in a neighborhood clinic setting.

FINANCIAL REQUIREMENTS

The funds necessary to operate an ambulatory care system may be obtained through the following payment methods: a) fee-for-service, whereby the patient reimburses the system for each of the itemized services he receives; b) third party payment, whereby the patient is insured by the government or by a private insurance carrier (depending on the plan, an insurance carrier guarantees full or partial reimbursement to the patient for the amount spent on ambulatory care services, or the third party payor pays an agreed upon amount directly to the ambulatory care system); c) health maintenance organization, whereby a specified number of comprehensive services are provided to enrolled members for a fixed, prepaid annual fee.

SUBSYSTEMS OF AMBULATORY CARE

There are several basic prototypes of ambulatory care delivery systems, each of which may constitute the subsystem of a larger ambulatory care system: hospital outpatient departments, private offices of solo practitioners, group practices, and health care providing organizations.

HOSPITAL OUTPATIENT DEPARTMENTS

Practically all community hospitals include an outpatient department where patients receive ambulatory care services from staff physicians. Generally, the most utilized hospital outpatient facility is the emergency room. However, large hospitals, especially those affiliated with a medical school, have extensive outpatient facilities for the provision of primary care, or for consultation services of a secondary or tertiary care nature.

PRIVATE OFFICES OF SOLO PRACTITIONERS

Until rather recently, solo practice was the most common method of primary care delivery in western countries. Solo practice is an entrepreneurial model which has the advantages of maintaining the physician's independence and personal autonomy, and preserving the one-to-one relationship between patient and physician. However, the physician working in solo practice is isolated from professional colleagues, is concerned with financing his own enterprise, and has difficulty in regulating his work hours to allow adequate time off for continuing education. As for the patient, he is faced with the inconvenience and expense of referral to a secondary facility if the physician's solo practice cannot perform laboratory tests and X-ray examinations.

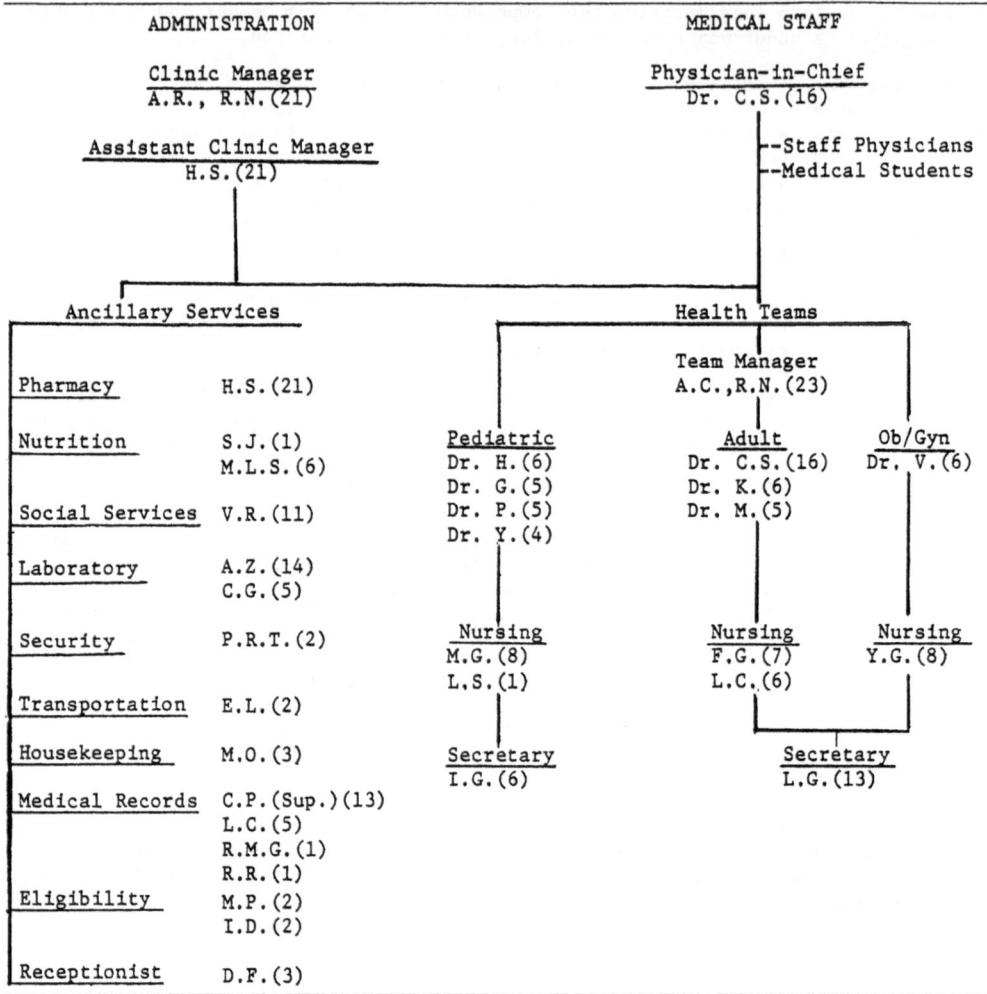

Figure 2.   Casa de Amigos Neighborhood Clinic Organizational Chart: 1974
        *The numbers in parentheses indicate the number of personnel with whom
        the respective person communicates, according to his own estimates.

GROUP PRACTICE

    Group practice is the formal organization of three or more physicians to provide
medical care, consultation, diagnosis, and treatment through the shared use of facilities, equipment and personnel, with the income from the medical practice distributed on a partnership basis. A large group practice relies on an administrative
staff to handle its financial matters. There are three basic categories of group
practice: single specialty groups, general or family practice groups, and multi-
specialty groups. A successful group practice is capable of delivering a large
volume of services and includes specialists on its staff to provide adequate backup
for the primary care physicians.

    It has been stated that physicians working in a group practice are more produc-
tive than solo practice physicians, they have less overhead cost, they rely more on
ambulatory care than on hospitalization of patients, and they engage in close peer

supervision with resulting high quality of services rendered. In addition, group practice physicians can control their work schedule much better than solo practice physicians, and thus they have more opportunity to attend post-graduate training courses.

In the U.S., the trend toward group practice has been growing steadily for the past 20 years, and at present, very few physicians in urban areas provide services according to the solo practice model.

HEALTH CARE PROVIDING ORGANIZATIONS

Some segments of the population cannot afford the cost of services rendered by private practitioners and must rely on publicly financed institutions. These institutions may be: a) totally owned and operated by the government, b) public health units, which in the U.S. are geared almost exclusively to provide preventive services, or c) comprehensive health care centers which provide both preventive and curative services to low-income persons. The neighborhood clinics of the Harris County Hospital District, financed by revenues from taxes levied on the citizens of Houston, are examples of comprehensive health care centers established to provide an adequate ambulatory care system to low-income residents of the community.

Some health care providing organizations are privately financed, and the best prototype is the health maintenance organization (HMO) which we have mentioned earlier.

Health Maintenance Organizations

HMOs are complete health care systems which provide both ambulatory and hospital care to individuals enrolled under a contractual arrangement whereby, upon payment of a pre-specified annual fee, the enrollee is entitled to receive free medical care of a preventive or curative nature in an ambulatory care setting or a hospital. In order to function effectively, HMOs must have a competent management vehicle, a fiscal intermediary that markets membership, collects premiums and spreads risk among large numbers of people, a sufficiently high enrollment (at least 30,000), a group or association of physicians who will deliver ambulatory and hospital services, and adequate physical facilities for the delivery of ambulatory and hospital care. The theoretical advantages of the HMO system over the traditional fee-for-service system include: a) the financial incentive for physicians to emphasize preventive care and avoid high hospital utilization, b) greater continuity of care, c) increased accessibility to and use of primary care services.

STRUCTURE DIFFERENCES IN WESTERN COUNTRIES

Characteristic of most European and Latin American countries is the strong intervention of the government in financing ambulatory care. However, in spite of varying degrees of government regulation, the modes of ambulatory care delivery described above can be found in practically all western countries.

INFORMATION FLOW WITHIN A SYSTEM

The flow of information is very heavy in any ambulatory care system, regardless of its size. Of course, the greater the complexity of the ambulatory care system, the greater the flow of formal information (e.g., written forms, medical records), whereas small systems maintain their flow of information, no matter how heavy, on an informal basis, with little reliance on elaborate medical record keeping. The informal flow is dependent on the size of the staff and on the lines of authority established in the clinic. We illustrate this point in Figure 3, which shows the total number of persons communicated with by the various Casa de Amigos Clinic staff members. It is clear that more clinic personnel communicate with the health team manager and the clinic manager than with the physician-in-chief or other staff physicians. The graph, of course, does not reflect on the importance of the communication, but merely indicates that more people report directly to the clinic manager (whose functions are assumed by a nurse in the case of Casa de Amigos Clinic) than with the physician-in-chief. The formal information flow takes place through a variety of forms which may or may not constitute part of the medical record.

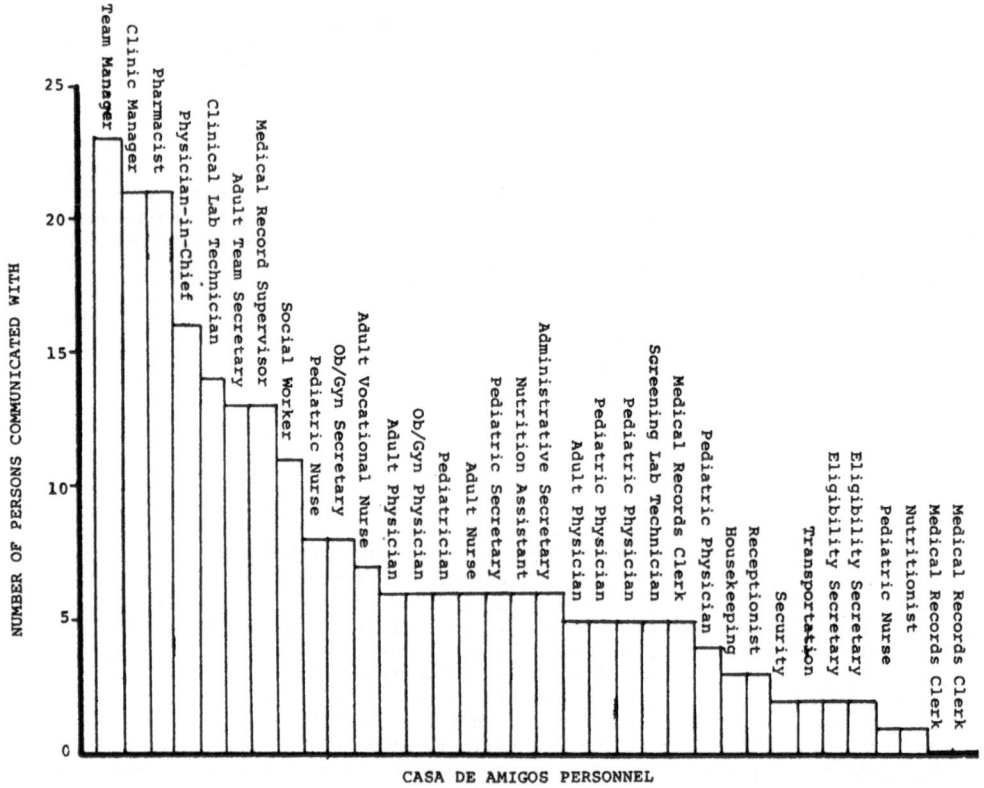

Figure 3. Total number of persons communicated with by Casa de Amigos Clinic personnel

VOLUME OF INFORMATION

In a typical ambulatory care setting, the volume of information may be judged by the number of forms that are used. Even in the relatively circumscribed setting of a neighborhood clinic, the number of forms used to guarantee smooth flow of formal information is overwhelming. Table 1 indicates the number of forms that have been used over the years in the Casa de Amigos Clinic. It should be noted that the introduction of a computerized information system did not result in a significant decrease in the number of forms used. This does not necessarily mean that the compu- terized system was not useful, since major advantages were derived from easy access to a widely retrievable data file, as we will discuss in detail later in this report.

TIME ASPECTS OF INFORMATION

Often, the reports available in an ambulatory care setting are not timely. In emergency situations the laboratory reports and recorded medical impressions are provided on an up-to-date and timely basis, but most commonly, the information is recorded with a significant time delay, thereby losing potential usefulness if the ambulatory care system has to respond rapidly to changes in the process or outcome of the system. An additional problem is the inaccuracy of reports when there is a long time interval between a reportable event and the recording of such event in the

Table 1: Casa Clinic Forms 1971-1974

SUMMARY OF DATA	CATEGORIES OF FORMS					
	A. Medical Data Forms	B. Administrative Information Forms	C. Forms Given to Patients	D. Patient Enrollment	E. Social Service	F. Special Programs
A. Actual Number of Forms Used from 1971-1974 for all Groups	64	40	29	27	8	4
B. Summary by Group:						
1. Groups of Forms Used in 1971 --						
Used 1971-1974 (still used)	20	5	1	4	0	4
Discontinued since 1971	1	3	1	0	0	0
Modified	10	2	2	0	0	0
Never used	1	0	2	0	0	0
Total groups of forms used in 1971	32	10	6	4	0	4
2. Forms Replaced since 1971 (Discontinued and replaced)	- 1	- 2	- 0	- 0	- 0	- 0
3. Forms still in use since 1971	31	8	6	4	0	4
4. New Forms developed since 1971 --						
Completely new	6	23	5	11	8	0
New - replacing discontinued form	1	2	0	0	0	0
Total new groups of new forms developed since 1971	7	25	5	11	8	0
5. Old and new groups of forms used from 1971-1974	38	33	11	15	8	4
6. Forms developed or introduced by the Computer Project n= 17	14	1	1	1	0	0

medical record. In systems terms, we could say that the feedback network is often much too slow to effect timely regulation, thus causing hysteresis in the system's response.

FLOW OF PATIENTS IN AN AMBULATORY CARE SETTING

In an ambulatory care setting such as a neighborhood clinic, the flow of patients is somewhat complex. We will not enter into the details of this issue, but the interested reader may examine the flow chart shown in Figure 4 which depicts the flow of patients in the Casa de Amigos Clinic. The chart illustrates very well the implications of patient flow in regard to the actual flow of information within the setting. It is important to analyze the time spent by patients and clinic personnel in the various steps of the clinic care process shown in Figure 4. Table 2 shows the results of an analysis of time spent in each service or function category by physicians, administrative personnel, nurses, clerical staff, and other personnel in the Casa de Amigos Clinic.

168

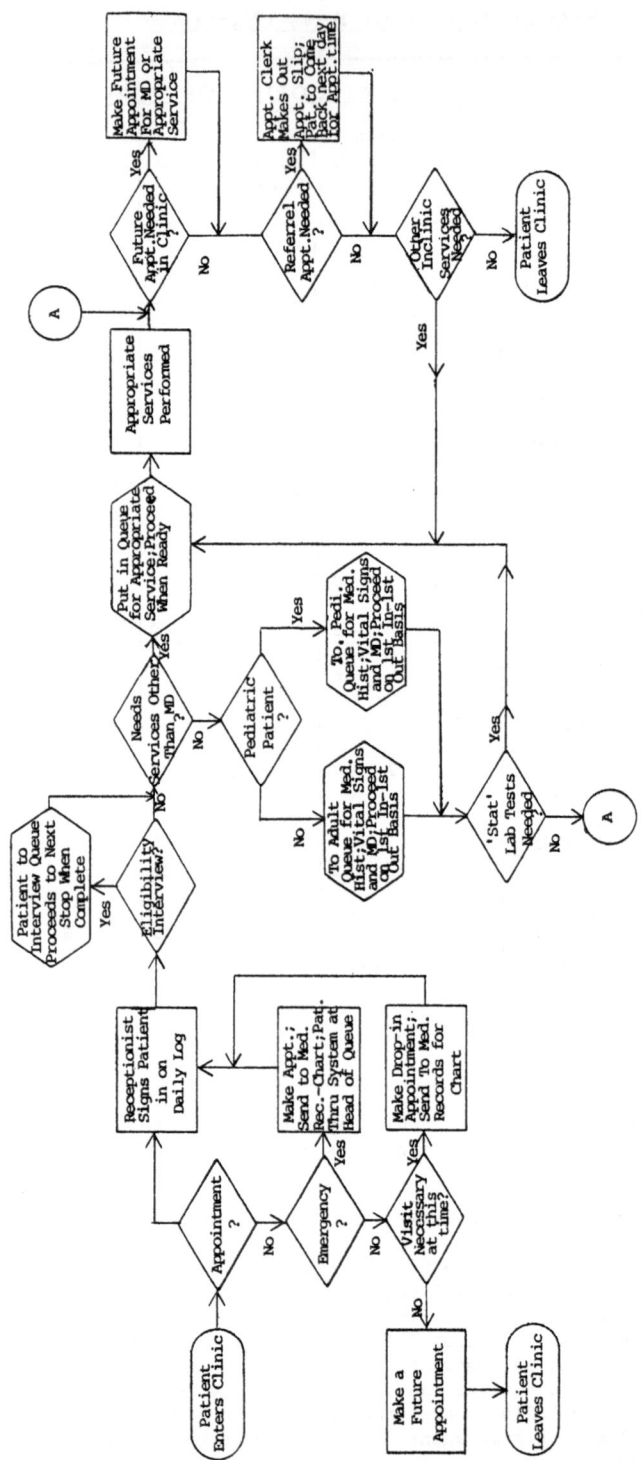

Figure 4. Patient flow through clinic

Table 2: Mean Percentage Time Spent in Each Service/Function Category
As Reported from March Through May, 1974

Summary of All Personnel

Service/Function*	Physicians	Adminis- tration	Nurses	Secretaries and Clerks	General Services	Technicians	All
1. Patient Evaluation	23.63	1.18	14.87	-	-	7.73	9.81
2. Physical Examination	25.65	0	5.92	-	-	-	7.06
3. Procedures and/or Treatments	13.02	.33	17.72	.08	-	0	5.95
4. Medication and Injection	2.41	.67	5.30	-	-	-	1.48
5. Health Screening	6.04	0	11.07	-	-	7.32	4.61
6. Health Counseling	13.02	0	8.48	-	-	11.32	6.32
7. Home Visits	.14	0	.42	-	-	.49	.18
8. Hospital Visits	.03	-	.02	-	-	-	.02
9. Clinical Laboratory	3.28	-	.07	-	-	13.68	3.15
10. ECG Laboratory	.24	-	.06	-	-	3.69	.69
11. Prescriptions	0	-	0	.28	-	7.53	1.37
12. Contact with Other Agency	0	1.15	4.40	-	-	3.71	1.45
13. Referrals to Other Facilities	1.33	4.83	3.45	5.75	-	0	2.98
14. Language Translation	.25	2.30	9.10	.58	.20	1.27	2.38
15. Reception and Registration	-	11.75	.07	4.30	-	-	1.99
16. Eligibility Interviewing	-	6.15	.18	15.31	-	-	5.05
17. Appointments	-	0	.96	9.52	-	-	3.07
18. Data Collection	-	0	1.15	3.58	.21	3.96	1.98
19. Medical Records	-	9.12	-	21.11	-	-	6.95
20. Inventory	0	.38	.93	.82	2.08	1.13	.74
21. Other Clerical Functions	0	5.95	1.63	13.95	.75	9.02	6.46
22. Staff Information Exchange	7.15	10.59	1.53	3.48	.98	8.08	5.02
23. Supervision and Evaluation of Staff and/or Medical Students	2.51	10.20	.81	.04	-	6.46	2.37
24. Community Involvement	.13	2.83	.35	.72	2.07	.55	.68
25. Housekeeping	-	-	.01	.89	42.75	-	2.72
26. Security	-	-	-	-	32.22	-	1.84
27. Driving Patients-Residence	-	-	-	-	0	-	0
28. Driving Pts.-Other Facilities	-	-	-	-	.10	-	.01
29. Delivery Service	-	-	-	-	16.42	-	.94
30. Gardening	-	-	-	-	2.22	-	.13
31. Data Processing-General	-	0	0	3.68	0	0	1.12
32. Vacation Leave-Holiday	0	8.17	10.44	5.38	0	12.69	6.21
33. Administration and Planning	1.17	24.40	1.06	.31	-	1.36	2.15
34. Data Coding	-	-	-	4.49	0	-	1.37
35. Keypunching	-	-	-	1.56	-	-	.48
36. Data Entry-Teleprocessing	-	-	-	3.62	-	-	1.10
37. Data Retrieval-Teleprocessing	-	-	-	0	-	-	0
38. Batch Processing	-	-	-	.55	-	-	.17
Total %	100%	100%	100%	100%	100%	100%	100%

Key: - indicates category is inapplicable to personnel type
0 indicates no time spent in category for this time period, but
category is applicable

INFORMATION FLOW BETWEEN SYSTEMS

FLOW BETWEEN LEVELS OF CARE

In a previous section we discussed three levels of care: primary, secondary, and tertiary. We stated that the care provided at each level is for different types of health problems, and that it requires different types of facilities and increasing degrees of specialization on the part of health care professionals as we move from one level to the next.

There is abundant information flow between the self care and the primary care levels, since the definition of primary care implies that patients and their families have easy and continuous access to an ambulatory care system. Fry's diagram (Fig. 1) depicts the broad base of interaction between the self care provided by patients and their families for minor and limited problems and the primary care delivered by physicians in ambulatory care settings for common problems which are sufficiently serious so as to require consultation with a physician or properly trained physician extender. The flow of information between these two levels is usually informal and does not require the use of records and communication forms.

There is also a constant flow of information of a more formal type between the primary and secondary care levels. Usually, the medical record which is stored in the ambulatory care setting is transmitted in part or in its entirety to the secondary care facility. In turn, the data collected at the secondary facility are referred back to the primary care level.

The flow of information to and from the tertiary care level is formal. Extensive records must be sent to the specialists working in a tertiary care center, and in turn, voluminous reports of their findings and/or recommendations must be sent back to the referring physician. Because of the participation of tertiary care centers in research activities, it is likely that a significant portion of the medical record will be kept in computerized data banks, some of which will contain information contributed by several tertiary care institutions.

FLOW BETWEEN THE AMBULATORY SETTING AND OTHER COMMUNITY AGENCIES

Provision of comprehensive care to patients requires attention to sociological problems which cannot be managed adequately by a primary care team and must be referred to an appropriate community agency. The channels of communication may be both formal and informal, depending on the type of agency to which the patient is referred, but in general, information flow is formal and impersonal. Bureaucratic barriers are insurmountable, and numerous forms have to be filled out by patients and health care providers alike. This problem reaches extraordinary proportions in neighborhood clinics serving low-income persons. Although these clinics have frequent interaction with social and welfare agencies, the flow of information is not easy, and there is a great deal of redundancy in data collection.

FLOW BETWEEN AMBULATORY CARE SYSTEMS AND THIRD PARTY PAYORS

There is formal and very heavy information flow in the case of health care systems financed totally or in part by third party payors. Although the flow of information serves strictly fiscal purposes, it still requires transmission of patient identification data, diagnoses and types of services rendered. The high volume of information is brought about by the need to transmit information regarding each patient on whose behalf a fee-for-service is being requested. In addition, there is a heavy flow of aggregate information collected over a period of time or for a certain number of people.

INTERFACE WITH OTHER HEALTH CARE SYSTEMS

Primary care systems must include facilities and personnel for the provision of care on a 24-hour basis. Emergency care systems have emerged as important primary care providers in highly mobile communities whose residents have not lived in a given location long enough to establish a continuous relationship with primary care providers. In addition, adequate provisions must be made to handle emergency situations resulting from sudden injury, such as automobile accidents. One of the major problems confronting physicians who work in an emergency care setting is the lack of adequate information available to them on the past and current health-illness condition of the patients who seek emergency care. In a large number of cases, the emergency condition can be handled adequately, but in some situations, especially if the patient is unable to communicate with the physician, significant problems may arise because of the physician's unawareness of a pre-existing condition which can influence the outcome of emergency treatment. We believe that one of the major contributions that information science can make to primary care delivery is the establishment of computerized medical data banks containing information which can be made available to authorized physicians in emergency situations.

The pharmacy system is an important component of primary care, although its role is often ignored. Of course, the pharmacy is an integral part of large ambulatory care institutions, especially those connected to a community hospital. Often, however, the pharmacy is run as a free enterprise system independent from the ambulatory care system. In this case, communication between the two systems takes place through a very formal channel, i.e. the transmission of a written prescription form signed by the physician. Such prescription is a legal document authorizing the pharmacist to dispense drugs, including those of a dangerous and restricted nature such as narcotics). Unfortunately, the information that can be conveyed by means of the prescription is extremely limited and relates only to the type of medication and the amount to be dispensed. If the pharmacist has received adequate clinical training, he is in a unique position to assess the extent to which adverse drug interaction may occur when a physician prescribes several drugs simultaneously. Nevertheless, the pharmacist seldom has enough knowledge of all the circumstances to provide solid advice to the patient or to warn the physician of the danger of drug interaction. A system for automatic detection and warning of drug interaction has been developed at Stanford University of Cohen and co-workers (6).

Some health care systems are directed by non-physicians. Practically all cultures have untrained "folk healers" who rely on empirical methods to handle medical conditions. There is seldom, if ever, any formal or informal communication between a medical ambulatory care system and a folk health, who always works on a solo basis. Some patients, especially those with a chronic illness, may seek the advice of both a physician and a folk healer. Often such dual consultation creates conflicts for the patient and may alter significantly the degree to which the patient complies with the recommendations of the physician.

Community nursing systems also relate with the ambulatory care system. Nursing organizations are in charge of carrying out home visits to patients who cannot visit the physician. Such organizations are of great importance in urban settings in the U.S. because the physician seldom, if ever, makes house calls to bedridden patients. The communication between the community nursing system and the physician may be formal or informal, depending on the community and on the type of nursing organization. A close relationship between the visiting nurse and the physician is essential. If the nurse works in the same ambulatory care setting as the physician, there can be adequate sharing of medical records, whereas there is less continuity of care when a nursing organization takes over home surveillance of the patient only for the time he is bedridden.

Funeral home systems interface with the ambulatory care system in the case of death. The flow of information is informal except for the need to report adequately the circumstances of death and to sign a death certificate. From the standpoint of community mortality statistics, the contribution of the funeral home system must not be overlooked.

ORGANIZATION OF INFORMATION

BASIC DOCUMENTATION

The ambulatory medical record is the basic document (or set of documents) used to record all the patient care transactions that take place in an ambulatory care setting. If the patient continually seeks care in the same ambulatory setting, the medical record is an excellent repository of information on both the patient's health status and his disease profile. However, if the patient seeks care in more than one ambulatory setting, the information in the medical record is fragmentary, and it is extremely difficult to analyze the evolution of the patient's problems.

It would be highly desirable to have a uniform medical records format in order to facilitate communication among physicians. In the U.S. such uniformity has not been achieved, and several approaches to the organization of medical records are currently being followed. The records may be organized by source (e.g., medical history data, laboratory data, medications data), by time (i.e. chronological sequence of patient visits), or by problem. The so-called problem oriented medical record has been widely used in the U.S. from the time it was originally proposed by Weed (7).

A computer generated summary medical record which we have developed for use in a neighborhood clinic will be described in detail later in this report.

REPORTS BETWEEN PHYSICIANS

We have discussed information flow between levels of care and among providers in the same setting. No matter how conscientious a physician is in transferring a patient's records to another physician, seldom, if ever, is the information transmitted sufficiently well organized and complete. Similar considerations apply to the transmission of laboratory reports or results of special functional studies.

COMMUNICATION VIA THE PATIENT

A well-educated patient is a good custodian of his own medical record, and through him the value of adequate record keeping to insure continuity of care could be demonstrated. However, many physicians feel reluctant to allow the patient to be the custodian of his own medical record, inasmuch as the fear of creating undue anxiety on the part of the patient or of being misinterpreted could deter the physician from recording all his impressions.

Issues of confidentiality and privacy of medical information take on great importance in the case of the patient as custodian of his own record. The same issues, of course, apply to the storage of information in a medical records department which does not make adequate provisions to prevent access to medical records by non-authorized persons.

INFORMATION SINKS

In a complex ambulatory care system where numerous forms are used to transmit information, information sinks must be used to discard seemingly irrelevant data. Unfortunately, criteria to distinguish relevant from irrelevant data are not clear, and consequently, data of potential importance in epidemiological studies or in health services research may be irretrievably lost.

EVALUATION OF AMBULATORY CARE SYSTEMS

It is clear that well-defined "outcome" objectives will provide the basis for an evaluation of the effectiveness of the ambulatory care system. Issues of cost-effectiveness are dealt with by considering the cost of providing certain services to accomplish a desired outcome. A system may be very effective, but if the desired outcomes are accomplished at a high cost, one may legitimately ask whether or not the same outcomes could be achieved at a lower cost by other means. Thus, in any evaluation of cost-effectiveness, alternative methods of obtaining the same outcome must be considered. Assuming equal outcomes, the system which appears less costly is the one to be chosen.

The efficiency of the system is usually measured in terms of "process" variables. An effecient ambulatory care system is one in which the productivity of the health care providers is very high and the unit cost of the services is kept to a minimum. In considering the effeciency of a system, outcomes are disregarded. Indeed, a system may be very efficient, yet not effective in modifying favorably the health status of the population served.

Figure 5 depicts the cyclic process of evaluation which involves the following

steps: identification of a mission congruent with societal values, establishment of
quantifiable objectives, selection of the variables that must be measured in relation
to each objective, development of measurement instruments, pre-establishment of
criteria for success or failure, data collection process, data analysis, and re-exa-
mination of objectives in view of the results.

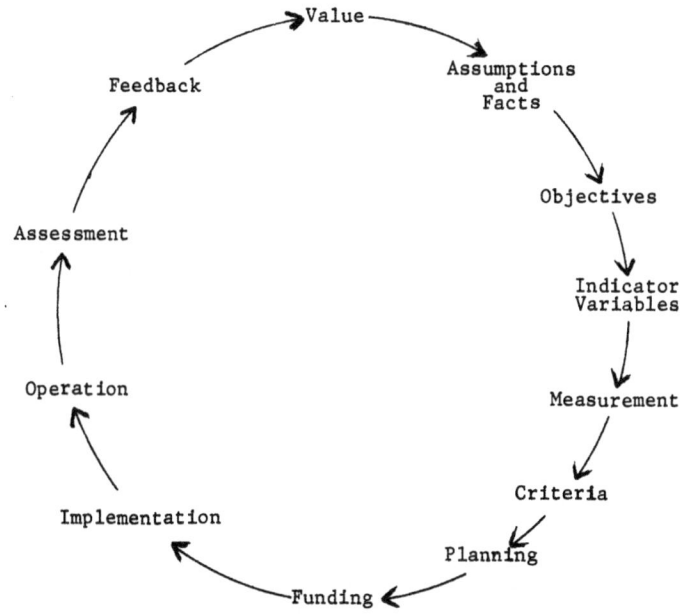

Figure 5. Cyclic process of evaluation of an ambulatory
care system

In evaluating an ambulatory care system, it is important to assess how the population served feels about the system. The level of patient satisfaction can be measured through the administration of attitudinal questionnaires. However, the results
of such studies must be viewed with caution, since a well designed methodology
involves selecting with statistical rigor the sample of patients whose opinions will
be sought, validating the consumer answers (i.e. does the patient actually answer
what he believes), and establishing their reliability (i.e. is the patient consistent
in his opinion if interviewed on two or more occasions by the same interviewer).

ASSESSMENT OF CARE QUALITY--PEER REVIEW

At present, great attention is given in the U.S. to the assessment of the quality of medical care rendered to patients both in ambulatory care settings or in
hospitals. Peer review is defined as the process of evaluating the quality of a
physician's medical services by other physicians who are peers of the physician un-
dergoing review. Many articles have been written about measurements of care quality,
and we have listed the most important ones in the bibliography.

CONCEPTS OF INFORMATION SYSTEMS

We believe that most health care systems, be they local or regional, have limited feedback properties, and as a result, it is difficult to monitor the process and
outcome of health care in these systems. The data base used for feedback is that
contained in medical and administrative records. Usually feedback capabilities are
insufficient to provide complete and timely reports to the persons who are responsible for directing the health care system. We contend that health care systems
with adequate provisions for timely feedback of information become more effective and

efficient than those which have limited feedback properties. In a previous publication we have discussed the important role that computerized information systems can play in facilitating patient and clinic oriented decisions in an ambulatory care setting (8). To illustrate this point, we have drawn an analogy between a physiological servomechanism and the process of care in a neighborhood clinic.

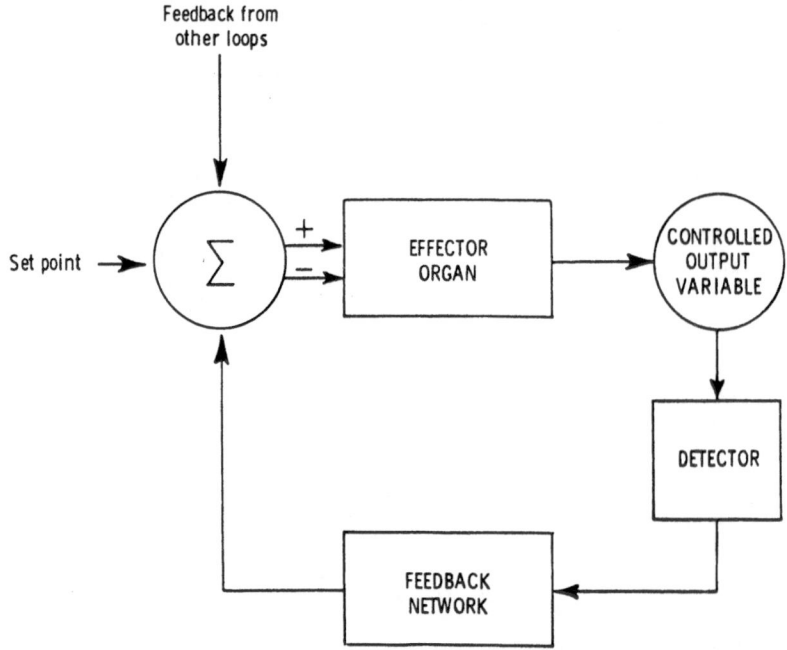

Figure 6. Model of the feedback process of a
cybernetic system (8)

A physiological system consists of a control or integrator center (Σ), an effector organ, a controlled output variable, a feedback network, and a set point of reference (Figure 6). For example, in the servomechanism that controls blood pressure, the vasomotor centers are the control organ, the arterial walls are the effector organ, the blood pressure is the controlled variable, the carotid sinus and other baroreceptors are the detector organ, the afferent autonomic fibers constitute the feedback network, and the "ideal blood pressure" is the set point of reference. The action of the vasomotor centers on the arterial wall is mediated via the efferent autonomic fibers and through them a positive or negative control is established on the level of activity of the effector organ.

In a neighborhood clinic system, the patients as members of the community are the input to the system. The objectives of the health care system serve as the set point of reference to assess the extent to which the clinic is able to control the output variable, i.e. the state of health of the community. A strong clinic feedback process can be established if the detector organ (physician extenders and other health team members) record adequately their observations and the results of laboratory tests, and transmit such information to a medical record data base. If such data base is computerized, we can then establish an adequate feedback network which provides useful and timely reports to the regulator center, constituted in the case of the neighborhood clinic by the physician-in-chief and the clinic manager.(Figure 7).

It is important to keep in mind that at the level of patient-physician interaction there is also a feedback process. Ordinarily the data collected in the medical record are the main feedback source. A reasonable goal of a computerized information

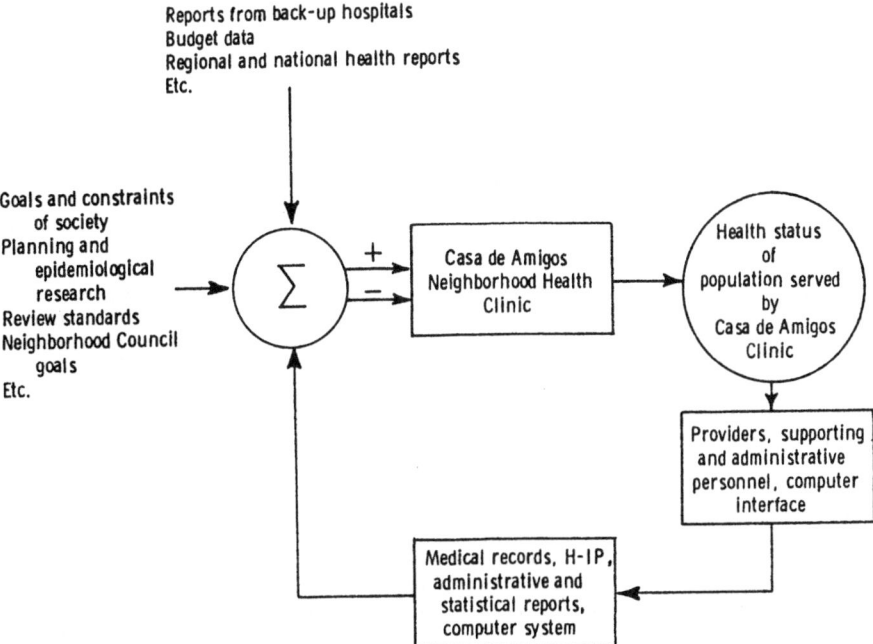

Figure 7. Model of the feedback process as applied to the Casa de Amigos Neighborhood Clinic (8)

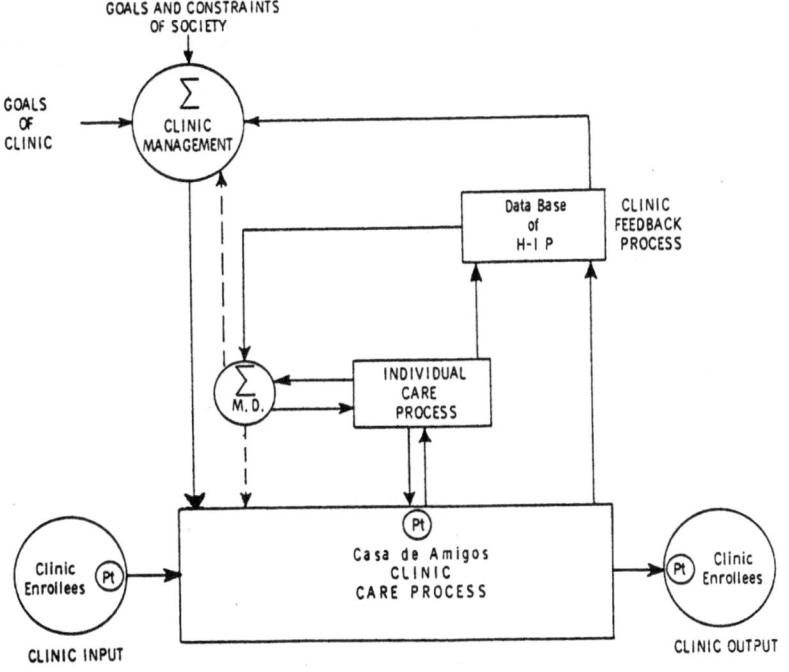

Figure 8. Feedback loops of the clinic care process: individual care process and clinic care process

system is to facilitate integration of individual patient care data into an aggregate file which can be used to provide feedback to the clinic directors. Figure 8 depicts the two basic feedback loops which must be taken into consideration in an ambulatory care system. The small loop applies to the patient-physician encounter when the physician acts as the integrator center that exerts a controlling influence on the patient's health problem. The large loop applies to the clinic director-clinic system interaction. In two neighborhood clinics in Houston, Texas, a computerized data base of medical records provides the major feedback for patient-oriented and clinic-oriented decisions.

CASE STUDY--A COMPUTERIZED INFORMATION SYSTEM FOR A NEIGHBORHOOD CLINIC

Throughout this report we have alluded to the successful implementation of an information system for a neighborhood clinic. The first stimulus to establish a computerized patient management system in a neighborhood clinic was provided by the awareness of Baylor's Department of Community Medicine that a complete, retrievable patient care data base was essential to: a) facilitate the patient-oriented decisions made by physicians of the neighborhood clinic, and b) allow the clinic directors to make appropriate decisions based on accurate projections of future needs.

Early plans for the computerized system resulted from the interaction of the principal investigator, Dr. Vallbona, with Ms. Susan Beggs-Baker, who was then a research associate at the Texas Institute for Rehabilitation and Research (TIRR), and Mr. Robert L. Baker, director of computer applications at TIRR and assistant professor of rehabilitation, computer science, and community medicine at Baylor. This group of investigators had worked together in the design, implementation, and evaluation of a computerized information system for a rehabilitation hospital (TIRR), which in 1959 began using electronic data processing techniques in the management of disabled patients. These investigators felt that the basic concepts of the TIRR system were applicable to an information system for a neighborhood clinic and that some specific modules of computer support were indeed transferable to a neighborhood clinic environment.

Based on their previous experience, the investigators formulated a theoretical model of information processing for ambulatory care, established general objectives for a computerized system, and identified potential areas of computer support. Most of this preliminary work was carried out as Ms. Beggs-Baker's Master of Public Health thesis (9), and the design model and plans were presented at the 10th IBM Medical Symposium held in June 1970 (10).

We have alluded earlier to the theoretical model of the clinic feedback process that guided the investigators of this project. The model is based on the assumption that a computerized patient information data base could enhance the feedback properties of the ambulatory care system. Having formulated a theoretical model, the following considerations reinforced the investigators' belief in the potential usefulness of a computerized patient management system:

1. A neighborhood clinic may be considered as a self-contained health care system whose performance must be assessed in terms of the volume and efficiency of the services rendered (process) and their impact on each patient (outcome).

2. A strong regulatory mechanism is needed to render the process of care as efficient as possible, with a subsequent favorable influence on the outcome.

3. Preventive and anticipatory care must be added to the routine delivery of episodic care to minimize the frequency and severity of acute or chronic problems (i.e. comprehensive care). Comprehensive care requires coordination of services among a variety of health care agencies, with a corresponding need for rapid and efficient flow of information among these agencies.

4. Insufficient physician manpower in the U.S. demands the assistance of physician extenders (e.g., nurse clinicians, physician assistants) in the
   delivery of comprehensive care, thereby compounding the need to provide updated and concise information to several health care providers.

5. A large retrievable data base of medical records could be useful in community health studies, in ambulatory care research, and in epidemiological surveys.

The opportunity to implement the computerized system in a neighborhood clinic
(Casa de Amigos Clinic) was provided by a contract between the National Center for
Health Services Research and Baylor's Department of Community Medicine (Contract
HSM-110-71-172). The project was conducted under this contract from July 1, 1971
through December 31, 1974.

Initial plans called for the development of several modules of computer support:
a) registration system (appointment system and patient identification system), b)
patient information file, c) clinic work-up support, d) health-illness profile, e)
home care management plans, and f) administrative statistics.

REGISTRATION SYSTEM

Appointment System

We developed successfully a computerized program, but it did not prove to be as
cost-effective for the Casa de Amigos Clinic as a simple manual approach (the ACME
visible record system) which provides essentially the same types of access and reports at a very low cost. We must indicate that the extension of the computerized
system to take maximum advantage of a computerized on-line system was restricted by
patient behavior. The drop-in and no-show rate is rather high (sometimes 40%) in a
neighborhood clinic environment. Because of this, computer scheduling may be quite
ineffective. We concluded that computer technology was inappropriate and too expensive as a means to provide the necessary data and accessibility in a clinic with
high volume, co-located resources, and inadequate number of staff.

Patient Identification System

The purpose of the patient identification system is to provide unequivocal identification of the patient for medical record retrieval, administrative statistics,
scheduling for services, family identification, and for community health studies.
Specifically, the objectives were intended to ensure accurate daily reports on visits
and patient identification information, accuracy of socioeconomic requirements for
eligibility information, and completeness of central file.

The problem of determining, from imprecise data, whether or not a patient has
been seen before at the clinic, or at any site of a central hospital/community clinic
network, is a significant one from several points of view. With respect to the institution involved, failure to properly identify a patient results in redundant efforts such as reinterview, financial clearance, and inaccurate managerial data.
Clinically, it can result in multiple charts for the same patient and consequent loss
of information obtained in prior encounters, with possible reduction in care quality.
Statistics regarding problem incidence and prevalence can be erroneous, and demographic and epidemiologic data can be inaccurate. Also, the procedural problem of identifying with certainty the chart number, given other data, is complex. Identification cards given to the patient do not entirely solve the problem. Automation offers
an efficient and prompt way of assigning chart numbers to new patients from a central
location, when facilities are geographically dispersed. For patients who have had
encounters with one of the facilities before, other facilities visited by the patient
have the benefit of access to the "institutional memory."

During the course of the project, a workable approach to identifying the chart
number, given less precise data, was developed which reduced the clerical time in-

volved. Thus, an automated system is possible and can provide a wide range of subjective and objective benefits. Problems arise in implementing the system in only
one clinic in the network, since the one module must somehow interface with the
information flows used elsewhere in the network. The integration of an automated
patient identification system in only of the many health care service facilities of
the Harris County Hospital District thus poses problems in ensuring accuracy, completeness, and currency of the automated file. It is best if the system is implemented universally. Indeed, interaction with staff of the central hospital was carried
out during the project. The Hospital District is now implementing an on-line patient
identification system on a District-wide basis. At this scale, the cost of automation, as a means of implementing the patient identification system, becomes even more
reasonable.

PATIENT INFORMATION FILE

The objectives of this module are to: a) provide an adequate health record
serving as a basis for the Health-Illness Profile (H-IP); b) provide a basis for a
tentative diagnosis after the patient presents himself to the clinic; c) provide
information that will be used by planners, epidemiologists, and administrators to
enhance the health maintenance of the referenced population.

The basic approach to the patient information file could be either a modular or
an integrated one. Both approaches were considered for our project at Casa de Amigos
Clinic. However, a modular file structure was ultimately chosen rather than a single
comprehensive data base. Reasons for this choice included the need to be responsive
to one of the basic principles set forth by the project staff, namely, that any given
module which found utility within this clinic might be implemented individually or in
conjunction with other modules in the same or different media in other clinics. An
integrated data base would increase the overhead of a single module. Therefore,
modular, but linked, files were used. With respect to file reorganization, both direct (indexed) and sequentially accessed files were implemented. Both organizations
are record-oriented rather than hierarchical by data item (i.e. rather than extensively inverted). Direct access techniques are used for the maintenance of the large
data base for the H-IP. The basic notion is the emphasis on simplicity.

The structure of the file is shown in Figure 9. Only one index (patient number)
is used. This index contains only a pointer to the first block of patient data.
Multiple data blocks may be used, and are linked via pointers. Each 756-character
data block contains multiple varying length records. These records are maintained
in order by type (e.g. problem statement, medication, basic patient identification
data). Records are dense, as blanks are deleted before filing and replaced during
retrieval. Few patients require more than on 756-character block, most being 580
bytes long. At the time a transaction is applied to the file, a number of sequential
files are updated in preparation for use by a variety of statistical reports and
summaries.

It appears that large, integrated data bases are unnecessary for use in a single
outpatient clinic. Their complexity requires the availability of sophisticated and
expensive supporting staff. Commercially available data base software likewise is
expensive. Through experimentation with one sequential and several indexed files,
we have found simple indexed files more appropriate for patient-specific data. A
combination of the two types of file organization proved to be most effective, and it
was found that at the time a transaction was applied to the patient data file, sequential files for use by other modules could be prepared. Anticipating the needs of reporting programs in this manner permitted the file access time to be reduced. It is
our opinion that this approach is less expensive (in terms of computer time and supportive staff) than large, complex, fully integrated data bases that must serve all
purposes.

CLINIC WORK-UP SUPPORT

The use of the computerized system to support the medical decisions in relation

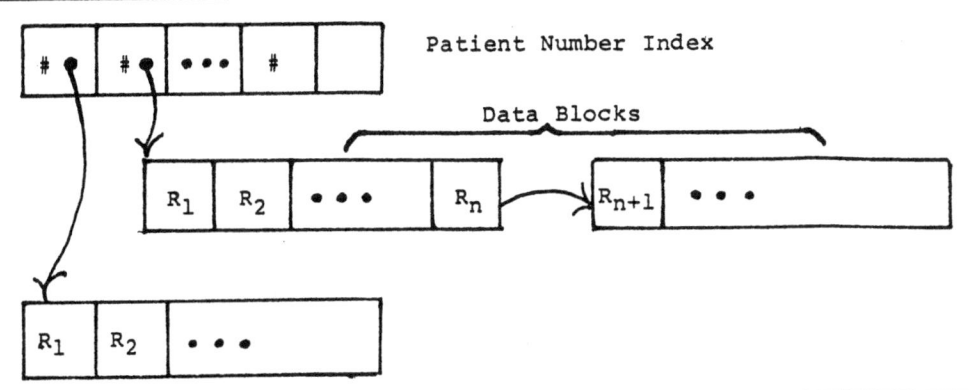

Figure 9. Indexed patient information file structure

to patient work-up or treatment was expected to affect care favorably in the general areas of acute episodic illness, chronic disease, and preventive care, primarily by increasing the efficiency or the effectiveness of the care process. In acute care episodes, efficiency would probably be improved because, in many cases, a paramedical person could readily learn to manage such problems almost independently of the physician. On the other hand, chronic care requires thoroughness; therefore, algorithms would more likely alter the effectiveness of the care process since extensive involvement of the physician would still be required. Both efficiency and effectiveness could be altered by algorithms targeted to preventive care.

Based on our own work, as well as the work of various other projects engaged in algorithm development, we explored the implementation of algorithms in a community clinic. Two modes of implementation were kept in mind; a) a manual technique involving flow charts of algorithm logic, and b) automation functioning interactive with the user. Our criteria for successful implementation involved the factors of need, acceptance, validity, and resources (space and personnel). Based on these criteria, Table 3 shows the status of algorithms that were developed or planned as part of the work-up support module of the computer project for Casa de Amigos Clinic. As the table indicates, only the "development" portion of the growth and development algorithm was implemented. The other algorithms failed to overcome one or more obstacles. Lack of resources, particularly space, precluded full implementation of most of them, even though there was a need.

Table 3

ALGORITHM IMPLEMENTATION CRITERIA

Algorithm	Need	Acceptability	Validity	Space	Personnel
URI	Yes	No	Partial	No	Yes
Growth	Yes	Unknown	Unknown	No	No
Development	Yes	Yes	Partial	Yes	Yes
Immunization	Yes	Unknown	Unknown	No	No
Vaginitis	Yes	Yes	Partial	No	Yes
Acute Gastro-enteritis	Yes	Unknown	Unknown	No	Yes
Diabetes	Yes	Partial	Yes	No	Yes
Hypertension	Yes	Partial	Yes	No	Yes
Family Planning	Yes	Unknown	Unknown	Unknown	Yes

With respect to automation, it was found that many algorithms, especially those for acute care episodes, may be implemented adequately in flow chart form. These can serve as teaching tools for medical students and paramedical staff. For chronic illnesses, some form of automation may be necessary, since care algorithms (e.g. nutrition, immunizations) also require history data and yield, therefore, to automation.

THE HEALTH-ILLNESS PROFILE (H-IP)

The most successful module has been the Health-Illness Profile. The H-IP is a computer-generated document which provides an updated summary report of the state of health and/or illness of every individual enrolled in the neighborhood clinic. The document is also a clear expression of the level of comprehensive care provided to a given individual and serves as the basis for peer review. The H-IP contains concise, pertinent information on the physiological, psychological, and sociological condition of the patient. The H-IP includes the following components: a list of active problems, inactive problems, current medications and their dosage, prior medications, past hospitalizations and procedures, and a health profile containing physical and anthropometric characteristics, results of laboratory tests, parity data in the case of women, immunization status, and growth and development status for children. An example of an H-IP is shown in Figure 10.

The H-IP has been fully implemented at the Casa de Amigos Clinic. The computerized data base of H-IPs at present contains information on more than 11,000 patients. The H-IP has also been introduced in the Sunnyside Clinic, and at present we have a data base of approximately 6,000 profiles on as many patients enrolled in the Sunnyside Clinic.

During the first three years of the project, the data for the H-IPs were extracted from the patients' medical records and entered on-line via CRTs to the medical school computer located seven miles from the clinic. On-line retrieval of the H-IP was possible. However, the cost of producing and retrieving an H-IP was too high for continuous on-line operation. For this reason, we decided to keypunch the medical record data and process the cards on a batch basis. The H-IP data of patients seen in the clinic on a given day are keypunched and processed that same day. The updated printouts are then returned to the patients' charts.

The requirements for updating and editing the H-IP documents make the use of automation valuable in that data editing and error checking can be carried out consistently by the machine, whereas people usually have variable attention spans when tasks are routine and monotonous. Updating a report such as the H-IP also requires retyping or reprinting. The speed of automation in achieving this saves time. Machine preparation of the reports also provides a report that is both dense and legible. In addition, since the data are in machine-readable form, many analyses reauired by management can be obtained at little increase in cost and effort.

An important aspect of the H-IP is the automatic encoding of the problem list. This is achieved through the utilization of a special encoding system developed by Drs Charles Schade and Carlos Speck of our department.

An evaluation of the value of the H-IP was carried out through a questionnaire administered to the staff of Casa de Amigos Clinic in October 1973 and in June 1974. All Casa staff members associated with the H-IP were asked to state opinions concerning their preference for the H-IP over the manual record system. There was an overwhelming testimony in favor of the H-IP. All physicians felt that the H-IP was of assistance to them, and similar comments were made by the nursing staff and by other allied health professionals.

HOME CARE MANAGEMENT PLANS

Home care management plans were intended to assist the patient in understanding his role in the management of his problems after clinic encounter, to provide medically oriented care plans for the patient chart, to provide patient oriented plans

HARRIS COUNTY HOSPITAL DISTRICT
CASA DE AMIGOS COMMUNITY CLINIC
HEALTH-ILLNESS PROFILE LEVEL III

```
= = = = = = = = =C U R R E N T   A C T I V E   P R O B L E M S = = = = = = = = =
  ACTION ONSET CODE STATUS                                        #VSTS LAST VST
#01 ... 02/19/74 44        HYPERTENSION                            09 07/24/75
#02 ... 02/19/74 B2        CHRONIC ANXIETY                         09 05/28/75
#03 ... 03/22/74           OBESITY                                 09 07/24/75
#08 ... 12/18/74 32        DEC VISUAL ACUITY                       01 12/18/74
#09 ... 12/18/74 7A        HYPERGLYCEMIA                           02 04/11/75
#14 ... 04/03/75 B6        ACUTE SITUATIONAL DISTRESS
#15 ... 07/24/75 FF        PAINFUL R FLANK ? 2ND TO SPRAIN
#.. ... ../../..   ....    ..........................................  (NEW)
#.. ... ../../..   ....    ..........................................  (NEW)
#.. ... ../../..   ....    ..........................................  (NEW)

= = = = = = = = = =I N A C T I V E   P R O B L E M S = = = = = = = = = = = =
  ACTION ONSET CODE STATUS                                        #VSTS RESOLVED
#04 ... 03/01/74           HYPEROPIA RX                             0 03/05/74
#05 ... 06/22/74           RT ROTATOR CUFF TEAR                    02 08/22/74
#06 ... 08/07/74 42        ARTERIOSCLEROSIS THORACIC AORTA         01 05/28/75
#07 ... 12/18/74 D1        URI                                     01 04/03/75
#10 ... 12/18/74 8B        BACTERURIA                              01 05/28/75
#11 ... 12/18/74 DA        OTITIS EXTERNA-BILAT                    01 05/28/75
#12 ... 12/18/74 9B        TRICH VAGINITIS                         01 05/28/75
#13 ... 04/03/75 1F        RASH                                    01 05/28/75

= = = = = = = = =C U R R E N T   M E D I C A T I O N S = = = = = = = = = = =
  START    REFILLED HCHD#                                     DOSAGE        DSP
12/03/74 12/18/74 50004 ACETAMINOPHEN   325 MG              2 TAB PRN      040
07/24/75  /  /    50448 BUFFERED ASPIRIN   10 GR (CAMA)     1 TAB Q6H      030
08/07/74 08/01/75 51723 DIAZEPAM (VALIUM)   10 MG           1 TAB PRN      030
05/28/75  /  /    51734 NUPERCAINAL OINTMENT                AD            001
02/19/74 07/24/75 53073 HYDROCHLOROTHIAZIDE (ESIDRIX)  50 MG 1 TAB BID     060
02/01/74 07/24/75 54430 METHYLDOPA (ALDOMET)  250 MG       1 TAB TID      090
05/28/75  /  /    59841 METAMUCIL                           AD            003
05/28/75  /  /    59942 SACCHARIN   32 MG                   AD            001

= = = = = = = = = =P R I O R   M E D I C A T I O N S = = = = = = = = = = = = =
  START    STOP    HCHD#                                    DOSAGE        DSP
12/18/74 05/28/75*51029 CEPACOL LOZENGES                    AD            020
12/18/74 05/28/75*51925 DIMETAPP EXTENTABS                  1 TAB Q8H      020
03/22/74 04/03/75*53201 IMIPRAMINE (TOFRANIL)   25 MG       1 TAB HS       030
12/18/74 05/28/75*54516 METRONIDAZOLE (FLAGYL)    250 MG    1 TAB TID      050
04/03/75 05/28/75*57104 TRIAMCINOLONE (KENALOG) CREAM       AD            002
12/18/74 05/28/75*58154 CORTISPORIN OTIC DROPS              AD            001
12/18/74 05/28/75*58492 AVC VAGINAL CREAM                   AD            001

= = = = =P A S T   H O S P I T A L I Z A T I O N   A N D   C A R E = = = = = =
DATE                                       PROVIDER(MD OR FACILITY)  RCD
06/74 #01 RT ROTATOR CUFF TEAR 2ND TO FALL  BTGH                      R

= = = = = = = = = =H E A L T H   I N F O R M A T I O N = = = = = = = = = = = =
------------SOCIOECONOMIC------------ :------------ANTHROPOMETRY------------
PREFERS TO SPEAK SPANISH              :WEIGHT: 192 LBS      HEIGHT: 60 IN.
OCCUPATION: HOUSEWIFE                 :WEIGHT/HEIGHT-SQ: 37.5  KG/MSQ
03 YEARS OF EDUCATION       GEO: 493G3 :------------HEALTH TESTING----------
BIRTHPLACE: PORT ARTHUR, TX           :QUESTIONNAIRE GIVEN: Y
MARRIED            FAMILY# 1736-02    :LAST MPS: 12/18/74
05 PERSONS IN HOUSEHOLD  ELIG CODE: 19 :VISION: ABNORM
------------HEALTH RISKS------------- :HEARING: ABNORMAL
FAMILY HX OF: DIABETES                :SCREENING LAB:     VDRL--NO DATA
ALLERGIC HX: NONE KNOWN               :HIGH SERUM GLUCOSE URINE MICRO-NO DATA
                                      :CYTOLOGY:  NO DATA
                                      :------------------PARITY---------------
C      M.                             :  17 PREGNANCIES    17 TERM BIRTHS
#06-85-10-0                           :     ABORT/MISC        PREMATURE
56 YR  M/F DOB: 07/05/19              :  15 LIVING CHILDREN
DR. SPECK                             ---------------------------------------
REPORT DATE:  08/05/75
                                      ELIGIBILITY EXPIRES: 12/11/75      C
```

Figure 10. Example of a Health-Illness Profile

for easy understanding of the instructions of the care providers, and to enhance the continuity of care between clinic and home. Operationally, they were to be generated from a set of standard plans for specific diseases and/or problems in which the selected instruction and comment subsets would be merged into a plan tailored for the particular individual. Similar plans had been used in the chronic care setting of the Texas Institute for Rehabilitation and Research, and it was hypothesized that they would have applicability in an ambulatory care setting as well. However, in the Casa environment, the need for verbal information exchange is more or less mandatory, since both language and literacy problems exist in the population served. In this situation, written information is of little value regardless of how it is generated. Even in settings where these problems do not exist, standard plans might be preprinted for those situations that occur most frequently. The preprinted plans might be supplemented with notes made by the clinic staff or by the patient. It does not seem necessary to automate the production of the documents in an ambulatory care environment. Instead, general health education programs, presented through audiovisual media can be (and were) used to achieve the same ends, especially when supplemented by concerned and communicative clinic staff.

ADMINISTRATIVE STATISTICS

The objective of statistical reporting is to provide indices of the performance of the clinic services, consumer satisfaction, and community health of the clinic population. It is possible to interrogate the data base of H-IPs to produce a variety of reports. These reports may be oriented by source, by time, or by problem.

Routine monthly reports prepared from our data base of H-IPs include: a tally of clinic visits according to age, socioeconomic characteristics and ethnic group of the patients, a summary tally of repeat visits, a "problem profile" which summarizes the number and frequency of specific problems diagnosed in the clinic during the month, and a "drug profile" which lists the classes of drugs dispensed in the clinic. Figure 11 shows and example of the monthly problem profile.

Ad hoc programs can be written to satisfy the user's request. A commonly used program is the "sick list" which produces a list of all patients who present with a specific problem and a statistical summary of the characteristics of these patients (Figure 12).

In summary, of the modules described above, the following have been fully implemented in two neighborhood clinics (Casa de Amigos and Sunnyside): patient identification, the Health-Illness Profile, and administrative statistics. The patient information file currently contains only the data base of Health-Illness Profiles.

PROBLEM PROFILE: NOVEMBER 1975

ENCOUNTERS FOR MOST FREQUENTLY NAMED PROBLEMS OR DIAGNOSES

PROBLEM	NUMBER OF ENCOUNTERS	FREQUENC⁻
HYPERTENSION/HYPERTENSIVE CARDIOVASCULAR DISEASE	127	6.9
UPPER RESPIRATORY INFECTION	109	6.0
DIABETES MELLITUS	90	4.9
PREGNANCY	90	4.9
OBESITY	74	4.0
MISCELLANEOUS MENTAL/EMOTIONAL PROBLEM	65	3.6
PAIN OR ACHE (ANY SITE)	49	2.7
URINARY TRACT INFECTION	43	2.4
ANXIETY	42	2.3
DEGENERATIVE ARTHRITIS/JOINT DISEASE	42	2.3
ACCIDENT/INJURY	36	2.0
OTITIS MEDIA	35	1.9
TUBERCULOSIS	33	1.8
POOR VISION/BLURRED VISION	32	1.7
IMPETIGO/ERYSIPELAS/PYODERMIA	30	1.6
VIRAL INFECTION (UNSPECIFIED SITE)	29	1.6
MISCELLANEOUS DERMATOLOGIC PROBLEM	29	1.6
MISCELLANEOUS EYE PROBLEM	27	1.5
DERMATIDES	26	1.4
SOCIO-ECONOMIC PROBLEM	25	1.4
CONSTIPATION	22	1.2
NON-VIRAL INFECTION (UNSPECIFIED SITE)	21	1.1
CORONARY ARTERY DISEASE	20	1.1
HEADACHES	19	1.0
CERVICITIS/CERVICAL POLYPS	18	1.0

Figure 11. Example of a Casa de Amigos Clinic "Problem Profile"

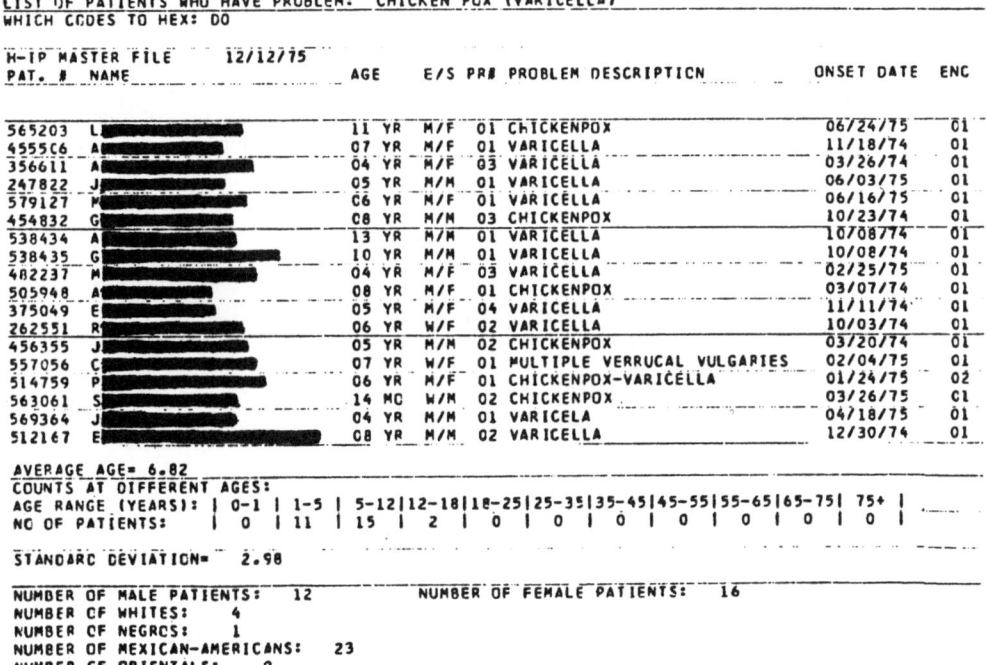

Figure 12. Truncated list of all Casa de Amigos patients with the diagnosis
of varicella

REFERENCES

1. Smith Muller, M.: National Health Expenditures, Fiscal Year 1975
    In Gibson, R.M.: Social Security Bulletin, February (1976) 3-20

2. Somers, A.R.: The Kaiser-Permanente Care Program--A Symposium.
    (New York: The Commonwealth Fund 1971)

3. Donabedian, A.: A Guide to Medical Care Administration, Vol. II: Medical
    Care Appraisal.
    (New York: American Public Health Association, Inc. 1969)

4. Fry, J.: Ambulatory Medical Care Data: Information for Patient Care in
    Office-Based Practice.
    Med. Care 11 (Suppl.) (1973) 35-40

5. Parker, A.: The Team Approach to Primary Care
    Neighborhood Health Center Seminar Program, Monograph Series Number 3.
    (University of California, Berkeley: University Extension 1972)

6. Cohen, S.N., Armstrong, M.F., Crouse, L., and Hunn, G.S.: A computer-Based
    System for Prospective Detection and Prevention of Drug Interactions.
    Drug Inform. J. 6 (1972) 81-86

7. Weed, L.L.: Medical Records that Guide and Teach.
    New Engl. J. Med. 278 (1968) 593-600, 652-657

8. Vallbona, C., Schade, C.P., Moffet, C.L., Speck, C.D., Osher, W.J., and Tristan,
    M.P.: Computer Support of Medical Decisions in Ambulatory Care.
    Meth. Inform. Med. 14 (April 1975) 55-62

9. Gotcher, Susan Beggs: A Computer Information System for an Ambulatory Care
    Facility. Master of Public Health Thesis.
    (University of Texas School of Public Health, Houston: June 1970)

10. Vallbona, C., and Gotcher, S.B.: A Plan for Computer-Aided Care in a Neighbor-
    hood Clinic. Proceedings of the 10th IBM Medical Symposium, Poughkeepsie, New
    York, 1970, pp. 79-88

BIBLIOGRAPHY

TEXT BOOKS

1. Giebink, G.A. and Hurst, L.: Computer Projects in Health Care.
    (University of Michigan, Ann Arbor: Health Administration Press 1975)

2. Collen, Morris F. (Edit.): Hospital Computer Systems.
    (New York, New York: John Wiley and Sons, Inc. 1974)

JOURNAL ARTICLES

Evaluation of Care Quality

1. Brook, R., and Stevenson, R.L.: Effectiveness of Patient Care in an Emergency
    Room.
    New Engl. J. Med. 283 (1970) 904-907

2. Donabedian, A.: A Guide to Medical Care Administration, Vol. II: Medical Care
    Appraisal.
    (New York: American Public Health Association, Inc. 1969)

3. Fessel, W.J., and Van Brundt, E.E.: Assessing Quality of Care from the Medical Record.
    New Engl. J. Med. 286 (1972) 134-138

4. Kroeger, H.H., et al.: The Office Practice of Internists. 1. The Feasibility of Evaluating Quality of Care.
    J. Amer. Med. Ass. 193 (1965) 371-376

5. Lembcke, P.A.: Medical Auditing by Scientific Methods.
    J. Amer. Med. Ass. 162 (1956) 646-655

6. Payne, B.C.: Continued Evolution of a System of Medical Care Appraisal.
    J. Amer. Med. Ass. 201 (1967) 526-540

7. Rosenfeld, L.S.: Quality of Medical Care in Hospitals.
    Amer. J. Public Health 47 (1957) 856-865

8. Sanazaro, P.J., and Williamson, J.W.: Physician Performance and Its Effects on Patients: A Classification Based on Reports by Internists, Surgeons, Pediatricians, and Obstetricians.
    Med. Care 8 (1970) 299-308

9. Starfield, B.: Health Services Research: A Working Model.
    New Engl. J. Med. 3 (1973) 132-135

10. Williamson, J.: Evaluating Quality of Patient Care: A Strategy Relating Outcome and Process Assessment.
    J. Amer. Med. Ass. 218 (1971) 564-569

11. Zemach, R.: Program Evaluation and System Control.
    Amer. J. Public Health 7 (1973) 607-609

Computerized Medical Information Systems

1. Ayers, W.R., et al.: Mobilizing the Emergency Room Record. A Case Study in the Capture of Technology Developed Elsewhere for Use in Health Care Delivery.
    Comput. Biol. Med. 3 (1973) 153-163

2. Bolinger, R.E., Price, S., and Kyner, J.L.: Computerized Management of the Outpatient Diabetic.
    J. Amer. Med. Ass. 216 (1971) 1779-1782

3. Cohen, S.N., Armstrong, M.F., Crouse, L., and Hunn, G.S.: A Computer-Based System for Prospective Detection and Prevention of Drug Interactions.
    Drug Inform. J. 6 (1972) 81-86.

4. Collen, M.: Automated Health Testing.
    In M. Collen (Edit.): Hospital Computer Systems.
    (New York: John Wiley and Sons, Inc. 1974)

5. Côté, R.: Use of Nomenclature of Medicine in a Medical Information Management System. Proceedings of MEDIS 73, Osaka, 1973, pp. 324-331.

6. Fries, J.F.: Time-Oriented Patient Records and a Computer Databank.
    J. Amer. Med. Ass. 222 (1972) 1536-1542

7. Griest, H.J., Van Cura, L.J., Kneppreth, N.P.: A Computer Interview for Emergency Room Patients.
    Comput. Biomed. Res. 6 (June 1973) 257-265

8. Grossman, J.H., Barnett, G.O., Kolpsell, T.D., et al.: An Automated Medical Record System.
    J. Amer. Med. Ass. 224 (1973) 1616-1621

9. Komaroff, A.L., Black, W.L., Flately, M., Knopp, R.H., Reiffen, B., and
    Sherman, H.: Protocols for Physician Assistants: Management of Diabetes
    and Hypertension.
    New Engl. J. Med. 133 (1974) 294-299

10. Lenoski, E.F., et al.: Computer Processing of Pediatric Emergency Room Data.
    J. Amer. Med. Ass. 204 (1968) 797-804

11. Levy, R.P., Cammarn, M.R., and Smith, M.J.: Computer Handling of Ambulatory
    Clinic Records
    J. Amer. Med. Ass. 190 (1964) 1033-1037

12. Vallbona, C., Quirch, J., Moffet, C.L., and Speck, C.D.: The Health-Illness
    Profile: An Essential Component of the Ambulatory Medical Record.
    Med. Care 11 (1973) 117-124

13. Vallbona, C., Tobias, P.R., Moffet, C., et al.: Computer Support for a
    Neighborhood Health Clinic: Design and Implementation.
    IEEE Trans. Biomed. Engin. 20 (1973) 180-184

14. Vallbona, C., and Speck, C.D.: An Experience With Computer Applications in
    Ambulatory Care. Proceedings of MEDIS '75, Tokyo, October 1975, pp. 124-131.
    (Osaka: Kansai Institute of Information Systems 1975)

15. Vickery, D.M., et al.: Computer Support of Paramedical Personnel: The Question
    of Quality Control.
    In Anderson, J., and Forsythe, M. (Edits.): MEDINFO '74, Preprints, pp. 281-287.
    (Amsterdam--New York: North-Holland Publishing Company 1974)

16. Warner, H.: Health Evaluation Through Logical Processing: HELP. Proceedings
    of MEDIS '73, Osaka, 1973, pp. 197-203.
    (Osaka: Kansai Institute of Information Systems 1973)

ACKNOWLEDGEMENTS

    The authors wish to acknowledge the collaboration of Drs. Charles P. Schade and
Carlos D. Speck and of Mrs. Alicia Reyes in the development and implementation of
the computerized patient information system for a neighborhood clinic. They acknow-
ledge also the contribution of Ms. Norma R. Cobb in compiling material describing
health care systems, and the assistance of Ms. Valory Pavlik in the editing and preparation of the manuscript.

INFORMATION SYSTEMS IN PUBLIC HEALTH

J. CHAPERON, C. CHASTANG, B. DOYON, M. GOLDBERG, P. GOLDBERG and P. LEBEUX

I. GOALS AND ORGANIZATION OF THE PUBLIC HEALTH SYSTEM

In the recent years the complexity of the health care system has considerably increased due to development of hospital technology. The cost of medical technology
can only explain the current   enormous increase in health   expenditures. Therefore, the government planners as well as the users of the health care system, and
more recently medical personnel are looking for better tools to analyse the health
care system, in order to set up plans for the future. By health care system, we
mean all the means working towards a change in a population's state of health. Up
to now, the system was not studied as a whole and notions of health, sickness,
supply, demand, need and efficiency ... were treated as if they were completely
unambiguous. This has led the advanced industrialized countries to face the following paradox : "How is it that life expectancy is no longer increasing, whereas
health expenses have gone up considerably ?". At the same time, there is currently
a growing tendancy to question the efficiency of modern medicine in every sphere[VII]

I.1. FROM "NEED" TO "STATE OF HEALTH"

As far as health is concerned, the term "need" is extremely vague and refers to
several different meanings :

a) the needs of the economic system : since medicine constitutes a means of maintaining the productivity of a population, need can be expressed, for example, by
   the desire to minimize the number of work days lost on account of illness.

b) the needs of the health system itself : the medical profession in particular,
   uses certain types of medical practices in preference to others and tries to justify their choice. Furthermore, it naturally tends to - more or less consciously -
   increase the need for medical services.

c) the individual's needs : here it may be a question of
   . a physiological necessity : pain, invalidism
   . a vague feeling, related to the definition of health established by the World
     Health Organization (WHO) : "Health is a state of complete physical, mental
     and social well-being and not merely the absence of disease or infirmity".
   . a reaction to conditioning, for example as the result of a television program
     showing the "miracles" accomplished by an extremely specialised type of medi-
     cine. This kind of conditioning reinforces the feelings mentioned above, and
     can go as far as to deny the very possibility of illness and of death.

This qualitative notion of need must therefore be defined more precisely by using
a more quantitative concept : the state of health, as a biological and social individual and collective phenomenon.

To be operative, this notion must take into   account a multidimensionnal description of possible states. During his or her lifetime, an individual, may go through
different states : he or she can return to an earlier state after a crisis, remain
in an intermediary state, etc ...

It is not the purpose of this paper to give a detailed description of these states, but three remarks can be made :

1) first of all, it is only possible to set up a normative typology of these states, which implies a certain hierarchy. The problem is to define this hierarchy and its purpose, in each particular case studied.

2) these states of health and the changes they under-go are not purely the product of medical activity ; they depend on a multitude of interdependant heterogeneous factors : heredity, environment, life style, socio-cultural level, and so on. For example, it is well known that the mortality rate of a population diminishes as literacy increases and the quality of its drinking water improves. It is equally well known that, statistically, executives do not suffer from the same diseases as workers.

   In some cases, non-medical factors are even used to define particularly "high risk sub-populations".

3) In the description of these states may enter the frequency and type of illnesses affecting the population. This is usually called "morbidity". But this term is itself ambiguous and at least three "levels" of morbidity can be distinguished :

   - "objective" morbidity : this is an ideal. It would refer to all morbid phenomena such as could be revealed by a multiphasic health screening of the entire population and taking into account all the medical knowledge at a given moment as well as the norms in use at that time.

   - diagnosed morbidity : this is revealed when the subject makes use of the health system. Two essential points should be stressed :

     . the population using the system is not a representative sample of the entire population ;
     . this notion reflects more the specificity and performance of the institution itself than the real state of health of a population. For example, morbidity diagnosed by the general practitioners is not the same as that diagnosed by highly specialized hospital services.

   - "felt" morbidity : this is the kind experienced by the patient in relation to what he considers as normal or abnormal. This notion obviously is not taken into account by previous ones, not only because there exist illnesses unknown to the subjects but also because, for example, a chronic illness will be so much a part of a person's life that he or she won't even be aware of it any more. In this domain there is no anthropological vital minimum.

I.2. THE GOALS OF THE HEALTH SYSTEM

The main goal of a health policy is to use and improve the system to maintain the majority of the population in a certain ideal state which is above a minimum level. The thresholds can vary considerably, according to whoever defines them and to the goals to be achieved. In particular, the thresholds will most likely differ according to whether one is interested in

1) the permanent overall functioning of the system : observation of the entire population on all fronts ;

2) the specific functioning of a sector concerning either a particular population (pregnant women for example) or a particular problem (such as cardiovascular pathology).

Finally, within the scope of a public health program, two strategies may be defined :

1) Improving the utilization of existing resources without changing the level of resources. For example : design a better organization of the hospital such that the greatest number of patients can be treated in the shortest amount of time.

2) Defining an objective expressed in terms of one or several indicators and estimate the new resources to be provided. For example : lowering of infant mortality

and estimating of the funds needed to meet this objective possibility, the first
stage won't be merely to fight the illness but to study the problem.

It should be noticed that these strategies   are not incompatible in practice, and
that the latter strategy is not necessarily the most expensive one. If a problem
is studied very carefully and if the solutions are properly implemented, a secondary
benefit be obtained by decreasing in other sectors.

I.3. THE RESOURCES OF THE SYSTEM

The system's resources may be broken down into 4 categories :

- intellectual : state of science, direction of research in progress
- material : medical centers, hospitals, doctors' offices ...
            consumable products (drugs for example)
            non-consumable products (equipment)
- human : medical, paramedical, and administrative personnel whose activity must be
          considered in three different areas :
            . daily service to the population
            . training of new personnel
            . research
- institutional : material and human resources are brought together and organized
                  in various institutions : hospitals, dispensaries, variously spe-
                  cialized prevention organizations, isolated individuals.

Their functions are regulated by all sorts of laws, in which are included health
insurance plans. The way they operate can sometimes have a great influence on the
development of one type of practice or another (For example, medical bills that are
covered compared with those that are not).

It was noted above that the population's state of health does not depend solely on
the health system. It is then a question of knowing whether or not to take into consideration as integral parts of the health system factors such as the fight against
pollution, research in city-planning, etc. If the analysis is to be at all useful,
a limit must be defined, but it is difficult to say where it should be and the
choice of such a limit is debatable.

II. THE HEALTH CARE SYSTEM'S NEEDS : DATA AND METHODS

A health care program can be defined as the set of means which enables the decision
makers to modify some characteristics of the health care system.

Whatever type of health care program is adopted, those responsible for putting it
into practice should procede as follows :

a) first of all, according to the needs and resources of the health system, objectives must be precisely defined (in economic terms, in terms of the level of
   health) and so must the means necessary for achieving these objectives.

b) Then, what may generally be called a "cost-benefit" analysis must be undertaken
   to provide an estimate of the results expected compared with the resources com-
   mited to achieving them. It must be stressed here that in the area of health, the
   notion of "benefits" is very broad, and, depending on the point of view, it may
   even go against the economic interest of the community. For example, detection
   of a particular type of illness may be more expensive (the cost itself of detecting the disease but also the cost of treating the patients who are affected)
   than a passive attitude : defining the benefit in such a case is therefore above
   all an act of a "political" nature. The conclusion of a preliminary study will
   lead either to undertaking the program as it has been defined in the first stage,
   or to modifying the objectives and/or the means.

c) Once the decision has been made, a fundamental step will consist in a follow-up evaluation of the results according to the objectives chosen earlier. Of course depending on the case, this evaluation can take place while the program is in progress or at once at the end of a timely program.

According to the results of this evaluation, it may be decided that the aims and/or the means need to be modified.

The general strategy described above can visualized in the diagram below :

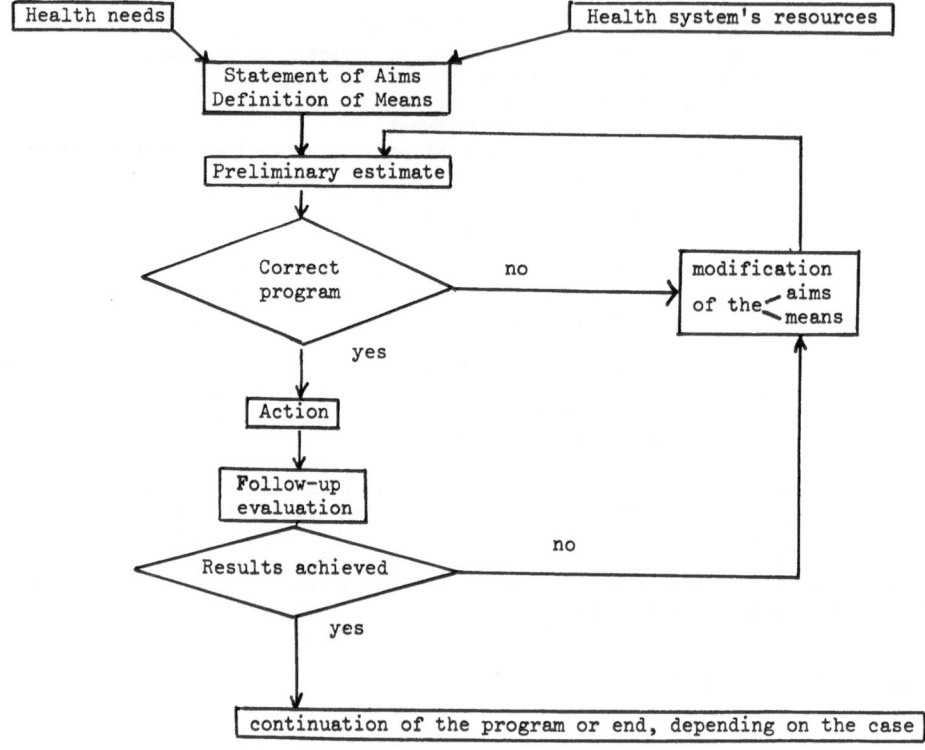

It will be noticed that this schema implies that at every stage of the process a certain amount of data as well as methods of processing such data be available.

The first stage – statement of goals, definition of means – requires that the states of health to be treated, as well as the health system's resources, be known. It is also necessary to have a precise definition of both internal relationships within the two sub-systems (state of health, resources) and the links between them.

The second and third stages – preliminary estimate and follow-up evaluation – also imply the knowledge of the same type   of data   and the use of appropriate evaluation methods. In other words, as far as methodology is concerned, every health program requires the use of a certain number of tools corresponding to the following needs :

1) Measure : it was stated that, in the domain of health, decisions are of a political nature ; but in this   framework, to make decisions as well as to estimate and evaluate their results, certain standards must be available. These are called health indicators [17, 18] . A health indicator may be defined as the value

of a variable which measures a phenomenon connected with health in view of making a _comparison_ : a temporal comparison (is a given pathological phenomenon increasing or decreasing and by how much ?), a spatial comparison (regional, national or even international), a social comparison (is a given phenomenon linked to a particular socio-professional category ?), etc.

A reliable health indicator which is usually composed of various basic data must have two essential qualities :

- it must reflect   as faithfully as possible the phenomenon it is supposed to represent.

- a health indicator is above all a criterion corresponding to a precise objective it is therefore first and foremost the use it is intended for,   which will orient the choice of such an indicator. A health indicator must therefore reflect its user's point of view : different indicator   will in effect be chosen to measure one and the same phenomenon according to the user's point of view. For instance, it is likely that an insurance organization will classify illnesses in function of the average cost of a treatment it will **have to** cover while a planner in charge of preventive medicine will classify them according to their causes, which he is responsible for fighting. In both cases, health indicators that reflect the frequency of various illnesses can be established, but they won't be identical. So, in order to define indicators, it is necessary to study the possible interactions between the various data which compose an indicator as well as the interactions between indicators.

Therefore, as far as methodology is concerned, the most important requirement to be **fulfilled** is the identification of measurable parameters which can be used as health indicators.

2) Once a health indicator reflecting a given phenomenon has been set up, the means for measuring it should be defined. Thus, for each of the data that enter into the indicator, it is necessary to define the statistical unit to which the measure refers (country, area, etc ...), the periodicity and the way to collect it. The second most important methodological requirement is therefore the implementation of the procedure to collect the data which make up the health indicators.

It should be noted that this requirement is considerably tied with the previous one : it is useless to define an indicator if its basic data components cannot be measured. The definition of an indicator and the study of the means to measure it must therefore be carried out concurently.

3) When the first two requirements are met they provide a means of obtaining the data necessary for a preliminary estimate and a   follow-up evaluation of the results of a health program. But it is also necessary to be able to use these data correctly. So methods of estimating and evaluating must be available.

To fulfill these three basic requirements of any coherent health program, a certain number of tools must be used or developed.

III. THE TOOLS

III.1. Identification of parameters affecting   health phenomena and their inter-relationship : definition of health indicators

There are two steps (1) observation of the health system in order to define hypotheses about useful factors and (2) statistical validation of theses hypotheses.

III.1.1. Classification of health indicators

It is possible to set up a broad classification of possible health indicators starting from a simplified diagram of factors affecting states of health:

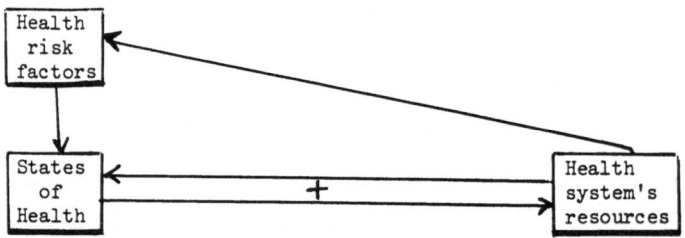

This diagram brings out interactions between the main elements which influence a population's level of health : various risks factors have a negative effect on states of health : this creates needs bringing into play the resources of the system, which should have a positive effect on the states of health and a negative one on risk factors.

According to the diagram, health indicators can be divided two categories : those which can be used in order to measure the states of health of the population, and those which measure the factors that influence these states in a negative or positive way (risk factors and resources).

a) Indicators measuring the factors affecting states of health

the risk factors can be divided into :

- environment-linked risks : transportation, work, housing conditions, various types of "addiction" (tobacco, alcohol, medicines, "hard" drugs) diet, pollution (air, water ...) climate ...

- individual risks : genetic characteristics, old age, obesity, high blood pressure, pregnancy ...

According to the objectives, various risk indicators can be established : for example, the average number of kilometers traveled per year in a car can be a risk indicator corresponding to the risk of highway accident.

Protection indicators (a name often given to resources indicators) : at first sight there are no specific problems involved in establishing indicators that would allow us to know the state of various resources described above (intellectual, material, human...). However, it must be pointed out how dialectic the definition of an indicator really is : for example, drug comsumption, is often considered as a protection factor in view of the therapeutic effect of drugs, but it is also a risk factor if side effects are taken into account. Similarly, the density of physicians in a population is often taken as a protection indicator but it can be considered as a risk factor, if the iatrogenic power of physicians is considered.

b) State of health indicators

They represent the biggest problem for at least two reasons : the first one is the difficulty in classifying states of health. At present, most state of health indicators - including mortality indicators - are based on classifications or nomenclatures such as the International Classification of Diseases (ICD) of the WHO [12] or the Systematized Nomenclature of Pathology (SNOP) [3, 14] , which are the most widely used in the world. ICD is a way of classifying diseases and causes of death according to their etiology for the system affected : for instance, the infectious diseases or the nervous system groups are found in ICD. SNOP is a descriptive classification of the illnesses whereby each is described by four types of keywords : T keywords designate the Topography of lesions : M keywords their Morphology, that is the type of lesion ; E keywords their Etiology and F keywords the Functional problems created by the disease.

The main problem with these classifications in their present state is that they only tell you whether or not people have a given illness ; they don't inform you as the true state of health of individuals. Only very partial indications can be deduced from these negative indicators - especially when the purpose is to evaluate the results of the use of the health system's resources. This is particularly true for chronic ailments, which an ever-growing proportion of illnesses in advanced societies. Knowing that an individual has, for example, chronic bronchitis, does not tell much about his or her state of health. Since in the present state of medical technology this individual will remain a victim of bronchitis, in spite of any treatment he or she may receive, the means of evaluating a treatment which might improve his or her state of health, are not provided by such methods. It is surely the lack of good state of health indicators that has led certain people to say that the healt system is inefficient if not harmful (see ILLICH [VII] in particular).

The ideal solution to this problem would probably be the use of data contained in individual medical records : but in the present state of the art it is practically impossible, except perhaps in a very few specific cases.

Some attemps, however, have been made to define health level indicators. CUYER, LAVERS and WILLIAMS [5] have proposed a two-dimensional indicator taking into account intensity and length of the illness. The intensity is itself broken down into two components : pain and restriction of activity, which provide a means of establishing a scale of intensity. The indicator set up in this way can theoretically provide a way of evaluating the efficacity of a given treatment on both dimensions either simultaneously or at different times. It can also be used to compare different illnesses, and in this way to express a population's state of health.

FANSHEL and BUSH [IV] have also defined an indicator using eleven states based on the restriction of activity imposed by the illness, and which go from feeling well to death. At a given moment, each individual is in one state and one state only, but with a certain probability of going into another (prognostic). A population can thus be represented by taking into account both how serious the illness is and what its probability of evolving is. This is a dynamic indicator which allows for making various comparisons.

The second major problem connected with health state indicators is the access to the data that goes into the composition of these indicators. As mentioned above, three kinds of morbidity can be distinguished, with respect to the source of information and to the various bias associated with these sources :

- felt morbidity : it is "encoded" by the individual himself and may consequently be different depending on his or her psychology and social position and the social and cultural background from which he or she comes.
- diagnosed morbidity : it is "encoded" by health professionals. So it may differ greatly according to level of specialization and to the different schools of thought especially at the national or international level. Medical personnel act as a filter and diagnosed morbidity reflects perhaps to a greater degree the development of the health institutions then the health level of a population. For example, it is a well-known fact that when a specialist physician set up his or her practice in a place where no specialis of the same pathology previously existed so that an increase of the diagnosed morbidity of this pathology will result in this area.

Morever, the evolution of medical knowledge and institutional structures make the interpretation of temporal comparisons of diagnosed morbidity very difficult.

- objective morbidity : an objective measure does not rely on the instruments of

measurement ; but in health systems it is known that means always depend on the
technical, cultural, social and political environment. What is defined as "objective morbidity" must reflect this environment. But the basic point here is that
the "encoding" of morbidity could be perfectly controlled   by use of systematic
data collection processes such as comprehensive health screening or specific
enquiries.

III.1.2. Epidemiological methods

When it is believed that certain factors affect a given aspect of health in some
way, these hypotheses must be confirmed and the relationship existing between these
factors must be clearly defined.

Let us take the following problem : we want to define an indicator   of the risk
related to pregnancy. One can think that factors such as the age, the number of
previous pregnancies, the existence of given diseases, the habitation place, the
distance to the nearest hospital, etc ... are important ones. But it is necessary to examine each of them, to search some possible correlations between them
- that would allow to take only a few into account - and to order them in respect
with some criteria, such as the nature of the risk for example.

This is the task of epidemiology backed up by statistical methods which are nearly
always based on multivariate analysis.

It is not the purpose of this paper to study multivariate statistical methods
(cf "Decision Making Methods"), but a simple example will be given considering
that there is a connection between people's age and the kind of illnesses they suffer from, is it possible to classify the population by age according to the types
of illness encountered ? The purpose of this investigation would be to define a
risk indicator which would   determine the probability of a person's being affected by such and such illnesses when he or she is a given number of years old.
The following example shows how a multivariate statistical method (Factorial correspondence analysis) provides a good basis for approaching the problem [10] .

Every year, a French Organization called IDREM conducts a survey based on a certain
amount of data collected by 1600 physicians every time they see patients. In this
 way it has been possible, using 74,000 medical consultations as a sample, to set
up a contingency table comparing the 39 most frequent illnesses with the patients'
age divided into 11 categories (less than 9 months old, from 9 months to 2 1/2
years, etc ...). It is interesting to study this table, not only to compare the
various illnesses with the different age categories but also to see the way each
illness spread out among the age categories :

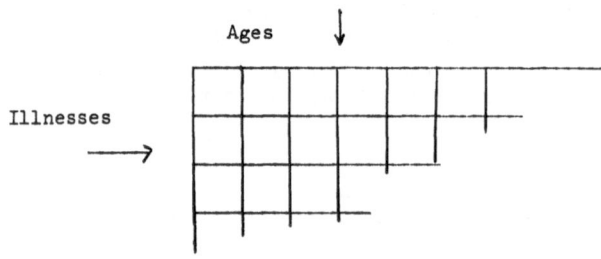

(see next page)

Correspondence analysis makes it possible to represent visually, in a sub-space
of small dimensions, the age categories and illnesses (see figure A).

In this sub-space, if two categories are close to each other, it means that the
same type of illness affects them ; conversely, two illnesses are close to each

195

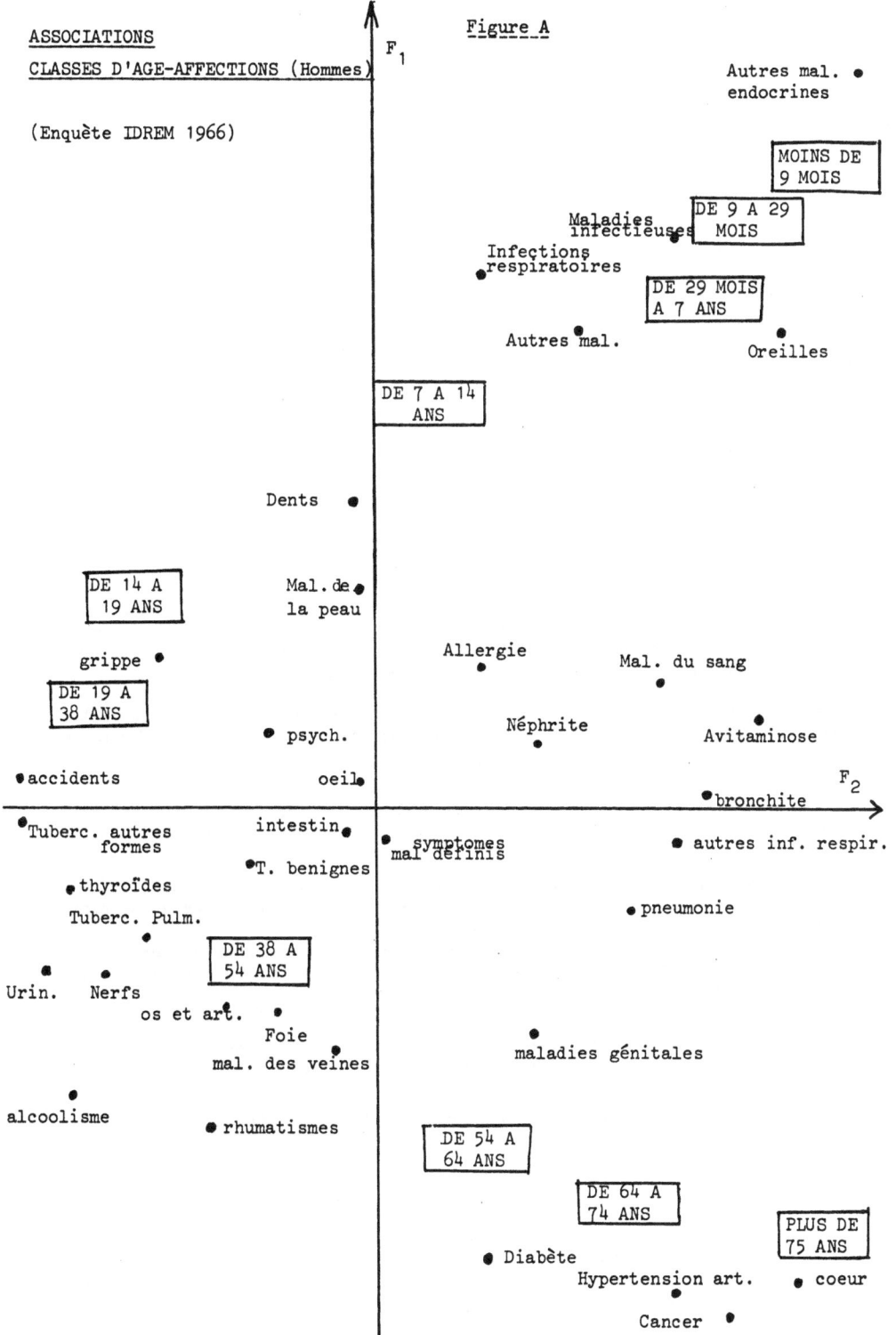

ASSOCIATIONS
CLASSES D'AGE-AFFECTIONS (Hommes)

(Enquête IDREM 1966)

Figure A

F_1

Autres mal. •
endocrines

MOINS DE
9 MOIS

DE 9 A 29
MOIS

Maladies
infectieuses

Infections
respiratoires

DE 29 MOIS
A 7 ANS

Autres mal.

Oreilles

DE 7 A 14
ANS

Dents •

DE 14 A
19 ANS

Mal. de •
la peau

grippe •

Allergie

Mal. du sang

DE 19 A
38 ANS

• psych.

Néphrite

Avitaminose

F_2

• accidents

oeil •

• bronchite

Tuberc. autres
formes

intestin •

• symptomes
mal définis

• autres inf. respir.

• T. benignes

• thyroïdes

Tuberc. Pulm.

• pneumonie

DE 38 A
54 ANS

•
Urin. Nerfs

os et art. •

Foie

mal. des veines

maladies génitales

•
alcoolisme

• rhumatismes

DE 54 A
64 ANS

DE 64 A
74 ANS

PLUS DE
75 ANS

• Diabète

Hypertension art.

• coeur

Cancer •

other when their age profile is close. Furthermore, the proximity of an age category and an illness has a specific meaning because an illness is surrounded by the age categories frequently affected by this particular type of illness and vice versa.

Naturally, the analysis of this figure reconstitutes the order of the age categories, each one being close to its immediate neighbors.

This kind of statistical analysis obviously represents no more than a first stage. But it shows the basic role played by multivariate methods in epidemiology.

III.2. Measuring parameters

III.2.1. Data collection

Once the appropriate parameters have been defined, the procedure of collecting data should be set forth : what subjects should data be gathered about ? How much time should be alloted for collecting the information ?

a. The spatial dimension

In a schematic fashion, exhaustive collections pertaining to the entire population are the opposite of samplings studying representative samples of the population.

a_1. The exhaustive collection

The exhaustive collection aims at collecting one or several parameters for all statistical units (individuals, families, country).

Thus official records provide information about the dates of birth, marriage, and death of individuals and their families. Similarly, the WHO's records of diseases (the outbreak of which must be officially declared) provides data on a daily basis about the progress of such diseases.

However, the exhaustive collection meets up with many problems which may make it inoperative as it is, insofar as determining morbidity is concerned. The main reasons are :

- health care structures are quite different from one country to another : in France for example, any patient may consult a doctor at his office or in a dispensary or in a hospital ; therefore it would be necessary to set up a multitude of data collection centers.

  This obligation entails certain consequences   for it will be necessary,
  1) to make the data to be collected as objective as possible by using simple criteria that every one agrees upon
  2) to produce a simple collection scheme so as not to overburden tha data collectors (but this simplification often robs the collected data of the interest it may have)
  3) to set up an organization to coordinate and gather the data

- moreover, an individual, within the same health care structure, may be counted several times (chronicity, morbidity) and this may bias the evaluation of the results.

  So, with respect to this type of exhaustive collection, the drawbacks seem to be numerous

  - the obligation to set up and maintain a complex system is costly ;
  - the data collected are necessarily reduced and approximative, and not always connected with the aimed-for objective ;
  - the results of such studies are arrived at only after long periods of time which are often incompatible with the nature of the problem being studied ;
  - finally, it often happens that some statistical units are not counted at all while others are counted more than once.

However, it shouldn't be concluded from this that such collections should be forbidden. In effect, the ability to collect data strikes us as one of the essential tasks of a health system.

For instance, it involves the obligation to report infectious diseases in order to rapidly detect potential epidemics. Similarly, it is the only way to detect rare phenomena.

So having the framework for an exhaustive data collection provides a health system with a general warning apparatus.

a_2. Samplings

A sampling may be defined as the study of a representative sub-group of statistical units, the purpose of which is to infer to the entire group of statistical units.

Every one knows about public opinion polls : their aims is to evaluate voters' attitude by using a small portion of the population, 2500 voters, for example, as a sample.

The statistical unit is not always the individual ; it can be families, living quarters, hospitals, regions, even countries.

The sampling methods require fewer data collectors and provide more precise information of a higher quality (owing to the specificity of the collection) for less money and shorter amount of time.

In some cases, the sampling methods is the only one possible due to the high cost of obtaining certain data (time consuming examinations) or to the underdeveloped nature of the existing health system.

The methodology of samplings is well known to-day. The following methods may be used : random sampling, are based on random selection of statistical units, which may be done once or any number of times. The simplest random sampling consists of randomly drawing from all the statistical units a sample of statistical units.

In the stratified sampling, the random selection is made within homogeneous sub-groups (strata) of the population, which allows for increased precision in the estimates made.

In the cluster sampling, groups of statistical units (clusters) are selected at random and the study focuses on all the statistical units of the clusters that were selected. Thus a particular hospital department can constitute a cluster of patients, statistical units to be studied. The cluster sampling therefore makes it possible to carry out at a lower cost a study of statistical units grouped together by function.

This various types of sampling can be used together in multilevel samplings. Other samplings are not based on random selection : the people conducting the sampling have to find the proper subjects so that the sample thus created resembles the characteristics of the population as a whole.

b) The temporal dimension

Sampling whose objective is a single collection of data on each statistical unit are called transversal samplings and are the opposite of longitudinal samplings which make it possible to trace the evolution of statistical units.

Official records of birth, marriage and death are exhaustive longitudinal collections whereas a referendum constitues a transversal collection.

Many forms of transition exist between these two types : a transversal collection can accomplish a longitudinal observation of the population if the collecting of data is undertaken on sub-groups of statistical units at various times. Similarly, repeating transversal samplings results in the obtention of longitudinal data.

In fact longitudinal samplings are rare because they are expensive and difficult to carry out. Only some samplings pertaining to chronic or malignant ailments can really be considered longitudinal at the present time.

III.2.2. Recording of health data

We have seen how data may be collected either in a specific way, by samplings, or in an exhaustive way. With respect to the former method, which corresponds to the needs of a specific health program, the problem of retrieval of the data hardly arises, because the data are usually collected and processed in a centralized manner during a brief period.

On the other hand, for the exhaustive collection method which correspond to a system of general observation over an indefinite period of time, the problems of spatial breakdown of data sources and their evolution in time arise again if the data is to be used.

It must be said at the outset that no satisfactory solution to this very broad problem exists at the present time. In various countries, however, (Scandinavia and West Germany in particular) attempts have been made to set up health data bases.

Two major approaches have been taken :

- the centralized approach involving the creation of a central data base : the organization in charge defines the data it considers useful as well as the means of collecting the data and the different sources that will provide it. This method would appear to be the only one possible when the various local data sources do not possess computer facilities. This is the way the WHO, for example, procedes for its morbidity and mortality statistics.

- the hierarchical approach presupposes the existence of local data bases which would already be putting together an exhaustive collection for their own use. Thus a central organization familiar with the contents of each of the local data bases can be connected - either directly or through intermediairy gathering centers - to the local bases and can obtain from them the desired data when necessary. A project of this type is currently being studied for use in the city of BERLIN.

Such data bases, relying on collections of personal data coming from individuals obvioulsy pose the problem of the privacy and safety of the data.

III.3. MODELISATION OF HEALTH CARE SYSTEM

In the previous chapter, the necessity of health indicators was stressed, and various methods of collection and storage were described. The next step is building of a model to study the dynamics of the system. This phase is indeed quite difficult but even if the model is only approximative, it can be used to study specific interaction or to evaluate several alternatives before implementation. In most of the cases, evaluation is done a posteriori by measuring indicators for example and by comparing them with the objectives.

The theory of modelisation is applicable to the design of large models such as the health care system is still at an early state of development.

III.3.1. System analysis

According to system analysis, a system can be viewed as a black box with several input flows (information, energy, resources ...). These inputs are expressed by quantified variables and relations between these variables. The outputs are also expressed by quantified variables such as levels, means, trends, which give the state of the system at a given time.

Usually, the system can be decomposed into several sectors which are interconnected by various flows and feedback loops. The goal of the system analysis is to build a model or the real system in which the output parameters are functions of the input parameters. It is therefore possible to compute the values of the output variables from the values of the . input variables. Ideally, such a model can be used to predict the behaviour of the real system when the inputs are modified.

For instance, a health care system can be viewed as a complex dynamic system [V] which can be described by several equations in which the system is represented by level variables and flow variables expressing the health resources, manpower environment ... and the output variables are given by the health status of a population expressed either by morbidity levels or by more sophisticated health status indicators [IV] .

III.3.2. Operation research models

Operation research models are used whenever the sytem or a subsystem can be described by a set of equations and inequations which express respectively the rules and contraints of the systems.

A given system can be analysed from different points of view and with each of these points of view it is necessary to define an objective function which measures the performance of the system according to the point of view chosen.

Once the objective function has been defined, the problem is usually to maximize or minimize this function to find the optimal solution under the contraints of the system.

A system such as the health care system can be viewed quite differently by the patients, the physicians and the insurance companies and it is therefore difficult to use this method because each model of the same system may have different constraints which might lead to different optimal solutions. However, some specific subsytems may be successfully represented by operation research models. In particular, this type of model is often more adapted to specific problems encountered in hospital management such as menu planning [2] or allocation of resources. For more complex systems such as health care systems, it is more appropriate to use simulation models.

III 3 3 Simulation models

Simulation models are used whenever the dynamics of a system cannot be studied analytically. In general, the scientific approach is based on the experimental observation of a system in the real world and a mathematical model is build to predict the behaviour of the system in the future.

Such an approach is usually decomposed in four steps :

- experiments and observations of the real system - this step presupposes that the experiments are reproducible ;
- formulation of hypothesis and laws about the system ;
- building of a model according to the hypothesis and laws discovered ;
- testing the validity of the model and comparing the results obtained by the experiments and those obtained by the model.

Once these steps have been completed, the model is considered operational until a new experiment invalidates the hypothesis of the laws used in the model.

Simulation models are justified each time one of the preceding steps is impeded by the complexity or the nature of the system.

For instance, it may be impossible or too costly to observe the real system (either because it is a living systel on which some experiments are impossible or because experiments are not reproducible : social systels). There may be too much hypothesis   laws and equation fully describe the system.

The model may be impossible to solve analytically or it may be impossible or too costly to do the experiments which would validate the model (social systems for instance).

The time involved to do the experiments or validation on the system might be to long. In these case, a simulation model can be used to perform experiments and test hypothesis on the model itself instead of the real sytem.

Therefore the goal of a simulation model is to study a representation of the real system by allowing experiments which would have been impossible to perform on the real system.

This types of model can be used to compare different scenarios and although it might not be possible to find an optimal solution, this method may be useful to choose the most satisfactory solution and help decision making process.

The implementation of such models can be done in two phases : the modelisation phase during which the model is designed and the simulation phase during which experiments are performed and analyzed.

The modelisation   phase can be itself decomposed in the following steps :
- observation and data collection on the real system
- formulation of model (inputs, outputs, relations and laws describing the model)
- estimation of the parameters' values
- evaluation of the model (consistency and logical structure of the model)

The simulation phase can be decomposed in the following steps :
- programming of the model
- preparation of the simulation experiments (choice of hypothesis, scenarios, results to be observed ...)
- analysis of the results of simulation experiments
- validation of the model.

Such models have been implemented for regional health system design [13] and to help decision making in large public health agency [15] .

The most important model of this type is currently developed by the MEDICIS project sponsored by the Ministery of Social Affairs in QUEBEC [VI] .

The model is a dynamic model with multiple feedbacks in which the results can interact with the inputs of the models. This is done by introducing delays and continuous flows in the model (funding, demand, personnel, materials, equipments, information, etc ...) such that each flow may modify the level of the inputs and the rate of each flow may be controlled by the levels of the input flows.

A model of this type is currently being used for planification and policy making in the health care system in Quebec.

IV. A CASE STUDY

The case we are about to expose here   was chosen for its relative simplicity, because it is related to a very limited medical problem. It is incomplete insofar as it does not go beyond the preliminary estimate of the results of a health program. In fact, despite the positive results of the preliminary estimate, the corresponding program was not carried out. However such as it is, it seems interesting enough for it provides an example of most of the methods described above.

The study was made by F. FABRE and J.M. GRANDMONT [6] in 1968. The purpose of this study was to find an answer to the following question : is early systematic detection of cervical cancer effective and economically possible, and, if so, what are the means necessary ? The point of departure for this study was the most recent medical knowledge about cancer detection and means of treatment as well as data on death rates linked to this disease.

IV.1. The medical problem

Putting it simply, it can be said that 5 different stages of cervical cancer can be observed, with the following percentages of cure after treatment :

$$
\begin{array}{llll}
S & 0 & : & \text{practically always cured} \\
S & 1 & : & 70 \% \\
S & 2 & : & 50 \% \\
S & 3 & : & 30 \% \\
S & 4 & : & 11 \%
\end{array}
$$

It appears from this data that the earlier the treatment, the better the chances of being cured.

The main difficulty comes from the fact that the stage 0, for which medical tech- nology is the most effective, gives no warning signals, that would lead the patient to consult a doctor : only a systematic examination can detect a stage 0 cervical cancer. There are in fact very simple methods of examination which can be done at Stage 0. Then,if necessary, they can be followed by more precise types of exa- mination.

This kind of systematic detection of cervical cancer will therefore appear useful because means of detection and appropriate treatment are available.

IV. 2. The method

The problem to be solved was to set up a system of detection which would be the most profitable in terms of health level and cost for the community. In particular, it should take into account the resources of the health system.

A similar model was build to evaluate the different solutions : this model was composed of :a model of the disease which will make it possible to estimate its evolution (and therefore its economic impact) with several hypothesis : without detection or with different types of detection ; a detection model which uses se- veral parameters that can be modified in order to obtain different types of detec- tion ; an indicator of results that makes it possible to evaluate the results when different types of detection are applied to the disease model.

IV. 2. 1. The disease model

The disease model is built with a certain number of hypothesis since, on the one hand, the natural progress of the disease is unknown (every diagnosis brings about a treatment) and, on the other hand, the most adequate statistical data is not avai- lable. In this study, the most complete set of data come from MEMPHIS (Tennessee, USA) where systematic repeated detection has been carried out since 1952. In 1957, when they first published, 151,000 subjects had been examined at least once. This makes it possible to determine objective morbidity in a primary detection by age (10-year categories) and at various stages of the disease. We know moreover the amount of medical care required annually by these same categories when no detec- tion is done on them [4, 8, 9] . These parameters can be used as indicators of states of health.

As the appearance and progress of the disease vary extremely from one subject to another, the simulation model uses a POISSON probabilist law in which the para- meters were computed from the MEMPHIS statistics. This model gives the probability in the event of cervical cancer detection, of a woman of a given age finding her- self in one of the possible states of health.

IV.2.2. The detection model

The medical technique of detection is already   established and is not open to question (PAPANICOLAOU test).

The choices to be made have mainly to do with :

- the frequency of examinations
- the priorities to be respected when the program is being put into practice, since it is impossible for the population as a whole to be subject to detection of this kind at once.

A certain number of choices related to secondary methods are not discussed in the present study : problems of getting information to the doctor and the population, the practical means (permanent centers or mobile teams), whether the examination is compulsory or not and how it will be paid for (social medical coverage).

The medical personnel and equipment involved will show up in the financial balance-sheet of the program and by the number of people to train for the future.

By varing the parameters of the detection model (frequency of the examinations, age of the subject at the first and last examination and by determining by Operational Research methods (linear programming) the priority that should be granted to the various categories when the program is set up (all the age categories are introduced gradually one by one), the disease model was used to determine the probable evolution of morbidity in the population. In particular, the following indicators were obtained : occurence of each stage by age category ; hence the number of annual treatments required; mortality ; the number of subjects who have had surgery, medical personnel required, etc ... This required that an estimate of expenditures could be computed for each year of the program.

IV.2.3. The result indicator

The best model was chosen according to a criterion based on financial cost, on the one hand, and benefits to health on the other. The criterion used in this study was defined by :

the sum of the benefits due to the program minus the costs of the program, compared to no program at all. The cost of the program could be determined by the disease model for each detection model proposed. The cost when no program exists was computed by means of statistics coming from various medical centers which revealed the frequency of the disease when no program exists. The result indicator was defined in terms of life-expectancy gained with a detecting program. This estimate based on studies done for highway, aviation and work safety [1] is minimal and corresponds to the minimum state of health in which normal work can be performed. The authors have therefore selected a life-expectancy criterion that takes into account women's work and a health index that has been computed somewhat arbitrarily in function of the handicap created by surgical operations necessitated by the illness. The life-expectancy table was calculated by using the detection model in conjunction with the disease model and comparing the results with those obtained when no program exists. The results pertaining to the lack of an existing program were also determined by using available statistical data.

IV.3. The results

Given the fact that a number of factors place limits on this study, namely the estimates, the approximations, the simplifications and .the hypotheses selected, the results can only be taken as an illustration and by no means definitive. It was nevertheless possible to select an optimal detection model following features :

- optimal age of the first and last examinations : 25-60 years old ;
- periodicity : 4 years   with 2 annual examinations at the beginning of the program ;

- length of time required to set up a program like this in France : 15 years ;
- age category to be tested first : 39 years old. The older age categories should be tested next and then the younger ones.

Then it was possible to study the results of the detection program defined by the optimal detection model and which would begin in 1975.

One of the first conclusion that was reached is that over a period of thirty years the financial balance-sheet was totally in deficit, as the money saved on treatments did not compensate the funds spent on the program. On the other hand, the estimated annual balance-sheet, taking into account the financial aspect as well as the benefits gained in level of health (expressed in terms of life-expectancy increase), showed a positive gain in 1988 and increased greatly from that year on. The other results obtained were :

- morbidity becomes stable in 2000 and in comparison with the absence   of such a program. The following decreases are observed :

$$
\begin{array}{ll}
34\ \% & S\ 0 \\
65\ \% & S\ 1 \\
75\ \% & S2,\ S\ 3,\ S\ 4
\end{array}
$$

- need of treatment increases until 1981 and then decrease by :

$$
\begin{array}{l}
41\ \%\ \text{for S 1} \\
72\ \text{to}\ 78\ \%\ \text{for S 2, S 3, S 4}
\end{array}
$$

- mortality increases slightly (by 4.5 %) in the first 5 years due to an increase in the need of treatment hence for surgery, and then goes down by 70 % in 2000.

- states of health expressed in terms of handicap due to surgical operations, shows a decrease until the year 2000 since the number of women requiring operations for S 0 increases and then this factor levels off.

Since the balance-sheet became positive, the authors have concluded that a policy of detection in this domain should be established and they indicated that a more precise analysis of the means (non-periodical examinations, for example) and of the techniques of cervical cancer detection would make it possible to make the system more profitable in the long run.

V. REFERENCES

    I. BARDEAU,J.
       La prévention
       Rapport annuel. Inspection Générale des Affaires Sociales 1973

   II. CHADWICK, J.
       Health service systems for a finite world
       SRI Working paper n° 3595-1

  III. COLLEN, M.F.
       Health   planning : problem of concepts and methods in Global System Dynamics
       ed. ATTINGER E.O. Basel S. Karger 1970

   IV. FANSHEL, S., BUSH, J.W.
       A health status index and its application to health services outcomes
       Operations Research Vol. 18, n° 6, 1970

    V. FORRESTER, J.W.
       Principles of systems
       Wright Allen Press, 1969

   VI. HURTUBISE, J.
       "MEDICS" : Rapport de la phase préliminaire
       Ministère des Affaires Sociales - Direction de la planification
       QUEBEC Sept. 1972

  VII. ILLICH, I.
       Némesis Médicale. L'expropriation de la santé
       Ed.   du Seuil. Paris (1975)

 VIII. LEVY, E., BUNGENER, M., DUMENIL, G., FAGNANI, F.
       Indicateurs de Santé et analyse du système français
       Rapport du Commissariat Général au Plan. Paris 1973

    1. ABRAHAM, C., THEDIE, J.
       Le prix d'une vie humaine dans les décisions économiques
       Rev. Française de Recherche Opérationnelle n° 16. 3e trimestre 1960

    2. BALINTFY, J.
       Linear programming models for menu planning
       in H.E. SMALLEY and J.R. FREEMAN : Hospital Industrial Engineering
       N.Y. REINHOLD N.Y. 1966

    3.BECKETT,R.S., RYAN, J.A., LAZOR, M.
       Medical nomenclature, coding and utilization review : facilitation by the
       Medical Records Department
       Journées Inf. Médicales. Toulouse 1971. IRIA Editor

    4. COLEMAN, S.A., RUBE, I.F., ERICKSON, C.C.
       Cytologic detection of adenocarcinoma of the uterus in a mass screening project
       Am. Journal Obst. and Gyn. St-Louis - Vol 92, June 15 - 1965

    5. CULYER, A.J., LAVERS, R.S., WILLIAMS, A.
       Social Indicators
       Health Social Trends n° 2,1971

    6. FABRE, F., GRANDMONT, J.M.
       Le dépistage précoce du cancer du col de l'utérus - Etude économique
       CERMAP Working paper. Paris, 1968

7. Health planning in USSR
   WHO chronicle (26) May 1972

8. KAISER, R.F., ERICKSON, C.C., EVERETT, B.E., GILLIAN, A.G., GRAVES, L.M.,
   WALTON, M., SPRUNT, D.J.
   Initial effect of community-wide cytologic screening on clinical stage of
   cervical cancer detected in an entire community
   Memphis - Shelby county, Tennessee. Nat. Cancer Inst. 25. p. 863. 1960

9. KASHGARIAN, M., FRICKSON, C.C., DUNN, J.E., SPRUNT,D.J.
   A survey of public awarness of uterine cytology in Memphis-Shelby county
   Acta cytologica Vol. 10, n° 1, 1966

10. LEBART, L.
    Recherches sur le coût de la protection de la vie humaine dans le domaine
    médical.
    CREDOC Working paper, 1970 - Paris

11. REICHERTZ, P.L.
    Hospital and Health care systems
    IFAC 75 august 1975, Boston, MASS

12. International classification   of diseases and causes of death
    WHO publications

13. SMALLWOOD, R.D., BONDIK, E.J., OFFENSED, F.L.
    Toward an integrated methodology for the analysis of health care system
    Operations Research vol. 19, n° 6, 1971

14. Systematized Nomenclature of Pathology
    College of American Pathologists Chicago

15. STIMSON, D.H.
    Utility Measurment in Public Health Decision Making
    Management science n° 16 - 1969

SOME ASPECTS OF
MEDICAL DOCUMENTATION

J. R. MOEHR, HANNOVER

1. Definitions

"Documentation" is used in medicine to denote acquisition of information and orderly storage in a manner that enables retrieval according to defined criteria, as well as presentation of this information (19). Even if we substitute data for information in this definition, it has to be observed that documentation in medicine is used in a more encompassing manner than in informatics. A documentation system comprises in medical usage of the term what an informatician would call an information system.

This terminology has evolved historically. Documentation is part of medical care at least since the times of HIPPOCRATES. Until the 17th and 18th century it consisted however overwhelmingly of a free style narrative account of individual patient's histories. During the development of the ontologic disease concept this was replaced by descriptions of 'diseases' (12). Attempts to standardize medical documentation with respect to format, contents and employed terminology, and the development of documentation systems in the sense of information systems as understood by informatics are characteristic for this century (5).

REICHERTZ (26) discerns three levels of documentation.

1 Recording of cognitive processes with maintenance of their inherent redundancy for conservation of a maximum in detail and resolution.
2 Abstracting of source information for synoptical presentation of a complex pattern at the expense of detail.
3 Classifying association with notions of defined semantic content in order to make processes comparable and retrievable at the level of these concepts or categories. This stage includes standardization of the elements of description and abstraction.

All three levels are part of conventional documentation in patient care. At the first level, symptoms and facts, observation orders and procedures are recorded and collected in a medical record, a case history. Second level activities include the critical summarization of the essentials of a case in the form of an epicrisis. The epicrisis also contains diagnoses that were arrived at. They constitute examples of the third level of documentation in that they are shorthand symbols of defined semantic content for characterizing a case within an accepted model.

It must be noted, however, that the requirements for documentation and documentation systems in medicine extend beyond the immediate requirements of patient care. The whole spectrum comprises
- patient care
- health facility management,
  administration and
- research.
Requirements for health facility management and research have resulted in special documentation practices which shall not be covered in the following. Examples are literature documentation, administrative bookkeeping or research laboratory documentation. The requirements

relate, however, to patient care oriented medical documentation, influence its contents and techniques as will be pointed out in the following.

2. Purpose and objectives:

The purposes of patient care and health facility management are closely related in most subsystems of medical care. Research aspects are particularly prominent in the environment of educational health care centers such as university hospitals, but have to be taken into consideration in other medical care subsystems as well. In the setting of the private physician's office the recording of medical transactions is immediately related to the system of reimbursement in most countries. In public health and social medicine it is an essential requirement for epidemiologic control of the society cared for. In hospitals it relates to financial aspects, resource allocation and planning, of the entire hospital as well as its function units such as operating theatres and laboratories. The spectrum of medical documentation in the sense of recording patient care related information does then include the following purposes:

  - recollection of past events
  - communication about the treatment process
  - education
  - scientific education
  - justification of measures taken as related to
    = medical
    = financial
    = legal standards and requirements
  - administration and management, in particular
    = patient management
    = facility management
    = administration of resources,
      personnel, finances.

Since perhaps some 90 percent of all persons are cared for by private physicians in a single patient - single physician relation, the recollection of past events is a major purpose of notes kept by these physicians. They are used during a particular treatment episode, and may be referred to if the future treatment requires particular caution. This fact that the notes are essentially used only by the note taker himself, makes highly individualized styles of documentation possible, where a small set of symbols may be used for note taking (c.f. figure 3). Usually, these notes are the only record of health impairment. This is important in the comperatively rare cases where a disease takes a turn which makes hospitalization necessary, or where a chronic disablity requires social help. In this latter case, a certificate concerning the development of the disability is frequently required from the physician.

Also in these instances of severe afflictions, the cooperation between specialists and the family physician becomes necessary, in which case the patient record serves as a basis for communication about the disease process. This type of purpose is the primary purpose of the patient record in the hospital care setting.

Closely related to these requirements are the educational aspects and the aspects of justification of the medical actions taken. As will be pointed out in more detail below, 'peer review' is an important measure for insuring high quality care. It serves to evaluate and correct the treatment process whether it is initiated by a student or by an experienced physician. The primary requirement for any assessment of medical care on an individual basis is the medical record. In the same manner, the reimbursement of the physician or hospital may have to be justified on the basis of the notes taken. This aspect is an important issue in Germany, where the physicians are paid on the basis of individual medical services rendered, and where a review system is installed in order to insure that individual physicians do not exceed certain limits considered sufficient for and consistent with good practice. Legal justification becomes increasingly necessary, particularly in countries like the U.S., where malpractice suits start to replace other sources of income for lawyers.

Scientific evaluation of medical records, in a way, is a subspecialty of the use of records in medical education. Since human disease cannot be produced in laboratory experiments and since - luckily - a great number of disease conditions which require scientific attention are very rare, records of disease conditions have to be kept in a way which makes scientific evaluation possible, if it should become necessary. There may be only a few single individuals in whom a certain condition was observed, and if it was documented inadequately the basis for scientific evaluation becomes very small.

Finally, the use of medical records as an administrative tool gains importance under the pressure of steeply rising costs of health care. The medical requirements of a patient have to be known and communicated to others in order to smoothe his treatment in complex medical care installations. Therapeutic and diagnostic procedures have to be standardized to insure maximum economy etc.

Evidently then, medical documentation has to suit a great variety of different purposes and there will be little surprise that some of these objectives may be in conflict with each other.

3. Problems

Among the problems of medical documentation, let us discern two classes,
          - conceptual and
          - technical problems.

3.1 CONCEPTUAL PROBLEMS

Conceptual problems may be traced essentially to conflicts between various kinds of objectives, which may entail conflicts between contents, techniques, methods and styles of documentation, and which give rise to the error problem which will be treated below. The primary conflict in patient care related documentation arises from the conflict between treatment and documentation itself. The more encompassing a type of documentation is strived for, the greater the possible interference with actual treatment. The act of documentation, of note taking, interrupts the direct rapport between patient and physician. This even more if check list type documents have to be elaborated in order to insure complete 'workup' of a case. On the other hand, if history taking and examination are carried out seperately from documentation of the findings, errors of omission are likely to increase. Especially in the environment of a busy practice or ward, a lot will be left undocumented. One usually has to be lucky that all

positive findings, indicative of disease are noted, let alone the
negatives. The act of documentation in itself may therefore initiate a
conflict within the scope of other medical objectives.
Other problems are the result of conflicting purposes of documentation.
E.g. for use of the document for patient care, for communication about
a disease process, for medical education by peer review techniques, a
medical record should be concise and possibly problem oriented, all
notes being indexed by the problem to which they refer. Such 'records
that guide and teach' (36) may be difficult to evaluate in many types
of clinical investigation. It is not surprising therefore, that the
traditional medical record, which evolved in the teaching and research
environment of academic hospitals, is not problem oriented but source
oriented and keeps documents of each source in chronological order. In
such records, laboratory results are kept seperate from x-ray reports
and from documents being generated on the ward, such as patient charts
letters of discharge etc. Just as medical practice may have to strive
for a different type of completeness, in order to achieve scientific
comparability, scientific patient records have to be complete in a
different way as solely patient care oriented records.

This type of problem is closely related to the effects of alternative
medical models applied, to a particular case (c.f. the chapter on
'medical information and related terminology'). Completeness of
information is relative to the medical models of disease taken into
consideration. Additional data may indicate that constellations
considered previously to represent an entiety have to be assessed
seperately. 'Stomach trouble' may be due to cirrhotic liver disease due
to a psycho social problem constellation with chronic alcoholism.
Further investigation may reveal that the cirrhotic liver disease has
resulted in carcinoma of the liver and this in turn may completely
change the attitude towards necessity of further diagnostics and
therapy.

Likewise, completion of the data base may reduce to an entiety what
seemed to belong apart. A patient's psychic depression, congestive
heart failure and bowel obstipation may turn out to be due to
hypothyroidism, insufficient function of the thyroid gland.

The advent of automation of medical procedures, in particular the
automation of the clinical chemistry and hematologic laboratories,
which produce increasingly vast amounts of data, have pointed out,
however, that complete interpretation of available symptoms within the
scope of accepted medical models is not always possible. With
increasing frequency of undirected testing, a growing number of such
tests proves to be found temporarily or persistently in a pathologic
range without being able to explain those abnormal findings by known
pathophysiologic phenomena.

The problems connected with the relativity of the completeness of a
medical record should point out that patient care related medical
documentation is by necessity highly subjective. The contents of a
medical record are profoundly influenced by the physician's reasoning,
even if they are not structured in a way to reflect the reasoning
process as in a problem oriented record. Items are selcted according to
their perceived relevance for a particular case. This even if they
represent facts that are offered spontaneously by the patient during
interview. They are interpreted, condensed, selected and summarized by
the physician or who else takes the notes. The greater number of facts
entered into the medical record have to be actively collected by the
physician - be it by direct observation or interrogation of the patient
or by initiation of special test procedures. This makes the record
subjective, and results again in a certain conflict between

subjectivity and objectivity.
Subjectivity is an essential prerequisite for economic, efficient and effective patient care. It increases intelligibility of the record where objectivity increases the bulk of data and may render the process of patient care inefficient and uneconomic. Objectivity may on the other hand be again desirable for better scientific comparability.

A last type of conceptual problems results from the fuzziness of the employed terminology and relates to the problem of errors discussed below. The reasons for this type of problem have been covered in the chapter on 'medical information and related terminology' and need not be repeated here. It should only be emphasized again in this context that the problem exists, particularly in comparison of documents originating in different medical subspecialties and in the context of differing medical objectives.

3.2 TECHNICAL PROBLEMS

Technical problems of medical documentation arise from a variety of conditions, such as

    - amount of data
    - availability with respect to
      = time
      = location
    - identification and record linkage
    - acquisition and presentation
    - qualities of data
    - security
    - confidentiability.

As pointed out above, the amount of data generated during a particular treatment episode will vary with respect to medical context, patient care setting and the like. Still, even in private physician's offices, a considerable amount of documents accumulates over time and makes measures for reduction and concentration necessary. In modern centralized maximum care facilities such as academic hospitals, the reduction of the volume of medical records becomes mandatory. At the Medical School Hannover, with its capacity of roughly 25,000 patient days of inpatient care and 100,000 outpatient visits per year, more than 100.000 different patient records, containing some 3,5 million pages of patient documents accumulate each year (20). This document load places high demands on technical support of data communication since the same documents may be needed in different locations for different types of patient care purposes or for research as well as patient care. Also, the documents must be easily and reliably retrievable from achieves and have to be communicated to the various users at various locations in time for their use.

This in turn increases the demands on data security as well as confidentiality since orderly control of record use and record movements becomes increasingly difficult with increasing complexity of the institution.

Confidentiality and security are also related to the problem of identification and record linkage. So far, in our experience identification errors represent the most important reason for loss or misplacement of data. Even if the identification number is, as in our institution, generated by a deterministic and therefore reproducible process, a comparatively high chance of error results from factors like misspelling of a name, change of name, e.g. due to marriage, or from the usual errors connected with the reproduction of numbers like the birth date. The resulting corrections usually come about as a chain of alterations necessary on a great number of identification carriers.

The problems of data acquisition and data presentation present in at least two different modes, depending on the recording media used (see below). Using conventional paper and pencil techniques for recording, data acquisition presents no problem, except at the bedside, as discussed above. The bulk of documents is produced by many different function units. On the contrary, if means suitable for machine processing of the data are employed, data acquisition immediately becomes a problem. This issue will be referred to below again. Data presentation, on the other hand, tends to remain a problem, irrespective of the media of documentation. Due to the bulk of data, it becomes difficult to maintain an overview of what is available. Techniques to arrive at synopses, abstracts and reviews are therefore mandatory. They are established part of conventional documentation. Letters of discharge or epicrises are prepared by physicians, complex findings summarized into diagnostic statements, charts are drawn to depict the course of treatment, the development of disease with alterations between remission and recurrence, laboratory findings obtained at different instances are summarized on review sheets etc. The automation of test- and monitoring procedures results frequently in the automatic generation of such charts and synopses. Through electronic processing of digital data this type of techniques has gained new dimensions, mainly because data originating from various sources may be compiled and linked in such activities which have to be counted among the techniques of second level documentation as defined by REICHERTZ (26).

3.3 THE ERROR PROBLEM

This section is intended to cover the problem of errors that influence the value of medical documentation and which arise before the data enter a document. Errors in transcription of data will not be covered.

Usually, two types of errors, the

        - error of omission
and the

        - error of commission

are differentiated. The first is self explanatory, arising from omssion of important facts, and relates to the problem of the relativity of completeness discussed above. The other, the error of commission, arises from false interpretation of available evidence. Apart from the conceptual problems arising from the relativity of medical model concepts, such factors as

        - intellectual capacity
        - scope of attention
        - experience
        - knowledge
        - preoccupation and bias
        - thoroughness
        - persistence

are importatnt determinants in this respect. They are of little

importance for the acquisition of measurement data they influence,
however, the initiation of a measurement and the interpretation and
processing of its results. For observational and related data on the
other hand, they are of great importance even during the phase of data
acquisition. Observational data still are of greatest importance for
medical action, in that they provide the basis for medical decisions in
the greatest number of cases (11).

Medical transactions may be viewed as a circle, in which signals are
perceived and apperceived by a physician and result in an
interpretation which leads to action, which in turn generates new
signals (25,29). The data entered into documents are a by-product of
this process, an extract of information processing, not only on the
part of the physician but also of the patient.

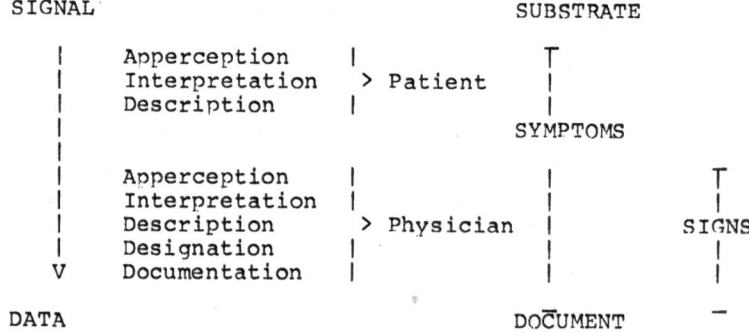

```
SIGNAL                                    SUBSTRATE

  |     Apperception     |        T
  |     Interpretation   > Patient |
  |     Description      |        |
  |                                SYMPTOMS
  |
  |     Apperception     |        |        T
  |     Interpretation   |        |        |
  |     Description      > Physician |     SIGNS
  |     Designation      |        |        |
  V     Documentation    |        |        |

DATA                              DOCUMENT      —
```

A long chain of processing steps may lead from signals in a substrate
to data in a document. It includes processing by the patient and the
physician in the case of symptoms in the English sense of the word,
while signs are processed only by the physician. At any of these steps,
errors of omission and commission may occur.

A number of measures may be taken to reduce errors on the part of the
medical professional:

  - training
  - standardization
  - redundancy.

One important objective of training is to achieve the ability for
efficient selection of relevant and necessary evidence within the
context of the current status of considerations. Closely related is the
training of perception and apperception. These rely nowadays
overwhelmingly on the visual senses and to a lesser extent on tacticle
and auditive senses. Individual sensory capacity is an important
limitation in this respect and limits what may be achieved by training
and experience. In order to optimize performance at this level,
adherence to the sequence of

  - description
  - denomination
  - interpretation

is advocated (7). This sequence is again intended to make the process
of medical reasoning transparent and to reduce errors due to bias and

narrowness of attention. If a consultant's advice is requested, FEINSTEIN (7) recommends to refrain from the frequent practice of offering at first the suspicion one has in mind. Instead it is advised, to present the case in an unbiased manner and let the specialist collect all the evidence necessary for his judgement. This emplies that all evidence is documented accordingly, i.e. by listing the complete description before arriving at an abstracting denomination and interpretation.

In particular, it is emphasized to note what was actually witnessed. This rule is frequently violated in medical documentation. Examples cited by FEINSTEIN are that one may note 'depression' when one sees tears which may actually be caused by joy or emotion, or that one may note 'mitral regurgitation' when one hears a certain type of murmer over the heart which may actually be accidental and not have a pathologic significance.

Certainly all these measures and recommendations do add to the volume of documentation and to the time and effort it takes to prepare it. An optimum between efficiency with respect to operational constraints and efficiency with respect to objectivity and correctness may be hard to obtain, and needs considerable attention, especially in the development of automatic support of documentation and reporting systems. The engineer and informatician should in the development of such systems be considered and act as a partner of the medical professional and not follow his recommendations or requests obligingly.

Standardization, as another means of reducing errors in documentation, may consist of following developing standardized procedures of documentation, such as outlined for the conventional procedure in the preceeding paragraph and such as will necessarily result from automated support of documentation. The necessity of defining the terminology used in a particular context and enforcing its consistent application is outlined in the chapter on 'information in medicine and related terminology'. If such definitions have been achieved, one should take care, that the common practice of noting only positive findings, is reduced. Negatives should also be documented. This makes it possible to achieve complete documentation for a given purpose under given circumstances. Medical requirements may, of course, still present a limiting factor. Certain findings are unobtainable under certain conditions. A biopsy cannot be performed if the patient has a bleeding disorder, certain labvalues, e.g. enzyme activities, are unobtainable in heavily jaundiced serum.

Notwith standing this, the definition of the scope of documentation provides the basis for another means of error reduction: The crossvalidation of data. This is possible through plausibility checks and redundancy. Plausibility checks are part of everyday medical practice - however, to a considerably varying extent. In this respect, the automation of documentation offers considerable advantages since plausibility checks may be incorporated as unconditional part of the routine. They may be executed on the syntactic level, but due to recent developments include to an increasing extent the semantic level of documentation (21,22,29).

Redundancy finally is provided if the findings obtained at the bedside by one physician, are confirmed by a consulting specialist (peer review) or by measurements. This process adds again to the volume of documentation, particularly since the confirming evidence is frequently not only redundant but complementary in detail as well as scope.

In all then, a number of means is available to increase the quality of medical documents by reduction of errors. Automation considerably adds in this respect in that it emphasizes standardization, consistent use of terminology and offers the possibilities for reliable and consistent execution of plausibility checks.

5. Contents of Medical Documents

The conventional medical record contains all documents pertinent to the treatment of a patient that accumulate in a given institution of the medical care system.

In the usual private physician's office, a patient record most commonly consists of a card board folder which contains patient identification and some personal data (e.g. name, birth date, address, telephone number). In West-Germany, the insurance company and insurance status (memberchip, relative of a member or pensioneer) are important.

On this card, all further items that the physician deems of value for further treatment or for billing are noted. Commonly it consists of two pages of size DIN A 5 (21 by 15 cm), folded on one of the longer edges so that other documents for this patient may be kept in the middle. Several forms have been suggested for this folder. Most contain patient identification on the uppper left hand corner. Frequently, the upper end may be marked by stickers or coloured tape to facilitate placement of the card in alphabetic order (or less frequently according to some number system) in the patient record file.

A detailed study of currently used documentation practices has recently been published (30). This investigation revealed that only the aspects of documentation enforced by the German system for paying the doctor, are documented fairly by German practitioners uniformly. These are the diagnoses and related services. Other aspects, such as a patient's complaints, physician's findings, kinds and quantities of drugs given, are documented less consistently. The extent of documentation may reach from zero to documentation in considerable detail, depending on the physician. Not surprisingly the forms suggested for the patient record in private offices vary considerably in their suggestions for formal documentation of medically relevant details. When such suggestions are made on a form adopted for a given office, it was still found quite frequently that they were not adhered to.

Also it was found that the patient chart is exclusively used by the staff of a particular office, overwhelmingly by the physician who made the notes. For external communication, a host of other forms is used, into which the relevant notes are entered, sometimes by extraction or transcription from the main chart, but never by reproduction techniques (except , of course, for identification data).

Apart from the main chart, there exists also a number of other documents, for use within the office. In some instances, history forms are employed, which are used by the patient to enter data pertinent to his past history or to the present illness. Sometimes special forms are used to instruct the patient, e.g. concerning drug therapy, diets or for scheduling further visits. This last example leads over to a number of forms or other documentation media used for office management. These comprise books for the scheduling of patient visits to the office, or of physician's visits to patient's homes, books and other forms for recording results of special investigations, (blood chemistry, x-rays, electro cardiograms etc.) which are frequently transcribed into the main chart or on some form kept within the chart, where the letters received from specialists or hospitals are also kept.

The reimbursement of the doctor in the Federal Republic of Germany is based on the 'Krankenschein' as a document. The patient obtains this form from his insurance company and is supposed to hand it out to his physician on the first visit of a quarter. All diagnoses and related services are noted on this form during this and the ensuing visits of a quarter. Diagnoses are noted in free text, services are coded according to one of several codes, depending on the category of insurance company. Insurance companies for compulsorily insured patients are applicable for about 80 percent of the patients, and require a certain type of coding. Most of the voluntarily insured patients are insured in companies requiring another type of code. In addition, some codes exist for some small groups of patients, especially if the employer has his own insurance agency (e.g. in case of the army).
In this way, the information relevant for billing is the most uniformly documented category. For the others, very liberal styles of documentation are sometimes practiced. They may rely on a small number of symbols as exemplified in figure 1.

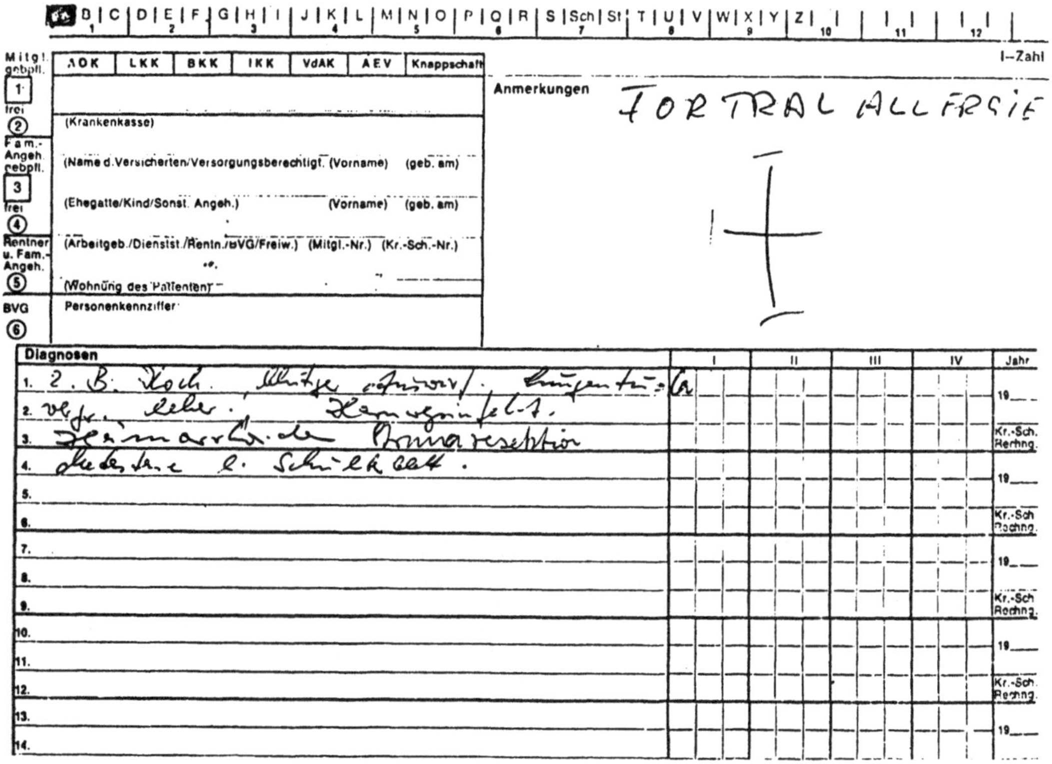

Figure 1
Patient record face sheet for practicing physicians, front side (developed by Arbeitskreis Praktische Medizin of the Deutsche Gesellschaft fuer Medizinische Dokumentation und Statistik). Patient identification in upper left hand corner is blotted out (here as in all following figures). Problemoriented documentation is enabled by listing diagnoses by numbers and marking their activity on right hand side. This suggestion is not adhered to, however.

BASISANAMNESE

Operationen:)nein

Unfälle: ja

Rente: nein

Eigene Vorkrankheiten:				Diabetes	Magen/Darm
Masern	Diphtherie	(Para-)Ty.	Tbc (wo?)	Schilddr.	Galle/Leber
Mumps	Scharlach	Ruhr	von — bis	Augen	Niere/Blase
Röteln	Mandelentzdg	Malaria	überwacht bis	Ohren	Nerven
Windp.	Rheum. Fieber	Zoonosen	Geschl. Kr.	Lungen/Rippenf.	Haut
Keuchh.	Gelbsucht			Herz/Kreislauf	WS/Gelenke

Sonstige Krankheiten:

Impfungen:

Früherkennung
(wann zuletzt)

Familien-Anamnese:		Geschwisterreihe:			
Krebs	Übergewicht	Venenleiden	Magen	Nerven-	Sonstige
Tbc	Herzleiden	Haut	Galle	Gemüts-	Krankh.:
Diabetes	Hirnschlag	Asthma	Niere	Anfalls-	
Gicht	Hochdruck	Rheuma	Steinleiden	Erbleiden	

Frauen:		Medikamente:	Langzeitbeh. (von—bis)	Alkohol:
Menarche	Fluor	Schlafm.		
Menses	Kont. Blutg	Abführm.		Nikotin:
Menopause	Fehlgeb.	Pille		Drogen:
Geburten	Totgeb.	Sonstige		

Vegetative Funktionen/soziales Milieu:

Schlaf:	Tageslauf:
Appetit:	Freizeit:
Durst:	Urlaub:
Stuhl:	Sport:
Miktion:	Berufl. Belastg
Vita sex.:	Famil. Belastg

Entwurf: AK Praktische Medizin der Deutschen Gesellschaft für medizinische Dokumentation und Statistik, Kassel.
Bezugsquelle: CEDIP-Verlag GmbH & Co, 8 München 13, Destouchesstr. 67.

Figure 2
Patient record face sheet for practicing physicians, rear side. Details
on history may be checked off. Very rudimentary use of this
possibility.

In hospitals, on the contrary, the patient record has to serve to a far
greater extent for communication between different physicians involved
simultaneously in the treatment of a patient. Billing aspects have had
secondary relevance in Germany, and are now entirely irrelevant since
the hospital billing system has been converted to remuneration on a
patient day basis in West-Germany. (A fixed fee exists for every
hospital which is paid by the insurance company for every day of a
patient's stay.) Within a patient record, as kept in a hospital, there
are usually several types of documents:

- charts
- letters of referral (and discharge)
- special investigation reports
- history and physical examination data
- prescriptions, certificates, authorizations etc.

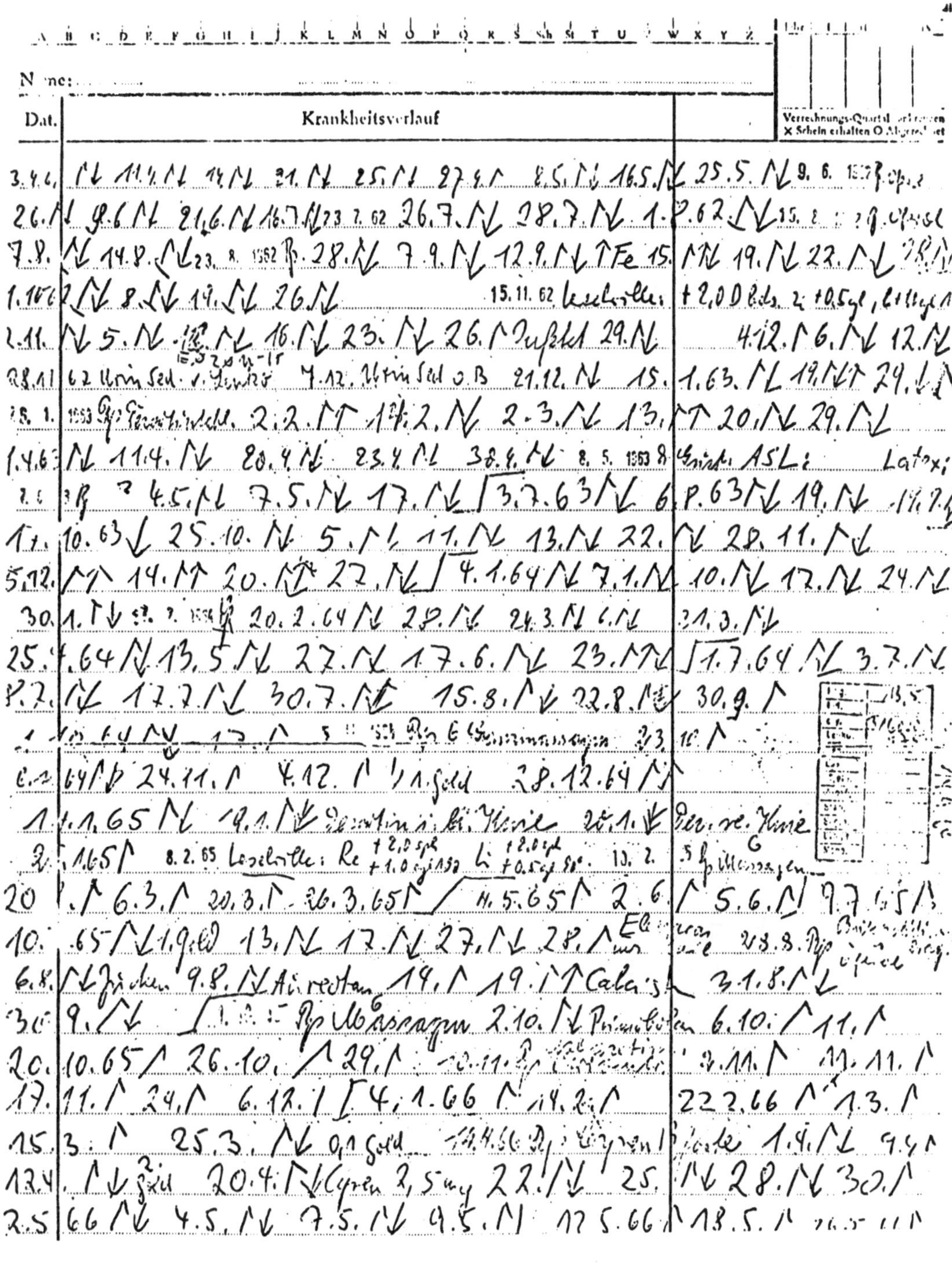

Figure 3
Patient record of private practitioner. 5 years of a patient's history are documented using a small set of symbols.

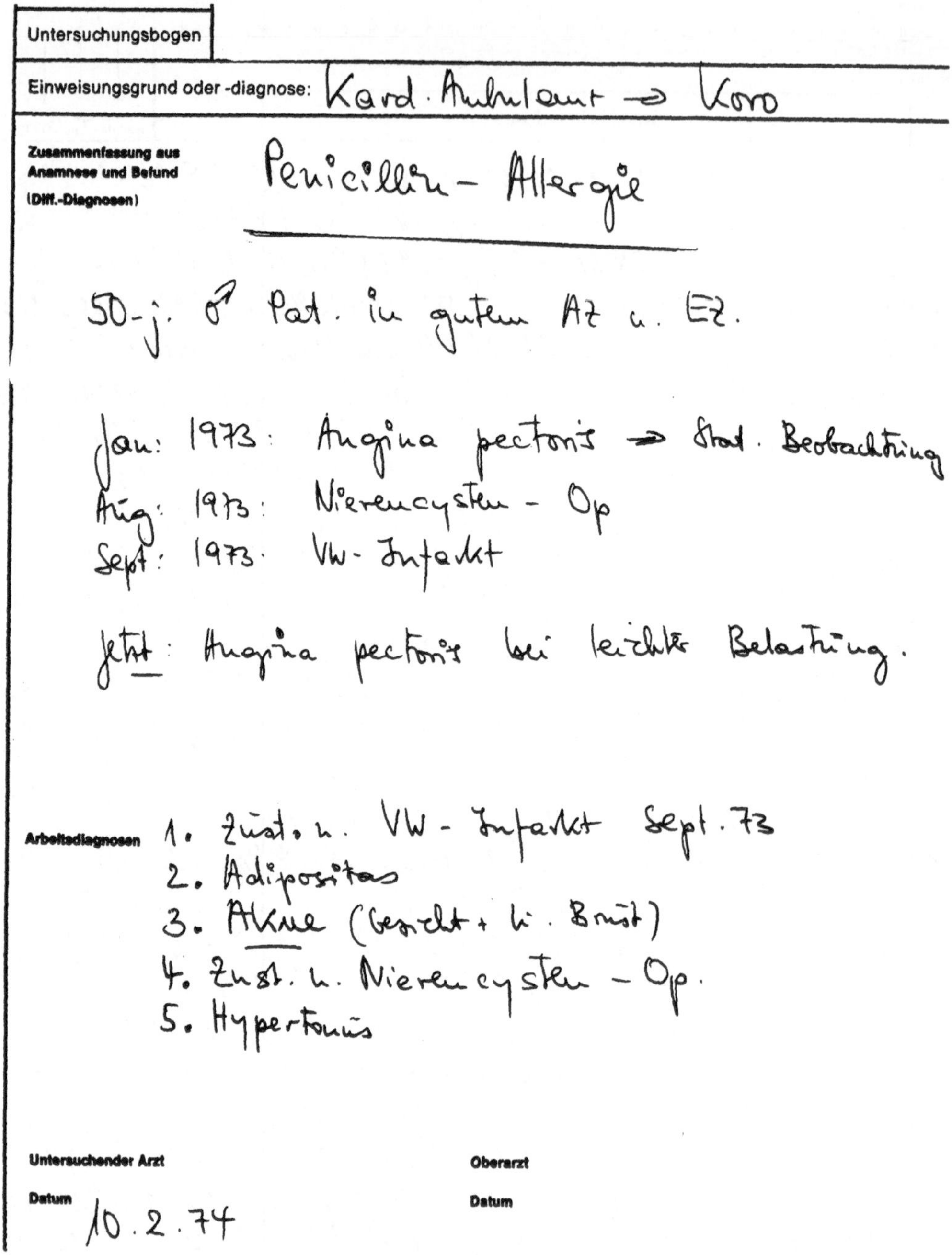

Untersuchungsbogen

Einweisungsgrund oder -diagnose: *Kard. Ambulanz → Koro*

Zusammenfassung aus
Anamnese und Befund
(Diff.-Diagnosen)

Penicillin – Allergie

50-j. ♂ Pat. in gutem Az u. Ez.

Jan: 1973: Angina pectoris → Stat. Beobachtung
Aug: 1973: Nierencysten – Op
Sept: 1973: VW- Infarkt

Jetzt: Angina pectoris bei leichter Belastung.

Arbeitsdiagnosen

1. Zust. n. VW – Infarkt Sept. 73
2. Adipositas
3. Akne (Gesicht + li. Brust)
4. Zust. n. Nierencysten – Op.
5. Hypertonus

Untersuchender Arzt   Oberarzt

Datum 10.2.74   Datum

Figure 4
Face sheets of history and physicial examination form of the Medical
School Hannover. Example of legible, clearly structured summary
including working diagnoses.

ANAMNESE der jetzigen Krankheit

Die Hauptbeschwerde Dauer Stärke Art und Ort Beziehung zu Funktionen	Angina pectoris bei leichter Belastung, bei Ärger. Nitro hilft.
Bisheriger Krankheitsverlauf und Begleitbeschwerden Benutzen Sie die System-übersicht (S. 3) als Gedächtnisstütze Im Rahmen des chronologischen Krankheitsverlaufs werden die Begleitbeschwerden dargestellt, die mit der Hauptbeschwerde zusammenhängen. Bei Rezidiven und chron. Verläufen mit dem ersten Krankheitsereignis beginnen. Bisherige Behandlung der jetzigen Krankheit erwähnen.	① Sept. 72 bei Anstrengung Schmerzen in der Brust mit Ausstrahlung in den li. Arm, auch nachts, ohne Luftnot. → HA, Besserung auf Nitro ② Jan. 73: Stat. wegen Angina pectoris in Stadthagen, Zunahme der Beschwerden, Gehstrecke: 150 m → Kur: Gewicht: 10 kg ↓ ③ Aug. 73: Nierencysten - Op. 4. postop. Tag VW - Infarkt. 9 Wo. Stationär. Nach Entlassung: Ruhe - Angina - pector. Langsame Abnahme der Beschwerden. ④ Vor 4 Wochen: Rhythmus - Störungen. Jetzt: Angina pectoris bei leichter Belastung Th. Visken 3×1

Figure 5
Present illness documentation, same case as in figure 4.

		Knoten		links		rechts	Druckschmerz	sonst.				
Klopfschall	unauffällig	links	vorn	oben	Mitte	unten		rechts	vorn	oben	Mitte	unten
		links	hinten	oben	Mitte	unten	Dämpfung	rechts	hinten	oben	Mitte	unten
		links	vorn	oben	Mitte	unten		rechts	vorn	oben	Mitte	unten
		links	hinten	oben	Mitte	unten	hypersonor	rechts	hinten	oben	Mitte	unten
Lungengrenzen	unauffällig	Verschieblichk. .... cm				fehlende Verschieblichk.		links		rechts		sonst.
Atemgeräusch	unauffällig	links	vorn	oben	Mitte	unten		rechts	vorn	oben	Mitte	unten
		links	hinten	oben	Mitte	unten	abgeschwächt	rechts	hinten	oben	Mitte	unten
		links	vorn	oben	Mitte	unten		rechts	vorn	oben	Mitte	unten
		links	hinten	oben	Mitte	unten	verschärft	rechts	hinten	oben	Mitte	unten
		links	vorn	oben	Mitte	unten		rechts	vorn	oben	Mitte	unten
		links	hinten	oben	Mitte	unten	bronchial	rechts	hinten	oben	Mitte	unten
		links	vorn	oben	Mitte	unten		rechts	vorn	oben	Mitte	unten
		links	hinten	oben	Mitte	unten	trockene RG	rechts	hinten	oben	Mitte	unten
		links	vorn	oben	Mitte	unten		rechts	vorn	oben	Mitte	unten
		links	hinten	oben	Mitte	unten	kleinblas. feuchte RG	rechts	hinten	oben	Mitte	unten
		links	vorn	oben	Mitte	unten		rechts	vorn	oben	Mitte	unten
		links	hinten	oben	Mitte	unten	mittelblas. feuchte RG	rechts	hinten	oben	Mitte	unten
		links	vorn	oben	Mitte	unten		rechts	vorn	oben	Mitte	unten
		links	hinten	oben	Mitte	unten	großblas. feuchte RG	rechts	hinten	oben	Mitte	unten
		links	vorn	oben	Mitte	unten		rechts	vorn	oben	Mitte	unten
		links	hinten	oben	Mitte	unten	klingende RG	rechts	hinten	oben	Mitte	unten
		links	vorn	oben	Mitte	unten		rechts	vorn	oben	Mitte	unten
		links	hinten	oben	Mitte	unten	Reibegeräusch	rechts	hinten	oben	Mitte	unten

Stärkegrade, sonst. Befunde u. Erläuterungen

Sonorer Klopfschall
Vesiculäratmung Grenzen –
und Verschieblichkeit in Normbereich

Kreislauf	RR links *190/100*		RR rechts *180/100*	Puls *84* /Min. Pulsqualität *regelmäßig*			
Herz	unauffällig	linksverbreitert	rechtsverbreitert	Pulsationen links parasternal	epigastr.	sonst.	
Herzspitzenstoß	unauffällig	nicht tastbar	hebend	verbreitert	innerhalb MCL	außerhalb MCL	(Erläuterung)
Herztöne	rein	leise	betont I	Grad 1	2	3	4
			betont II	Grad 1	2	3	4
			Spaltung I	Aorta	Pulm.	Erb	Trikusp.	Spitze
			Spaltung II	Aorta	Pulm.	Erb	Trikusp.	Spitze
Geräusche	fehlen	Systolik (Max.)	Aorta	Pulm.	Erb	Trikusp.	Spitze
		Diastolik (Max.)	Aorta	Pulm.	Erb	Trikusp.	Spitze	Reibegeräusche

Skizze pathol. Töne und Geräusche

I II | I II | I II | I II | I II
Aorta | Pulm. | Erb | Trikusp. | Spitze

Rhythmus	regelm.	Extrasystolen	absolute Arrhy.	Pulsdefizit (radial .... / zentral ....)

Sonst. Befunde an Herz und Kreislauf

Spitzenstoss 6 ICR ausserhalb MCL.
Töne o.B. Keine Geräusche!
LV: perkussorisch vergrössert

Figure 6
Documentation of physical examination findings (cardio respiratory organs). Same case as figure 4 and 5.

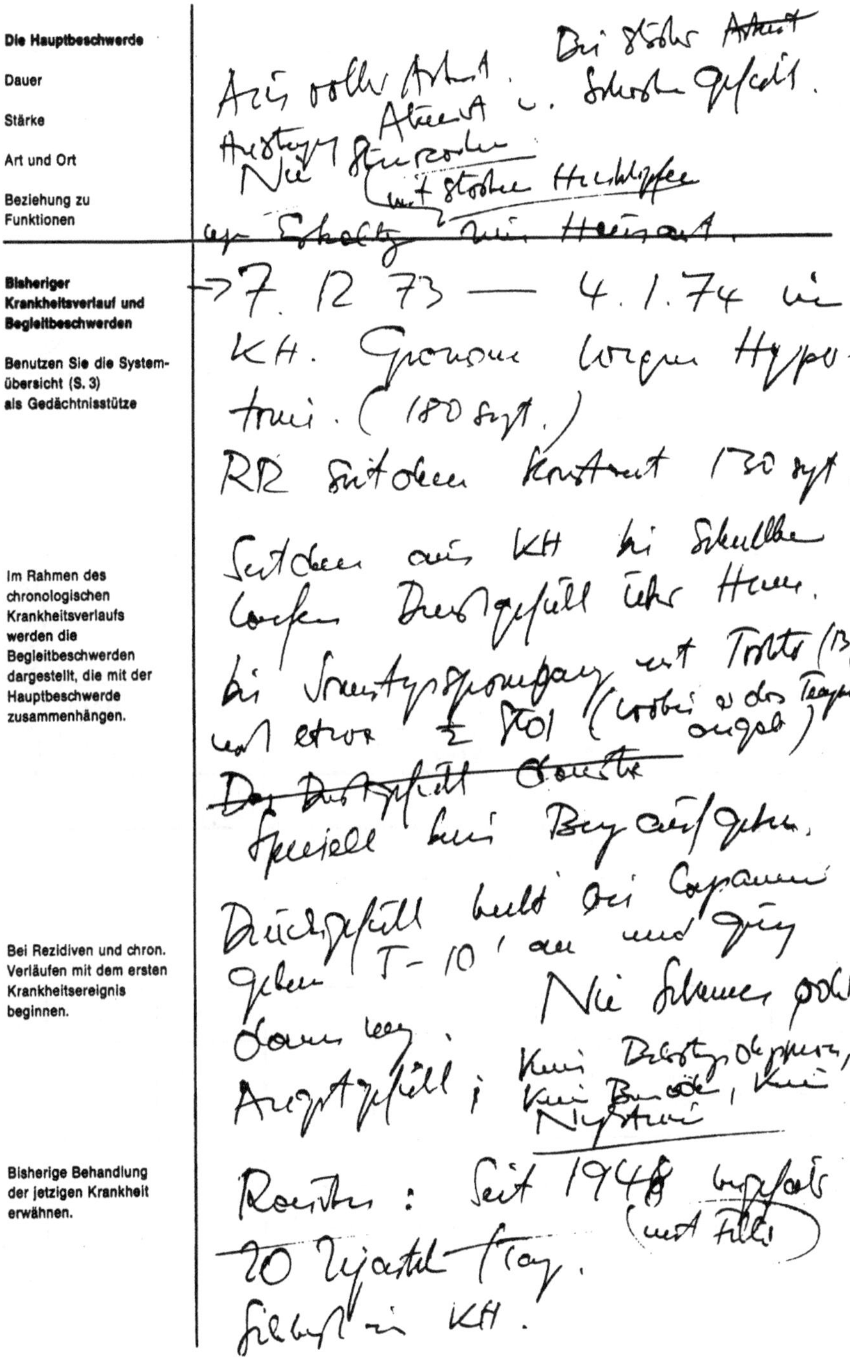

Die Hauptbeschwerde	
Dauer	
Stärke	
Art und Ort	
Beziehung zu Funktionen	
Bisheriger Krankheitsverlauf und Begleitbeschwerden	
Benutzen Sie die Systemübersicht (S. 3) als Gedächtnisstütze	
Im Rahmen des chronologischen Krankheitsverlaufs werden die Begleitbeschwerden dargestellt, die mit der Hauptbeschwerde zusammenhängen.	
Bei Rezidiven und chron. Verläufen mit dem ersten Krankheitsereignis beginnen.	
Bisherige Behandlung der jetzigen Krankheit erwähnen.	

Figure 7
Hasty unorderly summary of history, corresponding to figure 5.

FIEBERKURVE — Op. am 20.5.74

Datum/Krankh.-Tag	12.6 37	13. 38	25. 14.	.5. 40	27.	.7 42	29.

Therapie: 30g Eiweiß

d GX - Lsg 40% +   8 IE Alt-Insulin + 10 mval KCl   2×500,0 ml ...

Tutofusin HL10   500,0 ml

Lasix   500 mg   3×40 mg

3×1 Tbl Lefax

binotal 3+2g   Kalinor bra. 3×1

Lanicor 0,125 mg   Lanicor 2×1/2 Tbl.

Bisolvon   3×1 Amp

...   20 Tr. Novalgin

...   1000 ml   2000 ml

O_2-Zufuhr 2 L/min

Diagnostik: E'lyte H'stoff / BZ-Tg-Prof. H'stoff / BZ Tg Pr. H'stoff / H'st. E'lyte 4 st E'lyte / Röntgen Tho. EKG

BSG mm W / RR mm Hg: 110/80 120/70 130/80

P = • 120	T = ★ 39
100	38
Alter: 80	37
Größe: 156 60	36
Kost: 40	35

Stuhl/Erbrechen

Gewicht: 45,6   56,5   47,5   46,7   45,6

Einfuhr/Ausfuhr: 2000 / 1015   2700/10...   1900/... 118   1700/1010   1300/12

Fieberkurve

Blatt Nr.:

Figure 8
Patient chart with graphic representation of pulse and temperature;
medication and diagnostics indicated above, vital signs below curve.

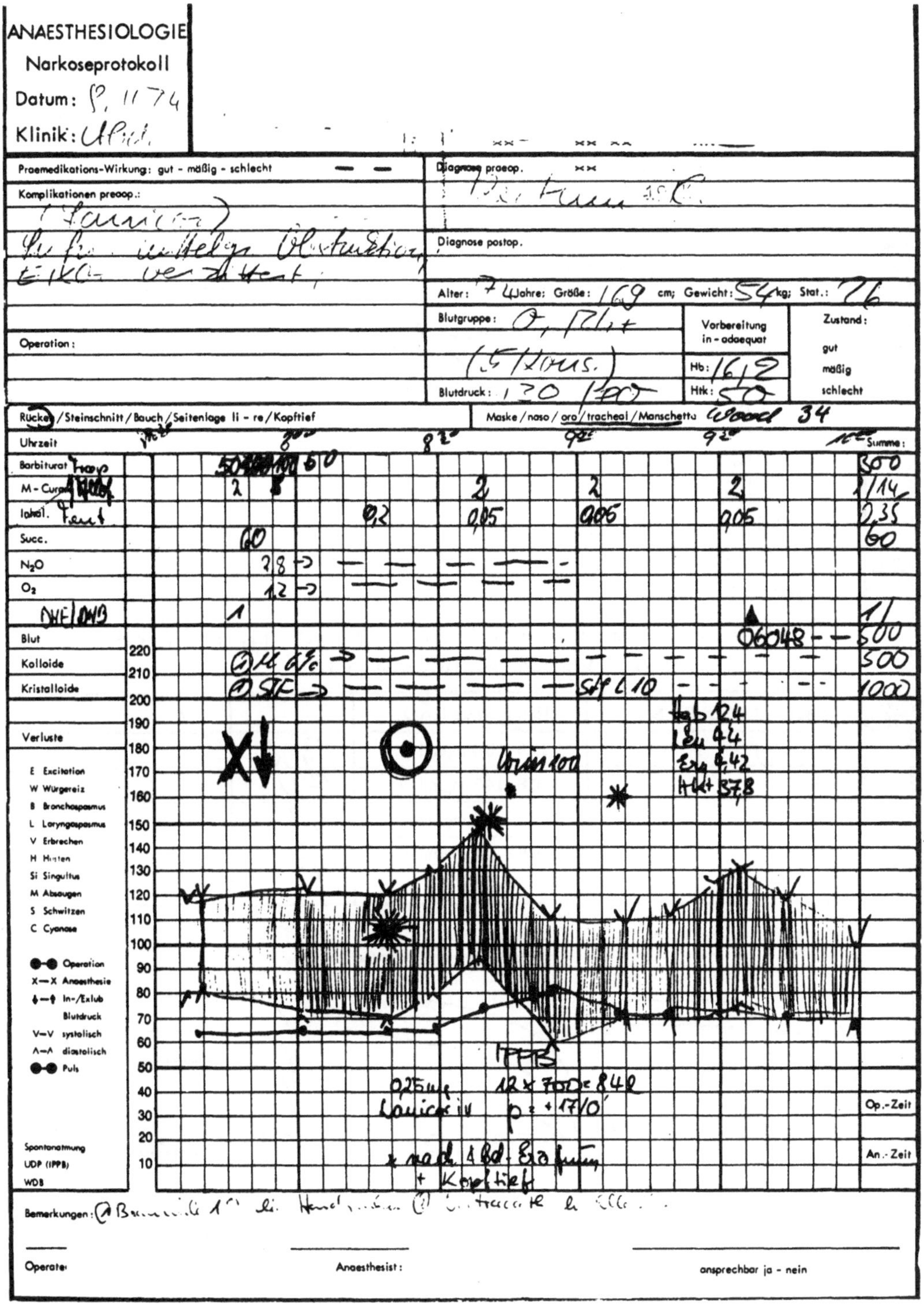

Figure 9
Anesthesia protocol. Combined use of numbers, special symbols and graphics to record course of anesthesia.

MEDIZINISCHE
HOCHSCHULE
HANNOVER
Medizinische Klinik
Abteilung für klinische
Immunologie und
Bluttransfusionswesen

D, V.

Immunglobuline Immunelektrophorese				
Hier ankreuzen	Stat.:	Datum: *5,1,74*	P06	
	Klin.:	Diagnose: *Plasmonyto*		KL

	Immunelektrophorese	Zusätzliche Wünsche:
	AS: Anti-Gesamt Anti-IgA Anti-IgM Anti-IgD Anti-K, Λ Anti-	
200 ml x 24h-Urin	Mikroglobuline i. Urin	

Ergebnis:

Jgg - (π) Parapokin mit schindären Antikörper-mangelsyndon norgeniesen!

IMMUNGLOBULINE i. S.	Normalwerte (Erw.)		
"Gesamt-Ig"	11,5 - 19,4 mg/ml	*17,2*	
IgG	8,8 - 14,7 mg/ml	*15,0*	
IgA	1,2 - 3,6 mg/ml	*1,3*	
IgM	0,6 - 2,4 mg/ml	*0,9*	

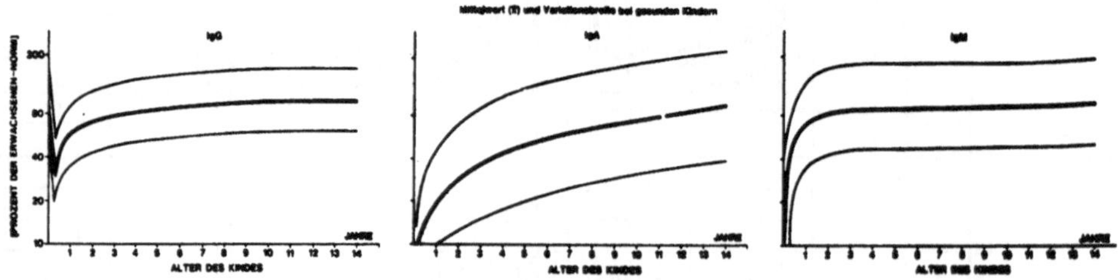

Figure 10
Special investigation report (immune globulin determination) using numbers and free text with graphics as reference for interpretation of results.

MEDIZINISCHE HOCHSCHULE HANNOVER
ARBEITSGRUPPE FUER KLINISCHE KARDIOLOGIE
EKG-ABTEILUNG ,D. ███████4

BETRIFFT: ███████████

FKG ANGEFERTIGT AM: 4. APRIL 1974.

GEWUENSCHTES FKG:
     STANDARD EKG *

     BEI   DER EKG-ANFORDERUNG SIND IM FELD 'MEDIKATION' KEINE
     ANGABEN GEMACHT WORDEN *

BFFUND:
     STEILTYP   * SINUSRHYTHMUS   MIT EINER FREQUENZ VON 61 - 100 PRO
     MINUTE * AV-RHYTHMUS *

BEURTEILUNG DES EKG:
     PATHOLOGISCHES FKG *

                    EKG-ASSISTENTIN: ███████████T

                                   BEFUNDER:

                                   (███████)

Figure 11
Special investigation report prepared by computer using AMAP (21) (ECG
evaluation).

PROF.DR.MED. A. GEORGII   3000 HANNOVER,DEN 1██████5
PATHOLOGISCHES INSTITUT   KARL WIECKERT ALLEE 9
MEDIZINISCHE HOCHSCHULE   TEL.(0511) 532 2921

HERRN
P████   ██████
HNO-KLINIK
MEDIZINISCHE HOCHSCHULE

3000 H A N N O V E R

KARL-WIECHERT-ALLEE

        +-------------------------------------+
        | BIOPSIE : |
        +-------------------------------------+

NAME: |]   EINGANGSDATUM: 1██████5
I-ZAHL. ███████████]   UNTERSUCHUNGSDATUM: 1█████5

UNTERSUCHUNGSMATERIAL:

PE HALS

    DIE PATHOLOGISCH-ANATOMISCHE BEGUTACHTUNG HAT ERGEBEN:
    ==

MIKROSKOPISCH:

VON DER LINKEN HALSSEITE ZWEI EXCISIONEN VON INSGESAMT
REISKORNGROESSE. HISTOLOGISCH NACH DURCHSICHT DER PARAFFINHISTOLOGIE,
WIE BEREITS NACH SCHNELLSCHNITTUNTERSUCHUNG TELEFONISCH DURCHGEGEBEN
KEIN PLATTENEPITHELCARCINOM. VIELMEHR ZWISCHEN BREITEN BAENDERN
EINES HYALINISIERTEN LYMPHKNOTEN ODER NARBENGEWEBE WACHSTUM VON
ATYPISCHEN KLEINEN ZELLEN, TEILS IN SCHMALEN STRAENGE, TEILS IN
SOLIDEN NESTERN. DIE ZELLEN ETWAS GROESSER ALS LYMPHOCYTEN, MIT
MAESSIGER POLYMORPHIE, MIT NUR SEHR GERINGEM ABGRENZBAREN CYTOPLASMA
UND AUFFALLENDER KERNVULNARABILITAET. DER BEFUND ENTSPRICHT EINEM
INFILTRAT EINES KLEINZELLIGEN ANAPLASTISCHEN, DAS HEISST WENIG
DIFFERENZIERTEN CARCINOMS.

ALS AUSGANGSPUNKT KOMMT EIN BRONCHIALCARCINOM ODER EIN
SCHILDDRUESENCARCINOM AM EHESTEN IN FRAGE.

BEURTEILUNG:

UNDIFFERENZIERTES CARCINOM.   /   _

    [\   P████████████████

Figure 12
Special investigation report prepared by computer using PBS (39) (Histo
pathology report).

Charts are usually prepared on the wards and contain vital signs, medications administered, diagnostic and therapeutic procedures initiated and performed etc. These data are entered on a day to day basis. Vital signs (temperature, pulse, bloodpressure, bowel discharge, fluid intake, urine output etc.) are noted and sometimes depicted graphically. Drug dosages may also be depicted graphically. A small set of symbols is used to document essential characteristics of the treatment process (e.g. for diagnostic procedures like biopsies, for operations, for first time out of bed, radiation treatment, removal of drains etc.). These charts then represent an entire treatment episode in the form of a graphic pattern.

Letters of referral and discharge are the main documents containing a summary of a treatment episode. These are primarily intended for external communication, between the various institutions succeeding each other in the treatment of a patient (family physician, specialist, acute care hospital, rehabilitation centre etc.) Equal importance has the operating report for surgical disciplines. All these free text summaries are also the main document referred to if the treatment is reinitiated in the same institution at a later time. Although its contents is individualized for a particular patient, the dominance of a small set of measures repeated over and over for most patients is such, that automation of the preparation of these documents has become rather common practice meanwhile (8,9,10,17,18,21,22,29,35,39,40). Some of the systems cited are used extensively for reporting in special function units. These include radiology, nuclear medicine, routine and special purpose laboratories, endoscopy and consulting specialists. The number of such reports, their variety and diversity in styles is increasing with the specialization of medicine in general and with the specialization of the institution in which a patient is treated. The styles of presentation reach from pictures like radiographs and scintigrams over the narrative description and interpretation of these pictures, to tracings prepared by recording instruments (e.g. electro cardiogram, oscillographic tracings of arterial pulses, tracings of monitors in intensive care) to tables of numerical results obtained in chemical labs. Frequently documents contain all these types of data at the same time.

In contrast to the great variety existing for these documents, which serve for communication between the different disciplines, only few forms are usually used for documenting the history and clinical findings of a patient. These are usually completed soon after admission of an inpatient or after initiation of treatment of an outpatient and provide the basis for initiation of therapy. They are therefore predominantly used internally, i.e. by the physician who prepared them and who is responsible for the patient. Their extent may again vary considerably from institution to institution. It may consist of a single page for free format entry of notes referring to
- history
- previous treatment
- present illness
- physical examination and
- suggested therapy.
Such condensed forms are frequently employed in outpatient care. The other extreme is encountered in specialties like pediatrics or internal medicine. In this case, sometimes equally elaborate, several page forms are maintained for

- nurses notes
- notes of the examining intern (student)

        - notes of the examining
          resident (ward physician).

These contain data on

        - summary of working hypotheses, (working diagnoses) initiated
          treatment
        - present illness
          = chief complaint and reason for referral
          = development
          = previous therapy
        - review of systems
        - psychosocial status
        - previous diseases
        - habits, diets, drugs
        - physical examination, e.g.
          = general appearance
          = sensory apparatus
          = neurological status
          = pulmo-respiratory system
          = cardiovascular system
          = digestive tract
          = genitourinary system
          = musculoskellettral system
          = skin and appendages.

For each section, a number of items and findings may be checked off
from formatted lists. A detailed description is frequently added,
especially if the description refers to the troubles the patient is
cared for.

This part of the medical record seems to be again subject to the
greatest variety, perhaps due to its predominantly internal use. It is
the part for which the cautioning remarks in the section on the 'error
problem' are of greatest relevance. Under the pressure of the work
load, note taking for internal use frequently takes on an aspect of
extra work since one may feel that the unsupported memory is reliable
enough for making the necessary treatment decisions. The problem of
insufficient documentation may come out only later when the patient
presents again after a longer interval or when an evaluation of
patient records is attempted by others, e.g. for scientific purposes.
Incorporation of a thorough review of documentation into peer review
techniques is therefore necessary, and usually the only means of
insuring common standards of documentation.

A number of mixed other documents are usually found in patient records.
These may be copies of the records of other medical care institutions,
copies of certificates prepared by the physician for the patient or the
paying party, or by the patient (e.g. the agreement to undergo an
operation). Prescriptions and instructions given to the patient also
have to be named in this category.

The variety of documents which may be found in a medical record of a
tertiary care installation may be illustrated by the sorting scheme
used at the Medical School Hannover. It lists:

0 Sorting scheme (the sorting scheme itself is contained in the record
  to facilitate orientation and because it may be changed)
1 Cover sheet, admission data
2 Letter of discharge, correspondence
3 Surgery documents (operating report, anesthesia protocol, anesthesia
  questionnaire)

4 Pathology reports (histology, cytology)
5 Letters of referral (from family physician, referring specialist, other hospitals, internal referrals)
6 x-ray reports (Radiographs are kept in a seperate archive).
7 Special investigation reports
      7.1 electro cardiograms, echo cardiograms, phono cardiograms, heart catheterization, tracings reports and related documents.
      7.2 Electro encephalograms, electro mygrams, nerve conduction elocity, echo encephalograms; tracings, reports and related documents
      7.3 Nuclear medicine (all related documents, requests for services, pictures, tracings, reports, protocols)
      7.4 Specialist reports
      Reports from consulting physicians, special lab reports (e.g. microbiology, lung function, ophtalmology investigations etc., except special chemistry lab results)
8 Autopsy report and death certificate
9 Clinical pathology results
      9.1 Clinical chemistry routine and emergency lab reports
      9.2 Hematology lab reports
      9.3 Mixed lab reports
      9.4 Bloodgroup determinations, transfusion protocols, and related documents
      9.5 Immunology results
      9.6 Other clinical chemistry lab results (e.g. endocrinology, gastroenterology)
10 History and physical examination forms
11 Nurses' notes, physical therapy
12 Radiation therapy reports
13 Patientcharts, vital signs, hemodialysis protocols, intensive care charts
14 Certificates
15 Results from external institutions, copies from other patient records, other documents.

There are several hundred different forms in use in the entire institution. A typical patient record contains some thirty pages of documents. For intensive care patients, a volume exceeding one hundred pages is quite frequent. In outpatient clinics, on the other hand, volumes ranging between 5 and 20 pages care more typical.

The cited example is a typical case of a source oriented patient record, which is still the type used most commonly. The characteristics of the widely discussed alternative, the problem oriented record, shall not be repeated here because they have been outlined in the context of a discussion of the treatment process in the chapter on 'medical information and related terminology'. It may have to be emphasized here, that the two concepts are not strictly exclusive, because the problem oriented concept could be used for the history and physical examination findings, and for follow up and progress notes, i.e. the part contained in position 10, 11 and 13 of the sorting scheme our medical records, while the remainder of the record could still be kept in source oriented form.

Apart from these records serving patient management, there is a variety of documents in use for facility management. There exist a number of note book type documentation media which serve to schedule the utilization of special function units like operating theatres, outpatient clinics, emergency rooms, endoscopy investigation rooms, ray investigation equipment, physical therapy etc. Other forms and note books are used in different departments to record doctor's orders during rounds which are then used to fill out request sheets and patient charts. In special function units, again several documents are produced to monitor the processing of specimens, for quality control and for internal statistics. In pathology, for instance, all specimens received are recorded in a book and notes concerning processing of the specimens, its results and the reporting activities are added. In clinical chemistry the results produced are recorded for every instrument and quality controls monitor propper accuracy. In the blood bank a file of blood donors is maintained, who are monitored medically and called upon to donate blood, either routinely or in special emergency situations. Examples for automated support of these documentation activities are found elsewhere in this volume (c.f. e.g. the contributions of WINGERT and SCHNEIDER).

5. Media used in Medical Documentation

This section is intended as a discussion of the relative characteristics and benefits of currently used means of documentation. The emphasis will be on conventional means and their extensions through new reproduction techniques. Their substitution through information systems based on digital computers will be excluded since this subject is covered comprehensively in several other contributions in this volume.

Conventionally, there exist few original size copies of every document. Mostly, one is contained in the patient record and another in the unit where the data were generated. I.e. the material used for communication between different services is kept sorted according to patients, usually within the institution responsible for the patient. A second copy is kept by the unit responsible for generating the data. In traditional institutions, many of the special function units, such as radiology, clinical chemistry lab etc. are themselves part of a medical specialty, e.g. the department of internal medicine or of surgery etc.. Large centralized patient care installations, where one special service unit like a department of radiology, nuclear medicine or physical therapy services all clinical disciplines are relatively new in Europe.

The conventional original size paper based copy of the patient record has some advantages and merrits which are recognized in routine use. The most important ones are that it is portable and may be taken wherever the physician needs it. In particular it may be used at the bedside. Furthermore, all documents are just as good as they have been prepared. No recording process which is often suspected of reducing the information content of a document is interposed. Since the quality of the original e.g. in the case of notes documented in physician's notoriously poor handwriting - is sometimes restricted, the confidentiality issue may also be considered taken care of. This may sometimes even be the fact, to the extent that even the physician who prepared the notes may have difficulties in recovering their meaning.

Another frequently recognized advantage is the ability to make notes, mark important facts etc., which increases the handiness of the document at the bedside.

Finally the property issue is seemingly clearly settled: the patient record as a document belongs to the service responsible for the patient. The results of special investigations as documented in the reports belongs to the service generating them. The overlap due to inclusion of the same report in the patient record passes unnoticed.

These advantages stand against a number of disadvantages. The key problem caused by conventional single copy paperbased patient records is that they may be used only at one place at a time. However, simultaneous use in different locations would be preferrable in many instances. Interpretation of results obtained in one service would frequently be easier if the record were available. Simultaneously it may be necessary to prepare special treatment measures in another unit. Again one might wish to be able to refer to the patient record at the same time for scientific puroses. This creates a situation where substantial fractions of available highly skilled man power are absorbed by the search for documents.

Besides the fact that only a single copy exists its bulk, which makes transportation difficult, interferes with the availability of the record. Many of our original records are too voluminous to be transported by the pneumatic tube system.

The problem of availability is even augmented in the case of scientific evaluation. Since different aspects can make scientific evaluation worth while in the 'interesting cases', and since it is known that who ever has a record once will have it for good, it may become very difficult to retrieve all records relevant for a given problem. We have witnessed searches for scientific purposes where 40 to 50 percent of the relevant records could not be made available from a conventional archive.

Also, the bulk of the record makes it hard to work with, especially in the case of evaluation of several records.

Finally the storage of such records presents a problem. In West-Germany, legal regulations require that many documents be stored for as long as thirty years. The patient records that would accumulate over such a period in our institution would require between 2600 and 5700 square meters of storage space if stored in mobile racks, to the height of approximately 2 m (20).

In order to compensate for these disadvantages, an ideal medical record should be retrievable by patient or categorically for use in clinical investigation or service management. Data should be presented in clear alphanumeric types, if not in the form of graphs or pictures. The data should be available immediately after generation and where or when they are needed by authorized users.

The full scope of these requirements cannot be fulfilled yet. Digital computers are an essential prerequisite for their fulfillment, which cannot be replaced by other means. However, the interface with the user still presents considerable problems, mainly with respect to data capture and data presentation. The solution will most probably lie in the application of hybrid techniques, using digital techniques mainly for record linkage and storage and display of alphanumeric data, and analog reproduction techniques for storage of the bulk of data and of pictures.

Analog reproduction techniques are available in several different forms, e.g.
- telecommunication of original size hard copies
- telecommunication by video display of originals (videophone, close circuit television)
- storage on microfilm
- storage on high density videotapes.

Especially intriguing are combinations of the cited techniques, particularly if linked to digital computers for control of search and file.

Apart from the considerable advantages of these techniques over the conventional procedure, analog reproduction techniques have a number of disadvantages in common:

- requirements of displays, terminals viewers etc.
- costs
- insufficient quality for colour and halftone reproductions.

In most instances one will depend on a visual display, a television screen or another kind of terminal. Currently these devices are not mobile enough to be used at the bedside and too expensive to be installed wherever they may be needed, especially in the case of television screens, or hard copy generating terminals. For microfilmed material, the devices used for reading micro copies are already available at reasonable prices. In this case, however, the reproduction and sorting procedure is too demanding to facilitate recording and documentation of material at the time of generation. Therefore microfilm techniques are only used at present to store material from discharged patients. This can be made available to different users simultaneously with almost total guarantee of availability and close to absolute data security (20). The essential bottle neck of availability during the actual period of patient care, however, is not solved in this fashion.

The achievement of sufficient quality of the reproduction of halftone or colour documents (e.g. radiographs, scintigrams) again is highly costintensive. For reproduction of radiographs on microfilm, several systems have been developed but have not yet gained full acceptance. Colour reproduction on microfilm may be acceptable as to the quality for most purposes, but does entail even more procedural and organizational concessions than halftone reproduction. Both kinds of reproduction may be achieved with television techniques, however, at considerable cost.

The broadest acceptance has been gained so far by microfilm techniques. Close circuit television is yet restricted to the use in special purpose application, mostly in radiology and nuclear medicine. An attempt to solve the communication problems in patient care by these techniques does not seem to have been made so far.

For microfilm storage, the fiche system is commonly used. Another alternative would be to store the documents of film reels. This is only available if the documents may be accessed by automatic search techniques on the reels. In the fiche system, the film strips of one patient are mounted in transparent aperture cards.

These 'microfiches' are kept in patient identification order (alphabetic or patient number). If a record is requested, a diazocopy of the microfiche is prepared and forwarded to the user. In this way a record is practically safe against loss, may be made available to several users at the same time, is safe from additions or deletions of material and can be handled with considerable ease.

One remaining disadvantage for the user is the need of a viewer for reading. Another is that the processing of the record is so time consuming that it is difficult to incorporate this reproduction and documentation system into the communication process accompanying medical care.

Considerable advantages could be expected from a system that indexes documents as they are microfilmed and makes them available through some kind of random access. Recent developments are very promising in this respect. One such system stores 3,2 million documents, and makes them available with access times of 10 seconds (1). These characteristics make this system recommendable at least for special purpose documentation subsystems. Basing a total medical record system on such techniques would require

- decentralized capture of documents
- decentralized display of documents
- storage capacities in the range of > 100 million documents
- access times in the range of seconds.

One considerable advantage of a microfilm based system would be that it is legally acceptable because it generates a permanent record of a document. High density videotapes which seem to represent the only currently available technique which may fullfill the above requirements, if linked with digital computers (26) would therefore have to incorporate microfilm techniques for the storage of security copies.

6. The MSH Medical Record System

The Medical System Hannover (MSH) is a computer based medical information system which evolves since 1969. It provides a number of service functions for

- patient care
- administration
- research activities.

These have been described previously (27,28). For patient care, the paper based conventional medical record is the central instrument for recording patient related information. So far it has not been attempted to achieve comprehensive computer processing of this information. The complexity of our institution will preclude such attempts in the near future. Instead, the emphasis was placed upon developing a concept which would make integration of the medical record into a computer based medical information system possible. This concept has three key elements:

- a centralized integrated patient data bank including data retrieval systems
- data acquisition systems
  = patient admission system (PAS)
  = basic documentation system (BDS)
- a central archive for patient records.

This system is fully operational for inpatients. Various parts are in use for outpatients. The following description will review the system for inpatients. Its application for outpatients will consist of an extension of the current system without major modification, provided, the necessary prerequisites in terms of hardware and machine capacity will be available.

6.1 FUNCTIONAL ORGANIZATION

On admission, a set of administrative data concerning the patient is acquired through computer dialogue (6). From these, a unique reproducible identification number is produced, which identifies the patient for the hospital. This number is used to identify and link practically all patient related data. During a patient's stay in the hospital, the paper based medical record kept on the wards receives all documents generated during treatment. A number of these documents are prepared through the use of computer based reporting systems, which have gained considerable importance for daily routine work (21,22,39,40). Report generation through computer based reporting systems speeds up the preparation of reports by eliminating the delay caused by dictating and manual typewriting. In some instances, regular reporting and documentation was made possible only through application of these reporting systems. In others, the major gain from use of these systems lies in the enforcement of better documentation through strict application of plausibility checks. Still however, these documents are available only in single or comparatively few copies and can in most practical situations only be referred to where the patient record is available. In this respect, the availability of the Patient Information Display System (PIDS) (38) constitutes a considerable advantage. It enables the user to access patient data stored in the patient data bank via videodisplay. In this way, patient data are available as soon as they have been stored in the data bank, at any terminal linked to the computer system. These functions are of course protected against unauthorized use. In summary then, the conventional patient record is the key instrument for communication and documentation at the time of a patient's treatment in the hospital. Computer based reporting systems speed up report generation and make the reports more versatile, reliable and legible. For these reasons, they are indispensable in many applications for clinical care. Their results are used in the same manner as other reports. Essential prerequisites for making patient related data available in a more desirable fashion for use at different locations independently of the patient record during the actual treatment period are operational. Their role in actual clinical routine, however, is still secondary.

After a patient is discharged from the hospital or transferred to the service of another department, the record is finalized. This procedure includes dictating final reports, letter of discharge, etc., and the completion of the face sheet of the medical record, for basic documentation.

Thereafter, the record is forwarded to the central archive and documentation unit (medical record library). Here it is registered in the central archive and transferred to clinical documentation. For basic documentation, the medical record librarian converts the items noted by the physician in free text on the face sheet into numerical codes which are then read into the computer and stored in the patient data bank.

The basic documentation data may be retrieved if the patient presents again for treatment at a later stage. Their use for categorical retrieval of patient records is, however, more important at present. Due to the basic documentation data, it is possible to list records of patients with a certain combination of medical administrative descriptors (13,14). These records may then be evaluated scientifically.

From the clinical documentation unit, the record is returned to the central archive. Here it is stored for approximately one year in original form. After this period, it is retrieved and copied on microfilm. Thereafter it is stored in the microfilm archive in the form of microfiches, and on a simultaneously prepared unaltered security copy of the microfilm. Whenever the record is requested thereafter, diazocopies of the microfiches are handed out. Thereby several users can be serviced simultaneously, and loss of the documented material is precluded.

Following this rough outline of the functional organization of the medical record system, some more details, concerning the performance of its components shall be given in the subsequent sections.

6.2 THE PATIENT DATA BANK AND THE INFORMATION RETRIEVAL SYSTEMS.

The patient data bank (32,33,34) integrates data on patients relevant for
- patient care
- administration
- scientific evaluation.

The main components of the patient data bank are based on IMS as data base management. Thereby it becomes possible to store data in integrated hierarchically structured variable length records. This is achieved by dividing the information to be stored into subsets which are stored in various types of 'segments' which are linked by pointers. Each segment may be repeated an arbitrary number of times within a logical record, depending on the occurence of the corresponding data. A root segment contains the essential data for patient identification and links the various segments of a data base. Several such hierarchically structured data bases exist. They are complemented by several data bases of various other types of organization.

Data of primarily administrative relevance (e.g. ward number, home address) are in this fashion stored together with data of primarily medical relevance (e.g diagnoses). For each patient, the data pertaining to several hospital stays are linked together. For each hospital stay several diagnoses may be registered, each of which may again be linked to several types of treatment.

The data base is transparent to the programmer. For each application the logical structure of the relevant data base is specially defined. It usually consists only of a subset of the entire segment structure. In this fashion, data protection is enforced at the level of the application programmer. A number of programs is used for retrieval of data, for online or offline processing. The reporting programs, for example, may retrieve such items as the family physician's address in order to generate reports ready for mailing. Other programs generate statistics for medical or administrative purposes. Such programs shall not be considered in this section.

In the context of the medical record system, some search programs are of primary importance which enable the user to state requests to the data bank in order to retrieve records from the central archive.

One such program (DBAUS, 13) allows the user to state a logical combination of basic documentation data, such as diagnoses, therapies or complications.

Thus a request might consist of a search for all documents of patients for which either of a set of diagnoses (e.g. various types of myocardial infarction) and none of a set of other diagnoses (e.g. various types of diabetes mellitus) are registered. The program yields a listing of all relevent records, in ascending order of identification number and displays a set of statistics, e.g. age distribution of the patient.

This program constitutes a key link between the central archive and the patient data bank for the retrieval of records.

Another program (PATWERT, 13) yields additional crosstabulation of the basic documentation and administrative data. E.g. crosstabulations of diagnoses, outcomes of therapy, age groups, lengths of stay or annual distribution of admission frequencies may be generated. This program therefore has a complementary role for certain types of investigations.

The Patient Information Display System (PIDS) (37) finally, is an online system of programs for the display of patient data. It may be called from any terminal connected to the MSH central computer. Several function modules exist, e.g. for the display of administrative or medical data. Among administrative data, such as previous hospitalizations, location of a given patient within the hospital may be listed. The patients being treated on a particular ward may be displayed etc.. Medical information includes basic documentation data registered during previous treatment periods. The system is protected by a hierarchical key word system, giving different users access to different sets of system modules. The data displayed may be obtained as hard copies from the terminal. The most important medical application of PIDS concerns the display of laboratory data (38). These are generated in the routine clinical chemistry lab which is fully automated and equipped with an independent EDP system (23,24). Data transfer from this system to the central MSH computer facility is achieved through transfer of tapes.

All updates of the data bank are executed in batch mode. Input is provided by several files which receive data from the various program systems.

6.3 DATA ACQUISITION SYSTEMS

Only the systems linked directly with the medical record system will be treated in this section. These are the Patient Admission System PAS and the Basic Documentation System BDS. The reporting systems will not be covered.

6.3.1 THE PATIENT ADMISSION SYSTEM (PAS)

The Patient Admission System (6) evolved since the medical school took up patient care activities in the central building complex within its campus. It is progressively developing towards a Patient Admission and Scheduling System (PASS). As most other systems, it contains batch and interactive modules and is designed to acquire all administrative data on in- and outpatients. Though most admissions and status oriented transactions are made centrally in one central administering office, the system can again be operated from any of the MSH terminals. For some hospitals located remotely, the admissions are done within these hospitals. In addition, an increasing number of transactions is transferred to the responsibility of ward secretaries who execute them on ward units. Thus the application of this centrally controlled system becomes decentralized.

The admission dialogue consists of up to 75 questions. The answers obtained from the patient or an accompanying person are subject to extensive formal, logical and contextual plausibility checking. Of special importance are the items

- name
- date of birth
- sex

which are used to generate a unique identification number. This serves as reproducible link for all patient documents as well as for sorting argument for most patient oriented files, in the centralized patient data bank, as well as in the central archive, archive for radiographs, etc..

The Patient Admission System monitors patient location, contains information on financial and insurance status and such items as home addresses and address of family physician.

The most important patient data are output on an aluminium foil which is used for transcribing this data on other documents by means of a small printig device. Since the patient identification is also represented in machine readable form on this data carrier, this reproduction system may be used to identify machine readable documents. This is extensively used in many applications of reporting systems, which use mark sense reader forms as input medium.

Since PAS is in operation since the first day of operation of the hospital complex, it may be used to produce various kinds of statistics for planning of hospital operations.

6.3.2 BASIC DOCUMENTATION SYSTEM BDS

The Basic Documentation System in its first version was already implemented in 1968, at a time, when patient care activities of the then newly founded Medical School were restricted to one municipal hospital, which served as teaching hospital at that time already.

The original design of the Basic Documentation System was based on recommendations of 1961 (4) concerning a common face sheet for medical records suitable for documentation purposes. This was designed for manual entry of all relevant patient data, many of which are made available through the Patient Admission System in the MSH. Recommendations for documentation of medically relevant data were restricted to diagnoses and risk factors.

Because of the redundancy of data in the admission and basic documentation systems, and because application of the original basic documentation system beyond the scope of Internal Medicine oriented disciplines revealed a different set of requirements, the basic documentation system was redesigned. This was put into effect in 1975.

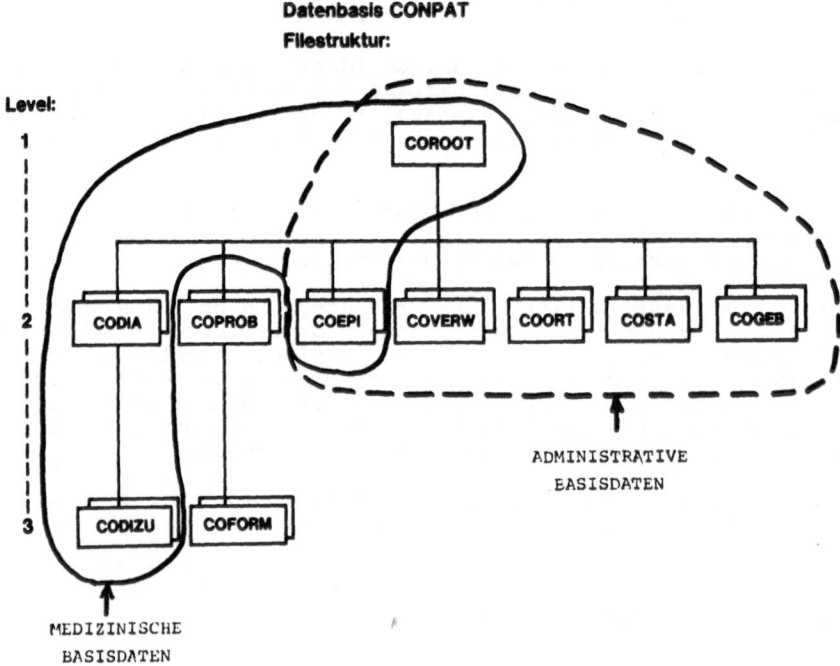

Figure 13
Example of logical structure of integrated patient data bank. File
CONPAT contains medical (plain line) and administrative (dashed line)
data in hierarchical relation.

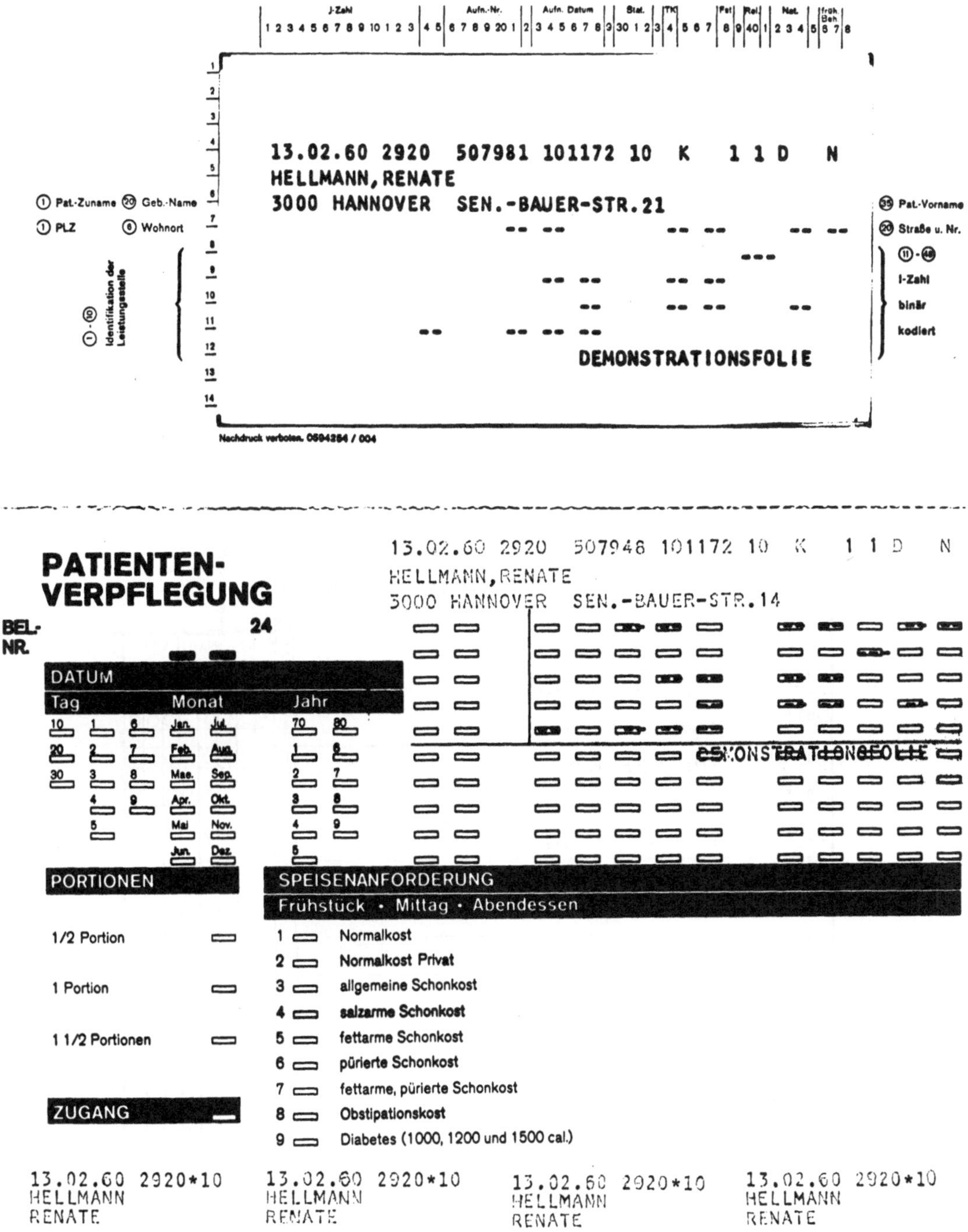

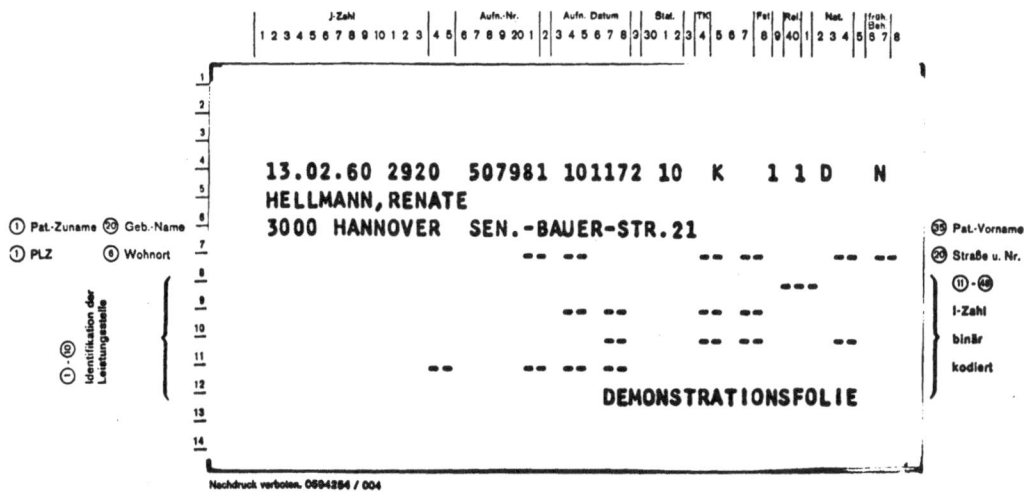

Figure 14
Patient Admission System data carriers. Patient identification data may
be transcribed from aluminium foil onto mark sense forms. Stickers with
name and identification number are also prepared.

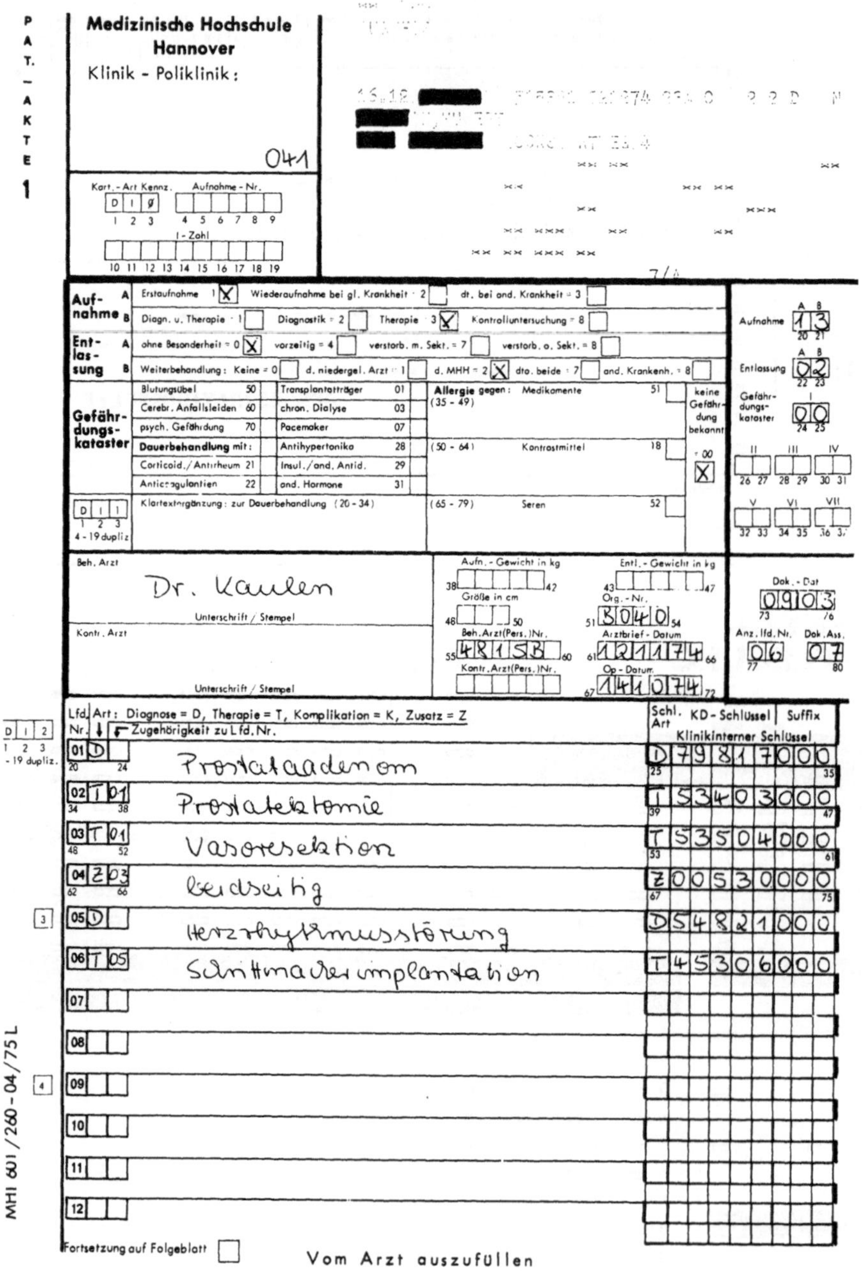

240

Medizinische Hochschule Hannover

Klinik - Poliklinik:

041

PAT.-AKTE 1

Kart.-Art Kennz. | D I Ø
Aufnahme-Nr.

1-Zahl

Auf- nahme A: Erstaufnahme 1 [X] Wiederaufnahme bei gl. Krankheit 2 · dt. bei and. Krankheit 3
nahme B: Diagn. u. Therapie 1 · Diagnostik 2 · Therapie 3 [X] · Kontrolluntersuchung 8

Ent- las- sung A: ohne Besonderheit 0 [X] · vorzeitig 4 · verstorb. m. Sekt. 7 · verstorb. o. Sekt. 8
sung B: Weiterbehandlung: Keine 0 · d. niedergel. Arzt 1 · d. MHH 2 [X] · dto. beide 7 · and. Krankenh. 8

Gefähr- dungs- kataster:
Blutungsübel 50 | Transplantatträger 01 | Allergie gegen: Medikamente 51 | keine Gefährdung bekannt
Cerebr. Anfallsleiden 60 | chron. Dialyse 03 | (35-49)
psych. Gefährdung 70 | Pacemaker 07
Dauerbehandlung mit: | Antihypertonika 28 | (50-64) Kontrastmittel 18
Corticoid/Antirheum 21 | Insul./and. Antid. 29
Anticoagulantien 22 | and. Hormone 31
Klartextergänzung: zur Dauerbehandlung (20-34) | (65-79) Seren 52

Beh. Arzt: Dr. Kaulen
Unterschrift / Stempel
Kontr. Arzt:
Unterschrift / Stempel

Aufn.-Gewicht in kg | Entl.-Gewicht in kg
Größe in cm | Org.-Nr. 3 0 4 0
Beh.Arzt(Pers.)Nr. 4 R 1 5 B | Arztbrief-Datum 1 R 1 1 7 4
Kontr.Arzt(Pers.)Nr. | Op.-Datum 1 4 4 0 7 4

Aufnahme 1 3 | Entlassung 0 2 | Gefähr-dungs-kataster 0 0
Dok.-Dat 0 9 0 3 | Anz.lfd.Nr. 0 6 | Dok.Ass. 0 7

Lfd. Art: Diagnose = D, Therapie = T, Komplikation = K, Zusatz = Z
Nr. Zugehörigkeit zu Lfd. Nr. | Schl. Art | KD-Schlüssel | Suffix / Klinikinterner Schlüssel

01 D Prostataadenom — D 79 81 70 0 0
02 T 01 Prostatektomie — T 534 03 0 00
03 T 01 Vasoresektion — T 535 04 0 00
04 Z 03 beidseitig — Z 00 53 0 00 0
05 D Herzrhythmusstörung — D 54 821 00 0
06 T 05 Schrittmacherimplantation — T 453 06 0 00

Fortsetzung auf Folgeblatt [ ] Vom Arzt auszufüllen

MHH 601/260-04/75 L

Figure 15
Basic documentation medical record face sheet. Patient identification in upper right hand corner; administrative data and risk factors may be recorded in middle section. Diagnoses, therapies and complications may be recorded with mutual relations in clear text and in coded form in lower half.

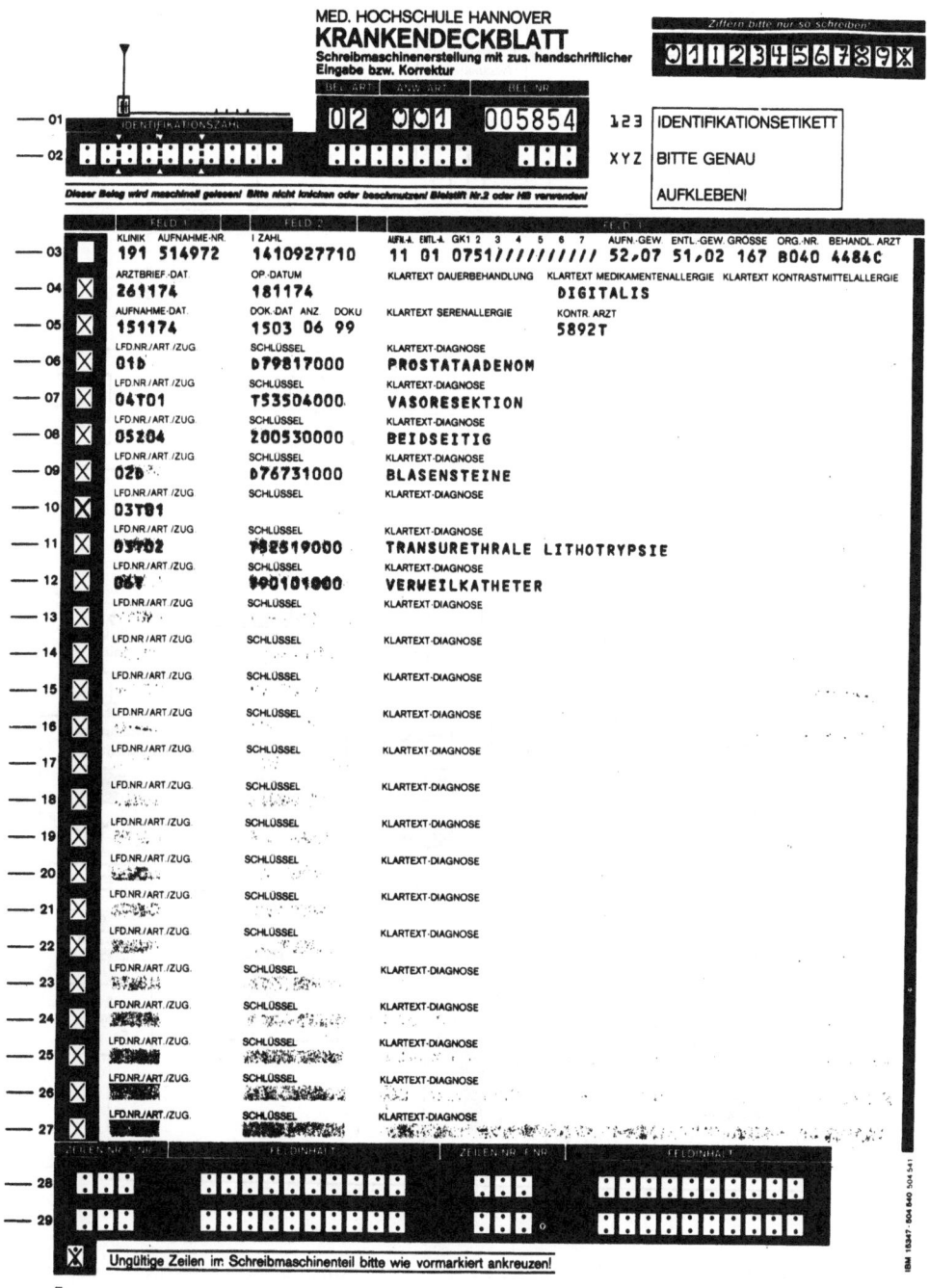

Figure 16
OCR Form used as input medium for Basic Documentation data.

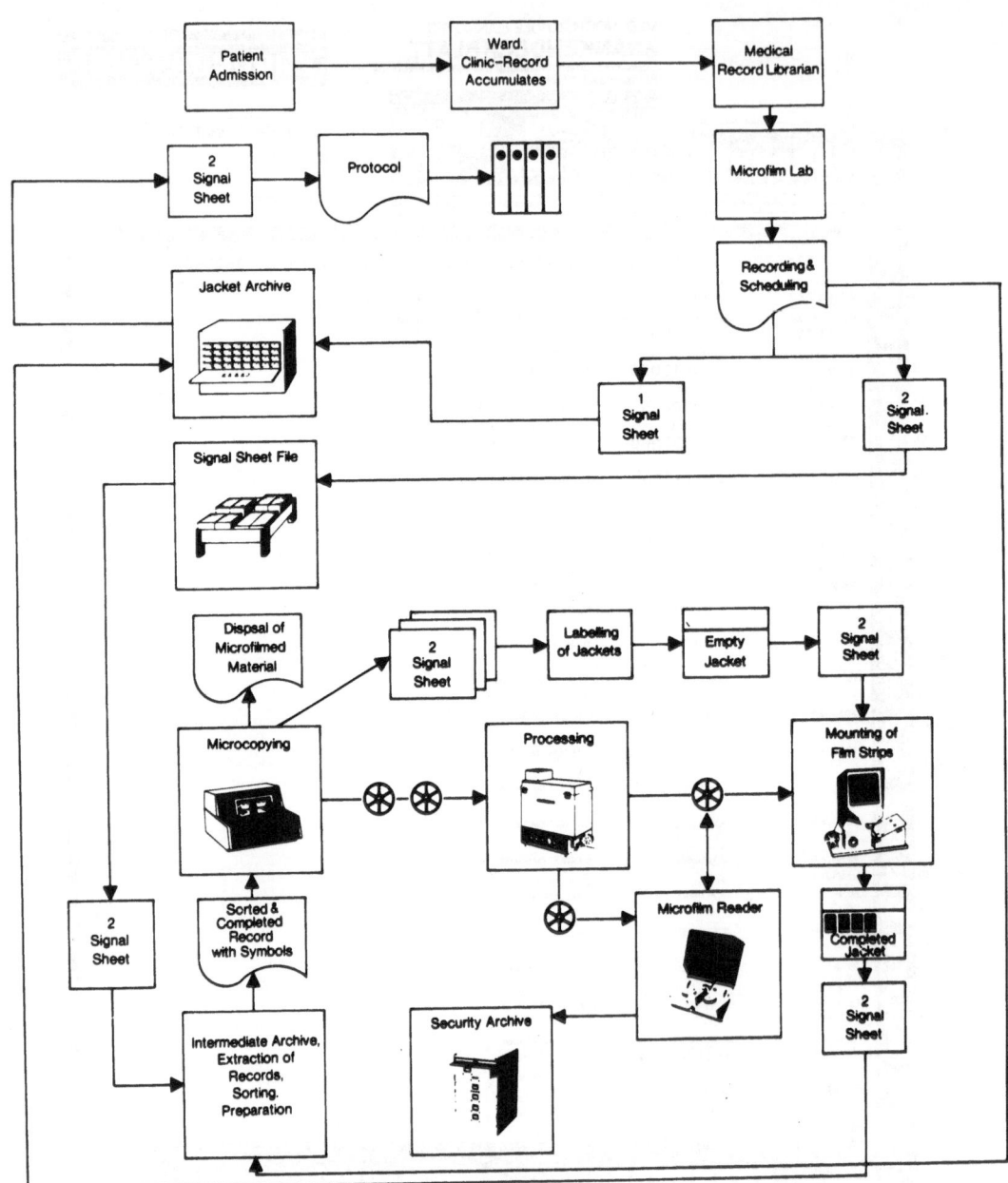

Figure 17
Central archive for patient record - Functional organization of microfilm lab. Refer to text for details.

The main characteristics of the redesigned system are (14,15)

- online and offline data acquisition facility
- greatly restricted set of administrative data covered
- greatly extended set of medical data, including
  = diagnoses
  = therapies
  = complications
  = modifiers
  = specification of risk factors and allergies in free text
- employement of dynamically adjusted coding systems
- coding of semantic relations between documented items
- extended automatic error checks
- extended feedback between central documentation and clinicians
- separation of responsibility for semantic content (physician) and its coding (medical record librarian).

Data acquisition is supported by the Data Interpretation and Evaluation System (DIES, 22) our most widely employed general purpose reporting system. Punched cards, optical character reader forms or CRT terminals are made available by this system for data entry. Especially the OCR forms and punched cards, after strict organizational regulations, did prove highly reliable.

Since the relevant administrative data are acquired by PAS, the data concerning modalities of admission and discharge could be greatly reduced in the basic documentation. For medical purposes, on the other hand, a considerably extended set of requirements could be served by the system's functions.

As a response to the considerations concerning medical information, the employed coding system was converted into an open ended system. Therefore the originally employed KDS code developed by IMMICH (16) was extended from 5 to 8 digits, thereby allowing for hierarchical subclassification of items contained in this diagnostic index. Also, several other diagnostic codes developed by such disciplines as Urology and Traumatology were compared to the KDS and incorporated into our extended system of keys by using previously unemployed codes, but strictly regarding the systematics proposed by IMMICH.

Also, diagnoses which could not be satisfactorily covered by the available spectrum of codes, are assigned new numerical codes (e.g. mitral ballooning, a diagnosis which is only possible since the use of echo cardiograph). This process of adaptation of the employed coding system is in continuous progress. Codes for therapies are predominantly needed by surgically oriented disciplines. The codes used in our institution are based on an extended and adapted code developed by SCHEIBE and GOEGELER (31). This requirement of the surgical disciplines passed unnoticed in the development of the original suggestions for the development of a common cover sheet for medical records (4).

Especially the purpose of monitoring newly appearing terminology did considerably influence the system design. For all items (diagnoses, complications, therapies), the medical record librarian notes the exact expression used by the clinician together with her translation of a numerical code. The system then retrieves the preferred term used for this code from a computer stored file and plays it back with the expression used by the physician. Both are reviewed by the physician responsible for clinical documentation in our department, or, in some cases, by a physician responsible for documentation in a clinical department. In this way, semantic errors in documentation are detected and identified for correction,and new notions are pinpointed if they have not been identified as such by the medical record librarian. If necessary, these are then assigned new code numbers within the coding system applicable (KDS for diagnoses or complications, or code of therapies/procedures). Generally the physician is supposed to act as specialist for the employed terminology, while the medical record librarian is responsible for correct employment of the coding systems.

Another feature of the system is that the relations between various items may be documented. Thus it is possible to link diagnoses and related therapies and complications. In some cases such links are even necessary for certain diagnoses. E.g. "meningitis due to mumps virus" may be documented by a link between the diagnoses 'mumps' and 'meningitis'.

In contrast to this extended use of dynamic coding systems, the use of codes for risk factors and allergies was considerably reduced in favour of the possibility to specify these items exactly in free text. These items are almost exclusively documented for patient care purposes and not for categorical retrieval. Therefore maximum precision is desirable and justified.

On the whole, the Basic Documentation System greatly increases the possible precision of categorical data bank inquiries as well as of patient care related information. In addition it provides a basis for more precise medical statistics.

With respect to the issue of precision, it has to be noted, however, that the demands proposed by clinicians have frequently been found to be impractical. Frequently, the precision of suggested catalogues of items is far greater than the actual user is willing to take into consideration. This results frequently in the fact that only some 20 to 50 percent of the items contained in such a catalogue are actually used. Precision may be such that the recall of documents is greatly reduced. The process of construction of code systems has therefore to be considered with great care. Frequently it is necessary and possible to arrive at a practicable spectrum of items in order not to sacrifice recall for precision.

It is our contention that the described system of using a common set of terms for the entire institution, which is adaptable to the requirements of changing medical needs, represents advantages such as consistent use of standardized terminology which make it preferrable over the use of rigid coding schemes although these may have a greater degree of comparability between institutions. We also hope to provide thereby a basis for sucessful application of automatic encoding techniques, such as through use of SNOP or SNOMED (2,3).

6.4 THE CENTRAL ARCHIVE FOR PATIENT RECORDS CAPR.

The Central Archive for Patient Records CAPR (20) is on its evolution from a storage facility for patient records that are hardly ever used into an essential component of our medical information system, which is used actively in the patient care process. The fundamental characteristics enabling this development are

    - use of microfilm as a storage medium
    - link to the integrated patient data bank system.

The link to the patient data bank makes it possible to base the retrieval of patient records on descriptors stored in the computer, and the use of microfilm as storage medium enables us to make the retrieved records available to several authorized users simultaneously. So far employment of archieved material in patient care is restricted to the use of data collected in previous treatment episodes. With the evolution of mass storage technology, it is, however, foreseeable that it will be possible to acquire material decentrally in some kind of analog copy and make it available by random access procedures during the actual treatment episode.

The central archive for patient records is composed of three subunits:

- the microfilm laboratory and microfilm archive
- the intermediate archive
- the security archive.

The microfilm lab's functions are

- registration of incoming records
- service of user's request for archived material
- maintenance of an archive of microfiches
- execution of all reproduction processes.

The functions of the intermediate archive include:

- storage of all patient records for one year before microcopying
- preparation of records for reproduction on microfilm
- maintenance of a small archive of documents which cannot be reproduced on microfilm.

The security archive, finally serves to

- guard and protect unaltered duplicate reels of microfilm (security copies).

The microfilm lab is therefore the central interface between the user and the actual archive, while the intermediate archive serves as buffer and the security archive serves as backup.

The main concern in the design of this medical record library was to render the stored documents

- safe and
- easy to use.

Safety is guaranteed for microfilmed material because of the availability of a backup copy and due to a strict organizational structure which highly precludes misplacement of a record in the microfiche archive as well as in the intermediate archive. The intermediate archive is particularly vulnerable to misplacement of records because no backup exists for the original records, and because the material may have to be handed out to the user in its original form. Despite of this, only 5 records are missing out of close to 80,000 records retrieved.

The key element for this degree of security is a signal sheet system. Two signal sheets identifying the record are prepared when a record is delivered to the archive. One is placed in the microfiche archive in the location where the microfiche will later be inserted. The other is kept in a special file, in the order of the incoming records. By using batches of signal sheets from this file, the records are later retrieved from the intermediate archive for micro copying. For all records handed out in original form, notes are kept in the intermediate archive by replacement of records with 'missing cards' and by maintenance of lists of requested records for every user.

A high degree of usability of the record is maintained by sorting all documents according to a common scheme for each treatment episode and by identifying each treatment episode with symbols which are legible without magnification. So it becomes possible for the user to locate a treatment period of interest within a microfiche which may contain several. Within each treatment episode, documents of a particular type are found always in a particular location relative to the others.

This form of a central archive has proven highly acceptable to the user. Recently, a commission of users was invited to review the central archive and to work out recommendations for further improvement. The resulting document turned out so posistive that it became valuable in convincing reluctant colleagues on the wards of the value of the archive. The work load has multipled since the installation of the archive and lies currently in the range of 6000 records being delivered and around 2000 records being retrieved for scientific or patient care purposes per month. So far, a link to the integrated data bank was mainly established through the patient admission system and the basic documentation system outlined above. These provide the data according to which records may be retrieved. Currently, another link is established by registering all incoming records through computer dialogue and monitoring all records movements within the archive as well as in and out of the archive. This patient record information system is based on another carrier system for medical reporting, the DAta DIrected Medically Oriented Programming System (DADIMOPS, 40). Use of this system is expected to result in reduction of the personnel requirements by one to two full time equivalents since the data gathered by this system will enable us to prepare
- working lists
- microfilm protocols
- microfilm jacket identification
automatically and since requests concerning archived material may be answered at least in part through lookup functions provided by DADIMOPS via MSH terminal system.

So far, maintenance of the current quality is highly personnel intensive. We calculated that we would need a minimum staff of 30 employees to maintain the essential functions of the archive for the full work load. Our ability to achieve it with 16 full time equivalents is due to the fact that an estimated 25 percent of records does not yet reach the archive, and to the fact that the intermediate archive has in fact a considerable buffer capacity. Within it records currently accumulate at the rate of 2000 per month, which is the difference between the input of some 6000 delivered records and the output for microcopying which is restricted to some 4000 due to lack of personnel.

So far, we are not able to solve this personnel requirement of our central archive. The key solution may lie in automatic random access by multiple users to documents on analog mass storage media. This, of course, would require propper indexing of documents and possibly decentralized acquisition. This would replace most of the current manual registration, preparation, book keeping processes in the central archive, which account for most of the cost intensive personnel requirements.

6.5 CONCLUSION

In summary then, it may be stated that the MSH medical record system is a hybrid system, comprising a hierarchy of integrated data carriers, such as

- conventional patient record
- microfilm stored patient record
- computer stored patient data.

Patient care is primarily based on the actual source oriented conventional record. It may be supplemented by material from the microfilm archive. Frequently used and highly abstracted information is kept in the computerized patient data bank. Computer stored medical data are less frequently used in actual patient care than for clinical investigations. The system provides a basis for further integrating the computerized medical record system into the actual care process.

Literature

1 ALLCOM: Computergesteuertes Informationssystem, MRS-90, Allcom Potter GmbH, Frankfurt Genferstr. 11a (1976)
2 COLLEGE OF THE AMERICAN PATHOLOGISTS: Systematized Nomenclature of Pathology (Chicago 1965)
3 COTE, R.A.: SNOMED - A Tool for the Computer Management of Medical Data. In: Intern.Symp.Med.Inf.Syst., Proceedings of Medin '75 66-75, Tokyo (1975)
4 DEUTSCHE GESELLSCHAFT FUER DOKUMENTATION: Ein dokumentationsgerechter Krankenblattkopf fuer stationaere Patienten aller klinischen Faecher (sog. allgemeiner Krankenblattkopf) Med.Dok. 5 (1961) 57-70
5 DUNN, H.L.: Hospital and Clinical Statistics in General (in BAHNE, G.W. (ed.)): Practical Applications of the Punched Card Method in Colleges and Universities. New York: Columbia University Press (1935) 241-270
6 ENGELBRECHT, R. et al: Patients' Dynamics and Functional Administrative Behaviour of a Multidisciplinary Medical Center. Meth.Inf.Med. 15 (1976) in press. Meth.Inf. Med. 15 (1976) . In press.
7 FEINSTEIN, A.R.: Clinical Judgement (Baltimore: Williams&Wilkinson, 1967)
8 GIERE, W., BAUMANN, H.: Zur Erfassung und Verarbeitung medizinischer Daten mittels Computer. 1. Mitteilung: Ein Erfassungs- und Speicherprogramm (DUSP) zur Dokumentation von Krankengeschichten. Meth.Inf.Med. 8 (1969) 11-18
9 GIERE, W.: Zur Erfassung und Verarbeitung medizinischer Daten mittels Computer. 2. Mitteilung: Die Fehlerpruefung durch das Datenerfassungs- und Speicherprogramm (DUSP) gespeicherter Daten. Meth.Inf.Med. 8 (1969) 197-200
10 GIERE, W.: Zur Erfassung und Verarbeitung medizinischer Daten mittels Computer. 3. Mitteilung: Decoding und Textausgabe Programm. Meth.Inf.Med. 10 (1971) 19-25
11 HAMPTON, J.R. et al: Relative Contributions of History Taking Physical Examination and Laboratory Investigation to Diagnosis and Management of Medical Outpatients. Brit.Med.J. 2 (1975) 486-489
12 HARTMANN, F.: Krankheitsgeschichte und Krankengeschichte (Naturhistorische und personale Krankheitsauffassung). Marburger Sitzungsberichte 87 (1966) 17-32

13 HILL, R.D. et al: The Data Bank Concept of the Medical System Hannover and the Analysis of Patient Data. In ANDERSON,J., FORSYTHE, H. (ed.): Medinfo '74, (Amsterdam: North Holland Publ. Comp., 1974) 399-406

14 HOLTHOFF, G.: Aufbau einer multidisziplinaeren zentralisierten medizinischen Basisdokumentation. Dissertation, Tieraerztliche Hochschule Hannover 1976

15 HOLTHOFF, G. et al.: Aufbau, Routineeinsatz und Weiterentwicklung einer computerunterstuetzten Basisdokumentation fuer die Medizinische Hochschule Hannover. Teil 1: Krankenblatt, Dokumentation, Mikrofilmverfahren. Arbeitstagung der Arbeitsgruppe Medizinische Informatik der GMDS, Hannover (1975) (Berlin, Heidelberg, New York: Springer, in press)

16 IMMICH, H.: Klinischer Diagnosenschluessel (Stuttgart: Schatthauer, 1966)

17 JACOBITZ, K., BOERNER, P.: Ein allgemeines System zur Synthese medizinischer Berichte aus Markierungsboegen (FTSS). Meth.Inf.Med 11 (1972) 163-172

18 KOEPPE, K. et al: Das System 'ORVID' , ein Beitrag zur programmierten Dokumentation in der Roentgendiagnostik. Fortschr.Roentgenstr.Nukl.Med. 112 (1970) 103-110

19 KOLLEGIUM BIOMATHEMATIK NW: Biomathematik fuer Mediziner (Berlin, Heidelberg, New York: Springer 1975)

20 MOEHR, J.R., TRAMP, H.J.: A Microfilm Oriented Central Archive in a Large Patient Care Installation. Meth.Inf.Med. 15 (1976) 74-82

21 POCKLINGTON, P.R.: AMAP, A General Optical Mark Reader Form Evaluation Program. Meth.Inf.Med. 12, (1973) 211-222

22 POCKLINGTON, P.R.: (DIES) The Necessity for Requirements of and Basic Design of a General Data Interpretation and Evaluation System (DIES). In ANDERSON, J., FORSYTHE, J.M. (ed.): Medinfo '74. (Amsterdam: North Holland 1974) 411-418

23 PORTH, A.J.: Ergebnisse und Moeglichkeiten der elektronischen Datenverarbeitung im Dienste der klinischen Chemie. Z.Klin.Cem.Klin.Biochem. 10 (1972) 478-482

24 PORTH, A.J.: Labordatenverarbeitung an der Medizinischen Hochschule Hannover. - Bericht ueber dreijaehrige Erfahrungen im Einsatz. In: REICHERTZ, P.L., HOLTHOFF, G.: Methoden der Informatik in der Medizin (Berlin, Heidelberg, New York: Springer, 1975) 56-61

25 REICHERTZ, P.L.: Hospital Information Systems. Concept and Implementation of the Medical System Hannover. In: MAROIS, M. (ed.): Man and Computer. Second International Conference Bordeaux 1972 (Amsterdam: North Holland, 1974) 153-186

26 REICHERTZ, P.L.: Probleme und Wege der EDV - Anwendung zur Dokumentation. Vortrag Systems '73, 30.11.73, Muenchen

27 REICHERTZ, P.L.: Medical School of Hannover Hospital Computer System (Hannover), in: COLLEN, M.F. (ed.): Hospital Computer Systems (New York: 1974) 598-661

28 REICHERTZ, P.L.: Informationssysteme in der Medizin (Bonn, Bad Godesberg: IBM Corporation 1975)

29 REICHERTZ, P.L.: Die zentrale Bedeutung textverarbeitender Systeme in der medizinischen Informatik. In: REICHERTZ, P.L. und HOLTHOFF, G. (ed.): Methoden der Informatik in der Medizin (Berlin, Heidelberg, New York: Springer, 1975)

30 REICHERTZ, P.L. et al: Struktur und Funktion der Allgemeinmedizinischen Praxis. Ergebnisse einer Analyse zur Untersuchung der Grundlagen fuer Computerunterstuetzung der Allgemeinmedizinischen Praxis. (Koeln: Zentralinstitut fuer die kassenaerztliche Versorgung in der Bundesrepublik Deutschland 1976)

31 SCHEIBE, GOEGELER,: Chirurgischer Therapieschluessel. (unpublished)

32 SAUTER, K. et al: Die zentrale Patientendatenbank in einem integrierten Hospital - Informationssystem. Meth.Inf.Med. 11 (1972) 91-96

33 SAUTER, K.: Structure and Functions of the Patient Data Bank in the Medical System Hannover. In: GUNTER, A., LEVRAT, B., LIPPS, H. (ed.): Proc. Int. Comput. Symposium 1973, Davos (Amsterdam: North Holland Publ.Comp., 1973) 585-589

34 SAUTER, K.: The Patient Data Bank in a Medical Information System - Tasks, Requirements, Planning and Design. Meth.Inf.Med. 12 (1973) 113-117

35 TEMPLETON, A.W. et al: 'Radiate' - Updated and Redesigned for Multiple Terminals. Radiology 92 (1969) 30-36

36 WEED, L.L: Medical Records that Guide and Teach. New.Eng.J.Med. 278 (1958) 593-600, 652-657

37 WEINGARTEN, W. et al: The Patient Information System and its user Reactions. Journees d'Informatique Medicale, Toulouse, 1975

38 WEINGARTEN, W. et al: Presentation of Laboratory Data in the Medical System Hannover. Journees d'Informatique Medicale, Toulouse 1975

39 WINGERT, F., RIES, P.: Pathologie-Befund-System. Meth.Inf.Med. 12 (1973) 150- 155

40 WOLTERS, E., REICHERTZ, P.L.: Problem-Directed Interactive Transaction Management in Medical Systems. Meth.Inf.Med. 15 (1976) 135-140

PROGRAM DOCUMENTATION

Gerhard Goos, Karlsruhe

0. Introduction

Program documentation is the information, available in writing, about a program; the
program text itself is part of the documentation. Documentation is a companion to the
different phases of creating a program. There exist different documentations describing
the state of the program at different stages of development. These different documentations are used by different people and for differing purposes.

Program documentation must be available. Hence, some sheet of paper on the desk of some
programmer even though it may be relevant to the purpose cannot be considered as
being part of the documentation. Secondly, there must be some standards stating which
information is part of which documentation. These standards also prescribe the form in
which the information has to be presented; without such standards it will be very
difficult to retrieve the information. Furthermore, the standards allow for checking
the completeness of the documentation, i.e., they guarantee that all relevant aspects
are covered.

Program documentation must be valid and up-to-date. There is limited interest only in
knowing the algorithms which somebody designed yesterday unless they are also used in
the present version of the program. It is no easy undertaking to guarantee the validity
of a documentation if many people are involved. The use of an automated documentation
system may greatly improve validity. But even then we must additionally care
for distributing the documentation, its updates and enhancements, to those people who
have no interactive access to the computer.

Program documentation must be understandable. It is often surprising to see the difficulties that even very good programmers have to express their thoughts in a coherent
and comprehensible way. Very often this is just a question of one's mastering of his
own language. Sometimes the lack of suitable formalisms considerably contributes to
the difficulties of understanding because it lengthens the presentation and makes
overview more difficult.

Software producing companies usually have voluminous handbooks defining the required
standards for documentation to every detail. It is not intended that this lecture
treats documentation in a comparable manner. Although these handbooks are doubtlessly

useful and for some purposes even necessary it must be stressed that only the form of a documentation can be prescribed that way. The quality and usefulness of a program documentation, however, depends on the information which we can derive from it and not so much on its form. We shall therefore try to survey the different needs for documentation and to show how we could increase its information content and practical usefulness without increasing its size too much. Finally we shall illustrate our comments by means of a (relatively) short example.

1. Objectives

Program documentation must give all the necessary information needed during

- development (design and implementation)
- testing
- maintenance
- installation
- operation
- use

of the program. From this list we may derive a broad range of questions which must be answered by help of the program documentation, including the following:

(a) What is the problem to be solved?

(b) What are the overall objectives of the programming project?

(c) Which basic model is used for achieving the goals (on the highest level of abstraction) and for subdividing the program into modules?

(d) What are the specifications to be met by these modules (functional, specifications, interfaces, qualitative properties)?

(e) Same question as (c) on lower levels of abstraction:

(f) What are the basic requirements for the environment in order to be able to run the program (configuration, basic software, program library, data files)?

(g) What is the meaning of the variables and data structures in the program?

(h) What is the status of the project?

(i) How can I use the program?

(j) What is the meaning of the error-messages?

Obviously the interests and the background of the people asking these questions may be highly divergent. Hence, it may be better to have different documentations for use by different people at different times:

(1) the conceptual description, (questions a, b, c, e, f, h),

(2) the design- and product- documentation (development description, a-h, j)

(3) the user's guide (f, i, j)

The conceptual description surveys the problem specification and the key considerations for the solution in technical terms.

The design-documentation describes the current state of the project during the design phase. It records the history of the design and provides the input for the implementation phase.

The product-documentation describes the current status of the project during the implementation and maintenance phase. The program itself constitutes a major part of the product documentation. Depending on the size of the program and the design methodology one may often elect not to distinguish between the design- and the product-documentation. These terms then merely exhibit two different aspects of the <u>development description</u>. We shall follow this view and not distinguish between these two documentations in the sequel.

The user's guide describes the user interface, i.e. all the information, needed for installing, using and operating the program. It is independent of the other documentation and it is often the only part of the documentation shown to the user.

Using any type of documentation is subject to the following conditions:

- Any question should be answered by the appropriate documentation in a minimum of time (in fact, the total sum of times used for writing and using a documentation is to be minimized).

- The answers must be complete. They must even reference related details which the reader had not asked for because he was not aware of their existence or relevance.

Furthermore there are some motherhood statements which must be observed in documenting programs, especially in providing for the development description:

- <u>Documentation will never be written if there is no authority insisting on it.</u> (Documentation basically is an aid for understanding and use of a program by others; the programmer does - at the moment of writing, - not see an advantage for himself in documenting a program although he himself may   later on belong to the group who wants to use the documentation.)

- <u>Documentation must be written during program development; it will never be written afterwards.</u> (Programmers tend to write documentation only after they have finished coding and testing the program. They fear that writing the documentation before

this will introduce the need for extensive changes, or the documentation may
become obsolete later on. However, experience shows that they will be assigned a
new task once they finished coding and testing, and hence they will never have
time for documentation afterwards.)

- It is very time consuming not to spend time on documentation. (Usually the number
of times and hence the amount of time used for retrieving information about a
program is orders of magnitude larger than the time spent on writing documentation. If retrieval time is increased because of lack of documentation or badly
written documentation the result is a much greater loss of time (and money) than
when a little bit more time had been spent for improving the documentation.)

2. The Conceptual Description

The conceptual description serves two different goals: It allows the user to grasp
the basic technical facts about the program without going too much into details. It
also allows the newcoming programmer or manager to get a quick survey about the project; he then should know enough about the context of the subproblem which he has to
consider.

The conceptual description is created during design and implementation. The first
version is that paper which the design starts from. It describes the problem and
the objectives in technical and formal terms. Together with the informal statement
of the problem in the user's guide this description should enable the reader to
convince himself that the formal statement of the problem meets the informal intentions.

The conceptual description especially specifies the constraints (minimal configuration, estimates about amount and frequencies of input data and external requests,
exceptional cases yet to be handled efficiently, reliability considerations etc.)
to which the program will be subjected. Whenever possible it must specify not only
the average performance but also the minimum performance which is absolutely required.

During the design of the program the conceptual description extends to a description
of the basic concepts and models underlying the design. It describes the decomposition of the program into modules and the basic concepts and objectives of each module.

Theoretically the conceptual description should be stable after the design has been
finished. Due to later changes of the design, adaptation to changing objectives or
repair of fundamental errors this happens very rarely.

3. The development description

The development description records all the information which could be useful during later phases of the development cycle, especially during maintenance. It is the basic document by which designers and programmers report on their work. It provides the means for communication in the team.

For understanding the internal working of a module one must know the module interface and, in addition, the internal algorithms and data of the module. If the algorithms are not obvious it is useful to comment in them by inserting the assertions which would be needed for proving the algorithm. Algorithms and data become understandable by simply recording the design-process in a top-down manner. In addition one should describe all the data structures and its elements. Especially those elements of records and other data structures which in the chosen programming language remain unnamed, e.g., because they are allocated dynamically or consist of only part of a computer word must be clearly described. Languages such as, e.g., PASCAL [3] are well suited for such a description even though the program itself may be written in assembly language.

Special attention must be paid to the problem of uniquely naming all program components (operations and data). It is useful to build a table containing all the names of modules of the program; naming of a module is only accepted if the name is entered into this table and checked for uniqueness. Even if the programming language allows for overwriting module names in case of nested modules this method is advisable for ease of reference. Next,one distinguishes between those names which are local to a module and those which appear in a module interface and may be used in other modules. While naming of local variables is free of constraints, every nonlocal name should begin with the name of the module containing its declaration. Special care must be taken to describe extensively all kinds of error-handling. It is this information from which the maintenance starts off in searching for errors and correcting them. Error messages are useless if it is impossible to trace them back to their source. For analogous reasons all the test cases (hopefully still) contained in the program have to be explained.

No program remains stable forever. Sometimes either the base system or the objectives or both change. In order to adapt a program to new requirements it is crucial that the documentation points out where to insert additional activities and most important, that the goals to be achieved by a given algorithm are not to be confused with the particular way by which this is done. Very often non-adaptability is a consequence of bad documentation because people must experiment in reconstructing the essentials

of an algorithm or a data structure instead of reading this information in the
documentation. Likewise, it is necessary to file the feasibility studies and discussion
records of the design period so that one may reconstruct at any time the reasons that
led to the rejection of certain solutions in order not to fall into the same traps
again.

Communication within the programming team requires that all module interfaces are
completely documented such that everybody who wants to use a module can easily see
what input data he has to provide, what other requirements he has to fulfill, and
what the module delivers in terms of output data, side effects etc. For quick use
this information must be highly concentrated. In addition it must be complete and
separated from the information on the internal workings of the module (principle
of information hiding, see [4]). Otherwise one can hardly avoid that other
modules will use internal information on the module and thus, modularity will be
destroyed if not already during development then during maintenance.

Managers of a programming project are primarily interested in evaluating the status
of the project, supervising the time schedule, finding out what the critical phases
of the project are that require special supervision or additional advice. For this
purpose the documentation must contain a condensed survey on each programmer's work.
This survey must show an up-to-date record of what has already been achieved and
what has still to be done.

3.1 A SET OF RULES

The previous discussion leads to the following set of rules for writing the conceptual
and the development description:

(1) State the problem both formally and in technical terms (a comparison with the
    informal description in the user's guide should show that the formal statement
    meets the informal intentions). State any limitations (minimum configuration
    etc.), other objectives (degree of reliability etc.) average and minimum per-
    formance expected.

(2) Describe the solution top-down on successive levels of refinement (use a pseudo-
    programming language). If no top-down description is possible describe the over-
    all strategy of your solution and how the solution is subdivided into modules;
    repeat this step for all larger modules.

(3) For each module describe the module interface (functions supplied, input and

output parameters, global data, side effects, error handling, test facilities).
Separate this description from the internal documentation of the module (otherwise you can be sure that modularity will be destroyed sooner or later).

(4) For each piece of program add the assertions needed in proving the program
correct.

(5) Explain the meaning of all data objects and data structures.

(6) Discuss how qualitative criteria and other limitations influenced strategic
decisions.

(7) File the design decisions including feasibility studies, discussion records,
reasons for choosing one solution and rejecting others.

(8) Make sure that the documentation is properly crossreferenced. (Not every
reader does really know all the questions relevant for his purpose.)

(9) File test data and test programs for later use.

(10) Organize the distribution of the documentation amongst the members of the
team.

(11) Sign every sheet by name and data both when you write it and when ever you
change it.

3.2 THE FORM OF THE DOCUMENTATION

The form and amount of documentation varies considerably depending on the size and
complexity of the program. Many parts of the documentation are relevant only for
programs from a certain size upwards. This remark especially applies to rules (6),
(7), (8) and (10) of the foregoing section. Also, in many simple cases the information required by rules (2), (3) and (4) can be derived immediately from the program
text. For obvious reasons programmers tend to decide in favour of the simple case
because this lightens their amount of work.

During system integration and maintenance the development description and the program
text are mostly used in conjunction. It is therefore preferable to include most of
the documentation in the program text as a comment. In this way the problem of cross
referencing between documentation and program text will disappear. The method has its
limitations, however, whenever the program text is blown up by too many comments and
program transparency is destroyed. For projects of a certain size upwards it is thus

recommended to include the assertions and the description of data in the program
text and to file everything else separately.

Updating and guaranteeing completeness of a documentation are especially difficult
problems. Updates must be distributed to all people involved. Hence, everybody has
the task of updating his private copy of the documentation, which is a time-consuming
and annoying task. Furthermore, since it takes some time to copy and distribute
updates it is possible to draw conclusions from parts of the documentation which
already are out of date (an interesting synchronization problem). To avoid this problem
of validity one either holds one central master copy of the documentation only. (In
addition one must have a backup copy to replace the master in case of damage or loss.)
Another solution is to put the documentation on the computer. In case of a time-sharing
system everybody can easily inspect the current version of the documentation. For large
projects, however, the documentation may consume much space although only very small
parts are accessed continously. In addition special care must be taken to mark changes
in such a way that everybody can easily detect any changes.

For controlling completeness of the documentation it is useful to set up a detailed
table of contents very early in the project. The table of contents contains for every
module a list of those topics that have to be treated by the programmer. The particular
topics may be treated at length or marked as less relevant but they may never be left
out. In case of a computer-based documentation the topics may be filled out in conversational mode by a program putting questions to the programmer. But note that even
such a conversation may only check completeness in a formal way. Conceptual completeness
cannot be checked automatically.

3.3 AN EXAMPLE

In the following example we show the most relevant parts of the development description
of a relatively simple problem. The example uses an ALGOL-like pseudo-language for
describing abstract forms of the program. This choice of description language does in
no way imply the programming language to be finally used. Therefore such questions as:
"what parameters are needed by the random-number generators involved?" cannot yet be
answered. Note that the description contains some implicit assumptions, e.g., that the
random number generators lead to the desired distributions. Such assumptions are un-
avoidable if the documentation shall not be blown out of proportions; every programmer
team must develop its own level of detail.

750815/Go

Producer - Consumer by FIFO queue

Problem: Given two processes P, C and a queue Q. P produces jobs J which he places into Q. C picks the jobs up from Q and processes them. C works on a first-come-first-served basis. The processing time T_J of job is known when J is placed into Q; it follows a distribution F_T. The arrival times A_J of the jobs in Q are distributed according to F_A. The queue has a fixed maximum length qmax.

Write a simulation program for studying the behaviour of the system in steady state. Particular studies are not yet included.

Solution: A simulation program with parameters:

R_T: a random-number generator producing processing times

R_A: a random-number generator producing intervals of arrival times.

qmax: maximum queue length.

timemax: time for which the simulation is going on

```
program : simulation (R_T, R_A, qmax, timemax)
           proc real : R_T, R_A
               int  : qmax
               real : timemax

  begin real : time
        data module : queue
        process : Producer
        process : Consumer
        create queue : Q
        initiate Producer : P, Consumer : C
        time := 0

        while time < timemax
        do simulate
  end
```

750815/Go

Functions and Interfaces:

1. Queue

   implements a queue with qmax places

   Input parameters:

         int : qmax   (global par., read only)

   Output parameters

            bool : empty   true if queue empty) public par.

                 full   true if queue full) read only

   Operations

       proc : injob (T, A); real : T, A

           Add a job with processing time T and arrival time A into the queue. T, A

           are input parameters. Must not be called if queue is full

       proc : outjob (T, A); real : T, A

           removes the first job from the queue. The processing time T and arrival

           time A of this job are output parameters. Must not be called if queue is

           empty.

   Error situations

   Break-down if empty = true and outjob is called or

                full = true and injob is called

2. Producer

   Process which, starting at time 0, produces new jobs in time intervals R_A. The
   processing times are given by (successive calls of) R_T. The produced job is
   inserted into the queue Q. If Q is full then the job is rejected and an error
   message and the parameters of the job are printed.

   Input parameters

           proc real : R_A, R_T random number generators

                                       (probably with some parameters;

                                       must be made precise later)

750815/Go

bool : Q . full	Is Q full? (read only)
proc : Q . injob (T, A);	inserts job with
real : T, A	arrival time A
	and processing time T into Q
real : time	model time (update variable)

Output parameters

    /

Error situations (message on standard output file)

JOB REJECTED ARRIVED AT time
            PROCESSING T. time

happens when Q is full.

3. Consumer

Process which, starting at time 0, takes a job from the queue Q. If T is the
processing time of this job then the process will be busy for a time interval T.
Subsequently it picks up the next job from Q or is idle if Q is empty.

Input parameters

bool : Q . empty	Is Q empty? (read only)
proc : Q . outjob (T, A);	takes job with arrival
real : T, A	time A and processing time
	T out of Q
real : time	model time (update variable)

Output parameters
    /
Error situations
    /

750815/Go

Modules:

```
process producer;
    begin            ( * possible initializations * )
         ( * here the simulations starts * )

    do forever
    begin if Q . full
          then
              print (" JOB REJECTED ARRIVED AT : ", time,
                    " PROCESSING TIME :", R_T (???))
          else Q . injob (R_T (???), time);
          wait until (time + R_A(???))

    end

    end
```

The modules consumer and queue are described simularly. The loop "simulate" of the
main program and the operation wait until are a little bit more difficult to design.

4. The User's Guide

The user's guide is subdivided into two or, if necessary, three parts:

- introductory manual
- the reference manual
- the operator's guide (if there is any activity of an operator implied).

The introductory manual serves three goals:

It gives an informal introduction and overview about what problems can be attacked by the program and what the limitations are. It is the part of the user's guide which should be drafted before the design of the program starts because it informally speci- fies the objectives of the program. But note that the final version of the introduc- tion describes the objectives one *has* achieved, not those one was trying to achieve when one started! The introductory manual mostly forms the descriptional basis for advertising and selling the program.

Secondly the introductory manual describes the "standard use" of the program. It is very useful to separate this part of the introductory manual from all other parts and to make it as short as possible because *every* user is expected to know these informations by heart or has them in this pocket. It eases the job of the user if he has not to select these basic informations from different parts of the introductory manual. A "cookbook" must be given describing the commonly used job control commands with only a few number of options; layout and order of input and output data are des- cribed mostly by examples. E.g., for an ALGOL 60-compiler the following information is given:

- Command for starting the compiler with listing of source text and standards core size.
- Command for starting the translated program using standard core size.
- Advice how to punch special characters ("(/" instead of "[" etc.)
- Rules for punching input data (separation of numbers by two blanks etc.)
- Remarkes concerning the available test facilities.
- Explanation of commonly occuring error messages.

Nothing is said about language restrictions or extensions.

Thirdly the introductory manual describes all possible applications of the program, informally and in common terms. In contrast to the corresponding description in the reference manual this description must be understandable for every potential user of the program. Previous programming experience or formal training of the user should be assumed only if the objectives of the program require it. In such cases, however, the informal description is superfluous and must not be supplied. E.g., an informal description of the interface between operating systems and assembly programs is not needed; the informal description of a compiler contains an informal description of the language as implemented. "Informal" means that sometimes a compromise must be made between readability and the rigidity required for describing *all* exceptional cases. The reference manual assumes that the reader has some familiarity with related publications and with the current state of the art how to solve a given problem. The informal description does not assume this. Therefore it should provide the user with some background information motivating him for the best usage of the program and telling hin which cases can be handled particularly efficiently.

The user's reference manual supplies complete information how to use the program. The formal level of the description must be such that clarity and completeness of the description can be achieved. In addition to the description of commands, format and content of input, output and error messages the following information is needed:

- How to install the program (minimal configuration required, operating system required, permanent files and other resources exclusibely used, how to read the delivered tape etc.)
- Time and space estimates as a function of input data.
- List of programs which might be useful for ameliorating the performance of the given one or for solving related problems.
- Possible changes or extensions for increasing the availablility, robustness, range of applicability etc.

The operator's guide is needed whenever operator's intervention is required by the program either for mounting devices or for reacting at the console. The operator's guide must describe the input stream (job control cards, data, tape files, disc files), the output stream (tape files, disc files, punched cards, printer output and its preparation) and the operation at the console, in particular for handling abnormal conditions.

LITERATURE

[1] Dijkstra, E.W.:
     Notes on Structured Programming, in:
     Structured Programming
     Academic Press, London 1972

[2] Goos, G.,:
     Documentation, in:
     Bauer, F. L. (Ed.)
     Advanced Course on Software Engineering
     Lecture Notes in Computer Science, vol. 30
     Springer-Verlag, Berlin-Heidelberg-New York, 1973

[3] Jensen, K. and Wirth, N.:
     "PASCAL-User Manual and Report"
     Lecture Notes in Computer Science, vol 18
     Springer-Verlag, Berlin-Heidelberg-New York, 1974

[4] Parnas, D.L.:
     A Technique for Software Module
     Specification with Examples
     Communications of the ACM
     May 1972, vol. 15, no 5, pp 330-336

[5] Walsh, D.:
     A Guide to Software Documentation
     McGraw Hill, N.Y., 1969

[6] Wirth, N.:
     Systematic Programming
     Prentice-Hall, Inc., Englewood Cliffs,
     N.Y., 1973

INFORMATION SYSTEMS: CONCEPTS, INTERFACES, TECHNIQUES

Peter C. Lockemann, Karlsruhe

1 Preliminary Remarks

1.1 OBJECTIVES

Information systems have grown into a major discipline in recent years. As an intersection of many seemingly diverse activities they have evolved into a truly interdisciplinary area of research and development. Today they include most aspects of computer science because of the multitude of problems in constructing large computer systems; they cover concepts of a wide variety of application areas from science to industry to public and business administration, from research to engineering to production; they have captured the interest of the legal and social professions because of their repercussions in everyday life.

Like all young disciplines, however, the information systems area suffers from the lack of a few, generally accepted and well-understood basic concepts. To name just one example, there is as yet no general agreement on the terms "information" and "data" or the relationship between them. Instead we observe the existence of several conceptual approaches to a theory of systems or a theory of data. Major efforts are still necessary to reconcile these and combine them into a single information system theory. A successful conclusion would also be of immense practical value to a number of issues, e.g.:

- The classical system development cycle proceeds in several steps: system analysis (analysis of the current state), problem definition (statement of objectives), system design and evaluation, system implementation and documentation, system installation. As yet there exists no consistent and systematic approach to system development. Large portions of the cycle, in particular system analysis and problem definition, are still based on verbal descriptions, check lists, fact sheets, interviews, observations, and estimates resulting in organizational charts, flow diagrams, decision tables, and form sheets which largely preclude the application of formal-deductive methods.

- Many institutions lack the facilities to design and implement computer-assisted information systems on their own. Instead they must select among commercially available systems. Neither are the interfaces of these systems standardized to any appreciable degree so that rational comparisons could become possible, nor is there any systematic way for determining which interface suits a given problem area best.

- Once a system has been designed or selected, a number of questions must be answered before instead of after the fact (of installing it): What effects does the system have on the organization, e.g. does it remove old bottlenecks or create new ones, does it require organization restructuring because of additional and perhaps unexpected capabilities, does it require additional resources that are already in short supply (witness the universally underestimated problem of data acquisition and input)?

The current series of lectures will certainly not overcome these difficulties. However, they attempt to establish a simple and transparent framework for a number of important aspects of information systems. The emphasis will be on the conceptual level for the purpose of designing systems and their interfaces. A number of examples will be discussed in depth in order to illustrate the interfaces of existing information systems as well as new approaches to interface design. The technical level will be touched upon only lightly and is intended mainly to demonstrate that the choice of technical solutions that are both efficient and economical depends in large degree on a thorough system analysis.

1.2 ASPECTS

Fundamental to the framework we are going to establish is the notion of dynamic system and organization. A _dynamic system_ is a collection of elements that are related to each other and whose concrete behavior varies with time. An _organization_ is a dynamic system in which the functions of the elements and relations can clearly be established from the overall objectives of the system. Moreover, we shall assume that the functional properties are established once and for all. Therefore, all temporal variations manifest themselves in an exchange of certain quantities among the elements. Information systems study exclusively the exchange of information, thus emphasizing the aspect of cooperation necessary to derive the desired behavior of the total system. In such a system the only activities of the system elements of interest are those of information processing.

The concepts necessary to describe information systems arise from three levels.

(1) Functions of the individual elements or groups of elements.
   The purpose and objectives of the system are considered. Tasks are split into subtasks and assigned to specific elements, or elements are designed to handle specific subtasks; the resources required by the various elements are determined.

(2) Interaction and coordination of the system elements.
   Issues on this level have to do with analyzing or planning the proper interplay of the various system elements so that the system objectives determined on level 1 are indeed met. The issues are described by catchwords such as information flow; resource management; deadlocks and bottlenecks; privacy and reliability; sequential, concurrent and alternative processes; interfaces; directives, orders and responses; hierarchical organization.

(3) Information structures.
   The concepts on this level investigate the particular forms of information that are to be exchanged in a particular situation so that the individual elements may function properly with regard to the system objectives. These objectives relate to the world outside the system, that is, what one might call the universe of discourse. Therefore, information structures are the reflection of a universe.

It should be noted that none of the concepts mentioned so far imply or demand use of a computer. Indeed, computers are but one out of many possible vehicles for the implementation of system elements, other possibilities being human beings, tabulating machines, conventional libraries, etc. Nevertheless, much of the remainder will be devoted to explications of the concepts as they have developed in connection with computers.

2 Coordination

2.1 DYNAMIC SYSTEMS

As mentioned above, the notion of dynamic system applies to any collection of elements that are capable of certain actions, where these actions depend on an exchange, between the elements, of certain quantities. The arrangement of the elements, and the characteristics of each individual element, shall remain unchanged so that the dynamic behavior manifests itself exclusively in variations in time and space of the quantities exchanged. Hence any system state is described by the (invariant) arrangement and characteristics of the elements ("system structure") together with a momentary distribution of the quantities ("system variables").

The dynamic systems that are of interest in connection with information systems are socio-technological organizations. In order for these organizations to function properly, they must be able to adapt to new requirements or technologies (just consider the introduction of a computer to a hospital). Hence their system structure cannot be considered invariant. Nevertheless we shall cover them by the definition given above since structural changes take place slowly and infrequently as compared to variations in the system variables.

Before a given dynamic system can be investigated more closely it must be modelled by means of abstract concepts. These should cover
- system structure (elements and their interrelationships),
- range of actions (system variables),
- functions (activities of the elements in a given situation),
- interactions (relationships between actions of elements),
- timing (temporal evolution of actions and interactions).

2.2 MARKED PETRI NETS [1,2]

Informal introduction

The simpler a model, i.e. the higher a level of abstraction, the more hope there is for formal-deductive analyses of system behavior. One of the simplest models for dynamic systems is known under the name of Petri nets. These may be characterized informally as follows.

a) System structure.

- All system elements are of one of two kinds: active elements called
  transitions, and communication channels called places. All
  transitions have identical functional properties, and so have
  places.
- The following conditions shall hold:
  (i)   Information is exchanged between transitions via places.
          Hence transitions may only be connected to places and vice
          versa.
  (ii)   Quantities to be exchanged can be exclusively observed on
          places, i.e. all activities within the system can only be
          studied indirectly via changes on the places.
  (iii)   Each place may hold information for any desired length of
          time, i.e. it may act as a store.
  (iv)   Places may hold any number of information items up to a given
          place-specific maximum.
  (v)   All connections between transitions and places are directed.
  (vi)   A place may receive information from more than one transition
          and, in turn, may be accessed by more than one transition.

b) System variables.

All information items exchanged are mutually indistinguishable, i.e.,
they have no structure. They are called tokens. A system state is
described by the distribution of tokens over the places (marking). A
system structure of transitions and places together with a marking is
called a marked Petri net.

c) Functions.

There is just one action defined on transitions which is called the
firing rule: A transition may fire whenever all of its input places
are marked, i.e. whenever it is activated. On firing, a transition
removes exactly one token from each of its input places and inserts
exactly one token on each of its output places. Consequently, firing a
transition may decrease or increase the total number of tokens within
a net.

d) Interactions.

Interaction exclusively takes place via the places. Total system
behavior as the sum total of the individual interactions within the
system is the subject of net theory.

e) Timing.

No time metric is introduced so that nothing can be said about the amount of time the firing of a transition may take, or a token may spend in a place. The only distinction possible is whether two actions must take place in a certain order (depend on each other) or may occur concurrently (independently).

Graphical representation

In order to study Petri nets by formal means, graph theory suggests itself. Because of the properties of places, the interrelationships between the active elements cannot simply be represented by edges. Instead, two kinds of nodes, transitions and places, are distinguished which are connected by directed edges. As a consequence, the structure of a Petri net is described by a directed bipartite graph. In the corresponding graphical representation, rectangles may symbolize transitions and circles places. Token may be shown as black dots within the circles. System behavior is then characterized by a sequence of markings, e.g.

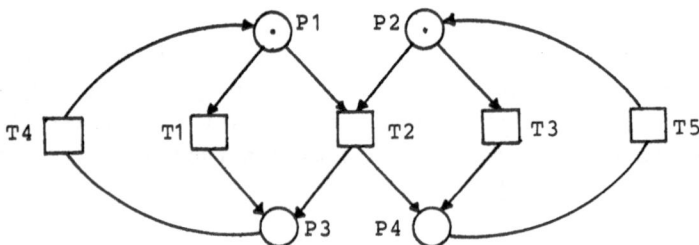

and after firing of either T2 or, alternatively, T1 and T3 concurrently

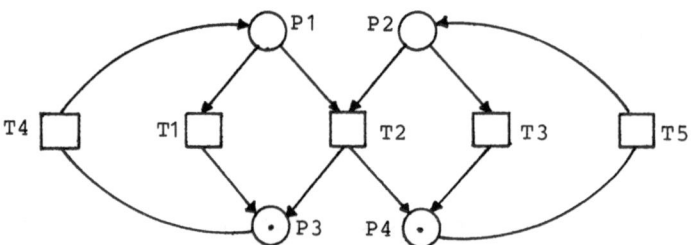

Most of the problems arise because the behavior of Petri nets is non-deterministic:

- If two transitions may fire independently they may fire in any order. Since the resulting markings may differ, all further behavior of the net may differ as well.
- If the same place is input place to two transitions and holds one token only, either one of them but not both may fire. In the example above, firing of T2 precludes firing of both T1 and T3.

System behavior

Given a Petri net and a marking M, and, consequently, a number of activated transitions. A marking that results from the concurrent firing of any subset of these transitions is called immediately reachable from M. Any marking resulting from a sequence of firings of the kind just described is called reachable from M.

Given a Petri net and an initial marking M, the following properties are of major interest.
a) Liveliness: A marked Petri net is called live whenever for each marking M´ reachable from M, each transition is or may still at some later time be put into a position to fire. In other words, at no time will a transition be forever excluded from all further activities. Alternatively, a weaker definition requires only that each marking M´ reachable from M has one marking reachable from it. In this case, at any time there exists at least one active transition.
b) Boundedness: Given a Petri net in which each place may hold no more than a certain number of tokens. A Petri net with marking M is called safe if there does not exist any marking reachable from M under which for any place, the number of tokens exceeds its bound.

As an example consider the following net

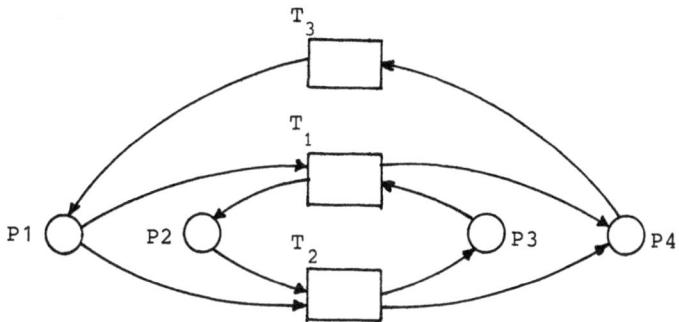

If one places a token each on Pl and P3 the only possible sequence of firings is: Tl-T3-T2-T3-Tl-...., i.e. one obtains a firing cycle that is repeated ad infinitum. On the other hand, if one places tokens on P2 and P3 the net is not live.

Formal considerations

The following section may be safely disregarded by readers with little formal background. We just wish to demonstrate what kind of formal deductive methods may be applied towards a theory of Petri nets.

Because of its non-deterministic nature, it is impossible even for a modest-sized Petri net to determine its behavior by constructing all of the markings reachable from it unless, of course, one detects simple cycles as in the example above. Instead, one may attack the problem by deriving its properties solely on the basis of the system structure and a given initial marking. For certain classes of nets this may be done by employing linear algebra techniques. These are based on the following considerations.

A Petri net is a quadruple $N=(P,T,pre,post)$, where P and T are finite non-empty disjoint sets (places and transitions), pre, post $\subseteq P \times T$ are binary relations (edges in the graph), field (pre, post) $= P \cup T$ and, usually, pre $\cap$ post $= \emptyset$.

A marking is a mapping $M:P \rightarrow \mathbb{N} \cup \{\emptyset\}$ with $M(p)$ the number of tokens on a place $p \in P$. A place $p \in P$ is marked if $M(p) > 1$.

A marked Petri net is an ordered pair (N,M).

The net structure may be represented by an incidence matrix C such that

$$C(p,t) = \begin{cases} -1 & \text{if } (p,t) \in \text{pre} \\ +1 & \text{if } (p,t) \in \text{post} \\ 0 & \text{else} \end{cases} \quad \text{and } p \in P, t \in T.$$

Likewise, the marking may be represented by a vector M so that a marked Petri net is represented as an ordered pair (C,M).

The firing of a transition t is defined as a transformation of a given marking M into another marking $\tilde{M}$ whereby
$\tilde{M} = M + C(*,t)$.
Let M and $\tilde{M}$ be markings. If there exists a system of linear equations with a vector x:
$M + C \cdot x = \tilde{M}$ where $x(i) \in \mathbb{N} \cup \{\emptyset\}$
then the component $x(t)$ indicates how often the transition t would

have had to be fired to transform the marking M into M̃. If there exists a corresponding firing sequence of transitions which transform M into M̃ then marking M̃ is said to be reachable from M. M together with all markings reachable from it form a set [M].

A marking M is called live (in the weaker sense) if
∀M̃ ∈ [M] : |[M̃]| > 1.
A marking M is called safe with respect to a bound B:P->N if
∀p ∈ P ∀ M̃ ∈ [M] : M̃(p) < B(p).

Besides linear algebra, another approach has been to determine additional rules that control the sequence of firings such that no deadlock (absence of live transitions) may ever result.

2.3 TIMED PETRI NETS [3]

A slightly lower level of abstraction is obtained by the introduction of timing into Petri nets in such a fashion that a transition executes for a fixed non-zero time called its <u>firing time</u>. This implies that again tokens may be held on places for an arbitrary length of time, including zero. Note that bottlenecks may not be modelled or discovered until timing is taken care of.

In formal terms: A timed Petri net is a quintuple (P,T,pre,post,Ω) where P,T,pre,post as before and Ω is a function that assigns a real non-negative number τ to each t ∈ T:
$\Omega : T \rightarrow R^{+}$
The number $\tau_t = \Omega(t)$ is termed the firing time of transition t. At any instant τ of real time, the net has a marking M(τ) (a vector varying in time). The initial marking is denoted by M(O). The number of tokens on place p at time τ is written as M(τ,p):=M(τ)(p). The firing rule is modified as follows: When a firing of transition t is initiated, a token is removed from each input place of t and t is said to be executing. The execution phase lasts for τ_t. At the end of this time duration, the firing of t terminates, and a token is placed on each output place.

Previous example as a timed Petri net

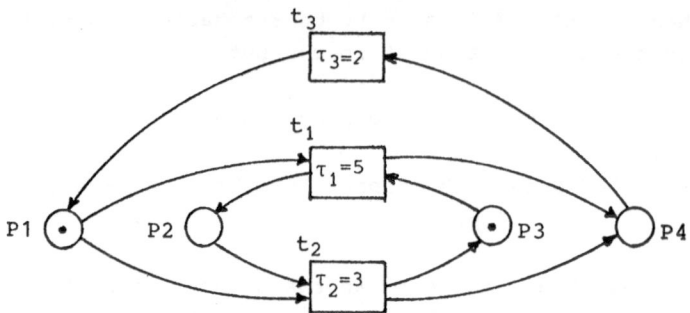

The time at which the firing of a transition takes place is recorded in a table known as a <u>firing schedule</u> which is a set of sequences of initiation and termination times for the transitions of a net. For the net and the initial marking shown above the following is a possible firing schedule which assumes that each transition fires as soon as it is enabled (note again the cycle).

no. of firings tran- sition	1	2	3	4	5	
t_1	(0,5)	(12,17)	(24,29)	...	...	. . .
t_2	(7,10)	(19,22)	(31,34)	...	...	. . .
t_3	(5,7)	(10,12)	(17,19)	(22,24)	(29,31)	. . .

A more realistic assumption for real world systems is that the execution time for activities depend upon the information to be handled. Thus it may be more reasonable for the model to assume that a transition firing time is a random variable.

2.4 INFORMATION NETS [4]

Petri nets overemphasize the aspect of proper coordination while neglecting the purpose of all that coordination. As soon as one turns to the purpose much more must be specified on the functions which, in turn, requires a host of additional concepts and a much heavier formal apparatus. Some of these concepts are sketched below.

a) System structure.

- The active elements, now called agencies, must be distinguished according to the type of activities they may perform. In the general case this is possible only by specifying more or less complex algorithms.
- In contrast to the communication channels of Petri nets, a sharp distinction is made between the parts which may hold information, and the access paths to and from these. Consequently, there are
  - Stores, with properties identical to (ii), (iii), (iv), (vi) of places.
  - Directed interfaces between stores and agencies for transporting information. However, since agencies are limited to certain activities, they impose certain restrictions on the kind of information upon which they may act or which they may deliver. Hence an interface has the additional property of letting pass only certain kinds of information.

b) System variables.

Correspondingly, information must now reflect structure
(i) typifying the information so that interfaces can have an effect;
(ii) providing specific and distinct information items in order to direct the concrete activity of an agency.

The simplest approach to information structuring is to assume the existence of a set of universally accepted primitive information items (atoms). An information item is a collection of atoms (requirement (ii)). Furthermore, the set of atoms is divided into a finite number of disjoint classes. Information is typified by a function that determines which classes are covered by the information (requirement (i)). Interfaces and functional properties of agencies may then be discussed in terms of these classes.

c) Functions.

Aside from the description of functional properties by algorithmic means, several additional characteristics are introduced.

- Removal characteristics: An agency may remove information items from one store but copy them from another.

- Conditioning: In order for an agency to be activated, the information on its input stores must meet the interface conditions. However, not all input places need carry information. It may suffice if any one input store or certain combinations of input stores carry the desired information.

- Activation: An agency is activated whenever at least one of the input store combinations of its conditioning carries informations that meet the respective interface criteria.

- Transfer characteristics: In place of firing, an agency removes or copies information from those of its input stores that correspond to exactly one activating combination (note the indeterminacy). From the input information new (output) information is derived according to the specified algorithm, and placed on one, all or certain combinations of output stores.

d) Interaction.

Again, interaction takes place exclusively via the stores and interfaces. Given the higher degree of complexity of nets, total system behavior is now described by a larger number of characteristics which should be the subject of a corresponding net theory.

e) Timing.

No time metric is introduced.

2.5 PRIVACY AND SECURITY

All the approaches to system modeling discussed so far presume a given predetermined system structure. All results obtained for system behavior hence are valid only as long as the system structure remains unchanged. In practice this is an unrealistic assumption:

(i)   The system objectives may change and hence necessitate restructuring.
(ii) Some system components may malfunction or break down.
(iii) Some agencies may malbehave deliberately.

While (i) will occur infrequently, (ii) and (iii) may take place any time and must be guarded against. The measures taken must either avoid (ii) and (iii) or at least keep their effects well localized. As a prelude one should study whether, without any additional measures, the effects are already local in nature. In such a case the cost of implementing the additional measures may extend the damage done without them.

Methods for avoiding or localizing malfunctions are known under the term security and their results as reliability. Basically, in the terminology of information nets they aim at duplicating (in a wider sense) communication channels (particularly stores) or agencies and, in case of error, switch from one to the other.

Methods for avoiding or localizing intentional malbehavior are governed by the assumption that malbehavior can only be based on access to information and will cause damage by providing information. Consequently, one attempts to contain malbehavior by intercepting unauthorized or erroneous information as close to the malbehaving agency as possible. This is done by imposing further restrictions on the interface, i.e. on the information that may pass to or from an agency. Measures of this kind are collectively known as privacy.

3 Information structures: Basic concepts [5]

3.1 MODELS

Structuring information by distinguishing among atoms and declaring classes over the set of atoms - as we did in ch.2.4 - is a simplistic approach that is almost too much for a formal investigation of systems but still too little to explain what is observed in real-life systems. Since informatics has attended to the question of information structuring much longer than to the question of system modeling, knowledge in the first area has extended far beyond the simplistic approach mentioned above. On the other hand, there is still insufficient consensus on what constitutes an information structure or a data structure or what are the primitive structural components. This section will explore a few concepts on which to base the description of information structures in data base systems.

Fundamental to the discussion of information structure is the notion of modeling the universe. In this regard the notion of Petri net, besides being a useful tool for the investigation of system behavior, has been an excellent example for a modeling process: A Petri net is a model of a dynamic system, a transition a model of a department or person performing certain tasks, a token a model for a memo, letter or medical record. Petri nets, timed Petri nets, information nets are, to various degrees, abstractions of a universe consisting of dynamic systems.

It is generally accepted that data bases, in particular, are to be considered models of certain physical or conceptual realities. Each attempt at modeling a given reality starts out from an abstraction base which we shall call a modeling system. Such a base must provide tools
a) for the abstraction of elementary objects, their properties, and relationships, i.e. for the abstraction of states of a universe (e.g. a Petri net and its marking);
b) for the abstraction of the processes that take place in the universe, i.e. for the abstraction of transitions between states (e.g. producing a new marking in a Petri net).

The reader should be aware that models are a source of conflict between the user of an information system and its manufacturer or designer:
- A user is always interested in one particular problem area and hence

in one well-defined universe: Only certain objects, relationships and processes are considered relevant, and in particular only certain ways in which objects and relationships are composed to new more complex objects and relationships, or processes into new processes, are of interest.
- The informatician, on the other hand, must design systems that may be applicable to a wider range of problem areas. Hence he must simultaneously deal with a variety of universes, most of them still unknown to him at the time of design. However, he must impose some restrictions in order to build a viable system. These restrictions are defined with respect to the structural properties that the models may assume.

Hence we regard a data base system interface as a set of tools that determine which abstractions are possible for universes. Since the informatician deals with sets of models he requires concepts that are more abstract than those of the user: Essentially he must be able "to model models". We shall demonstrate how these concepts will allow us to systematically describe various data base system interfaces.

3.2 ABSTRACTION OF STATES

In a first step some concepts pertaining to structural properties will be introduced.
- A mode is an abstraction tool.
- A model is an abstraction of a given state of a universe by means of given modes.
- Models may be part of other models. In particular, the same model may be part of several other models. Any occurrence of some model is called a model object, and the model itself the value of the model object.

In particular, we introduce the following terminology.
- An elementary mode is an elementary concept for abstraction that cannot further be defined. Examples: Object, property, attribute, relationship.
- A complex mode is a rule of composition that determines how given model objects (called components) may be combined into new models. In particular, a complex mode may limit its components to models based on specified modes. Examples: Tree, set, network, record.
- An elementary model is an abstraction by means of an elementary mode.
- A composite model is an abstraction by means of a complex mode.

- We shall call an <u>instance of a</u> (given) <u>mode</u> both a model obtained by means of that mode and a model object with such a model as its value. (The ambiguity can always be resolved in context).

In a second step we shall study the effects of restricting all models to one particular universe. This is reflected in the following premise:
- For a given universe, all models can be enumerated.

Hence new concepts must be developed for the enumeration of models.

- A <u>class</u> is a set of models that are instances of the same mode. A class may be named by a <u>class name</u>. The set of models is called the <u>value set</u> of the class.
- An <u>instance of a class</u> is (depending on context) an element of the value set of the class or a model object whose value is an element of the value set of the class.

Concerning the constructivity of classes, the following distinction is made.
- An <u>elementary class</u> is a set whose elements must be explicitly stated. The elements may all be either elementary models or composite models. The value set may be explicitly specified, e.g. <u>bool</u> = {<u>true</u>,<u>false</u>}, or it may be "known" and then be implied by the class name, e.g. <u>int</u> is the set of all integral numbers.
- A <u>complex class</u> is a procedure for recursively constructing a set. It is defined on models, classes (constituents), and a complex mode such that each element of the value set (i.e. each instance) has the following properties:
  a) For each model encountered in the definition, the element includes exactly one component to which the model is assigned. (Example: All hospital admission forms agree in their field names.)
  b) For each constituent class k, the element receives between m and n components whose values are instances of the constituent class. (Example: In a file of records m=0, n some large number.)
  c) The components are combined according to the mode.

3.3 ABSTRACTION OF TRANSITIONS

Evidently, if a transition is defined between states, its abstraction must be defined between model objects. We are interested in procedures that construct a new model object (target) from a given model object (source). Furthermore, if only certain parts of a model are involved in the transition, we shall limit the application of the procedure to just these parts.

Strictly speaking, a source object and a target object cannot both exist at the same time. Under certain conditions, however, it is convenient to view the replacement of a model object by a new one as the replacement of the value of a given model object. Consequently, we shall allow some source and target objects to be identical, that is, that a new model may be assigned to a given model object.

The following concepts are explained rather cursorily (readers interested in more detail are referred to ref. [5]):
- An <u>activity</u> is a procedure that creates new objects "out of nowhere", drops objects, and/or rearranges existing objects.
- An <u>operator</u> is a procedure that covers all other functions. In particular, it establishes a defined relationship between the values of source and target objects.
- A <u>mode activity/operator</u> is defined on modes such that its arguments are instances of the respective modes. In particular, if a model object is both source and target it must be an instance of the same mode both before and after executing the procedure.
- A <u>class activity/operator</u> is defined on classes such that its arguments are instances of the respective classes. In particular, if a model object is both source and target it must be an instance of the same class before and after executing the procedure.

3.4 SELECTORS

A <u>model selector</u> identifies a model object to an activity or operator. Various selectors are conceivable.
a) The value (or part of the value) provided the model object is the only occurrence of the same model.
b) Properties that the object has by virtue of being a component of a model object.
c) An <u>object name</u> which one may assign to the model object, in particular if identification by means of a) or b) does not apply.

3.5 TYPES

So far there have been no restrictions as to the activities or
operators applied to a model object as long as the mode or class
remains intact.

Further restrictions are conceivable, however:
a) Not all procedures that qualify under the condition may be applied
   to the model object.
b) Not all procedures that qualify under the condition may be applied
   to the components.
c) Only certain selectors for components may be used in conjunction
   with certain procedures.
d) Procedures and/or model selectors may be used only in certain
   prescribed sequences.

In order to account for the fact that users may wish to impose such
restrictions (which they do more often in programming languages than
in data base systems) the notion of type is introduced. The following
definition covers activities only:

- A mode type is a mode together with a set of restrictions a), b), c)
  and/or d) on mode activities and on selectors.
- A class type is a class together with a set of restrictions a), b),
  c) and/or d) on class activities and on selectors.

Notice that different sets of restrictions may be defined for the same
mode or class. We shall call an instance of a (given) type a model
object that is an instance of the mode or class in the type, and that
may be subjected only to the activities of the type.

3.6 REPRESENTATION

A model is no more than a mental affair. In order to express a model
to ourselves or to the outside world we must find a physical
representation for it. We briefly introduce the following notions.

- A symbol is a representation technique. An elementary symbol
  represents an elementary model, a complex symbol a complex mode, and
  a composite symbol a composite model.
- A representation is a symbolization of a model.
- A representation object is an occurrence of some representation.

It is quite conceivable to have many different representations for the same model. However, one must at least demand that a given representation be interpreted unambiguously, i.e. by one and only one model object. The reverse need not be true because we may wish to represent the same model object more than once. In this case, however, the identity must be apparent from the representation.

Whereas representations are a means for communicating the results of a modeling process to the outside world, another subject of communication may be the process of modeling itself including the mapping between models. In particular, if communication is with a computer, the following terms are used:
- Data manipulation language: Application of activities and operators to model objects identified by selectors.
- Data definition language: Description of classes and types. A description of a particular class or type is called a schema.

3.7 DATA STRUCTURE SYSTEMS

In summary, a modeling system is a set of modes, classes, activities and operators subject to the following rules:
a) Mode activities and operators are defined on modes.
b) Class activities and operators are defined on classes.
c) Each mode participates in the definition of at least one mode activity or operator.
d) Each class participates in the definition of at least one class activity or operator.
e) All instances of a class are instances of the same mode.
f) A model object remains an instance of the same mode or class over its lifetime.

A representation system is a set of symbols that are related to a modeling system according to ch. 3.6.

We define:
- A data structure system is a pair (modeling system, representation system).
- A datum is a pair (model, representation).
- A data structure is a triple (model, representation, type).

Given a modeling system one must find a representation system that satisfies the requirements above. Paper and pencil or printed paper

will usually do, core storage never except under the most trivial
circumstances. Hence the concept of representation must not be
confused with the concept of realization. A _realization_ is a mapping
from one modeling system to a second, lower-level one.

4. Information structures: Examples

4.1 IMS [6]

In order to apply the concepts to data base system interfaces we shall start out with a comparatively simple but instructive example.

Elementary modes
- Segment
- Field

Note: The contents of a segment are irrelevant with the exception of those fields whose values may serve for identification. Consequently, segment must be treated as an elementary mode.

Complex modes
- Key: A pair (segment, field) indicative of the physical relationship between a segment and its identification field.
- Data base record: A set of segments on which a hierarchical order is defined.
- Data base: A set of data base records of identical class (note that the general notion of class, though not a particular class, is needed to describe a mode). Data bases need not be disjoint, i.e. they may share the same instance of a segment.

Elementary classes
E.g. C (character). These are already prespecified by the system.

Complex classes
Complex classes may be defined by the user via a set of macros. The following example defines:
a) A data base class in terms of a single record class (DBD-DBDGEN).
b) A data base record class in terms of a number of segment classes. For each of these the n (sec.3.2) are specified (FREQU); m =0. The hierarchical ordering is defined on segment classes (PARENT).
c) The segment classes (SEGM). BYTES must be considered a rule determining the value set (namely all segments of the length specified). One may argue that a segment class is not an elementary class since it may be constructed. However, construction is in terms of bytes which is a concept alien to the logic of the IMS interface and indeed is an aspect of realization.
d) Key classes (FLDK/FLD with NAME and START).
e) Field (TYPE, BYTES). The remark under c) above applies here similarly.

```
DBD   NAME = PROFESSIONS-DATABASE
SEGM NAME = SKILL, PARENT=0, BYTES=40, FREQU=500
FLDK NAME = SKILL-TYPE, TYPE=C, BYTES=3, START=1
SEGM NAME = PERSON-NAME, PARENT=SKILL, BYTES=70, FREQU=1000
FLDK NAME = PERNO, TYPE=C, BYTES=8, START=1
FLD  NAME = FAM-NAME, TYPE=C, BYTES=24, START=8
SEGM NAME = EXPERIENCE, PARENT=PERSON-NAME, BYTES=63, FREQU=15
FLDK NAME = JOB-TYPE, TYPE=C, BYTES=2, START=1
SEGM NAME = EDUCATION, PARENT=PERSON-NAME, BYTES=100, FREQU=10
FLDK NAME = EDU-TYPE, TYPE=C, BYTES=2, START=1
DBDGEN
```

Notice that the macro keyword NAME denotes two things: an object name
(as in DBD, FLDK, FLD), a class name (as in DBD (singular class),
SEGM).

Mode activities (DL/1)
GU (get unique): Access to a uniquely identified segment.
GN (get next): Access to the next segment within a subset.
GNP(get next parent): Access to the next successor segment of a
    uniquely identified segment.
REPL: Replace the value of a given segment.
ISRT: Insert a new segment into a record. In particular, a new root
    segment defines a new record in the data base.
DLET: Delete the segment previously accessed by GU, GN, or GNP. If
    this is a root segment, the record is deleted from the data base.

Note that ISRT and DLET are explicitly defined on segments and
implicitly on records as well. There are no activities defined
explicitly on records. Implicit definitions of this kind must be
considered very unfortunate since they deny some of the controls one
may wish to exercise on instances of certain modes (here records).

The activities listed above can be considered class activities as well
insofar as they do not alter class membership of records or segments.
No operators are provided.

Model selectors
- Field: Field name; must be unique only within a segment instance.
- Segment: Value of a field preceded by segment class name since the
   field name is ambiguous:
   (<field name>=<field value>)
   e.g. PERSON-NAME (PERNO=53742).
   In case the selector does not identify a segment uniquely,
   expressions are constructed identifying a path from a uniquely

identifiable segment (e.g. the root segment) to the desired
segment. Example: PERSON-NAME (PERNO=53742), EDUCATION
(EDU-TYPE=65).
- Sets of segments:
  a) Segment class name for all instances of a segment class.
  b) Condition to be met by field values.
     e.g. PERSON-NAME
          selects all PERSON-NAME segments;
          PERSON-NAME, EDUCATION (EDU-TYPE=65)
          selects all PERSON-NAME segments leading to the desired EDU-
          TYPE;
          PERSON-NAME (PERNO=53742), EDUCATION (EDU-TYPE >10)
          leads to all EDUCATION segments for the given person that
          meet the stated condition.
- Data base: Data base name.

Types
No provision is made for types.

Representation of classes
The definition of class PROFESSIONS-DATABASE is an example of a class
representation by means of a data definition language. More clarity,
though less detail is provided by graphical representations such as

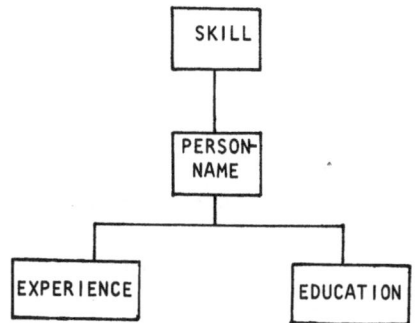

Representation of models

Graphical representations that meet the conditions of sec.3.6 are
widely in use for IMS models. They are based on the graphical
representation of classes shown above and include the name of the
class of which a model object is an instance.

Example:

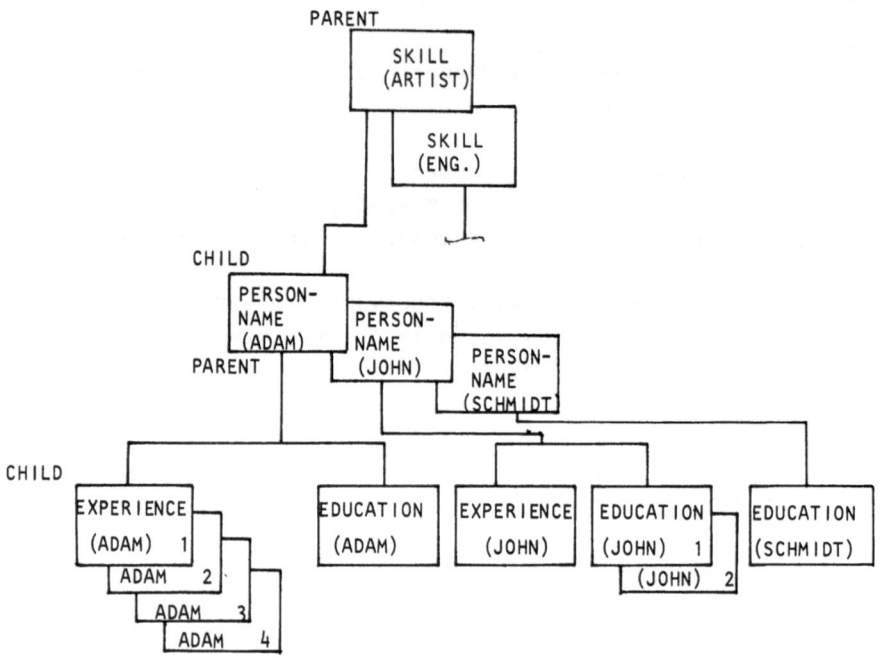

4.2 DBTG [7,8]

Among the attempts to standardize data base systems interfaces the CODASYL Data Base Task Group (DBTG) Report has had the largest effect on the planning of commercially available data base software. However, it is by no means unchallenged and still the subject of considerable discussion. Again, only a brief and incomplete outline shall be given below.

Elementary modes
- Data item
- Attribute

Complex modes
- Vector: Linearly ordered set of data items of identical class.
- Data aggregate: A set of ordered pairs (attribute, component) where a component may be an instance of data item, vector, data aggregate, or repeating group. (Notice the recursive definition which allows to build up data aggregates to any arbitrary number of levels!)

- Repeating group: Linearly ordered set of data aggregates of identical class.
- Record: Data aggregate which is not a component of a data aggregate.
- Area: Set of records such that each record is assigned to exactly one area.
- Data base: Set of areas.
- Coset: A one-to-many binary relation defined on records such that
  a) all pairs agree in their first coordinate (owner record),
  b) the pairs, or simply the second coordinates (member records) are linearly ordered.
  (Remark: In the DBTG proposal cosets are referred to as ´sets´. In order to avoid confusion we shall use the term ´coset´ which has been proposed by various authors.)

The only restrictions imposed on these relations are that owner and member records must be elements of different classes. However, the same record may be a member record in one coset and an owner record in another coset (giving rise to "hierarchies") or may be a member record of more than one coset (giving rise to "networks").

Examples:

owner	member
customer	articles-on-order
department	employees
company	departments

Hierarchies: company --> departments --> employees
Networks: company --> departments ↘
                          payroll   --> employees

Elementary classes

- Various classes of arithmetic items, bit and character strings.
- Database key.

Complex classes

- Record classes: Composition of records in terms of classes of data items, vectors, data aggregates and repeating groups, and of instances of attributes.
- Coset classes: Composition of cosets in terms of owner record class (n=1) and member record classes (m=0, n arbitrary) together with an ordering.
- Area classes: Composition of areas in terms of record classes. At any one time there is exactly one instance per area class.
  An area class is a list of record classes; this determines which

record instances may make up the single instance of the area class.
Technically, however, the schema does not include such a list;
instead each record class contains a clause specifying the area or
areas within which its instances may occur.
- Data base class: Defined in terms of area classes and coset classes.
At any one time there is exactly one instance of the data base
class.

Mode activities

No activities are defined on elementary modes, vectors, data
aggregates, and repeating groups. Hence the DBTG interface violates
the definition of modeling system in ch.3.7. Indeed, these modes serve
exclusively the purpose of determining the structure of records for
identification purposes. Since attributes are unique within a record,
a list of (attribute, item)-pairs would be entirely sufficient. This
is borne out by practical examples of DBTG schemas.

Quite similar to IMS, mode activities are defined explicitly on
records but sometimes implicitly on cosets, and no activities are
explicitly defined on cosets.

STORE: Create a record in an area. The record value is determined by
   the contents of the working storage area. Among the side-effects on
   cosets: If the record is of owner record type a new coset is
   created. Under certain conditions the record is inserted into a
   coset.
INSERT: Insert an existing record in order into a coset instance.
REMOVE: Remove an existing record from a coset instance.
DELETE: Remove an existing record from the data base. All cosets of
   which the record is a member are affected. If the record happens to
   be an owner record, the side-effects are most spectacular and
   almost unpredictable: Cosets may be deleted, perhaps recursively,
   as well as a number of additional records.
MODIFY: Replace the value of a record.
GET: Access the value of a record.

Since the activities attempt to maintain the class membership of the
objects involved, they may also be regarded class activities. To that
end, class names must be supplied with each invocation of an activity.
No operators are provided.

The interface does not provide activities for the creation of data
bases and areas. These are invoked instead by special facilities
outside the interface.

Model selectors

- Data base: Data base name.
- Area: Area name.
- Record:
  a) Within data base: Database-key.
  b) Within area: Value of one or more data items (usually unique within area).
  c) Within coset: Value of one or more data items (usually unique within coset).
  d) Within data base: Various current records. Basically, a current record is the last record subjected to an activity.
- Record components: Attribute value.
- Coset: Identified by its owner record which, in turn, is selected according to the rules above.

Basically, the subject of an activity is the current record. A special procedure, FIND, is provided for relating the current record to a record instance identified by an arbitrary selector.

Types

Class types may be defined as classes together with a set of restrictions on the applicability of the activities. No separate definition of classes is possible. Typical restrictions are:
- Use of selectors;
- applicability of INSERT, REMOVE;
- ordering of member records.

Representation

Aside from rules governing the string forms of data items and attributes, the DBTG report does not address itself to the question of representation.

Type description language

A DBTG-schema is comparatively complex, in part because there existed no agreed-upon set of basic concepts at the time of design, in part because a highly verbal COBOL style is used, in part because aspects of realization, interaction and privacy are included within the schema. Below the syntax of schemas is outlined in a considerably simplified form. This presentation is mainly intended to convey a feeling for DBTG-schemas; for detailed explanations the reader is referred to refs [7,8]. Basically, the meaning of the various clauses

is as follows:
- Class names: SCHEMA, AREA, RECORD clauses.
- Privileged access to the schema (!): PRIVACY clause in SCHEMA entry.
- Protection against simultaneous access by other users: PRIVACY clause in AREA entry.
- Privacy of data: All other PRIVACY clauses.
- Constituent classes: WITHIN, OWNER, MEMBER clauses.
- Record structure: PICTURE, TYPE, OCCURS clauses.
- Selectors: LOCATION, SEARCH, SELECTION clauses.
- Coset ordering: ORDER, KEY clauses.

Schema Entry Skeleton
SCHEMA clause
   PRIVACY clause
General Format of Entry
SCHEMA NAME IS schema-name-1

$$\left[;\underline{PRIVACY}\ \underline{LOCK}\ \left[FOR\ \left\| \begin{matrix} \underline{LOCKS} \\ \underline{DISPLAY} \\ \underline{COPY} \\ \underline{ALTER} \end{matrix} \right\| \right]\ IS\ \left\{ \begin{matrix} \text{literal-1} \\ \text{lock-name-1} \end{matrix} \right\} \right]$$

Area Entry Skeleton
AREA clause
   PRIVACY clause
General Format of Area Entry
AREA NAME IS area-name-1

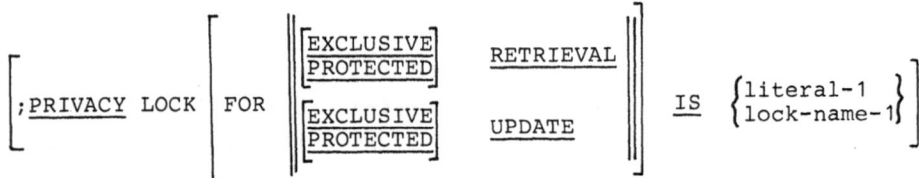

$$\left[;\underline{PRIVACY}\ \underline{LOCK}\ \left[FOR\ \left\| \begin{matrix} \left[\begin{matrix}\text{EXCLUSIVE}\\\text{PROTECTED}\end{matrix}\right] & \text{RETRIEVAL} \\ \left[\begin{matrix}\text{EXCLUSIVE}\\\text{PROTECTED}\end{matrix}\right] & \text{UPDATE} \end{matrix} \right\| \right]\ \underline{IS}\ \left\{ \begin{matrix} \text{literal-1} \\ \text{lock-name-1} \end{matrix} \right\} \right]$$

Record Entry Skeleton
Record Subentry
   [Data Subentry] ...

Record Subentry Skeleton
RECORD clause
   LOCATION clause   (selection in area)
   WITHIN clause   (corresponding area)
   PRIVACY clause

<u>Data Subentry Skeleton</u>

data-base-data-name clause

   <u>PICTURE</u> clause

   <u>TYPE</u> clause

   <u>OCCURS</u> clause

<u>General Format of Record Subentry</u>

<u>RECORD</u> NAME IS record-name-1

$$
;\underline{\text{LOCATION}}\text{ MODE IS}\left\{\begin{array}{l}\underline{\text{DIRECT}}\left\{\begin{array}{l}\text{data-base-data-name-1}\\\text{data-base-identifier-1}\end{array}\right\}\\[6pt]\underline{\text{CALC}}\;[\text{data-base-procedure-1}]\;\underline{\text{USING}}\text{ data-base-identifier-2}\\\quad[\text{,data-base-identifier-3}]\ldots\underline{\text{DUPLICATES}}\text{ ARE }[\underline{\text{NOT}}]\text{ ALLOWED}\\[10pt]\underline{\text{VIA}}\text{ set-name-1 SET}\end{array}\right\}
$$

;WITHIN area-name-1 $\bigl[$,area-name-2 ... <u>AREA-ID</u> IS data-base-data-name-2$\bigr]$

$$
\left[;\underline{\text{PRIVACY}}\text{ LOCK}\left[\text{ FOR }\left\|\begin{array}{l}\underline{\text{INSERT}}\\\underline{\text{REMOVE}}\\\underline{\text{STORE}}\\\underline{\text{DELETE}}\\\underline{\text{MODIFY}}\\\underline{\text{FIND}}\\\underline{\text{GET}}\end{array}\right\|\right]\text{ IS }\left\{\begin{array}{l}\text{literal-1}\\\text{lock-name-1}\end{array}\right\}\right]
$$

<u>General Format of Data Subentry</u>

[level-number-1] data-base-data-name-1

$$
\left[;\underline{\text{PICTURE}}\text{ IS }\quad"\left\{\begin{array}{l}\text{character-string-picture-specification-1}\\\text{numeric-picture-specification-1}\end{array}\right\}"\right]
$$

$$
\left[;\underline{\text{TYPE}}\text{ IS}\left\{\begin{array}{ll}\left\|\left\{\begin{array}{l}\text{BINARY}\\\text{DECIMAL}\\\text{FIXED}\\\text{FLOAT}\\\text{REAL}\\\text{COMPLEX}\end{array}\right\}\right\|&[\text{integer-1}[,\text{integer-2}]]\\[10pt]\left\{\begin{array}{l}\text{BIT}\\\text{CHARACTER}\end{array}\right\}&[\text{integer-3}]\end{array}\right\}\right]
$$

$$
\left[;\underline{\text{OCCURS}}\left\{\begin{array}{l}\text{integer-4}\\\text{data-base-identifier-1}\end{array}\right\}\text{ TIMES}\right]
$$

<u>Set Entry Skeleton</u>

Set Subentry

  [Member Subentry]   ...

Set Subentry Skeleton

SET clause

    OWNER clause

    ORDER clause

    PRIVACY clause

Member Subentry Skeleton

MEMBER clause

   KEY clause

   SEARCH clause

   SELECTION clause

General Format of Set Subentry

SET NAME IS set-name-1

 ;OWNER IS $\left\{ \begin{array}{l} \text{record-name-1} \\ \text{SYSTEM} \end{array} \right\}$

 ;ORDER IS $\left\{ \begin{array}{l} \text{FIRST} \\ \text{LAST} \\ \text{NEXT} \\ \text{PRIOR} \\ \text{IMMATERIAL} \\ \text{SORTED} \quad \text{[INDEXED [NAME IS index-name-1]]} \\ \left\{ \begin{array}{l} \text{BY DATA-BASE-KEY} \\ \text{BY RECORD-NAME} \\ \text{WITHIN RECORD-NAME} \\ \text{BY DEFINED KEYS} \end{array} \right\} \end{array} \right\}$

$\left[\text{;PRIVACY LOCK} \left[\text{FOR} \left| \left| \begin{array}{l} \text{INSERT} \\ \text{REMOVE} \\ \text{FIND} \end{array} \right| \right| \right] \text{IS} \left\{ \begin{array}{l} \text{literal-1} \\ \text{lock-name-1} \end{array} \right\} \right]$

General Format of Member Subentry

MEMBER IS record-name-1

$\left[\text{; [RANGE]} \; \underline{\text{KEY}} \; \text{IS} \left\{ \begin{array}{l} \text{ASCENDING} \\ \text{DESCENDING} \end{array} \right\} \; \text{data-base-identifier-3} \right]$

$\left[\text{;SEARCH KEY IS data-base-identifier-5} \right.$

$\left. \quad \left[\text{USING} \left\{ \begin{array}{l} \text{CALC} \\ \text{INDEX[NAME IS index-name-1]} \\ \text{PROCEDURE data-base-procedure-1} \end{array} \right\} \right] \right]$

 ;SET SELECTION [FOR set-name-1] IS
    THRU set-name-2 OWNER IDENTIFIED BY

```
┌                                                                        ┐
│  CURRENT OF SET                                                        │
│  ┌─────────────┐         ⎧data-base-identifier-7⎫                     │
│  │DATA-BASE-KEY│[EQUAL TO ⎨data-base-data-name-1 ⎬]                    │
│  └─────────────┘         ⎩                       ⎭                     │
│                                                                        │
│ ┌─────────┐            ⎡         ⎧data-base-identifier-8⎫⎤             │
│ │CALC-KEY │            │EQUAL TO ⎨data-base-data-name-2 ⎬│             │
│ └─────────┘            ⎣         ⎩                       ⎭⎦             │
│                                                                        │
│  MEMBER record-name-2 SELECTION                                        │
└ THEN THRU set-name-3                                                  ┐
  ┌  WHERE OWNER IDENTIFIED BY data-base-identifier-10                 │
  │    ┌─────┐    ⎧data-base-identifier-11⎫⎤           ⎫...│...
  │    │EQUAL│ TO ⎨data-base-data-name-4  ⎬│           ⎬   │
  └    └─────┘    ⎩                       ⎭⎦           ⎭   ┘
```

Example of a schema (incomplete)

```
SCHEMA NAME IS               DISTRIBUTION-ORGANISATION.

AREA NAME IS                 SUPPLIER-AREA.
AREA NAME IS                 ARTICLE-AREA.
AREA NAME IS                 CUSTOMER-AREA.

RECORD NAME IS               SUPPLIER-CONTROL;
    LOCATION MODE IS         CALC
                             USING CALC-KEY
                             DUPLICATES ARE NOT ALLOWED;
    WITHIN                   SUPPLIER-AREA.
    CALC-KEY;                PICTURE IS X(30).
    SUPPLIER-COUNT;          PICTURE IS 9(6).
    PURCHASE-ORDER--COUNT;   PICTURE IS 9(6).
    ARTICLE-COUNT;           PICTURE IS 9(6).

RECORD NAME IS               CUSTOMER-CONTROL;
    LOCATION MODE IS         CALC
                             USING CALC-KEY
                             DUPLICATES ARE NOT ALLOWED;
    WITHIN                   CUSTOMER-AREA.
    CALC-KEY;                PICTURE IS X(30).
    CUSTOMER-COUNT;          PICTURE IS 9(6).
    SALES-ORDER-COUNT;       PICTURE IS 9(6).

RECORD NAME IS               SUPPL-SALES-ORDER-CONTROL;
    LOCATION MODE IS         CALC
                             USING CALC-KEY
                             DUPLICATES ARE NOT ALLOWED;
    WITHIN                   CUSTOMER-AREA.
    CALC-KEY;                PICTURE IS X(30).
. . . . . . . . . . . . . . . . . . . . . . . . . . . . . .
SET NAME IS                  SUPPLIERS;
    ORDER IS                 SORTED INDEXED BY DEFINED KEYS
                             DUPLICATES ARE NOT ALLOWED;
    OWNER IS                 SUPPLIER-CONTROL.
```

```
MEMBER IS                        SUPPLIER;
    ASCENDING KEY IS             SUPPLIER-ID,
                                 SUPPLIER-SEQ-NO;
    SET OCCURRENCE SELECTION IS  THRU CURRENT OF SET.

SET NAME IS                      CUSTOMERS;
    ORDER IS                     SORTED INDEXED BY DEFINED KEYS
                                 DUPLICATES ARE NOT ALLOWED;
    OWNER IS                     CUSTOMER-CONTROL.
MEMBER IS                        CUSTOMER;
    ASCENDING KEY IS             CUSTOMER-ID,
                                 CUSTOMER-SEQ-NO;
    SEARCH KEY IS                CUSTOMER-NAME
                                 DUPLICATES ARE ALLOWED;
    SET OCCURRENCE SELECTION IS  THRU CURRENT OF SET.
SET NAME IS                      SUPPLIABLE-SALES-ORDERS;
    ORDER IS                     ALWAYS LAST;
    OWNER IS                     SUPPL-SALES-ORDER-CONTROL.
MEMBER IS                        SALES-ORDER;
    SET OCCURRENCE SELECTION IS  THRU CURRENT OF SET.
```

. . . .

Schema diagrams

As shown for IMS, graphical forms are a particular conspicuous way of portraying schemas. On the other hand, graphical schemas are always restricted to the description of classes (rather than types). For coset classes the following kind of graphical schema is widely used.

- Each record type is represented by a box containing the record type name.
- Each coset is represented by boxes for each record type involved, and arrows that connect the owner record box with each member record box. The arrow is labelled by the coset name.

Examples.

a) One member record type

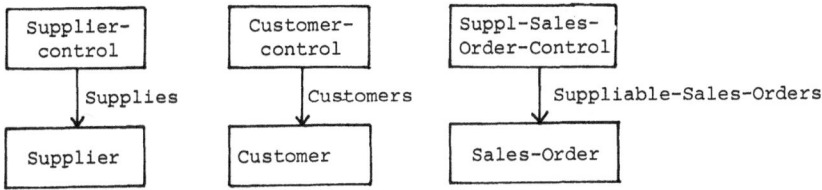

b) Two member record types in a coset type.

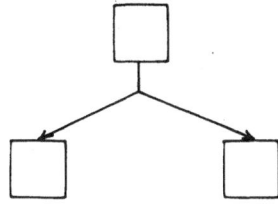

c) Identical member record types in two different coset types.

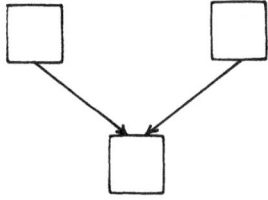

d) Two coset types with identical owner and member record types.

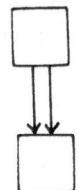

e) Hierarchies of coset types

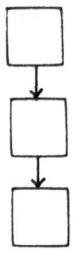

4.3 RELATIONAL MODEL [9-12]

In large part the community of data base experts is deeply split between the hierarchical view of the world as exemplified by DBTG and the so-called "relational view" of the world as exemplified by the relational model below. Although the latter has not yet reached the level of commercial availability we shall cover it briefly since it is as widely discussed as the DBTG report.

Elementary modes
- Data items
- Attributes

Complex modes

- Tuple: A set of ordered pairs (attribute, data item) where no two attributes are identical.
  It is standard practice to define an order on the attributes and then treat the Tuple as an ordered pair ((ordered n-tuple of attributes), (ordered n-tuple of data items)) together with a mapping from attributes to data items and vice-versa based on position within the n-tuples.
- Relation: A set of Tuples that agree in their n-tuples of attributes. Hence the n-tuple of attributes may be directly associated with the relation.

- Data base: Set of relations.

(Remarks:
a) The capital 'T' is used in order to avoid confusion: 'Tuple' is a mode whereas 'tuple' refers to a standard mathematical term.
b) Note that the elementary modes are identical for both DBTG and relational model. Nevertheless, the complex modes are vastly different.)

Elementary classes

Standard classes are provided like CHAR strings, numbers (NUM) with a given precision. In addition, classes may be introduced by explicitly naming them and enumerating their value set.

Complex classes

- Domain: An ordered pair (attribute, item class).
- Relation class: An ordered set of domains. The relation may then be interpreted in the mathematical sense (defined on the item classes under the domains).
  At any one time there is exactly one instance of a given relation (m=n=1) so that relation name and relation class name coincide.
- Data base class: Set of relation classes.

Example (taken from ALPHA [10]).

```
Domains:      DOMAIN   S# CHAR(5)
                       SNAME CHAR(15)
                       LOC CHAR(20)
                       P# CHAR(20)
                       PNAME CHAR(30)
                       COLOR STATE(1='BLUE',2='RED'....)
                       WEIGHT NUM(3,1)
                       QOH NUM(4,0)
                       J# CHAR(4)
                       JNAME CHAR(10)
                       E# NUM(6,0)
                       SHIPDATE DATE(YEAR,MONTH,DAY)
                       QUANTITY NUM(3,0)
Data base class:       RELATION SUPPLIER(S#,SNAME LOC) KEY S#
                       RELATION PART(P#,PNAME,COLOR,WEIGHT,QOH) KEY P#
                       RELATION PROJECT(J#,JNAME,E#) KEY J#
                       RELATION SUPPLY(W#,P#,J#,SHIPDATE, QUANTITY)
                                KEY (S#,P#,J#,SHIPDATE)
```

Comments:
(1) For KEY, see below.
(2) In the schema above, a relation is simply defined in terms of
    domain names. The attribute of a domain serves as its domain name.
    As a consequence, domain names must be unique within a relation so
    that there sometimes is a need for several domains with identical
    item classes.
(3) If the same domain name appears within different relation classes
    it refers to the same domain.

Model selectors

(i)   Data base: Unspecified.
(ii)   Relation: Relation name.
(iii) Tuple: Selection in a relation by one or a sequence of keys of
       the form <attribute> = <data item>.
(iv)   Data item: Selection in a tuple by attribute.

Mode activities

Originally, the relational model was defined in the form of a
"relational algebra" with a set of operators mapping a relation or the
direct product of two relations into a relation. Thus it would be our
first example of an interface based on operators. However, the
relational algebra is not known as a user interface. Instead,
interfaces have been proposed that are based on a "relational
calculus" within which one may again distinguish mode activities.
These refer to relations, tuples or just data items as their model
objects. The corresponding models are accessible in a ´workspace´.

(declare): Declare and establish a relation in the data base by giving
    its name and listing its domains (DOMAIN, RELATION).
DROP: Remove a relation from the data base.
PUT: Insert the Tuple provided in work space into a relation.
DELETE: Remove a Tuple from a relation.
GET: Fetch the value of one or more data items into workspace.
HOLD: Fetch the value of one or more data items to workspace for
    subsequent modification.
UPDATE: Replace the value of one or more data items previously
    referred to by HOLD by the contents of work space. No primary keys
    must be modified.

Logical expressions

Since the relational calculus has been shown to be equivalent in power
to the relational algebra, one starts wondering how activities could
replace n-ary operations. Indeed, the equivalence is reflected not in
terms of the activities but in terms of logical expressions on the
value of model objects that take the place of model selectors. These
expressions specify data items to be extracted from the data base and
placed in a workspace.

Simple example:
```
GET W (SUPPLIER.S#, SUPPLIER.SNAME, SUPPLIER.LOC):
                    (SUPPLIER.LOC = 'NEW YORK')
```
where W is a workspace, the parenthesized list is a target list
designating the data items of a Tuple to be fetched, and the condition
is a qualification indicating which Tuples to select.

Representation

The most common representation of relations is by means of tables. In
fact, one of the arguments put forward in favor of the relational
model is that it is natural for a human being to think in terms of
tables. Example:

```
SUPPLIER       (S#      SNAME        LOC)
                1       Jones        New York
                2       Smith        Chicago
                3       Connors      Boston
                4       Thompson     New York
```

4.4 ABSTRACT MACHINES [13]

By contrast to activities, operators establish constructive
relationships between model objects. New model objects never arise out
of nowhere but can always be traced to existing ones. As a
consequence, one can construct sequences of operations such that the
source objects in each operation existed beforehand or are the result
of a previous operation. A logical expression of the relational
calculus may be reduced to a sequence of relation algebraic
operations, and thus is indicative of the higher complexity possible
for user requests in case of operators.

For these cases the concept of abstract machine has proven useful as a
description tool. In short, an abstract machine is a set of modes

and/or classes, a set of operators for manipulating model objects and defined on modes and/or classes, plus a control mechanism that allows to construct and execute seouence of operations.

The concept is illustrated below by means of the set theoretic machine of the KAIFAS system which models a universe in a property-oriented way rather than the object-oriented way of the previous examples.

Elementary modes/classes
I   elementary objects (individuals)
Z   numbers
D   measures: ordered pairs (number, unit expression)
B   truth values

Complex modes
M   sets: list of individuals
R   relations: list of ordered pairs of individuals
F   measure functions: list of ordered n-tuples whose last
    components are measures.

Operators
On retrieval the machine is supposed to function in the following way. Set, relation, and function names refer to objects in permanent storage. In order to manipulate the objects they must be transferred into unnamed registers of which an unlimited number is thought to exist. Hence all operations except for the load operations are register-to-register operations. The following retrieval operators are of interest.

Load operators
Mw, ev, en, ef   Load a set, a relation (ev, en), and a measure
                        function, respectively.

Set operators
MU: MxM→M   Union
M∩: MxM→M   Intersection
Km: MxM→M   Relative complement $\{x \mid x \in M_1 \wedge x \in M_2\}$
Kz: M→Z   Cardinality

Binary relation operators
Ko: R→R   Converse relation
Rb: RxM→R   Restriction $\{(x,y) \mid (x,y) \in R \wedge x \in M\}$
Rp: RxR→R   Product $\{(x,y) \mid \exists z : (x,z) \in R_1 \wedge (z,y) \in R_2\}$
Ru: RxR→R   Union

Reduction of binary relations

Vo:	R→M	Domain $\{x\,|\,\exists y:(x,y)\in R\}$
Na:	R→M	Range $\{x\,|\,\exists y:(y,x)\in R\}$
Vg:	RxI→M	Individual domain $\{x\,|\,(x,I)\in R\}$
Ng:	RxI→M	Individual range $\{x\,|\,(I,x)\in R\}$
VgU:	RxM→M	Restricted domain $\{x\,|\,(x,y)\in R\wedge y\in M\}$

Reduction of measure functions

Fw: FxI→D   (n=2)

Logical operators

e:	IxM→B	Test on set membership
c:	MxM→B	Test on set inclusion

In addition, the standard logical operators are available as well as the standard arithmetic and comparison operators for numbers and measures.

Control mechanism

Sequencing of operations

"Programs" for the set theoretic machine are expressed in a functional notation. Operations are performed from left to right and, for each nested argument, from inside out. Example:
$c(Mw(M_{city}), VgU(en(R_{birthplace}), Mw(M_{engineer})))$
("Are cities birthplaces of engineers?")

Loops

Loops are introduced by the use of bounded quantifiers which have three arguments:

1) An expression resulting in a set of objects (range).
2) An expression for the condition resulting in a truth value (scope); it may be regarded as the loop body.
3) The name of a bound variable; each of its substitutions defines an invocation of the loop.

Important quantifiers are
AL: MxB →B   all, every
EI: MxB →B   some

```
DB: MxB ->M    which
ZB: MxB ->Z    how many
```

with the left-hand M the bounding set and the left-hand B the condition. Example:

$$DB \ (x_1,$$
$$\quad Mw(M_{manuf}),$$
$$\quad ZB(x_2,$$
$$\qquad Vg(en(R_{prod}),x_1),$$
$$\qquad DB(x_3,$$
$$\qquad\quad Mw(M_{ailment}),$$
$$\qquad\quad e(x_2, \ Vg(en(R_{medic}),x_3))))))$$

with the meaning of "How many products of which manufacturers are medications for which ailments?"

Formal expressions and, in particular, the use of quantifiers is highly typical for abstract machines and, in fact, gives them all their power. A bounded quantifier may be thought of to work in the following way: Take the first object from the range and check whether it satisfies the condition. Depending on the outcome take appropriate action, e.g. if the condition is satisfied AL continues, EI terminates with "yes", DB saves the object, ZB increases a counter. Unless terminated, pick up the next object from the range and repeat. Continue until the range has been exhausted. On termination provide the result, e.g. "yes" for AL, "no" for EI, a list for DB, a number for ZB.

4.5 CONCLUDING REMARKS

All the examples given so far are approaches to or concrete cases of interfaces of computerized data base systems. These systems are the ultimate objective of our discussion. However, the principles of ch. 3 are much more general and are supposed to cover arbitrary problem areas as well, e.g. hospital administration, diagnosis and therapy, patient care, drug inventories, pharmacological research. As a matter of fact, we hope that the concepts introduced so far may serve as a useful tool for systematically describing a given problem area before a concrete data base system is designed or selected.

After such a systematic problem description has been derived, one must translate the given data structure system into a new one that is determined by the data base system to be selected or designed. The amount of effort that goes into such a translation, and its success will be an indication of the effectiveness and efficiency that may be expected from the data base system.

5 Functions

5.1 INTEGRATION OF FUNCTIONS

A request to a computerized information system usually consists of up to three parts:
(1) Retrieval of certain objects according to some more or less complex selection criteria.
(2) Combination and evaluation of the objects retrieved.
(3) Modification of the data base on the basis of the results obtained in (2).
Parts 1 and 3 have well-defined objectives and thus are easily systematized by the means mentioned in ch. 3. By contrast, part 2 may serve any purpose and hence is much more difficult to systematize. As a consequence, one major problem in language design is integrating part 2 with parts 1 and 3. Three approaches are possible:

(i)   Host language systems.
        Part 2 is stated in a conventional programming language such as COBOL, PL/I, ALGOL. Parts 1 and 3 are interfaced with part 2 by means of subroutine or macro calls. In other words, the data manipulation language (DML) is embedded within the programming language used for part 2 (host language). The subroutines, on their part, make use of the schemas which are described by the data definition language (DDL). Contrary to the DML the DDL is usually not embedded but self-contained. Examples for this kind of approach are DBTG, IMS, ALPHA.
(ii)   Subroutine packages.
        Sometimes the programs required to perform part 2 already exist. This is especially true in the area of statistical analysis where several extensive subroutine packages have been developed. The problem, then, becomes one of interfacing two software systems, a data base management system and a subroutine package.
(iii)   Full integration.
        Data base management functions and processing functions are provided on the same level and may be freely combined. Experience shows that so far information systems of this kind are highly inflexible with respect to the addition, deletion or modification of functions or types. As a consequence, full integration is usually reserved to systems whose total function is well-understood, well-defined and fixed, e.g. reservation systems or inventory control.

5.2 CLASSIFICATION OF COMPUTERIZED INFORMATION SYSTEMS

Agreement on formalized approaches towards coordination, information structures, and classification of functional properties in agencies seem to evolve only slowly. Hence there is still terminological chaos as far as a characterization of information system types is concerned. For the purpose of this discussion we shall classify information systems into the following four categories. The first three categories refer to information systems that contain a data base that is an immediate model of the outside world. They differ with respect to the possible usage made of the data base.

- _Fact-retrieval system:_ Provides activities only; as such it is restricted to parts 1 and 3.
- _Question-answering system_: Provides activities and operators; however, operators are limited to performing composition and decomposition of objects (i.e. no new elementary values may be derived), and logical comparisons. One may argue that such a system covers part 2 as well, though in a limited way. Since the operators are intimately tied to the data base we shall still count them towards part 1. Nevertheless, while fact-retrieval systems are of little value unless combined with other programs, interactive question-answering systems may already be valuable on their own.
- _Strict information system_: No limits on the operators; hence, in particular, the operators may perform arbitrary computations. Consequently, such a system includes all three parts; internally it may be composed of several subsystems, among these a fact-retrieval or question-answering system.

By contrast, the fourth category is based on a different kind of data base:
- A _document-retrieval system_ is used in cases where the outside world is too little understood or too complex to be modeled according to the rules of a data structure system. Instead, there are only descriptive views of the universe in the form of documents. A document-retrieval system contains a data base that is a model of a universe consisting of documents (and in many cases contains the documents as well). This model may be treated by means of a fact-retrieval or a question-answering system.

5.3 FACT-RETRIEVAL SYSTEMS: EXAMPLE [7,8]

Evidently, the DBTG data structure system of sec. 4.2 conforms exactly
to the definition of a fact-retrieval system. Its interface consists
of a DDL for type description and a DML for mode activities, the
latter being invoked by subroutine calls. Hence DBTG has been designed
for incorporation within a host language system. The entire system
organization is illustrated by the following diagram.

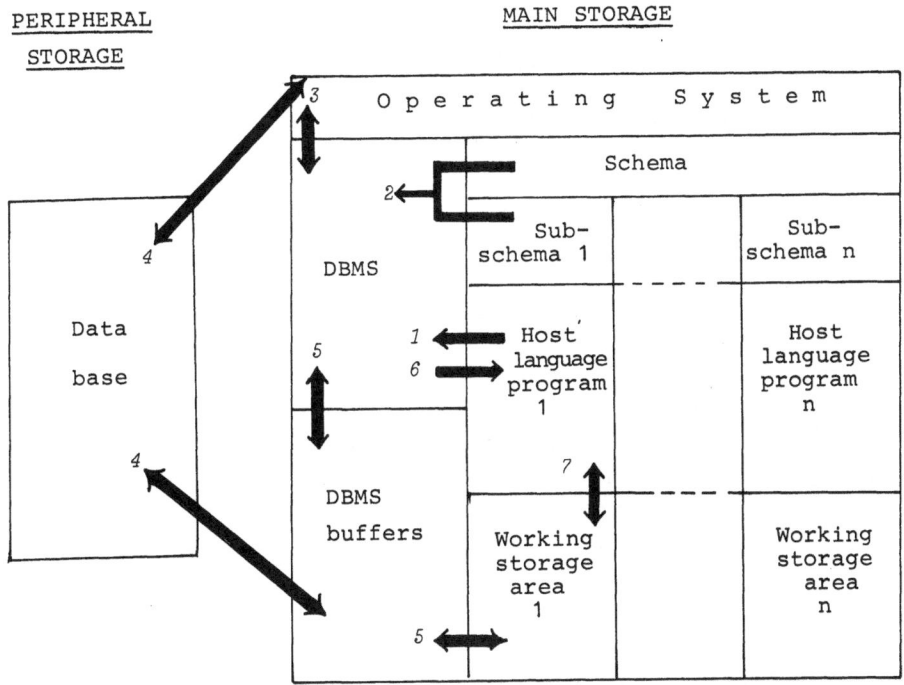

All activities are performed by a Data Base Management System (DBMS).
There may be n concurrent host language programs accessing the same
data base. The data base is described by the schema, however each
program may have an individual view of the data base as expressed by
its sub-schema. In case of retrieval the following phases take place:
1 Host language programm calls on DBMS by means of a DDL statement.
2 DBMS evaluates the call on the basis of schema and sub-schema.
3 DBMS calls on operating system to perform the necessary input/output
  chores.
4 Operating system controls the data transmission between peripheral
  and main storage.
5 DBMS transfers record from buffers to working storage area subject
  to modifications that are mandated by the differences between schema

and sub-schema.

6 DBMS informs host language program of success or failure or processing the request.

7 Host language program manipulates record in its own working storage area.

The communication between host language program and DBMS is illustrated below by a small portion of a COBOL program (activities are underlined).

```
UPDATE-SET-SALES-ORDERS.
    IF SALES-ORDER-CAN-BE-DELETED
        THEN PERFORM DELETE-SALES-ORDER
        ELSE PERFORM STOCK-UPDATE THROUGH END-STOCK-UPDATE
        PERFORM UPDATE-SALES-ORDER.
    MOVE OTHER-OPERATION TO OPERATION.

UPDATE-SALES-ORDER.
    FIND OWNER RECORD OF SALES-ORDER-CONTENTS SET.
    MODIFY SALES-ORDER.
    IF DELIVERY-CNT IN SALES-ORDER EQUALS O
        THEN INSERT SALES-ORDER
        INTO SUPPLIABLE-SALES-ORDERS.

DELETE-SALES-ORDER.
    DELETE SALES-ORDER.
    FIND CUSTOMER-CONTROL.
    GET CUSTOMER-CONTROL.
    SUBTRACT 1 FROM SALES-ORDER-COUNT IN CUSTOMER-CONTROL.
    MODIFY CUSTOMER-CONTROL.
    MOVE NOT-DELETABLE-SALES-ORDER TO SALES-ORDER-STATUS.
```

The concept of sub-schema merits a few additional words. A type and hence a schema reflects a certain view of the universe. However, it is quite possible that different users or different functional components (such as programs) may take somewhat differing views of the same universe, i.e. use different notations, eliminate or include certain relationships, exclude or incorporate certain objects. Hence a schema may be interpreted as a global model of a universe, and each sub-schema as an individual or restricted model of the same universe. In other words, the schema represents something like the union of all individual models. As a consequence, the data base in the diagram above reflects the global model, while each working storage area holds a restricted model. The DBMS, via the buffers, maps the two from one another.

The following differences may be observed between a schema and a sub-schema.

- Privacy locks may be supplied in the sub-schema where none have been

specified in the schema, and vice-versa, or the locks may differ. Privacy locks in the sub-schema, unless missing, take precedence over those in the schema.
- Certain data items, data aggregates, records, areas, or cosets from the schema may be missing in a sub-schema. (Note that this provides for additional privacy of data.)
- The types of data items, data aggregates, records, areas, or cosets may vary between schema and sub-schema.
- Areas, cosets, records, attributes may be renamed.

5.4 QUESTION-ANSWERING SYSTEMS: EXAMPLE

The KAIFAS system of sec. 4.4 is a typical instance of a question-answering system. The relational model of sec. 4.3 may also be counted towards question-answering systems on account of its logical expressions which, in effect, hide an abstract machine. There are several other experimental question-answering systems reported in the literature. All appear to have in common the following characteristics:
- The "machine" level is well formalized.
- All rely on quantification as a means for building complex expressions.
- All tend, incidentally, towards a second, natural-language interface for the user (see 5.5).

This was already demonstrated by the few examples for the KAIFAS system which is a self-contained system without data evaluation facilities. In this section we shall explore the expressions in the relational model. The corresponding expression language, ALPHA, is designed to be interfaced with further evaluation facilities and, consequently, to be embedded within a host language.

As indicated before, a retrieval query is composed of the name of an activity, a work space name, a target list and a qualification. Generally, a target list consists of elements each of which is of one of the forms
- relation name.attribute name
- Tuple variable.attribute name
- relation name
- Tuple variable
In the last two cases, complete Tuples are to be elicited from the corresponding relation.

Example:

GET W (PART.P#,PART.PNAME,PART.QOH) : (PART.QOH<25)

("Find the part numbers, part names and quantities on hand where quantity on hand is less than 25.")

The set of distinct PART Tuples (P#,PNAME,QOH) satisfying the requirement is copied into workspace W which may subsequently be regarded as a ternary relation named W with attributes P#,PNAME,QOH.

If frequent reference is made to the relation PART, a range declaration

RANGE PART P

may be made which introduces a bound Tuple variable P whose range is the relation PART. Hence the request takes the form

GET W (P.P#,P.PNAME,P.QOH) : (P.QOH<25)

The RANGE statement can be considered as being equivalent to a universal quantifier.

This example supports the claims made above on the role of quantification. In fact, a closer inspection of the very first example indicates that even there PART must be considered a Tuple variable since attributes may act as selectors only within Tuples. Hence, for reasons of transparency it is recommended to insist on the use of RANGE statements.

Now that the format of quantification in ALPHA has been established we may proceed to a more complex example:

RANGE   SUPPLIER S   (ALL is implied)
RANGE   SUPPLY   Z   SOME
GET   W S.SNAME:(S.S#=Z.S#) ∧ (Z.P#=3)
("Find the supplier names of those suppliers who supply the part with part number 3.")

Two variables may have the same range but must be distinguished in the query:

RANGE   SUPPLIER S
RANGE   SUPPLIER T SOME

GET W S.S#:(T.SNAME = JONES´) ∧ (T.LOC=S.LOC)
("Find the supplier numbers of those suppliers who have the same location as supplier Jones.")

Readers may have noticed by now that use of the RANGE statement is equivalent to formulating a query in prenex normal form (which, incidentally, is also required in KAIFAS). (In prenex normal form, all quantifiers appear to the left of all other logical operators.) Unfortunately, this is not always the natural form of a query. For example, a first translation on paper of the request "Find the supplier numbers of suppliers who do not supply part number 3." resulted in

GET W S.S#:¬ ∃ Z((S.S#=Z.S#)∧(Z.P#=3))

There is a formal rule for transforming the qualification above into a logically equivalent expression which is in prenex normal form:

GET W S.S#:∀Z¬((S.S#=Z.S#)∧(Z.P#=3))

so that the use of RANGE statements is again possible:

RANGE SUPPLIER S
RANGE SUPPLY Z ALL
GET W S.S#:¬ ((S.S#=Z.S#) ∧ (Z.P#=3))

The target list may make use of more than one relation:

RANGE PROJECT J
RANGE SUPPLIER S
RANGE SUPPLY Z SOME
GET W (J.J#, J.JNAME, S.LOC):(J.J#=Z.J#) ∧ (Z.S#=S.S#)
("For each project obtain as a triple the project number, project name and supplier location for all suppliers who supply that project.")

These examples should suffice to illustrate some of the salient features of ALPHA. A few more shall be mentioned: Ordering of Tuples in workspace, limiting the number of Tuples in workspace, using workspace as just another relation, piped (sequential) access to Tuples in place of concurrent construction in workspace. However, we conclude with a single example for primary key update:

GET W PART: (PART.P#=3)
DELETE PART: (PART.P#=3)
W.P#=4   (host language)

PUT W PART

("Change the primary key of the part with part number 3 to 4.") GET
retrieves the entire PART Tuple with key 3 (PART as a Tuple variable).
DELETE deletes that Tuple from the data base relation PART but not
from workspace W (in the target list PART acts a relation name, in the
qualification as a Tuple variable). The host language statement alters
the key in the Tuple to 4. Finally, PUT inserts the new (actually
modified) Tuple into the data base relation PART (PART as a relation
name).

5.5 NATURAL-LANGUAGE QUERIES [13,14]

It was mentioned in sec. 5.4 that question-answering systems tend
towards natural-language interfaces, at least when used
conversationally. By now the reason should have become obvious: Few
users will feel at ease with the highly stylized languages such as
ALPHA or the set theoretic expressions in KAIFAS. In particular, few
will have the formal training to appreciate and follow some of the
requirements such as quantification or prenex normal form.

It is only a logical next step to design languages which correspond
more closely to the natural habitat of a user. By implication, many
designers take this to mean natural language. As a consequence, many
of the experimental question-answering systems include an additional
processor for the translation of natural-language queries into formal
expressions of the kind discussed above. This is not quite as
difficult as it may sound: By necessity the query language is a highly
restricted form of natural language since its semantics, and hence its
syntactic forms, can be no more than what may ultimately be reduced
to, in the KAIFAS case, a set theoretic interpretation. On the other
hand there are disadvantages, too: The degree of query complexity
achievable is much less than in stylized languages; indeed one can
often find circumstances that cannot be expressed in natural language
at all although they pose little problems in a mathematical notation.

An example of a question-answering system with a natural-language
processor is the KAIFAS system of sec. 4.4 which permits queries in
natural German. Below a few examples of queries and their
corresponding set language expressions are given:

"Welche Firmen sind Hersteller tablettenfoermiger Medikamente?"
$DB(x_1, Mw(M_{Firm}):, \in (x_1, Vg \cup (en(R_{Herst}), M\cap(Mw(M_{tabl}), Mw(M_{Med})))))$

"Welche Medikamente sind Tabletten?"
$M \cap (Mw(M_{Med}), Mw(M_{Tabl}))$

"Welche Produkte welcher Hersteller sind Heilmittel gegen welche Krankheiten?"
DB $(x_1,$
   $Mw(M_{Herst}),$
   $ZB(x_2,$
      $Vg(en(R_{Prod}),x_1),$
      $DB(x_3,$
         $Mw(M_{Krankh}),$
         $e(x_2, Vg(en(R_{Heilm}),x_3)))))$

The additon of natural-language interfaces must be carefully weighted. Much time must be spent on developing an adequate grammar that accounts for the numerous syntactic aspects to be observed even for restricted natural language, especially so for German with its wealth in morphems. By comparison, the time expended on translating a query is negligible.

Likewise, attempts are under way to provide a natural-language interface for the relational model. On the other hand, it is quite possible to devise interfaces that are still stylized but do not impose formal requirements of the same rigidity as ALPHA. For an example of the relational model, see SEQUEL whose constructs are reminiscent of programming languages.

5.6 DEDUCTIVE QUESTION-ANSWERING [15]

To many users, even those with some knowledge of its inner workings, a question-answering system will seem a highly sophisticated instrument with which "to feel one's way" through the maze of relationships in a model. The more so users become frustrated when they detect that the system, despite its sophistication, seems to lack even the most trivial capabilities for making inferences.

For example, in the relational model one could not simply ask for all suppliers of a given project since in this case the system would have to know that there is exactly one intervening relation, SUPPLY, in which both supplier number and project number happen to occur as attr·outes. Instead, the user himself must be aware of the fact in orde· to formulate the request:

```
RANGE   SUPPLIER S
RANGE   SUPPLY Z
RANGE   PROJECT J SOME
GET  W S.SNAME: (J.JNAME='A125') ∧ (Z.J#=J.J#) ∧ (S.S#=Z.S#)
```

More famous is the example of the families data base in which all
married couples are stored as well as for each female person her
children. Unless one lists the children of each male person, too, the
system is not able to deduce the father of each child (even when unwed
mothers are excluded!).

Apparently, what is needed are additional rules that specify the
intervening relation SUPPLY and how it is to be used, or that each
child of a woman is a child of her husband as well, respectively.
Furthermore, algorithms must be specified which formally derive truth
or falsity of a question from both the original information stored and
these rules.

Algorithms of this kind have been known for a long time in formal
logic. The original information and the rules are considered to be
logical axioms. The algorithms attempt to prove a given question from
these, that is, to prove that the question is a theorem.

Example:
Suppose the following information has been stored:

MAN (Smith)	"Smith is a man."
ROBOT (Rob)	"Rob is a robot."
$\forall x\{MAN(x) \rightarrow ANIMAL(x)\}$	"Man is an animal."
$\forall x\{ROBOT(x) \rightarrow MACHINE(x)\}$	"Every robot is a machine."

The following question is proved not to be a theorem:
$\forall x\ ANIMAL(x)$ "Is everything an animal?"
which would result in an answer like "No, Rob isn't."

In order to implement logical deduction on computers, special
automatic theorem-proving methods have been developed. Although these
have been the subject of intense study, and are supported by heuristic
strategies, they are extremely time-consuming even for very small-size
data bases. Their practical application, consequently, has so far been
virtually nil. In addition, as the example shows, data input must be
formalized in some form of classical logic notation which results in
cumbersome input procedures and high demand on storage space. Future
research should address itself to the question of how to integrate
some limited deductive capabilities into systems that are otherwise
based on standard retrieval techniques.

5.7 DOCUMENT-RETRIEVAL SYSTEMS: EXAMPLE [16-19]

Ge̲n̲e̲r̲a̲l̲ c̲h̲a̲r̲a̲c̲t̲e̲r̲i̲s̲t̲i̲c̲s̲

Given the definition in sec. 5.2, one would expect the interfaces of
document-retrieval systems not to differ appreciably from those of
fact-retrieval or question-answering systems. However, this is not
entirely true, as becomes apparent when we list some of the
consequences following from the different definitions in sec. 5.2.
- Fact-retrieval systems deal with immediate models of the universe
  while document-retrieval systems approach a universe in two levels,
  one being descriptive and the other modeling an internal universe of
  documents.
- This is usually reflected by a two-level interface: In a first step
  ("primary selection") documents are retrieved on the basis of some
  logical expression, in a second step ("refinement") the document
  text is inspected in order to eliminate irrelevant material.
- Other systems make only some rather general assumptions in the form
  of modes, on the structure of the universes they are prepared to
  model. Within this framework all universes are to be accepted. By
  contrast, the internal universe of document-retrieval systems is
  specific and well-defined.
- As a consequence, no types may be defined, i.e. no DDL is provided.
- Once a document has been entered into the system it undergoes no
  changes (aside from corrections), and rarely ever is it deleted
  again. Moreover, since a document is descriptive data, no evaluation
  by algorithmic means is conceivable so that the retrieval system
  need not be interfaced with a host language. Hence modern
  document-retrieval systems tend to be conversational systems for
  query purposes, while data input is strictly separated and usually
  relegated to batch processing.
- Refinement obviously makes use of the meaning of document texts. In
  order to relate primary selection to refinement, primary selection
  must make reference to the meaning as well. This is done by
  "indexing" a document: A document is assigned a number of index
  terms which correspond to semantic concepts that the document is
  thought to deal with.

These principles shall be briefly illustrated by means of Siemens
document-retrieval system GOLEM.

Classes

Elementary classes (refinement):
- Text word.
- Punctuation mark.

Elementary classes (primary selection):
- Semantic concept.
- Attribute.

Complex classes (refinement):
- Sentence: A linear sequence of text words and punctuation marks.
- Text segment: A linear sequence of sentences plus, possibly, a privacy lock.

Complex classes (primary selection):
- Simple descriptor: A semantic concept.
- Composite descriptor: One or more concepts (called bound descriptors) qualified by an attribute (called aspect), usually for disambiguation of different concepts with identical names or for establishing a context.
- Indexed descriptor: A descriptor augmented by one or more integral numbers. Each individual number identifies a set of descriptors whose collective occurrence is to be considered especially significant.
- Descriptor segment: A linear sequence of indexed or non-indexed descriptors plus, possibly, a privacy lock.
- Document description: A collection consisting of a linear sequence of up to 32 text segments, a linear sequence of up to 127 descriptor segments (the total number of segments not exceeding 128), and a privacy lock.

Example:

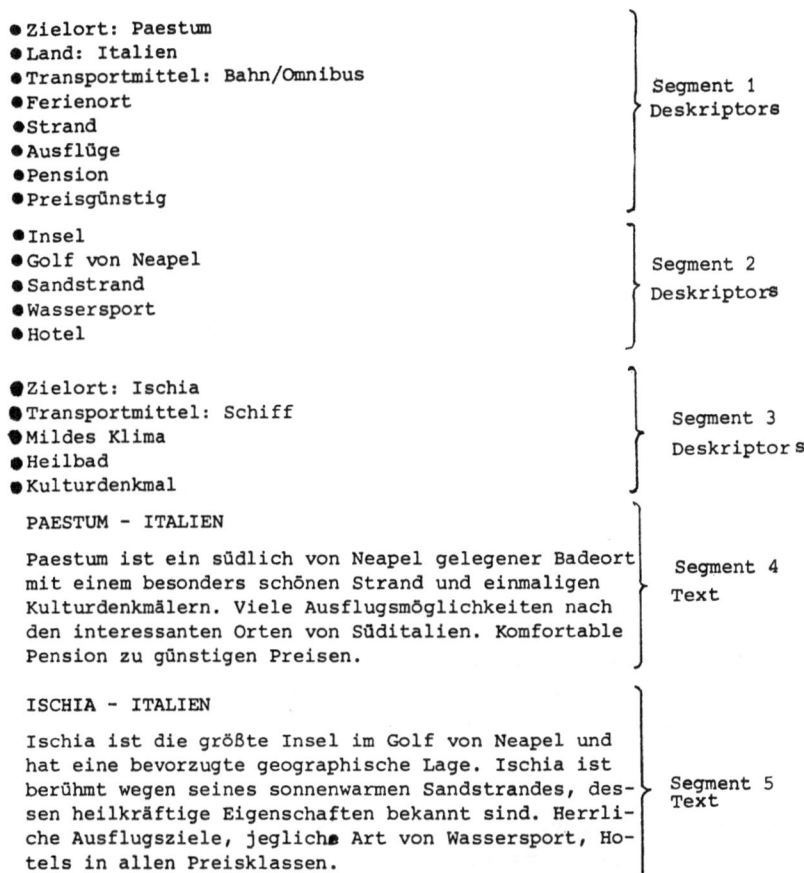

●Zielort: Paestum
●Land: Italien
●Transportmittel: Bahn/Omnibus   Segment 1
●Ferienort   Deskriptors
●Strand
●Ausflüge
●Pension
●Preisgünstig

●Insel
●Golf von Neapel
● Sandstrand   Segment 2
●Wassersport   Deskriptors
● Hotel

●Zielort: Ischia
●Transportmittel: Schiff   Segment 3
●Mildes Klima   Deskriptors
●Heilbad
●Kulturdenkmal

PAESTUM - ITALIEN

Paestum ist ein südlich von Neapel gelegener Badeort
mit einem besonders schönen Strand und einmaligen   Segment 4
Kulturdenkmälern. Viele Ausflugsmöglichkeiten nach   Text
den interessanten Orten von Süditalien. Komfortable
Pension zu günstigen Preisen.

ISCHIA - ITALIEN

Ischia ist die größte Insel im Golf von Neapel und
hat eine bevorzugte geographische Lage. Ischia ist
berühmt wegen seines sonnenwarmen Sandstrandes, des-   Segment 5
sen heilkräftige Eigenschaften bekannt sind. Herrli-   Text
che Ausflugsziele, jegliche Art von Wassersport, Ho-
tels in allen Preisklassen.

Conversational_activities

For conversational retrieval a procedure SUCHEN is invoked. The
various options and the sequence of their invocations may be inferred
from the following diagram.

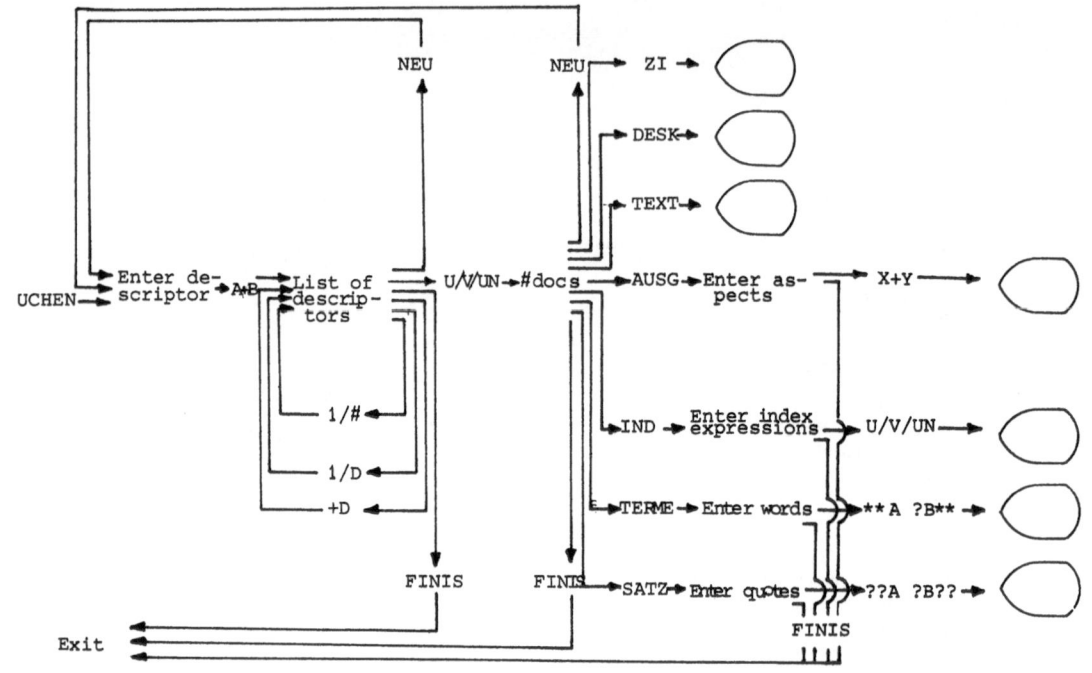

Comments:

1) Left-hand half: Primary selection.
2) +D, 1/D, 1/#: add, replace, delete descriptor.
3) U,V,UN: logical expression (see below).
4) ZI, DESK, TEXT: display of documents for visual inspection ("browsing").
5) AUSG: condensed display.
6) IND, TERME, SATZ: refinement.

Logical expressions

Descriptors are numbered serially in the order of their entry. Primary selection is on the basis of Boolean expressions on serial numbers with the binary operators U, V, UN, where U indicates that both operand descriptors must be part of the relevant document description, V that at least one must be, UN that the second operand must not be. Since each descriptor may be interpreted as a set of all documents to which it was assigned, U, V and UN may be interpreted as set intersection, set union and set difference, respectively.

Example:

```
DESKRIPTORENLISTE
 1. LAND: ITALIEN (9)
 2. ZIELORT: MERAN (1)
 3. FERIENORT (27)
 4. SCHWIMMEN (2)
 5. TENNIS (12)
ENDE DER DESKRIPTORENLISTE
NAECHSTE ANWEISUNG
 1 U3U(4V5)UN2
ANZAHL DER ZIELINFORMATIONEN:2
```

Thesaurus

Whoever tries to index a document will soon discover a few difficulties:

(i)   Not all index terms (semantic concepts) circumscribe the contents of a document with the same degree of precision.

(ii)   There are many terms that may be adequate for a given aspect of a document; some of them may be more precise than others. Chances are that many of them will be overlooked unless one checks with an appropriate dictionary.

(iii) The user may employ other, unanticipated terms than the indexer to specify a given aspect.

These difficulties may be overcome to some extent by one of the following methods.

(a) Assign exactly one "standard" index term to each semantic concept. Given a list of index terms, reduce these to the corresponding standard terms.

(b) Given a list of index terms, generate all terms related to them.

Reduction (a) is usually performed on data input of the document descriptions and, by necessity, for the query terms on retrieval time. On the other hand, generation (b) is usually left entirely to retrieval time and need only be done for the query terms. In either case, however, a list of all index terms and their relationships is required. Such a list is called a thesaurus. Typical thesaurus relations are synonyms, broader and narrower terms, used for, cause/effect, etc.

Example (from Thesaurus of Engineering and Scientific Terms)

```
DIENE RESINS     1109 1110              (descriptor, classification)
   Homopolymers and Copolymers          (scope note)
   UF  Nitrile rubber                   (used for)
       Polydiene resins
   BT  Addition resins                  (broader term)
   NT  ABS resins                       (narrower terms)
       Butyl resins
       Chloroprene resins
       Polybutadiene
       Polychloroprene
       Polyisoprene
   RT  Thermoplastic resins             (related terms)
       Thermosetting resins
```

The construction of a thesaurus is a major and expensive linguistic project. Once a thesaurus is available it may be incorporated within the data base of document-retrieval systems provided these include the necessary facilities. This is the case with GOLEM where the thesaurus is applied towards generation in the following way:

(i)   For a given descriptor, the user may ask for a display of its entry in the thesaurus. All related terms will be shown together with a serial number for each.

(ii) By choosing the corresponding serial numbers, related terms may be included in a logical expression in the same fashion as any descriptors that were originally entered.

(iii) Synonyms are automatically included.

Example:
1. DEUTSCHE BUNDESBAHN * (198)
   2. SYNONYM: DB * (10)
   3. SIEHE AUCH: BUNDESBAHN * (17)
                 EISENBAHN * (251)
   4. UNTERBEGRIFF: VERKEHRSMITTEL * (20)

Refinement

Whereas primary selection in GOLEM is exclusively based on semantic concepts, refinement makes use of the document description which, as mentioned before, may include the document text as well. As a consequence, two kinds of refinement operations may be distinguished:

IND followed by a logical expression makes use of the descriptor segments and chooses, among the documents retrieved on primary selection, those whose descriptor indices meet the condition expressed.

TERME, SATZ followed by a list of (perhaps incompletely spelled) words or sentence fragments, respectively, choose among the documents retrieved on primary selection, those whose text segments contain the words or fragments.

Automatic indexing [20,21]

Assigning index terms to documents in a dependable and meaningful way requires highly qualified personnel and is expensive both in time and money. Hence efforts have been under way for a long time to substitute them by automatic means, that is, computer-based methods for content analysis. These methods are based on the exact wording of the text. They extract nouns, adjectives, verbs and other words of significance from the text and, in general, reduce them to a standard form, e.g. nominative singular form in the case of nouns. Even this turns out to consume an inordinate amount of computer time especially for German texts because of morphemic analysis and composite nouns. Some manual intervention is still required. Furthermore, a dictionary for the control of the analysis must be constructed prior to or concurrent with the automatic analysis. For example, a special software system PASSAT that functions in the described fashion constructs descriptor segments for GOLEM documents, however excluding aspects and indices.

More ambitious forms of automatic analysis have been investigated that take into account multiple or collective occurrences of words, or assign index terms derived from but not spelled in the text. They all fail universally because of unrealistically high execution times.

Performance

Primary selection is based on terms for semantic concepts that, taken singly or collectively, approximate the contents of a document to varying degrees. Furthermore, the terminologies applied by the user or the indexer may vary considerably. Consequently, a user must not expect the system to select all documents in the data base that are relevant to his request, nor only these.

At best the quality of a document-retrieval system may be measured by how much of the relevant material is retrieved, and how relevant the material retrieved is with regard to the query. The simplest performance model of this kind may be illustrated as follows.

Suppose

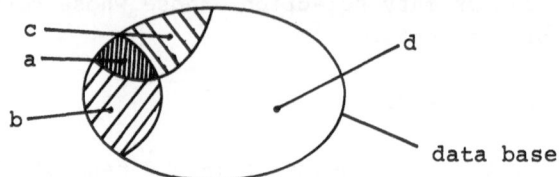

material judged by user to be

where for a given query || relevant | irrelevant

===

	retrieved ||	a	b
documents	--------||------------|-----------------		
	ignored ||	c	d

In this case the two performance criteria mentioned above may be expressed as

precision: $p = \dfrac{N_a}{N_a + N_b}$

recall: $r = \dfrac{N_a}{N_a + N_c}$

(N=number of documents)

Note the difficulty in calculating the recall since N_c or N_d remain unknown unless the entire data base is inspected. There are, however, some techniques to find an approximation to N_c.

By repeatedly calculating pairs (p,r) for different queries and plotting them in the p,r-domain one obtains a set of points whose position reflects system performance. The closer the set is to the upper right-hand corner the better are the retrieval characteristics. The points are always stretched out from upper left to lower right: For higher recall, i.e. more relevant material from the data base, more material must be selected in general. This in turn increases the amount of irrelevant material as well.

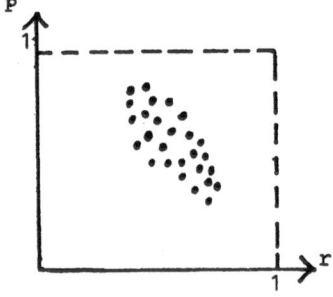

5.8 STRICT INFORMATION SYSTEMS: EXAMPLE [22]

Interfaces

In a strict information system a request may consist of up to three parts: retrieval, combination, and/or storing or update. Some queries may invoke only the first one or two, or the last one or two. Nevertheless, a few general rules concerning the interface may be observed.

(i)   All three parts should be fully integrated. A user should not be concerned with the question to which extent and at what stage in request processing any of the phases retrieval, combination or modification take place, unless he wishes so. Otherwise, from a user's point of view the system still behaved as a composite of two or more distinctive systems, each with its own idiosyncrasies.

(ii)   We should view an information system as an agency in the sense of ch.2, that is, an element with circumscribed responsibilities. Hence the functions provided by a strict information system must be dedicated to certain kinds of problems. Furthermore, one can only provide for a finite and limited number of modes, classes, and algorithms in an information system.

(iii)   Because of the combination phase, facilities for user-specific declaration of output formats are of importance.

(iv)   In many strict information systems the entire set of functions is prespecified and not subject to any addition, modification or deletion by the user. Examples are airline reservation systems, inventory control systems, hospital administration systems, accounting systems. Since these systems can be preplanned in their entirety, they may achieve a high degree of internal efficiency.

(v)   Other information systems allow for more flexibility on the part of the functions. The example discussed in this section, SPSS (Statistical Package for the Social Sciences), is of this kind. It should be noted, however, that SPSS does not rely on extensive data bases.

Modes and classes

Elementary modes:
- Data items
- (Statistical) Variables
- Labels

Elementary classes:

Among data items there are numeric values, alphanumeric values, and missing values. Variables and labels may signify classes as well, since the corresponding set of models is not further subdivided.

Complex modes:

- Labelling: A set of pairs of variables and labels, the latter being a verbal description of the variable mainly for output purposes.
- Case: A set of pairs of variables and values.
- File: A named set of cases that agree in their variables (as a consequence, classes may be defined for cases and files).
- Subfiles: A file may be subdivided into named subsets of cases. The subset sizes may differ.

Symbols

Representations are of interest to the extent to which values must be passed across the interface from the user world to the system (input) or vice versa (output). A rule for assigning symbols to values is called a format. Output formats are, for the most part, specific to a statistical function and need rarely be influenced by the user. Input formats, however, must be specified if data are fed to the system in the form of punched cards, typewriter input, and the like.

- Numeric symbols: Fw.d, where w indicates the total number of characters including sign and decimal point, and d is the number of digits to the right of the decimal point.

Example: Format	symbol	value	remarks
F3.0	100	(100)	-
F3.1	100	(10.0)	dec.point need not appear
F3.1	.1	(0.1)	-

  If n symbols with identical format are to follow each other, the resulting format is written as nFw.d.
- Alphanumeric symbols: Aw, where w is the total number of characters.
- Variable names: Up to 8 characters of which the first one must be alphabetic.
- Missing values: Specified numeric symbols.
- Labels: An arbitrary string.

Input

If data are to be provided by cards the following must be specified:
(i) Case class: A list of variable names (VARIABLE LIST); the item classes are taken from the input format (see (iii)).
(ii) Case instances: A list of values. Pairs of variables and values

are constructed by combining the i´th elements of both lists (i=1,...,list size) (READ INPUT DATA).
(iii) Symbols: A list of formats. The i´th format corresponds to the value of the i´th variable name (INPUT FORMAT).
(iv) Labelling: A list of pairs of variable names and variable labels (VAR LABELS).
(v) Number of cases (N OF CASES).

Example:
```
VARIABLE LIST      AGE, SEX, RACE, INCOME
INPUT MEDIUM       CARD
N OF CASES         5
INPUT FORMAT       FIXED (F2.0, 2F1.0, F7.0)
VAR LABELS         AGE, AGE OF THE RESPONDENT / SEX, SEX OF THE
                   RESPONDENT / INCOME, YEARLY FAMILY INCOME IN
                   DOLLARS
```

```
READ INPUT DATA
3011   9000      (age=30, sex=1, race=1, income=9000)
3113   7500
4022   8300
2713   12500
5411   13250
```

Mode activities

There is a considerable number of operators that are exclusively defined on files.
SAVE FILE: Cases, subfiles, and all the file-defining information (e.g. variable lists, variable labels, case numbers) are retained in binary form at the conclusion of processing.
FILE NAME: Assign a name to a file.
GET FILE: Access the specified file.
Modify a file: By accessing a file through GET FILE, supplying a number of definition cards, and SAVing the file again, the user may add to or change any of the following: File name and label, variable labels, subfile structure, missing value codes.
DELETE VARS: Delete selected variables from a file.
KEEP VARS: Retain selected variables in a file.
ADD VARS: Add variables to a file.
MERGE FILES: Merge all or a subset of the variables from two to five existing files.
ADD CASES: Add new cases to an existing file.
ADD SUBFILES: Add entire new subfiles to the end of a file.
DELETE SUBFILES: Delete all cases comprising one or more of the subfiles in an existing file.

delete cases: Cases may be specified by means of a SELECT IF operation (see below). The deleted cases are those ones which have not been selected.

REORDER VARS: Reorder the sequence of variables in a file.

SORT CASES: Modify the sequence of the cases in a file.

SUBFILE LIST: Define a subfile structure for a file which previously had no subfile structure or define a new subfile structure to replace the existing subfiles, by specifying a (new) subdivision.

RECODE: Replace one, some, or all values of the variables in a file.

COMPUTE: Unconditional variable transformation.

IF: Conditional variable transformation.

All modifications are also possible on a temporary basis, i.e., during a particular run.

```
Example:
RUN NAME        DEMONSTRATION
FILE NAME       STUDYA
VARIABLE LIST   AGE, SEX, RACE, INCOME
N OF CASES      5
INPUT FORMAT    FIXED (F2.0, 2F1.0, F7.0)
VAR LABELS      (see previous example)....
READ INPUT DATA (see previous example)....
SAVE FILE
FINISH
RUN NAME        MODIFICATION
GET FILE        STUDYA
ADD VARIABLES   NEWCASNO, INCOME2, LOCVOTE
INPUT MEDIUM    TAPE
INPUT FORMAT    FIXED (F3.0, 2F1.0)
FILE NAME       STUDYA, SECOND VERSION OF STUDYA
VAR LABELS      INCOME2, SUPPLEMENTAL INCOME/LOCVOTE, VOTE IN
                LAST LOCAL ELECTION
. . . . . . . . . . .(statistical analysis)      ①
READ INPUT DATA
DELETE VARS     NEWCASNO
SAVE FILE
FINISH
```

Model selectors

- Files: By name (see example above).
- Subfiles: By name, or all of them in order (ALL).
- Random sample of cases: SAMPLE.
- Cases by specific reference, logical or mathematical criteria: SELECT IF.
- Variables: By name.

Functions

The calculations to be performed are controlled by task definition cards of which there are the following.
- Procedure cards: Each statistical procedure has its own card:

CONDESCRIPTIVE	PARTIAL CORR
FREQUENCIES	REGRESSION
AGGREGATE	ANOVA
CROSSTABS	ONEWAY
BREAKDOWN	DISCRIMINANT
T-TEST	FACTOR
PEARSON CORR	CANCORR
NONPAR CORR	GUTTMAN SCALE
SCATTERGRAM	

The procedure name is followed by the variables to be entered into the calculations as well as further parameters needed.

- OPTIONS card: It supplies to the system further information to be used for the control of a calculation activated by a procedure card, or of its output.

- STATISTICS card: It enables the user to select among a number of available statistics (e.g. mean, standard deviation) to accompany the calculations and to be reported on the output.

Example: In the example above, the following cards may be inserted at ① :

```
FREQUENCIES    GENERAL = CHECKVAR, INCOME2, LOCVOTE
STATISTICS     ALL
```

6 Storage and retrieval techniques

6.1 INTRODUCTORY REMARKS

The emphasis in this paper is on user interfaces and the concepts that underlie these. This approach appears justified in view of the intended audience which we assume to be more or less sophisticated users of information systems but rarely ever designers or implementers of such systems. Still, the suitability of an information system is decided not entirely on the merits of its functional characteristics and interfaces but also on the quality of its implementation which includes, among others, the transparency and modularity of the design, the elegance of the technical solutions, the reliability of the software and hardware. This is hardly the place to present a comprehensive survey of all techniques that have proven useful in connection with information systems, especially since the number of these techniques is legion. Rather, this chapter shall provide a few typical and important examples and thus give a feeling for the issues observed on implementation.

The notion of implementation includes what was called "realization" in sec. 3.7, that is, the mapping from one modeling system to a second one. More than realization is involved though, for example multi-user operation, data transmission, peripheral input/output, interfacing with the operating system, data security. For this discussion, however, realization will be the main theme.

6.2 BLOCKS, RECORDS, AND FILES [23,24]

Once the data is in main storage, manipulating it is a fairly simple task from a computer scientist's point of view. By necessity, however, whatever is in main storage is only a miniscule part of a data base. Hence one of the foremost realization problems is organizing and storing a data base on peripheral storage, selecting portions of it, and transmitting it between peripheral and main storage.

In order to adjust a data base to these requirements, a data base is physically packaged into blocks which are units of transmission, and often correspond to storage units determined by the physical characteristics of a storage device. Usually two kinds of blocks are distinguished:

- Fixed-length blocks whose sizes do not differ within the space occupied by a data or a file, and whose individual sizes, consequently, remain unchanged over time. These blocks make for easy selection and management.
- Variable-length blocks whose size varies within the space of a data base or file and, in some systems, is also permitted to vary in time. These blocks make for an easier mapping between modeling systems. Variable-length blocks are usually prefaced by a length count field.

Blocks must be distinguished from records. The latter is one of the most widely used but nevertheless vaguely defined terms. The following definition is adequate but hardly precise: A record is a model object (in some modeling system) that (approximately) maps into a block. Quite naturally, there are also two kinds of records:
- Fixed-length records whose representations in terms of storage cells do not vary in time, and do not differ within the composite object of which they are components.
- Variable-length records for which the opposite is true.

Fixed-length records usually map into fixed-length blocks while variable-length records may be realized both by fixed-length or variable-length blocks. Since block sizes cannot exclusively be made to depend on record lengths but are to meet certain conditions imposed by the hardware and the operating system, it is quite usual to assemble several records into one block (in this case the number of records in a block is called the blocking factor). Under rare circumstances a record may also occupy more than one block.

Example:
(a) Fixed-length record and block, blocking factor=1

| Record | P |

(P = parity bits)

(b) Fixed-length block (Blocking factor = 3)
    Fixed-length records:

| record 1 | record 2 | record 3 | P |

Variable-length records:

$(RL_i$ = length of record i)   unused space

(c) Variable-length block and record (blocking factor = 1)

BL	RL	record	P

(BL = block length)

(d) Variable-length block and records (blocking factor = 3)

BL	RL_1	record 1	RL_2	record 2	RL_3	record 3	P

A file is a complex mode whose components are records (as viewed from
one modeling system) or blocks (as viewed from a more device-oriented
modeling system). Various composition rules are in use resulting in
several distinct file organizations that are discussed in sec. 6.6.

6.3 FILE COMPRESSION

With evergrowing data base sizes, and with large capacity stores with
simple and fast access mechanisms still several years away one is
often interested in reducing the storage requirements for a given
information structure even though this may entail higher processor
time.

In the area of model data bases a number of techniques for the
reduction of storage requirements have long been known: keeping
attributes only with the schemas but not with their instances,
eliminating empty fields (i.e. attributes for which no data items have
been specified), encoding attributes or frequently used words or
strings, storing arithmetic values in binary coded form, reducing
8-bit codes to 6-bit codes, employing variable-length blocks. These
may be used either alone or in certain combinations.

In the case of textual data bases, attention has been paid to the use
of codes which are specially designed for the purpose of reducing
storage. Systems of this kind have three objectives:
(i)   analyze the data in order to decide on a coding which reduces
       the storage requirements,
(ii)   compress the data using the codes produced in (i),
(iii) recover the data in its original form by decoding or expanding
       the compressed representation of it.

Encoding involves the elimination of redundancy from the data.
Basically, data contains redundancy if some symbols or groups of
symbols in it occur more frequently than would be the case if all the
symbols were randomly generated. Therefore one may devise automatic

methods that scan the file to be compressed noting which characters and sequences of characters occur most frequently, and then assign short codes to characters or groups which occur frequently, and longer ones to the others.

Example: What is needed is a set of symbols that are to be the units to which a code will be applied. The set contains the basic alphabet of the data and is augmented by a set of cords (where a cord is a string of two or more characters) that are chosen because of the frequencies with which they occur in the data. In order to determine the cords one must program an analyzer (a nontrivial algorithm!) which automatically scans a representative sample of the entire textual material. The analyzer may also be given the task to assign binary codes to the elements of the augmented alphabet, e.g. variable-length minimum redundancy codes. For the basic alphabet and German text one possibility would be

␣	000	d	1010	o	11100	k	1111110
e	001	t	10110	m	111010	p	11111110
n	010	u	10111	b	111011	j	111111110
s	0110	h	11000	w	111100	x	1111111110
i	0111	l	11001	z	111101	q	11111111110
r	1000	c	11010	v	1111100	y	11111111111
a	1001	g	11011	f	1111101		

Using this technique, storage savings of more than 50% have been claimed for textual material.

6.4 LINEAR SEARCH, INDEXES AND B-TREES [24-26]

Manufacturers usually provide file management systems as part of their system software. File management systems are characterized to the programmer by interfaces (albeit complicated ones). Consequently, we may repeat the approach of ch. 3 to the description of interfaces, and we shall indeed do so in sec. 6.6. At any rate, files, records and even blocks may then be considered conceptual entities, i.e. modes.

The kind of model selector most widely used for blocks or records in a file is keys. Almost universally, the first elementary object in a record or block serves as the key so that no attribute is needed. On the other hand, the representation selectors universally are addresses, e.g. in case of a magnetic disk they are of the form cylinder no./rel. track no./rel. block no. Assuming that each model object is represented exactly once, a one-to-one mapping σ from keys to addresses is required. While σ could be implied by inspecting each record for the existence of a given key, σ is usually maintained in explicit form as a set of pairs (key, address). Because of additions and deletions the corresponding mapping varies with time:

$\sigma (t) : N(t) \rightarrow A$

where N(t) is the set of keys which changes with time, and A the set of addresses. $\sigma(t)$ must be realized as a set of pairs $\sigma(t) = \{(n,a)\}_t$.

In order to choose one of the methods for organizing σ, these must be compared with respect to the basic operations

(a) given n, find (at a particular time t) the pair $(n,a) \in \sigma$, evaluate σ at n;

(b) insert a new pair into σ if it is not yet there;

(c) delete a pair from σ.

Linear search

The simplest arrangement of σ is that of a linearly ordered table. Unless $|\sigma|$ is small, however, choosing just any arbitrary order will result in an excessive number of steps to determine $\sigma(n)$. There are several techniques to reduce the number of steps; all of these are based on a lexikographic ordering with respect to the keys. Two of the simpler techniques are:

(i) Multiway search.

Suppose $|\sigma|=p$, divide the table into q segments of length p/q. Given n, check the last key k in segment 1. For n=k we are finished. For n<k inspect the entries of segment 1 in order until the correct entry is found. For n>k advance to segment 2 and repeat the procedure, etc. It can be shown that the number of steps is a minimum for $q=\sqrt{p}$, i.e. p should be a square number. The multiway search may be illustrated by the following diagram.

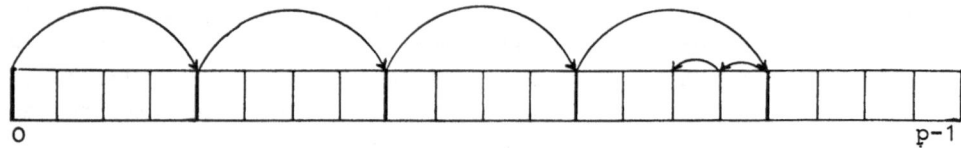

0   p-1

(ii) Binary search.

Start with the entry in the middle of the table (key k). For n=k we are already finished. For n<k inspect the entry in the middle of the segment to the left of k, for n>k the entry in the middle to the right. In either case repeat the procedure, etc. It can be shown that the number of steps is approximately equal to $ld|\sigma|$. However, $|\sigma|=2^{m-1}$, $m \in \mathbb{N}$ is required. Binary search may be illustrated by the following diagram (m=4).

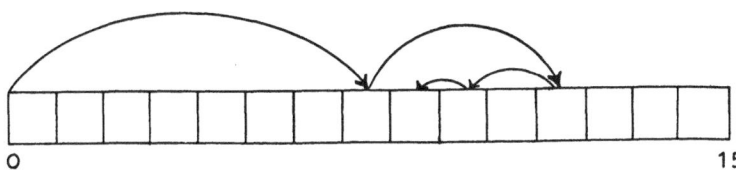

One may now ask how well linear search techniques do with respect to the criteria listed above.
a) Search times are good. Even in case the conditions on $|\sigma|$ in (i) or (ii) cannot be met, techniques with only slightly longer search times are available. Difficulties arise, however, as soon as σ becomes too large to fit into main memory.
b) Each individual insertion requires a large amount of effort for maintaining the order. Therefore, linear search is appropriate only if all records are available from the very beginning, or in case a file need be updated only periodically (say, once a day or a week). In either case, the table must undergo a lengthy process of ordering ("sorting") or reordering ("merging").
c) Deletion is nontrivial unless the corresponding entry is left in the table and simply marked as unused. With a large number of unused entries, however, the table size, and hence search time, grows beyond what is needed.

Indexes

Once σ must be kept on peripheral storage it must be mapped onto a set of blocks. If we keep with a linearly ordered table the multiway search may be extended in the following way.
- Segments are chosen such that each segment is exactly covered by one block.
- Since progressing from one segment to the next becomes too much time-consuming, a new linearly ordered table $\sigma'=(n',a')_t$ is constructed such that the n' correspond to the keys of the last entry in each block (thus effectively becoming the keys of the blocks) and the a' are the addresses of the blocks.

The previous example for multiway search now takes on the form

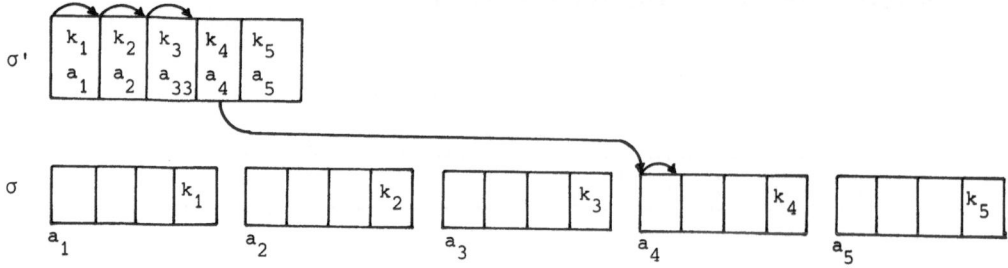

For very large |σ| even σ´ may not fit into available main memory. Thus the construction may be extended to additional levels σ", σ'''. For example, in connection with disk files one may observe indexes for tracks (σ), for the tracks in a cylinder (σ´), for the cylinders occupied by a file (σ") and, if σ" exceeds a block, a master index (σ''') that permanently resides in main storage. On evaluating σ (n) exactly one block per level is linearly searched. This may be done sequentially, but multiway or binary search is perfectly possible within a block.

Since indexes do not differ fundamentally from linear search techniques, they should meet the criteria similarly well or bad:
a) Search times are a little bit below the optimum since storage device characteristics preclude a complete control over segment sizes. Of course, large time delays occur on moving from one level to the next because of the input/output operations that take place. However, these are unavoidable on large |σ| no matter what the technique chosen is.
b) c) Insertion and deletion are as difficult as before, or even worse because several levels may be affected.

B-trees

It has been known for a long time that all three, retrieval, insertion and deletion, may be solved efficiently by balanced trees. These are tree-like arrangements of keys in which for each node in the tree all of its subtrees are of identical size. It turns out, however, that the balancing requirement must be relaxed somewhat: The better a tree is balanced the fewer the average number of retrieval steps but the higher the effort to maintain the balancing criteria under insertion and deletion. Various forms of trees have been suggested for striking a compromise between these two.

All these trees fail as soon as σ must be maintained on peripheral
storage since there is no natural way for mapping them into blocks,
the one exception being B-trees. These trees are perfectly balanced
multiway trees. Each non-leaf (except for the root) has g successors
with m≤g≤2k+1, the root itself can have 2≤g≤2m+1 (m≥2). All nodes
except for the leaves are blocks that contain, in alternation, a
sequence of (g-1) pairs (n,a) and g pointers to blocks except for the
leaves where the pointers are missing. This is illustrated in the
following example with numerical keys (m=2):

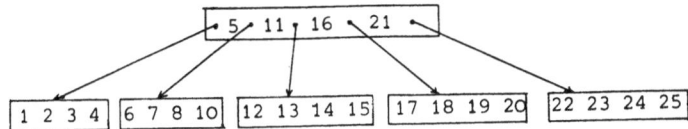

a) Retrieval.
   Inspect the root node in order (e.g. sequentially, by multiway or
   binary search, etc.). If the desired key n is found stop. Otherwise
   take up pointer between successive keys k_1 and k_2 with $k_1<n<k_2$,
   proceed to corresponding node and repeat procedure, etc.
b) Insertion.
   Given a key n, proceed as in a). If n is found we are finished.
   Otherwise a leaf has been reached which is the node to receive the
   new pair (n,a). If the node is not yet filled, insert the pair into
   the node at the appropriate place. If the node is already filled
   proceed as follows:
   - Suppose the node were inserted in the appropriate place
     (resulting in 2m+1 pairs).
   - Generate a new node which is to receive the last m pairs, while
     the first m pairs are left to the old node. (Notice that both
     nodes are now fifty percent filled.)
   - Attempt to insert the (m+1)st pair together with the pointers to
     the two nodes into the predecessor node, and repeat the
     procedure.
c) Deletion.
   Similar to b), except that contraction may take place.

For example, in adding ´9´ the tree shown above is transformed into
the following tree.

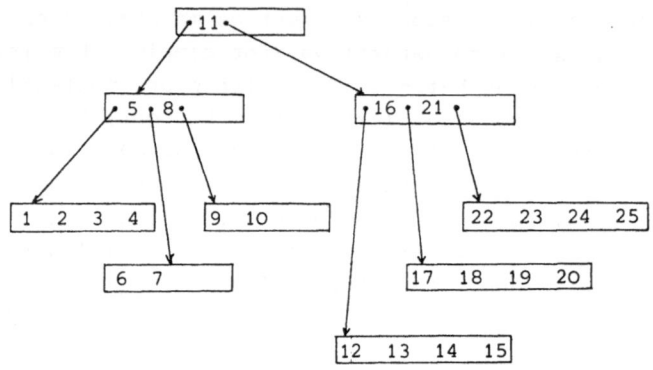

6.5 ADDRESS CALCULATION [26]

The selection of an object is a frequent process that takes place
whenever an operation is to be performed. Consequently, it pays to
minimize the time for evaluating σ. The techniques from sec. 6.4 are
not optimal in this regard: The best method available is the binary
search with a time delay of approximately $ld|\sigma|$, and times deteriorate
drastically as soon as one must resort to peripheral storage. Further
improvement is possible only if inspection methods are replaced by
address calculation.

Strict_address_calculation

These are one-to-one mappings between selectors and addresses. In
order to devise methods of this kind two preconditions must be met:
(i)   The set of selectors must be computable. Typically in this case,
      the set of selectors is the set of natural numbers up to some
      limit, hence implying a linear ordering of the model objects.
(ii) The set of addresses must be computable. Typically, the set of
      addresses is an interval in the set of natural numbers, perhaps
      multiplied by a fixed number. This implies
      a) sequential allocation of storage units,
      b) representation objects of identical size.

Example: Suppose a file that occupies a certain number of contiguous cylinders on disk storage. In case of fixed-length blocks and fixed-length records (arbitrary blocking factor) one may immediately calculate an address of the form (cylinder no./rel. track no./rel. block no./rel. address in block) for a given record no.

Hash techniques

In the case of arbitrary keys as model selectors, condition (i) cannot be met. Regardless of the particular algorithm applied there will always be situations in which two or more different keys map into the same address ("collision"). Under these circumstances one may employ a method that combines linear tables and address calculation in the following manner.

Let $[1:H]$ be the interval of natural numbers from 1 to H, N_p the set of potential keys such that $N(t) \subseteq N_p$, then a hashing function h maps N_p into the relative addresses $[1:H]$ of a hashing table. n, $n' \in N(t)$ are said to collide if $h(n)=h(n')$. For each $w \in [1:H]$ we define the collision class
$$K(w) = \{(n,a) \mid (n,a) \in \sigma(t) \wedge h(n) = w\}$$

Ideally $K(w) \leqslant 1$, but for large $|N_p|$ or $|N(t)|$ this is not always possible. Loosely speaking a hashing technique then works as follows.
(i)   Create a table whose size exceeds the expected maximum of $|N(t)|$. The table will receive σ. Choose a suitable hashing function h (of which there exist a number).
(ii) For a given n, apply $h(n)$.
(iii) - To find (n,a), search through $K(h(n))$.
      - To insert (n,a) into σ, insert (n,a) into the class $K(h(n))$.
      - To delete (n,a) from σ, delete (n,a) from $K(h(n))$.

Consequently, besides choosing h there is also the problem of organizing the collision classes. The methods fall into two categories.
a) Collision classes not explicitly specified.
   Suppose key k is given, $w=h(k)$. Inspect $(n,a)_w$. If $k \neq n$, $w:=w+ \Delta w$, repeat the inspection.
   - Linear probing: Δw constant.
   - Random probing: Δw a random number.
   - Quadratic probing: Δw a function of i where i is the number of entries inspected so far.
   On probing, entries may be inspected that are not part of a collision class. This may even be true for the starting point $(n,a)_{h(k)}$. Suppose two keys n and n' collide, the first one is

placed at w=h(n) and the second one at w´. Suppose a third key n"
is to be inserted such that w´=h(n"). Then a place w"=w´ must be
found for n" although there was as yet no collision for n".

b) Collision classes explicitly specified.

This implies $(n,a)_w$ -> $(n,a) \in K(w)$.

- Chaining: Starting with $(n,a)_w$ a linked list is constructed into
  which all elements of K(w) are collected. At most the elements of
  a list must be inspected.
- Bucketing: Up to p pairs $(n,a) \in K(w)$ may occupy a table entry w.
  In case $|K(w)|>p$, overflow techniques are available. At most the
  elements in the entry must be inspected.

The various methods differ in the amount of effort required for
retrieval, insertion and deletion.

6.6 FILE ORGANIZATION

File management systems are an integral part of most system software.
Most computerized information systems make use of the services
provided by file management systems (e.g., DBTG areas are realized as
files). As a consequence, file management systems offer user
interfaces in the same sense that information systems offer user
interfaces, the only difference being that the users of the former are
supposed to be programmers. One might expect that the methods of ch.3
for describing interfaces may as well apply to file management system
interfaces. Unfortunately this is not entirely true, since these
interfaces mix logical aspects (e.g., records), aspects of physical
representation (e.g., blocks, selector mappings), and operating
considerations (e.g., buffering). Some examples of mode types are
given below. In all cases the record is the only elementary mode.

Sequential organization

A sequential file is a linearly ordered set with the activities:
- write: Insert a new record at the end. This activity defines the
          order as being based on arrival sequence.
- read: Access the current record and advance the current position
          by 1.
- replace:Access the current record, modify its value and write it out
          again, then advance current position by 1.
- start: set the current position to 1.

Key-sequential organization

A key-sequential file is a linearly ordered set with the activities:
- write: Insert a new record with key n such that key(predecessor)
              <n<key(successor)   (special cases: empty and singular
              file). This activity defines the order as being
              lexikographic on keys.
- reads: Access the current record and advance the current position
              by 1.
- readk: Access the record with a given key. It follows that
              records of key-sequential files may be read sequentially
              or selectively.
- replaces: Access the current record, modify its value and write it
              out again, then advance current position by 1.
- replacek: Access the record with given key, modify its value and
              write it out again.
- start: Set the current position to 1 or to the sequence number of
              a record with a specified key.

In place of "key-sequential" the term "index-sequential" is widely
used because indexes predominate as selector mappings.

Random organization

A random file is an unordered set of records with the activities:
- write: Add a new record to the set.
- read: Access the record with a given key.
- replace: Access the record with a given key, modify its value and
              write it out again.
The name is derived from the realization of the selector mappings by
means of hash techniques. These do not imply any specific ordering.

Direct organization

A direct file is an ordered set of records. Activities are:
- writer: Insert a new record at the end.
- reserve: Insert an empty record at the end.
- writeg: Add a value to the empty record at a specified position.
              (Note that the user may retain complete control over the
              order.)
- reads: Access the current record and advance the current position
              by 1.
- readp: Access a record at a specified position. It follows that
              records in a direct file may be read sequentially or
              selectively.

- replaces: Access the current record, modify its value and write it
out again, then advance current position by 1.
- replacep: Access the record at a specified position, modify its
value and write it out again.
- start: Set the current position to a specified position.

6.7 INVERTED FILE ORGANIZATION

The selector mappings of secs 6.4, 6.5 are based on model names or
keys as model selectors. The examples of secs 4.3/5.4 (relational
model) and 5.7 (document retrieval) are indicative of selections that
are based not on a single unique model component but on a logical
combination of model components. Since these are usually not unique, a
mapping $\tau(t):N(t) \rightarrow \mathcal{P}(A)$ takes the place of σ. $\tau(t)$ must be realized
as a set of pairs $\tau(t)=\{(n,\{a_1,\ldots, a_n\})\}_t$. τ is called an inverted
file. In systems such as the relational model where the $n \in N(t)$ are
qualified by attribute, or as GOLEM where they are qualified by
aspect, a separate inverted file is defined for each individual
attribute or aspect.

The realization is divided into two levels:
(i) Implement the sets $\{a_i\}_t$. Problems arise mainly because of the
set sizes that vary with entry and time and for which no upper
bound can be given. Numerous techniques have been devised,
ranging from variable-size blocks of address lists to condensed
bit vectors. Further difficulties are due to the sorted order in
which addresses are to be kept.
(ii) Define a new mapping
$\sigma(t)=\{(n,\alpha)|\alpha$ is address of $\{a_i\} \wedge (n,\{a_i\}) \in \tau(t)\}$.
In other words, a new table of substitutes for the entries of
$\tau(t)$ is constructed. It may be implemented by any of the methods
discussed in 6.4 or 6.5.

Selection in the relational model and in document retrieval is based
on logical expressions. These are implemented by the standard set
operations defined on the $\{a_i\}$ whereby union $(\cup)$ corresponds to
disjunction $(\vee)$, intersection $(\cap)$ to conjunction $(\wedge)$ and difference
$(-)$ to negation $(\neg)$. The algorithms for the set operators are
simplified if the $\{a_i\}$ are kept in sorted order, as illustrated by the
following flow diagram.

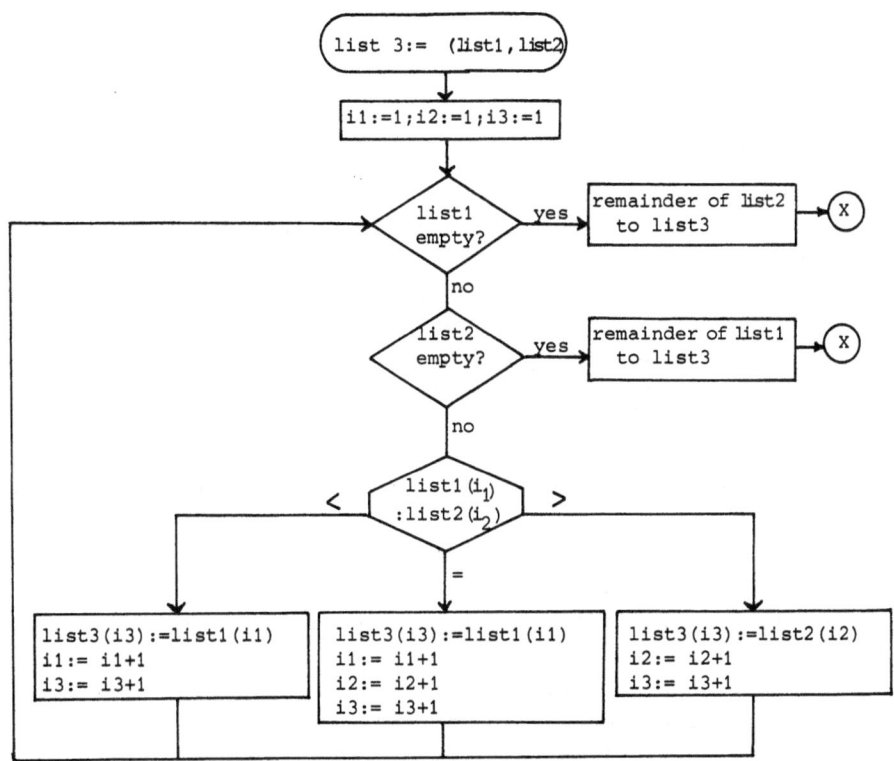

7 Data input and reliability

7.1 DATA INPUT [27,28]

The emphasis placed so far on the description of interfaces and the evaluation of implementation techniques seems to suggest that adequate planning of these will determine the success or failure of an information system. One easily overlooks the fact that even the best interfaces and techniques are useless unless they are related to an appropriate data base. Only too late many users detect that most of their financial and personnel resources and much of their time must be devoted not to system hardware and software but to data base construction. Two phases should be distinguished.

(i) Construction of an initial data base to exceed the critical mass needed for the system to be useful. This implies a high volume of input data in as short a time as possible.

(ii) Maintenance of an existing data base by updating it to the extent necessary to reflect the current status of the universe. Two extremes are conceivable.

  a) High degree of authenticity: Little time delay between observing a change in the universe and updating the model.

  b) Limited degree of authenticity: Some time delay (e.g. a day, a week, a month) between change in the universe and update.

Situations (i) and (iib) are similar in that one may collect a certain volume of information and then input it as a single batch. Situation (iia), however, requires real-time technical solutions. We shall briefly examine how the systems discussed in chs. 4 and 5 will handle the situations.

- IMS, DBTG
  Both systems are characterized by
  a) store and update activities,
  b) host languages,
  c) records as the subjects of the activities.
  These systems are suitable under both situations. Real-time update is possible by programming, in a host language, suitable procedures that may even be used interactively. Batch store or update is reasonably efficient since records represent a good-sized volume of data.
- Relational model, KAIFAS.
  The relational model provides for store and update activities and a host language as well. However, the subjects of activities are

Tuples which, by comparison, represent a very small volume of data. Consequently, the relational model interface is suitable for real-time situations only. For batch situations means must be developed to bypass the interface. Very little has been reported on this subject in the literature.

For KAIFAS, sec. 4.4 does not specify any store and update operators at all. These are known to exist but are on the level of single elements or pairs. Thus the remarks for the relational model apply here as well.

- Document retrieval.

Modern document retrieval systems are generally characterized by conversational access (no host language) and no store/update activities as part of the interface. Hence no real-time data input is possible (turning even a minor correction of erroneous text into a major headache), and batch input must be processed by means of a completely separate interface. Unfortunately, hardly anybody seems to pay much attention to a systematization of batch input interfaces. These usually are highly complex, based on scores of intermediate tapes, and offer little transparency so that their application tends to be error-prone.

Problems of data input arise not only on the technical level discussed so far. In fact, by the time data reach this level much of the work has already been done. Below is a list of earlier steps.

- Data acquisition.

An organizational framework and guidelines must be established which information must be collected and reported to the information system and how this is to be done. The information to be collected is usually called the "raw data".

- Translation of a particular world view into the structure (modes, classes) prescribed by the system interface.

For fact-retrieval, question-answering and strict information systems one may devise a separate printed form sheet for each class. These forms are divided into fields and subfields carrying printed fieldnames or explanations. The representations of the raw data are filled into the fields.

In document-retrieval systems there are two kinds of raw data: The document itself, and the document description. The latter may in part be derived from the document itself (bibliographic information), the remainder must be added manually (e.g., index terms). Both kinds of data must again be structured according to the system interface. This is usually done by manually inserting special control characters into the document and its description. For example, in preparing documents for GOLEM each aspect, descriptor, index, text segment, descriptor segment and sentence must be marked as such.

- Transcription of the raw data into machine readable form.

  Some raw data, e.g. in traffic control, clinical laboratories, intensive care stations, arise in a form that may immediately be fed into a computer. Usually, however, raw data must be collected manually or is available in printed form only. The advantage in collecting raw data in a form suitable for human inspection is ease of human control. On the other hand, this is definitely not the form suitable for computer storage. Two major kinds of transcription may be distinguished.

  a) Combination of translation and transcription within a single step.

  Examples: Punched cards with forms printed on them, mark sense forms, typewriters that punch paper tapes or write magnetic tapes simultaneously with the typewritten pages.

  b) Separate transcription.

  Raw data that is presented in printed or handwritten form is punched into paper tape, punch cards or written onto magnetic tape. In particular, raw data for document-retrieval systems cannot immediately be read in its printed form but must be retyped in special size and font (OCR-A, OCR-B). This includes the control characters mentioned above. Further control characters may be needed, e.g., to mark an umlaut as such or to distinguish between small and capital letters.

For all these steps a variety of technical equipment with widely varying price tags are available. At the same time, data input is as much an organizational problem as it is a technical one. Each combination of organizational and technical means draws on certain resources, hence it should be carefully evaluated with regard to volume, maximum permissible time delays, error rates, and quality control. In particular, under certain conditions a decentralized organization may offer advantages while under others transcription and perhaps even translation should be done in a central department.

7.2 RELIABILITY [29]

Two important topics are protection of the existence of a data base, and resolution of conflicts due to simultaneous access of a data base by several users.

a) Protection.

A data base must be protected against the effects of system failure that may leave a data base in an undefined and inconsistent state, against physical damage to the storage media, or against physical destruction. Following is a list of common recovery procedures.

- Rollback and recovery
  At certain points in time, called checkpoints, a copy of the data base is made on magnetic tape. During an intercheckpoint interval a chronological record, called the audit trail, is kept of all transactions which modify the data base. A data base is reproduced in two steps:
  (i)   Copy the data recorded at the most recent checkpoint.
  (ii) Update the data base (i) by reprocessing the audit trail in chronological order.
- Simple rollback.
  Only the checkpoints are generated. Protocolling the changes is left to the users.
- Duplicate data bases.
  The data base is continually maintained in duplicate form (master and backup). In cases of emergency the system switches from one data base to the other, and as soon as possible reconstructs the erroneous data base from the intact one.

b) Resolution of conflicts.

When a process updates a data base concurrently with another update process, the integrity of the data base is threatened. Similarly, the integrity of a reading process is threatened by a concurrent update process. A lockout mechanism is introduced. Lockout is a process of mutual exclusion; it assigns a part of the data base exclusively to at most one update process at any one time. For a reading process, however, a weaker form of lockout is preferable: Concurrent processes are permitted to look at the corresponding part of the data base but not to change it. The question, of course, arises what is meant by "part of the data base". Many conventional systems define lockout on the file level. However, this may be too much in case a few records or even just a few items are needed at a time, so that a number of processes are locked out unnecessarily or at least unnecessarily long. Unfortunately, lockout on coarse data base units is technically much simpler to handle than lockout on the lowest levels of resolution.

Lockout may lead to deadlocks, that is, two or more processes block each other by each waiting for the other to release certain resources.

Therefore, mechanisms for detecting or preventing deadlocks must be included in an information system. The strategy universally applied in information systems is to preclaim exclusive control of all needed resources before using any of them. For example, in DBTG there is exactly one OPEN statement per user process, in which all areas to be accessed must be listed simultaneously. Unfortunately, a priori knowledge of resources is usually possible only on a coarse level of resolution.

References

[1] K.Lautenbach, Exakte Bedingungen der Lebendigkeit fuer eine Klasse von Petri-Netzen, Bericht der GMD no.82, 1973 (in German)

[2] K.Lautenbach, H.A.Schmid, Use of Petri-nets for proving correctness of concurrent process systems, Information Processing 74, North-Holland Publ.Co 1974, 187-191

[3] Ch.Ramchandani, Analysis of Asynchronous Concurrent Systems by Petri Nets, Rep. MAC TR-120, Massachusetts Inst.of Techn., 1974

[4] H.C.Mayr, P.C.Lockemann, Entscheidungs- und Aktionsnetze, Bericht d. Fak. f. Informatik 10/75, U.Karlsruhe 1975 (in German)

[5] P.C.Lockemann, H.Visel, Interfaces for Data Base Management Systems: The Concepts Behind Them, to be submitted

[6] IBM: Information Management System/360, Version 2, Application Description Manual

[7] CODASYL Data Base Task Group Report, April 1971, available from: IFIP Data Processing Group

[8] CODASYL DDL Journal of Development, June 1973, available from: IFIP Data Processing Group

[9] E.F.Codd, A Relational Model of Data for Large Shared Data Banks, Comm.ACM 13(1970), no.6, 377-387

[10] E.F.Codd, A Data Sublanguage Founded on the Relational Calculus, IBM Research Report No.RJ 893, July 1971, also in: ACM Workshop on Data Description, Access and Control, Nov 1971, 35-68

[11] H.Wedekind, Datenbanksysteme I, Reihe Informatik vol 16, B.I.-Wissenschaftsverlag 1974 (in German)

[12] R.Rustin (ed), Data Base Systems, Courant Computer Science Symp., Prentice-Hall, Inc. 1972

[13] K.-D.Kraegeloh, P.C.Lockemann, Hierarchies of Data Base Languages: An Example, Information Systems (in print)

[14] R.F.Simmons, Natural Language Question-Answering Systems: 1969, Comm.ACM 13(1970), no.1, 15-30

[15] N.J.Nilsson, Problem-Solving Methods in Artificial Intelligence, McGraw-Hill 1971

[16] I.Steinacker, Dokumentationssysteme — Dialogfunktionen und Entwurf, Walter de Gruyter 1975 (in German)

[17] SIEMENS: GOLEM II: A General Purpose System for the Documentation and Retrieval of Information (data praxis), Form No. D 14/4186-101

[18] B.C.Vickery, Techniques of Information Retrieval, Butterworths 1970

[19] E.Lutterbeck (Hrsg), Dokumentation und Information, Umschau-Verlag 1971 (in German)

[20] G.Schott, Automatic Analysis of Inflectional Morphems in German Nouns, Acta Informatica 1(1972), 360-374

[21] SIEMENS: PBS 4004 PASSAT, Beschreibung, Form no. D14/40324 (in German)

[22] N.H.Nie, et al., SPSS — Statistical Package for the Social Sciences, 2nd ed, McGraw-Hill, 1975

[23] I.Flores, Data Structure and Management, Prentice-Hall, Inc. 1970

[24] H.Wedekind, Datenorganisation, Walter de Gruyter 1973 (in German)

[25] R.Bayer, E.McCreight, Organisation and Maintenance of Large Ordered Indexes, Acta Informatica 1(1972), no.3, 173-189

[26] R.Bayer, Storage Characteristics and Methods for Searching and Addressing, Information Processing 74, North-Holland Publ.Co, 1974, 440-444

[27] H.Duerr, Datenerfassung in der kommerziellen Datenverarbeitung, Walter de Gruyter 1973 (in German)

[28] C.-O.Mertin, Datenerfassung — Eine Uebersicht, R.Oldenbourg 1971 (in German)

[29] D.Tsichritzis, Reliability, in: Advanced Course on Software Engineering, Lecture Notes in Econ. and Math. Systems 81, Springer-Verlag

Further readings recommended:

J.W.Klimbie, K.L.Koffeman (eds), Data Base Management, North-Holland Publ.Co. 1974

D.E.Knuth, The Art of Computer Programming, vols 1 and 3, Addison-Wesley Publ.Co. 1968, 1973

F.Ahrens, H.Walter, Datenbanksysteme, Walter de Gruyter 1971 (in German)

F.L.Bauer, G.Goos, Informatik, Zweiter Teil, Heidelberger Taschenbuch 91, Springer-Verlag 1974 (in German)

L.J.Hoffman, Computers and Privacy: A Survey, ACM Computing Surv. 1(1969), no.2

SOME ASPECTS OF SYSTEM PROGRAMMING

M. Griffiths
Université de Nancy, France

1. INTRODUCTION

It is only recently that the programming profession has been able to make a serious effort to characterise its various activities and to try to structure them into a coherent discipline. Many observers believe that, now that structured programming, top down analysis and step-wise refinement exist, the necessary revolution has taken place and that the rest of the problem is merely education and application. This is, of course, not so ; the revolution has merely indicated the right way to start. It gives us the opportunity to set programming off on a sound base on which we can build conceptually acceptable mechanisms and also brings our way of thinking back towards that of mathematicians, with its emphasis on axioms, hypotheses and proof methods. These methods will only become applicable after some time, when sufficient work has been done to allow the use of high-level primitives which would serve the same purpose as the more sophisticated theorems of mathematics.

The results of current research are much more applicable to individual algorithms than to systems, and this for two reasons. There is firstly a problem of sheer size. As we shall see later, the analytical treatment of even a small problem rapidly becomes mathematically complex ; on the scale of a large, or even medium-sized, system, analytical methods are at present outside the capacity of the people involved. In this case we must resort to engineering-like methodology, with rules, guide lines and craftsmanship. The second problem is the influence of time. Even a small problem which involves real-time concepts, in particular when there is interaction between parallel processes, leads to problems to which we are not yet able to give satisfactory analytical solutions. We see that programming methodology has several aspects, depending on the scale and the type of the problem.

Let us first consider the problem of time-dependency in terms of an example. In a patient-monitoring system which studies waves from an electro-encephalogram in order to study heart-beat rhythms, sampling methods are often used to warn the doctor of any degradation of the standard PQRST cycles of the wave-form :

Degradation may be of form, of frequency or of amplitude. The system programmer's viewpoint of this problem is the following. He wishes to know the frequency and magnitude of the signal. In this case he will receive the vertical coordinate of the wave, after analog-digital conversion, every 10 ms, say. He in fact does not care whether these signals represent the number of cars passing a certain point, the temperature of a bar of steel being rolled or a measure of cardiac activity. He then wishes to know to which program to give the information and how long this program will require to perform the treatment. He can then organise his work and in particular set limits on the number of patients which can be monitored in parallel, and so on.

In the case of a dedicated computer system which handles only patient monitoring by sampling, the system aspect is very simple, and the capacity of an equipment is calculable. This situation changes when other methods are used which involve the arrival of signals of varying complexity at arbitrary intervals, for example when initial screening is done by specialised peripheral equipment which sends a signal only when certain limits are exceeded, and in particular when the computer is handling different problems at the same time. In this case the system problem is much more complex and we must consider questions like response time, possibilities of interference, maximum capacity, and so on. These calculations will be statistical in nature, since otherwise we would apply worst case methods, in supposing, for example, that all the monitored patients could have a heart attack at exactly the same moment. Worst case analysis will often lead to unacceptable waste of computer capacity. Sensible limits may well be implicitly known to the hospital system : how many emergencies can the doctors themselves cope with in parallel ?

We have already seen the need, in system evaluation and analysis, to have available knowledge as to the time spent to execute particular algorithms. This topic will be discussed separately in a later chapter. Of course, time is not the only problem, since the central processor time is only one of the resources of a computer system. We must also consider resources like channel time, main and peripheral memory capacity, and so on. General resource allocation is usually considered to be the kernel of system programming activity.

In a small number of hours, it would not be possible to give a complete course on system programming. What follows is therefore a discussion of a number of selected topics which, it is hoped, may prove to be of use in medical applications.

2. TIME DEPENDENCY

Problems involving time are found in operating systems, data collection systems, and process control, as well as being conceptually present in simulation models. The problems vary considerably in complexity depending on the type and number of competing processes, and in particular their degree of cooperation and any requirements for sharing resources.

2.1. Interrupt Systems

In systems like the patient monitoring system outlined in the introduction, that is to say in most data collection systems, the arrival of information is indicated by a signal, called an interrupt, which draws the attention of the central processor. After recognition of the source of the signal, control is passed to the relevant handling routine, at the end of which control returns once more to the system. The number of items read per interrupt varies with the type of peripheral, but this is irrelevant to the present discussion.

The first question we may ask is 'what was the processor doing before it was interrupted ?' In the simplest systems, the answer is 'nothing', where this may of course mean that it was twiddling its thumbs in a standard, short, useless waiting loop. When this is true, the system is dedicated to the treatment of a set of interruptions arriving in a controlled manner, that is to say that :
- the delay between two successive interrupts is always greater than the handling time
- the computer has nothing else to do between-times.

Relaxing either or both of these conditions requires more thought.

If central processor time and memory space are unused, they may be absorbed by a background job, which may, for example, be calculating the pay-roll. A background job which is time-independent and which uses no resource required by the foreground presents little difficulty. It is sufficient that the interrupt routine save the 'state of the interrupted program' on reception of a signal. This state is then restored after the handling of the signal. The state of a program is that information which will allow it to be restored in order that it may continue where it left off. The information concerned is found in different hardware registers like the location counter, arithmetic and logical registers, memory limits, and so on. If there exists commonality of resources between background and foreground, for example common data, common peripherals or memory locations, we must then consider them as co-operating processes. This problem will be treated later.

Since it is possible to interrupt a process in course of execution, restoring it at a later date for continuation, it becomes possible to accept an interruption before the end of the treatment of the preceeding one. The treatment of the arrived data takes the place of the background job in the preceeding paragraph. The two parts of the process, data arrival and data treatment, have been separated, arrival taking priority over treatment. Let us say that the interrupt for case B arrives while the computer is treating case A. The data for B is read immediatly, but there is no reason to start the treatment of B before termination of that for A. (Of course, in particular systems this may not be true, but we will suppose it to be so for the moment). The data for B must be stored in a buffer, in the form of a queue, and will be treated in its turn. We have the following situation :

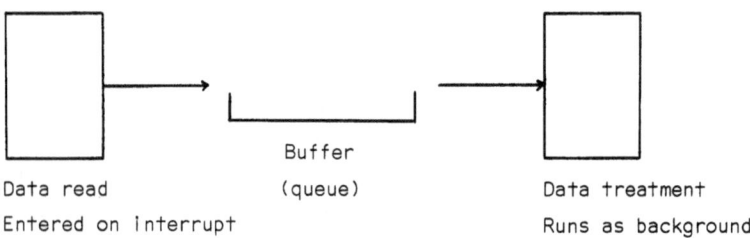

Data read   (queue)   Data treatment

Entered on interrupt   Runs as background

The two processes must cooperate, since they work on the same buffer, which is thus common data. However, they can never mutually interfere, since the module of treatment is only entered when no reading is being done.

The above structure allows us to smooth out bunched arrivals of data by interruption of one process by another. However, there is still a problem, since a new interruption does not necessary need to be so polite as to arrive only during the data treatment phase, but may arrive during the immediate response to the preceeding interruption. The simplest solution to this problem is to inhibit interruptions during interrupt-handling. The interrupt signal will be taken into acount when control is returned to the treatment module.

Let us now try to write the two programs. Data treatment has become a continous loop :

```
while true do
begin if nonempty (buffer)
        then begin take next data item ;
                   calculate
              end
  end
```

We see that if the buffer is empty, the program loops while doing nothing. Arrival of new data will interrupt this loop, put new data into the buffer, and change the condition. This is typical of parallel processes, the program above being complete nonsense in isolation. The read module could look like the following :

```
Inhibit interruption ;
Save interrupted program state ;
Read into buffer ;
Permit interruption ;
Return to interrupted program
```

If we consider the last two instructions, we may well ask what will happen if an interrupt arrives between the execution of the first and that of the second. The control counter of the interrupted program will be lost, since the interrupt will be taken into account before the address is reached. It is for this reason that many machines have an instruction which is the logical union of the two instructions : 'jump to address α with state change (allowing interrupts)'.

Of course, the above presentation of an interrupt system is a considerable simplification, since it is unthinkable to have only one type of interrupt. In particular, output will certainly be handled in the same way as input. However, the idea of working on a buffer space which is filled, or emptied, on receipt of an interruption, is basic to all time-dependent system work. In the next section we will consider, at least conceptually, some of the problems which may arise when the simple system seen above is generalised.

2.2. Generalisation to Several Processes

In non-dedicated systems, when the buffer is empty, we cannot afford to let the data treatment program loop while doing nothing. Control must be passed to another program, called the background task, so as to use the central processor while the data treatment routine is idle.

We get the following form of program for data treatment :

```
while true do
      if empty (buffer)
      then return control to suspended background task
      else calculate
```

How can the loop regain control when a new item comes into the buffer ?
The flow of control must, at least in some sense, become explicit. One form of the
resulting programs could be, ignoring the interrupt-handling book-keeping :

```
consumer loop : while true do
                if empty (buffer)
                then begin wait for chars ← true ;
                          return to system
                      end
                else calculate
producer : (entered on interruption)
      read into buffer ;
      if wait for chars
      then begin wait for chars ← false ;
                 goto consumer loop (putting the background program to sleep)
            end
      else return to interrupted program (which will be the consumer loop)
```

This duality of producer/consumer is the standard implementation of buffered input/
output by interruption. The program supposes that data treatment is more important
than any other interrupted program. This supposition may not be true, and in any case
our program is an implementation of a particular situation. In general, each program
should be independent, and should not have explicit returns to different modules. One
of the precepts of good programming in system work is that modules should not know
who called them nor should they know to where control will be returned at the end of
their execution. Thus it may be that one module of the system must look after the
flow of control. Not only will this new structure improve the security of the system,
but the program is also shorter and cleaner :

```
consumer : (as above)
producer : (entered on interruption)
              read into buffer ;
              wait for chars ← false ;
              return to system
```

The system will decide to whom control should be passed at this return. Programs built in this way do not have to be changed when the system is extended to include many processes. When the consumer loop 'goes to sleep' because the buffer was empty, the system will need to store the reawaken condition, so as to give back control when the condition is satisfied by action of the producer.

Of course, the program above is a long way yet from being satisfactory. First of all, we must consider not only the effects of the buffer being empty, but also that of the buffer being full. At this point, we may also generalise the problem, since producer/consumer pairs can be studied without reference to particular problems. We will also not consider external factors concerning the flow of control, and will therefore no longer consider whether the routines are entered by direct call or by interrupt. We will thus consider two continuous loops :

```
consumer : while ⌐ empty (buffer) do        producer : while ⌐ full (buffer) do
              begin take an object ;                     begin bring an object ;
                    n ← n - 1                                  n ← n + 1
              end                                        end
```

n represents the number of objects in the buffer at a given moment.
We can thus rewrite the tests, and obtain :

```
consumer : while n > 0 do                   producer : while n < buffer size do
              begin take an object ;                     begin bring an object ;
                    n ← n - 1                                  n ← n + 1
              end                                        end
```

Control may be lost by one of the loops either because the condition after while is not satisfied, or by interruption. When control is lost through interruption, the return is automatic when the interruption has been treated. The same is not true when the loss of control is due to non-satisfaction of a while condition, and the return must be explicit. Some program must look out for changes which would make the condition true. We may express this in our programs by writing :

```
consumer : do forever                producer : do forever
            begin waitfor n > 0 ;               begin waitfor n < buffersize ;
                  take an object ;                    bring an object ;
                  n ← n - 1                           n ← n + 1
            end                                  end
```

The new keyword waitfor has the effect of holding the process at its current position until the condition becomes true. The system is assumed to be able to cope with the necessary examination of conditions.

Incidentally, the same formalism would allow us to describe the fact that, for example, the producer works on interruption. In this case, the statement
    bring an object
can only take place when the object is available. This becomes
    waitfor interrupt ;
    transfer object to buffer

The parallel makes us realise the similarity between waiting for an interruption and waiting for a change in the value of n. Both should be considered to be events, which are thus directly signalled.

The reader should note that, although we have deduced a series of apparently acceptable programs, in fact, even this last version should be considered unsatisfactory in at least two different ways. First of all, as he will certainly have realised, the system will not normally be able to cope with waitfor followed by a general condition. Secondly our program structure is not necessarily time-secure. We will consider these problems, and their solutions, in the following section.

2.3. Synchronization and Security

The use of the special key-word waitfor in order to signal to the system that at that point there may be a temporary break in the execution of the program is a good idea. However, it is unreasonable to suppose the system to be capable of keeping track of the value of the condition after waitfor, which needs arbitrarily frequent recalculation. The system needs a flag. Changes of the value of the flag must also be indicated to the system by special key-words. Many different methods of indicating this information exist ; a discussion of some of them is to be found in [1].

A second problem suggested above was that of security. Let us consider what would happen if there were more than one producer. The result of an interruption from a producer is to cause the execution of the three statements.

```
if n < buffersize
then begin transfer object ;
          n ← n + 1
     end
```

Suppose another producer interrupts this execution between the test
   n < buffersize
and the assignment

   n ← n + 1

This second producer will in its turn believe that it can test the value of n, and will obtain the 'wrong' value, since the object being transferred is perhaps the one which fills the buffer. We see that it is useful to be able to link together the two actions of testing the value of a counter and of changing this value.

These two considerations were considered formally by E.W. Dijkstra, who invented the semaphore. Space does not allow us to give a full development, for which the reader should consult the original paper [2]. In order to solve the multiple producer-consumer problem we will use the concept of the integer semaphore, on which we may perform the following operations :

```
Declaration with optional initialisation :   sema s ← buffersize ;
Take :            P(s)      Equivalent to      waitfor s > 0 ; s ← s - 1
Release :         V(s)      Equivalent to      s ← s + 1
```

The operations P and V are indivisible. The solution of our problem would require two integer semaphores, and we obtain :

```
sema spaces ← buffersize, objects ← 0 ;
```

```
consumer : do forever                      producer : do forever
          begin P (objects) ;                       begin P (spaces) ;
                treat one object ;                         bring one object ;
                V (spaces)                                 V (objects)
          end                                        end
```

We see that the consumer loop will wait on

    P (objects)

until there is an object in the buffer (objects > 0). Similarly the producer loop
will wait on

    P (spaces)

until a space is available (spaces > 0). The programmer does not need to think further
about the coordination of the two routines.

        The use of synchronising primitives to control concurrent processes is a
form of programming which requires an apprenticeship. Some classical examples are
treated in [27]. The criteria that the programmer will apply to his solutions include

- fairness. Can all competing programs advance in function of the priority algorithm
  which the programmer wishes to impose ?

- security. As outlined above ; are all resources and all mutually exclusive sections
  protected, whatever the time-distribution of signals and events ?

- deadlock. Can the system stop as the result of some logical deadlock (deadly
  embrace) ?

We will treat this topic in the next paragraph.

        The classic example of blockage is that of the banker's algorithm [2].
Suppose that a banker disposes of a fixed sum, say 1 Million dollars, of capital to
invest in two companies. After some time each company has received 500,000 dollars,
and then requires another 100,000 dollars of investment in order to start making a
profit. Each will thus wait for the other to produce the money which will allow itself
to advance. In computer terms the resource may be memory which is shared between two
programs, which may get to the same deadly embrace because each requires more memory
and waits for the other to release it, nobody advancing. A relatively complete

treatment of problems of this sort may be found in [4] or [5], and we will not go much
further here. The user should note that solutions to this problem may be found either
in keeping enough spare (unallocated) resources so as to avoid the problem, or by an
energency procedure when the problem arises. Examples of these would be the banker
who keeps a reserve of capital (unallocated resources), or an operating system which
can empty a process onto backing store if necessary (emergency procedure).

2.4. Implementation

The preceeding paragraph has shown us some of the simpler tools and techniques
for handling cooperating sequential processes on at least a conceptual basis. We must
also consider what these tools will produce at the level of the machine.

Semaphores are obviously implemented as counters, and, if they are to be
implemented efficiently, require some special hardware instructions to access them
(TST in IBM 360, for example). When a program executes P(s), and s is non-zero, the
implementation is easy. The only problem arises when s is zero and the task must wait.
Waiting for a semaphore means being put into a queue which depends on that semaphore.
When V(s) is received, the first in the queue (or another, if the priority system so
requires) is released, or, if the queue for s is empty, s is increased by 1. Any system
of resource-sharing, cooperation and synchronisation will, in the end, be implemented
in terms of queues or an equivalent. A good practical knowledge of queue mechanisms
is essential for the system programmer.

One point in the above description which requires clarification in the
concept of process or task. Without wishing to go into too much details, we wish
nevertheless to introduce some simple ideas concerning this 'object' which may wait
in a queue. Let us call it a task for the purposes of this section. The most
satisfactory method of programming these problems is to dispose of a language which
furnishes an adequate model. Synchronising primitives like semaphores form only one of
the constituents of the model, which should permit at least two others ; satisfactory
control structures and clear data access.

Since different tasks require both individual and common data, the language
must provide some block structure in order to separate these. Each task must also be
a well-defined set of code in order to achieve this. The task must have a definite
beginning and a definite end, thus forbidding certain instructions like a goto which
would leave the task. Space does not allow us to consider these points in detail, the
important thing for the user being to realise that the choice of language and tools
is both delicate and important.

3. SECURITY, PROTECTION, RELIABILITY

Medical information science is one of the fields in which the related topics of security, protection and reliability are of the utmost importance. If we consider medical records systems, we come up against problems of professional secrecy, and, even if the necessary sharing of information amongst members of the medical profession becomes accepted, we will still be left with problems of access by other than those persons who have a normal right to know. In this situation, it is not the author's aim to decide what level of protection is required. This must be, and is being, considered by medical and legal experts. The reader may wish to consult the proceedings of conferences like [7] for this type of discussion. What the computer scientist must clarify is the limits of current technical possibilities in order to allow the user to make his choice on the basis of valid information.

A second problem to be faced is the degree of confidence which we may have in information systems. We may well wish to ask ourselves questions about the physical reliability of circuits, or whether we can be sure that software or applications programs perform the task for which they are built. Nobody can eliminate human error, and programmers and electronic engineers are human. Since no system can offer 100 % reliability, we should give ourselves more reasonable aims. The first would be to undo all the myths about computers, so that we may talk about a technology amongst others. This encourages us to treat computer disasters like aircraft accidents (and also, perhaps, to aim at a similarly low failure rate !). We should be able to consider, calmly and objectively, what the cost of a failure might be, give some estimate of frequency, and compare these figures with those of non-automatic systems. The profession will have reached maturity when this becomes the natural thing to do.

3.1. Reliability

We will not discuss techniques for hardware reliability, which fall outside the scope of this course. Current hardware, in practice, gives sufficient service, with no permanent problems, in all cases except those in which complete real-time performance is required.

Software reliability is altogether another problem. Everybody has heard horrific, and mostly true, stories about the thousands of found errors in operating systems, or about numerical errors discovered after months or even years. The surprising thing, for the computer scientist, is that so many programs seem to give satisfactory service. It is not sufficient that most users manage to live with present day programs, since the risk of error increases more than linearly with complexity, and we are forced to rely more and more on the computer. This problem is one of those which causes the most concern in computer circles, since progress, although sure, is slow. Improvement depends on the rigorous application of better programming techniques, which are being developped. In more detail, we should be considering all the following points :

- Methods of program construction. The keywords here are structured programming, top-down construction, program proving, stop wise refinement, and others. [8] gives a good set of guidelines. Control at this stage allows greater understanding and control of the result.

- Specification of problems and algorithms. Tighter specification of problems, algorithms and the data they use allows us to know to what situations standard algorithms apply and under what conditions programs are guaranteed to work. See [24] for a discussion of some of these problems, which imply a greater degree of formalisation than that which is currently applied.

- Education. Writing bad programs is unfortunately easy, and so many people do it. Writing good ones is difficult, and requires intelligence, education and experience. Although education is improving, it is not yet good enough, and anyway many employers have not yet become convinced of the necessity.

3.2. Protection

Here we are mainly concerned with information at different memory levels of the computer : preventing mutual interference between users of a multiprogramming system, preserving secrecy in file systems at the same time as preventing their destruction by different kinds of accident, or even design. Memory protection in operating systems is an interesting technical problem, but which depends on hardware considerations outside the scope of the course. We will concentrate on the protection of information stored in files, which is an important problem in medical record handling.

The contents of files must be protected against many different forms of possible depredation, access or mis-use :

- Hardware breakdowns causing physical destruction
- Operator error
- Programmer error
- Unauthorised access by accident
- Criminal action

- Abuse of power.

The basic mechanism by which we protect against physical destruction is that of redundancy. Copies must be kept of all files, and this in a manner which allows automatic reconstitution. This mechanism also permits recovery from certain types of programmer error. Access problems require that with each file be associated specific information concerning the type of access which may be allowed and to whom this access is applicable. This means that, each time a user is connected to the system, he can be identified. This identification will be the basis for all accounting and access problems, and thus represents a weak point in present-day systems.

With a well-built system, and by following strictly the required conventions, protection at the level required is possible within a community of users who are of good faith. This statement is not true when we consider protection against malevolent agencies. There is no computing solution to the problem of protection of information against criminal access, nor can there be. Here we are in a situation analogue to that of the protection of defense secrets in war-time. Protection comes from layers of physical screening and physical security conventions.

The real-world situation is presently the following. Few reasonable file systems are available, although the techniques are well-known. Few computer centres apply rigorous and useful discipline to assure protection. Finally, the author knows of no civilian computer centre in which the problem of physical security is satisfactorily handled, although there do exist some interesting, partial experiments.

3.2.1. Access Limitation

Information is stored on different peripherals in the form of files. The user should not need to know the physical location of the file, nor even on what type of peripheral it is stored. All he knows is that he owns a file, to which he gives a name. When he needs to recover the information he uses this same name. One of the system tasks is thus to provide the link between the name of the file which occurs in the program and its physical location. This information is stored in a catalogue, which is simply a file table. It is obvious that the catalogue is a particularly sensitive part of the system, since its destruction means that files, even if they exist, cannot be found.

Control of access rights is usually at the level of the catalogue. Let us consider the example of a medical records system in which information concerning a particular patient can only be recorded by his own doctor (that is to say that nobody else can order treatment) but in which the file corresponding to the patient may be consulted by any member of the same medical team (thus allowing the nurse to apply the relevant treatment). It could well be that, in such a system, statistics are kept in a separate file, which must be accessible to the whole hospital staff. To understand the equivalence of this structure in computer system terms, we must consider the different degrees of protection from the computer scientist's point of view.

We may consider three basic types of access, read, write end execute. The type of access involving writing may be divided in two, depending on whether or not the priviledge of writing includes the possibility of destroying past information. As examples of these types we may give :

- reading. A nurse may need to read the instructions left by a doctor, without being allowed to write on the files

- writing without change. The nurse may be allowed to add information to a file (temperature at 7.00 a.m, ...) but not to change preceeding information, or even perhaps to read

- writing with change. A doctor may wish to change a course of treatment

- execution. It may be reasonable to allow others to use a program without them being able to read its text, and hence not allowing the making of a copy, for reasons of copyright.

The four types of access, read, add, edit and execute, can be represented by four bits for a given user, the bit indicating whether or not the type of access is allowed.

In order to provide different access rights at different levels, the catalogue will probably have a structure which is that of a tree. A typical structure will have three levels, although there is nothing magical about this figure :

- programmer
- his group (or project number)
- the rest of the world.

When a programmer writes a compiler, he alone will be able to write on the corresponding file. Members of his project may be allowed to read, and any attached user be allowed to execute the program, that is to say use the product to compile their program. For any given file, access rights are thus divided in three levels, with four bits/level. In the compiler example, the file would be protected as follows :

	Read	Add	Edit	Execute
Programmer	1	1	1	1
Project	1	0	0	1
World	0	0	0	1

This organisation also helps in using the catalogue.

3.2.2. User Identification

We have seen that it is vital to identify the person who is connected to the computer in order to impose the relevant access rights, and also to help the accounting routines. In the absence of purely physical means of identification, present systems rely on passwords. The typewriter console will be programmed so that the password never appears in print, which gives a reasonable degree of security, especially if each console is associated with a list of its authorised users. The risks involved in this system are human, since, at least in the author's experience, users do not take seriously the degree of secrecy necessary in order to protect the password.

Future systems will use physical devices for identification purposes, such as the magnetic cards used in automatic banking machines. These cards will last until some economic method is developped allowing, for example, automatic fingerprinting or voice recognition.

Whatever method is used to identify the user at his console, the ultimate decisions are taken by stored programs in the operating system. These programs use tables containing passwords, access rights and accounting routines. The current degree of physical protection of this information, and of the programs and peripheral support units, is a long way from being satisfactory, mostly because users are not yet aware of the necessity. The protection will come from controlled entry of persons into the computer centre, the sealing of important programs in circuitry, use of codes and ciphers to store sensitive tables, and so on. Most of this is in interesting contrast to the fact that, on all the computers we have used, it has been possible to make a complete memory dump without any control from the computer centre management.

3.2.3. Archives

To avoid the permanent loss of information after accident, whether of hardware, software, operator error or programmer error, copies may be made of the

contents of the file system, usually on magnetic tape, at intervals which depend on
the average rate of change of the contents of the files. The process of recopying
also allows the recovery of space on the peripheral devices used to store information.
The aim is the automatic implementation of a hierarchical storage system in which
information under treatment is in main memory, files which are frequently consulted
are on disk or drum, while archives and rarely consulted information are kept on
magnetic tape.

For each file in the system, a note is kept of the date of the last access
and of the last time its contents were changed. At fixed intervals, the system copies
onto magnetic tape all files which have been changed since the preceeding copy was
made. In addition, those files to which no access has been made over some given period
are deleted from the system (and hence exist only in archives).

Users are encouraged to keep the listing corresponding to all changes for
at least the delay between successive recopies. In case of necessity, the system
recovers the preceeding version of the file, and signals the user that he must re-edit
from a certain date and time. The programmer may also avail himself of this facility
if he makes a wrong manoeuvre.

This technique leads to rapidly increasing numbers of magnetic tapes, which
must be recovered after a certain delay. At this recovery, the old tape is reconsidered,
and a copy is made onto the new tape of only those files of which there is no more
recent version in the archives. There will be few such files.

A further detail concerns the recopying of the main catalogue, which is
itself normally a file. It is usual to be able completely to restore the catalogue if
it is destroyed, and this requires the saving, on a different peripheral device, of
all changes in the catalogue since the last copy was made. In addition, as a second
line of defence, each peripheral device will contain its own catalogue, which indicates
the set of files on the particular device. This allows reconstitution of the main
catalogue from these secondary catalogues.

We have given some idea of one way of storing, recovering and protecting
files. The reader may wish to continue in studying [9], [10] and [11], amongst others.
The important point is that the system should be entirely automatic, leaving none of
the day to day protection to the individual user.

3.3. Power and Privacy

In parallel with other professions, the medical fraternity is faced with the difficult questions implied by the stockage of large amounts of information, often confidential, in data banks accessed by computers. We have discussed above some of the immediate problems and the limits of the known technical solutions. It is not the duty of the computer scientists to decide what degree of privacy should be required by the medical profession, the members of which must make up their own minds in function of the technical details of which they dispose.

This discussion would not be complete without considering the problem of security at the next level up. The centralisation of data, whether it be medical, judiciary, economic or educational, can put enormous power into the hands of he who controls the information. Rightly or wrongly, some computer scientists have formulated considerable reserves about the use of large data banks, in much the same way as some physicists have doubts about different applications of atomic physics. It would be unfair not to indicate the existence of these opinions when talking to prospective large-scale users.

The problem is partly one of confidence in the non-manipulation of the data. Consider, for example, the fact that bank accounts, and indeed all money, may well become simple entries in a computer data bank. We must not neglect the possibility that some unscrupulous politician or civil servant change the contents of these memories in order to eliminate adversaries, or to obtain power. It is not suggested that any particular present-day holder of a responsible position would be liable to do this, merely that we have created one more tool for the unscrupulous. The reader will certainly have considered the equivalent problem in medecine.

4. EVALUATION

Algorithms or programs may be evaluated on several different levels, using many different techniques. At the most abstract end of the spectrum we find the difficult, and not immediately useful, subject of the theory of complexity, which we will not study. At a more practical level we may wish to compare the efficiency of two algorithms, or to compare two programs which may even represent the same algorithm. Different evaluation methods include analysis, measurement and simulation, all of which should receive our attention.

4.1. Program Execution Time

We follow the method of [12] on an example in order to show some of the basic techniques of the evaluation of the number of operations which will be involved in the execution of a program. Consider the following simple piece of program, which counts the number of strictly positive and strictly negative elements in a vector :

```
for i ← 1 step 1 until n do
begin if a [i] ≠ 0
        then begin if a [i] > 0
                    then pos ← pos + 1
                    else neg ← neg + 1
              end
    end
```

In order to do calculation on a program it is useful to work on a corresponding graph, which many will recognise as being essentially a flow diagram. It is worth repeating at this point that, whereas a flow diagram represents possibly the worst tool ever invented for creating or explaining programs, the graph of a program is universally used in program analysis, whether for optimisation, evaluation or transformation, which are all related topics. The graph of our program is :

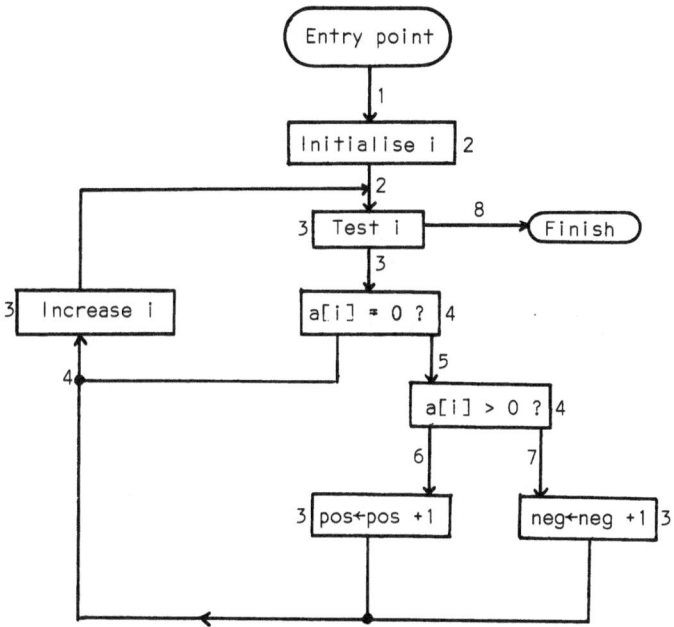

We do not use the normal flowchart representation, since we are only interested in possible paths, and not in why these paths are taken. The entry arcs to the different nodes have been labelled with integers. The nodes themselves are marked with an integer which represents the cost of executing this node. This cost corresponds to the number of machine code instructions that a compiler might generate for the node.

It is more convenient for our purposes to take the dual of this graph, which means transforming nodes into branches and branches into nodes. The integer labels we gave to the branches will become nodes in the following diagram :

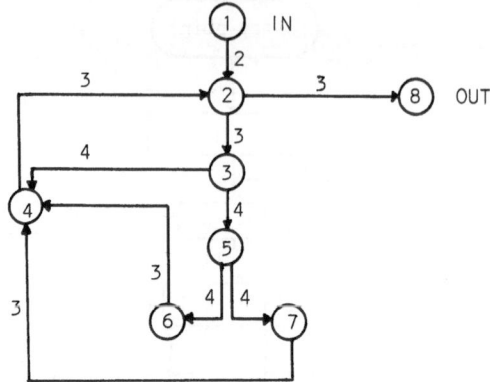

Each branch is labelled with the cost of taking the branch, figure which appeared on the node of the preceeding diagram. In order to decide the total cost of executing the graph, we need to know the probability of following each branch. Let a typical value of n be 99, and the probability of a zero entry be 1 in 10, the probability of a negative value being the same as that of a positive one. We may now decorate the graph with these probabilities, leaving the cost function unchanged :

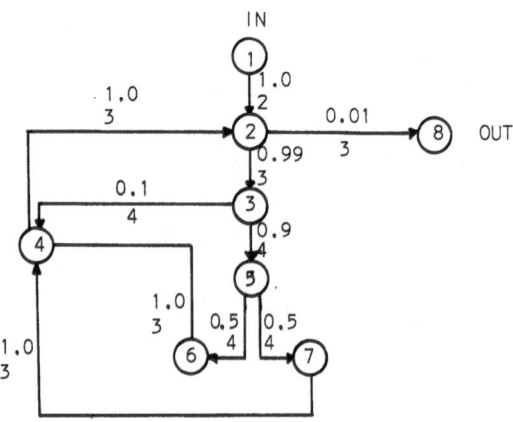

The sum of the probabilities of the branches leaving a node must be one. We will now try to eliminate the various nodes between IN and OUT in order to discover the total cost. The following rules allow this elimination :

(i) Given several branches from one node to the next :

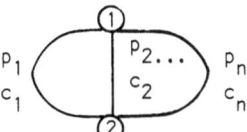

p_i = probability for branch i

c_i = cost of branch i

These branches become one branch by addition :

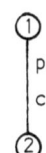

$$p = p_1 + p_2 + \cdots p_n = \sum_{i=1}^{n} p_i$$

$$c = \frac{p_1 c_1 + p_2 c_2 + \cdots p_n c_n}{p_1 + p_2 + \cdots p_n} = \sum_{i=1}^{n} p_i c_i / p$$

(ii) Given a node with a set of independent inputs and independent outputs :

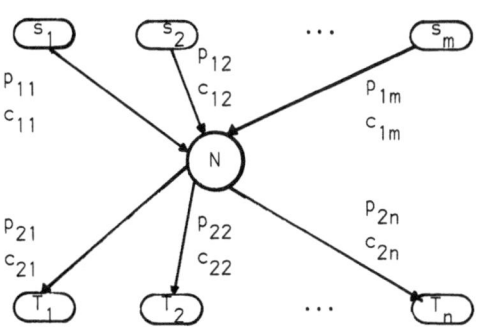

N may be eliminated by connecting each S_i to each T_j with the following calculation

$$p_{ij} = p_{1i} \times p_{2j}$$

$$c_{ij} = c_{1i} + c_{2j}$$

In this sense, independence in the set S means that the members of S are different, as are those of T.

(iii) Given a node on which there is a loop :

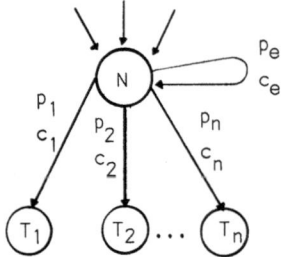

Insert a new node between N and the T_i, of the following form :

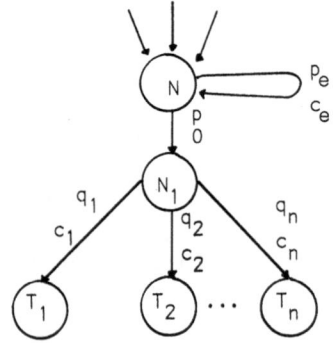

The new probability functions are :

$$p = p_1 + p_2 + \dots + p_n = \sum_{i=1}^{n} p_i$$
$$q_i = p_i / p$$

[confirming that $\Sigma q_i = \Sigma(p_i/p)$
$= (\Sigma p_i)/p$
$= 1$]

The loop may now be eliminated :

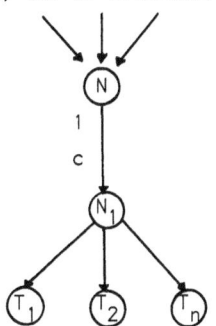

The new cost function is

$$c = (p_e/p) * c_e$$

A more intuitive presentation of this is to be found in the example.
Let us apply these rules to the example :

Elimination of ⑥ and ⑦ :

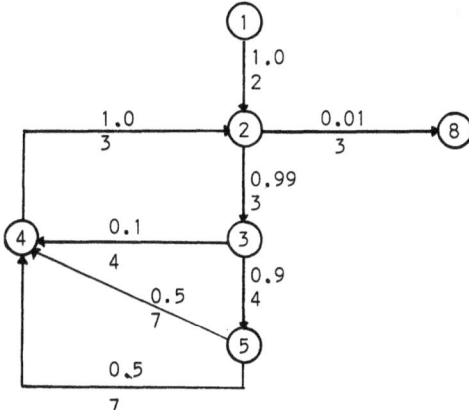

Join of branches between ⑤ and ④ :

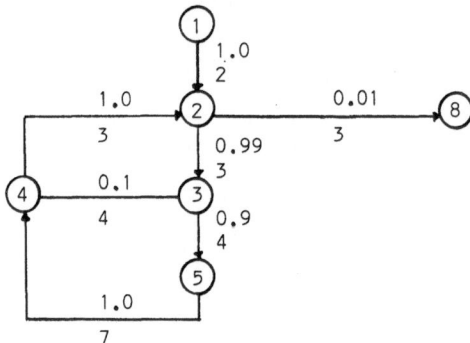

Elimination of ⑤ :

(A)

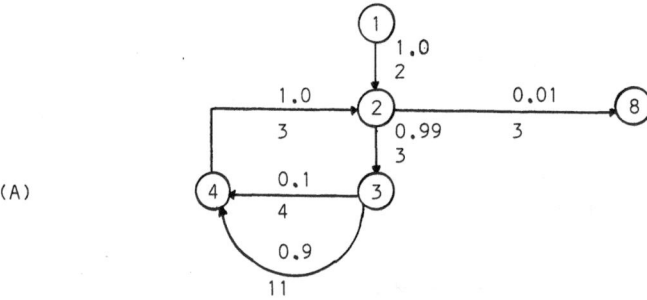

Join of branches between ③ and ④ :

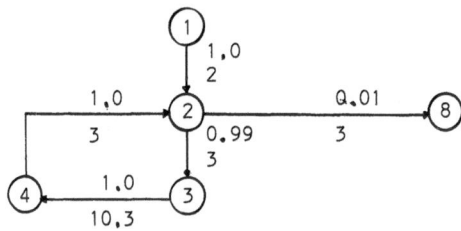

(10.3 = 0.1 × 4 + 0.9 × 11)

Elimination of ③ and ④ :

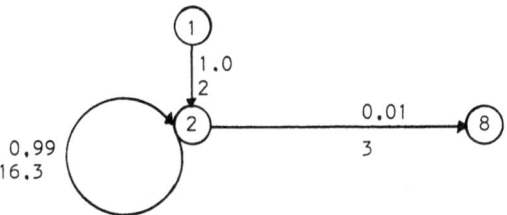

For the loop, we consider that we will loop 99 times and then quit, giving :

(1616.7 = 99 × 16.3 + 3)

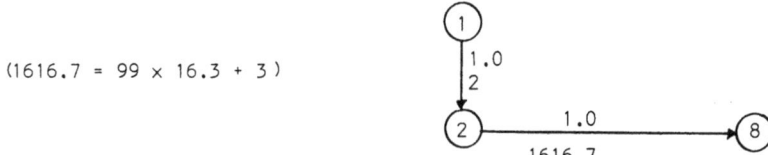

Note that it was not necessary to introduce a new node, since ② had only one other output.

The toal cost from ① to ⑧ is thus 1618.7.

It would also have been possible to consider the result as an analytical function of n and of the probability p of a zero entry.

The total cost function would then be, taking diagram (A)

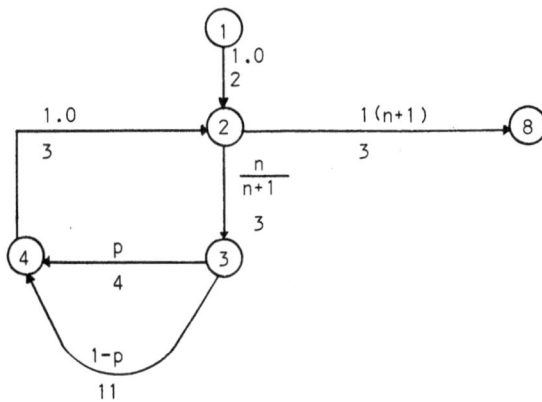

Successive diagrams are :

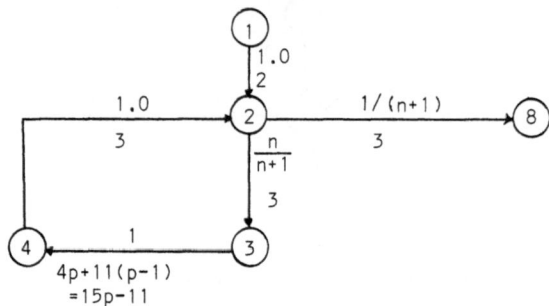

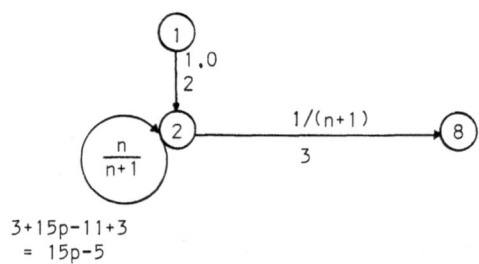

$$3 + 15p - 11 + 3$$
$$= 15p - 5$$

Total cost = 2 + n(15p-5) + 3
= 5 (1 + 3pn - n)

The decision as to whether we apply analytical or numerical techniques will depend entirely on the circumstances.

4.2. Algorithm Analysis

In the preceeding section, we have shown how to do a frequency analysis on a given program. This allows us to compare, at least in some sense, the efficiency of different programs. We distinguish between this type of analysis and the analysis of classes of algorithms, which may lead to theoretical bounds for the execution of processes, hence discovering whether or not a given algorithm approaches the theoretical minimum in execution time. Knuth [13] gives a good description of the two types of analysis, which he calls type A and type B.

Analysis of classes of algorithms would seem to be more interesting than the analysis of particular programs, since it solves an infinity of cases at once. However, in practice, much less use is made of the technique, for several reasons :

- the mathematics involved rapidly become complex, and so the process is usually impractically difficult ;
- the results may not be of direct practical application. For example, it is no use knowing that there exists a theoretical optimum if we do not know how to achieve it ;
- it is often difficult to decide on a measure.

Thus, we consider complexity analysis to be a more formal topic which interests theoretical computer scientists, but is not yet accessible to practical programmers, although they may well need to understand some of the achieved results.

4.3. Influence of Real-Time

The situation changes radically when the process to be analysed is not strictly sequential, since we have to consider the rates of arrival of external signals. The sort of question to which we are expected to be able to give an answer includes :

- how many patients can be monitored in parallel in the system ?
- what is the avarage reaction time of the system in reply to a trivial request ? What is the maximum reaction time ?
- what is the mean length of the queue of processes waiting for a given service ? And what is the standard deviation from the mean ?

The calculations involved in answering these questions are often outside the capacities of present-day system programmers, either because of mathematical complexity, or because the author of the question could not give a precise specification of what he meant. One of the more obvious questions in this latter class is that of the efficiency of an operating system. Manufacturers sometimes give figures indicating the percentage use of the central processor, which is no measure at all since it is simple to change any system to get 100 % use of the processor. This will not necessarily increase the throughput. One measure would be to compare practical throughput with the maximum possible on the configuration, but unfortunate the latter is an unknown figure. We consider some techniques which may help.

4.3.1. Worst Case Analysis

Consider the monitoring system in chapter 1. It may be that the medical staff may be able to give some upper limit to the rate of arrival of exceptional cases requiring immediate treatment, for example, not more than five cases of loss of rhythm in any one minute. The limit may be based on the doctor's experience, or simply on the fact that more could not be treated anyway, given the number of available doctors. This last point is more important than it appears. The computer system must be an integral part of the operation, and be subject to the same limits as the rest of the system. These limits are often not explicited, leading to surplus capacity, or, worse, insufficiency under emergency conditions. The good systems programmer will put these limits into his program and confirm that they are met, thus protecting himself, his program and the system environment.

Given well specified and reasonable limits, worst case analysis is simple. The maximum execution time of the program resulting from one signal can be calculated by frequency analysis, and this multiplied by the relevant factors to obtain what must be a guaranteed result. The technique is useful in the case of systems which must reply within a given interval. Such systems are necessarily incompletely used during their lifetime, although the slack may be taken up by a non-urgent background task.

4.3.2. Simulation

This technique may be used when decisions concerning hardware have to be made, since choice of hardware configuration is often a once for all decision of financial importance. The first thing to note is that simulation is expensive in computer time, and must only be used when necessary. In this case it is both useful and directly practical, giving good results when used by competent specialists.

Examples of successful simulation have been in traffic circulation, either in the air to test different types of radar cover, or on roads, to compare traffic-light algorithms ; in selecting page sizes or cache sizes in computer systems, and many others. Their common factor is that experimentation would be too expensive, or simply impossible.

The two main aspects of a simulation, apart from the interpretation of the results, are the construction of the model and the production of reasonable input data. The model depends entirely on the problem tackled, and there exist a certain number of special-purpose programming languages which help (see, for example [14] and [15] ; there are many others). Coding the model requires clear thought when simulating the passage of time.

We give an example of the simulation of a system of traffic lights at a multiple crossroads. There are n roads which feed the critical point, one of which has a green light at any moment, the others being red. The lights change at a fixed interval, and in strict rotation. The programming language is not one of those quoted in the references, but used simply for illustration :

```
procedure change lights ;
begin while true do
      begin delay (delay time on green light) ;
            lights [current] ← red ;
            current ← current + 1 ;
            if current = n+1
            then current ← 1 ;
            lights [current] ← green
      end
end ;
procedure car arrival ;
begin while true do
      begin delay (random (limits)) ;
            q ← random (some other limits) ;
            queue [q] ← queue [q] + 1
      end
end
procedure car departure ;
begin while true do
      begin if queue [current] ≠ 0
            then begin queue [current] ← queue [current] - 1 ;
                       delay (time to disengage one car)
                 end
            else delay (1)          comment try again soon comment
      end
end
```

The main program will be of the form :

```
begin integer array queue [1:n] ← 0 ; lights [1:n] ← red ;
      integer current ← 1 ;
      lights [current] ← green ;
      activate (car arrival) ;
      activate (change lights) ;
      activate (car departure) ;
      delay (time of experiment)
end
```

This program is not meant to be practical, but merely to give the flavour of a simulation of this type. Three parallel procedures regulate the traffic lights, the arrival of vehicles and their departure. The main program provides the initial conditions and activates the different tasks.

We see in this example some of the functions required in a simulation language, of which an incomplete list would be :

- to be able to define and activate parallel (simulation) tasks
- to be able to indicate delays in time, or waits for outside signals
- the definition of statistical data collection routines (not included in the example) in order to obtain and analyse results
- provision of a battery of random number generators for different statistical distributions.

The language may also include special data types, like queues and priority systems for task control.

The reader will easily transpose this example to the analysis of the queues waiting for medical or laboratory service of all kinds, and it is the concept of the control of random events and queues which characterise simulation.

Producing reasonable input data is often a real problem. The choice lies between theoretical assumptions based on experience or intuition, for example supposing that the arrival of signals has a poisson distribution about an average rate of n, or the use of live data, when this is available. The former method requires a battery of random number generators with different properties. These are usually supplied with the programming language. This method can lead to nasty surprises if the initial assumptions were not valid. The second method, which is obviously preferable if input data can be found, depends on a certain consistency in time.

4.3.3. Analytical Models

When the input data used in problems concerning queues, like that shown above, corresponds to some mathematical function, it is tempting, and more economical, to try to find analytical solutions. At the present time, systems of practical size are not susceptible to analytical treatment because of the mathematical complexity involved. However, amongst others, simple queuing problems have been treated, and we give an example from [3], again following [12].

Consider a first-come, first-served queue, into which arrive objects (patients for the doctor, demands to a laboratory, jobs in an operating system, ...) at an average rate of λ objects per unit time, according to a Bernoulli distribution. We suppose that the probability S_n of the treatment of a given element be n units of time is given by a geometric distribution :

$$S_n = (1-\sigma) \; \sigma^{n-1} \quad \text{for } n = 1, 2, \ldots \quad \text{and } 0 \leq \sigma < 1$$

The average execution time required per unit of time is given by

$$\rho = \frac{\lambda}{1-\rho}$$

The average length of the queue is

$$E = \frac{\rho \; \sigma}{1-\rho} \; .$$

We do not prove these results, and interested readers should consult the original paper [3] .

An analytical model of this kind is obviously more useful than a simulation model, if it covers the same ground. Unfortunately it is unusual to dispose of sufficient models, and their widespread use must remain a pious hope. The present state of the art may be found in [6].

5. SOFTWARE ENGINEERING

Bauer [16] tells us that this catchword was created to provoke response from the computing world, given that there was widespread discontent amongst users as to the software that was delivered. The more important publications on the theme are [17], [18],[19]. After an initial period of discussion, the term has become a reasonable description of a trade in which work engineers under the usual rules. By this we mean that the production of software should resemble the production of roads, bridges, aeroplanes or motor-cars, and in particular in the following respects :

- performance. The user should be able to evaluate the product in terms like 'forty miles to the gallon', 'supports a charge of ten tons'.
- Cost. Production cost should be known beforehand, as should be running costs.
- Security. The product must conform to given specifications, and the producer be held responsable for non-respect of them.

Few users would suggest that these criteria are respected at the present time, but we hope that few producers of software would doubt the importance of working towards them. We will discuss some of the techniques which are in the process of application and which may help.

5.1. Organisation of Large Programs

As Dijkstra [2] points out, the biggest problem we face is one of complexity. This problem can only be met by the application of strict technical control and discipline. We are trying to create the relevant techniques at the same time as learning how to apply them. Perhaps the most relevant references are [8] for the techniques, and [22] for their application.

Several catchwords help in the resolution of the complexity problem. The first must be top-down analysis, which implies breaking down a problem into logical, constituent parts. Each part is then treated independently as a new problem. Written down like this, top-down analysis sounds obvious and trivial, but in.fact is not universally applied. The advantages are the following :

- allow independent proof and/or testing of modules ; each one will assume that lower-level modules work. This possibility depends on the rigorous specification of each module, the module being on a human scale and not a complete program.
- stop programmers knowing too much about other parts of the program. This is one of the major sources of unclean programming : use of information which is under another

module's control. If the other module changes it, a separate module stops working. This phenomenon is one of the manifestations of side effects, which are nearly always bad programming.

- Increased understanding at each level. What each person needs to understand is clearly defined, as is his interface with the outside world and the environment in which he works.

What is delicate in this type of analysis is choosing what should constitute a module. It is here that the experience and knowledge of good programmers become pre-eminent.

Once an algorithm or a problem is well-specified, it becomes, at least in theory, a simple exercice to write the corresponding program. This is where the catchword "structured programming" comes in, although it may well also have been of importance at the specification level. Like most professional teachers, the author believes that the biggest need is of education, and that good programming practice can be taught. It is at this level that the programmer comes into direct contact with some programming language and with the underlying computer. It is also here that we realise that existing languages are completely unsatisfactory, and we will consider this point in the next section.

Over the last few years, methods have been developped for 'proving' programs, and the structured programming movement lays stress on the use of constructions which allow confirmation of the exactness of the program. Proof, in this context, means showing that the program performs the transformation on the data that is indicated by the mathematical formulation of the same problem. The technique dates from [23]. Many programmers never use sufficiently exact mathematical specifications of their problem, never mind proving the program afterwards, and we consider the existence of such models to be of paramount importance. Less obvious is the degree of explicit proof that should be given. Present opinion tends to the view that, instead of proving the equivalence of the mathematical specification and the program, the latter should be deduced from the former, thus avoiding the proof problem. Examples of this are given in [24]. The details remain open, but we have already learnt much from the discussion.

These few comments give only a small view of some of the techniques involved in the conception, construction and exploitation of large programs. The subject is much wider, and we have made no mention at all of subjects such as documentation. In practice, we find that there are not only technical problems, but also human and administrative problems, which will often be more difficult. The architecture of a

big program is usually such that its decomposition into modules at different levels
is very close to the hierarchical structure of the group producing the program. A lot
of thought and effort must be spent if reasonable control and discipline are to be
applied to the communications between people and the testing of finished products.

5.2. Choice of Language

Language is the basic tool of programming, and so has a considerable
influence on resulting products. We hope that nobody at this school will doubt the
wisdom of getting rid of assembler and using some high-level language, even if he has
to design it himself. The problem is which language to choose. We will discuss
different points which may be of interest.

Many programmers are completely unaware of the difference between language
and implementation. This is partly due to the influence of major computer manufacturers,
who use the confusion in defence of their particular policy. This means that we should
get rid of preconceived notions that one given language is always better than another.
On the computer available, the choice is often directed be the quality of the compiler,
which includes points like run-time efficiency, size of object code, diagnostics and
painful restrictions, as well as security, documentation and other practical details.
We all know missionaries who defend their favorite language against all comers.
Whether or not they are right in theory, practice requires living with unsatisfactory
compilers, amongst which we will choose the least painful.

If we consider only language aspects, we should consider separately problems
of flow of control and those of data structure and data access. Flow of control is
the easier, since, with reasonable programming technique, even FORTRAN is usable.
The point is that the programmer will create his program in a higher-level, abstract
text, translating it by hand to the ugly, linear style of FORTRAN. This method has
been very successful in teaching [25]. At this level, program creation is not seriously
affected by the poverty of the language, but program communication is seriously affected,
and is indeed very difficult. The original, elegant program should be given as
documentation. These techniques can be taught without difficulty to programmers at
any level.

This is not true when we talk about data structures and data access. A good
programmer is capable of creating, at little cost to himself, the primitives necessary
for the program he wishes to write. Less experienced, or less gifted, programmers find
this difficult and need more primitives in the language. To some extend, we are thus

opposed to the view that sophisticated languages like ALGOL 68 should only be put
into the hands of sophisticated programmers. The opposite view may well apply in many
cases, it being the less sophisticated programmer who needs to have his primitives
provided by the language.

In the particular field of system programming, many professionals criticise
general-purpose languages as keeping them too far away from the computer. Using
arguments involving matters like efficiency, direct control of special circuitry
(interrupts, input/output, ...) and particular programming style, a new generation
of specialised languages has come into being, variously called 'machine-oriented
languages' or 'systems implementation languages'. After a conference [26] confronting
these new ideas, a new IFIP working group, some of whose results are available in [21],
is studying these languages. It may well be that one of them will be the answer in
particular cases.

One important point is that of portability, since possible future transfer
of a program to (probably unknown) future equipment has often to be envisaged. The
subject is discussed in [19]. It is particularly unfortunate that the only languages
which allow any real portability are FORTRAN and COBOL, and even then it is necessary
to observe stringent precautions. This should not be read to mean that any portable
program should be written in one of these two languages, but that the simple and
obvious way of achieving portability, by use of standard languages, is not yet
satisfactory. Other methods do exist and have been applied. It is at this point that
we perceive most clearly the difference between language and implementation, and of
the fact that there is no satisfactory connection between the definition of a language
and its compilers.

6. CONCLUSION

Systems programming is a very large and relatively ill-defined subject, from which we have chosen some aspects which may be of general interest. The course should be taken as introducing a limited number of ideas, rather than as a survey, or even as a set of recipes. Correct training of a system programmer is a task which requires some years of education and practical experience.

It would seem that the computing world is now aware of its programming needs, and even possesses solutions, albeit insecure and unsatisfactory ones, to those needs. Current work is on the refinement and recasting of these solutions in order to create some sort of cohesive, reliable body of knowledge with professional standards. The process will take some years yet, and methods will undoubtedly continue to evolve. This is just one more reason to consider this course as something less than a permanent record of methods.

The human problem which we face is also considerable. Of the many thousands of professional programmers on the market, very few are educated in the sense that we now understand education in programming. The rapid application of experimental techniques which should have been further developped has led to a situation in which the people, the tools and the methods involved have all become obsolescent, and we do not really know how to change this situation. As one example, how can we get rid of FORTRAN ?

REFERENCES

[1] P. BRINCH HANSEN
     A comparison of two Synchronising Concepts
     Acta Informatica I, 3, 1972.

[2] E.W. DIJKSTRA
     Cooperating Sequential Processes
     in Programming Languages, F. Genuys (ed.), Academic Press, 1968.

[3] L. KLEINROCK
     Time-shared Systems : A Theoretical Treatment
     JACM, 14, April, 1967.

[4] A.N. HABERMANN
     Prevention of System Deadlocks
     CACM, 12, 7, 1969.

[5] R.C. HOLT
     Some Deadlock Properties of Computer Systems
     Comp. Surveys, Sept. 1972.

[6] E.G. COFFMANN, P.J. DENNING
     Operating Systems Theory
     Prentice Hall, 1973.

[7] G. BRAIBANT, Le Secret de Données Médicales
     J.M. CARROLL, Medical Informatics : Trial and Travail
     in Communications des Tables Rondes, Journées d'Informatique Médicale,
     Toulouse, March 1975.

[8] O.J. DAHL, E.W. DIJKSTRA, C.A.R. HOARE
     Structured Programming
     Academic Press, 1972.

[9] R.W. CONWAY et al
     Security of File Systems
     CACM, April 1972.

[10] R.C. DALEY, P.G. NEUMANN
A General-Purpose File System for Secondary Storage
AFIPS, FJCC, 1965.

[11] D. BARRON, FRASER, D. HARTLEY, LANDY, NEEDHAM
File Handling at Cambridge University
AFIPS, 1967.

[12] R.M. GRAHAM
Performance Prediction
in [19].

[13] D.E. KNUTH
Mathematical Analysis of Algorithms
Proc. IFIP Congress 71, Ljubljana, Aug. 1971.

[14] IBM
General Purpose Systems Simulator
IBM Form 7090 - CS - 05 X

[15] O.J. DAHL, K. NYGAARD
SIMULA - An ALGOL based Simulation Language
CACM, Sept. 1966.

[16] F.L. BAUER
Software Engineering
Proc. IFIP Congress 71, Ljubljana, Aug. 1971.

[17] P. NAUR, B. RANDELL (eds)
Software Engineering
NATO Conference, Garmisch, Jan. 1969.

[18] J.N. BUXTON, B. RANDELL (eds)
Software Engineering Techniques
NATO Conference, Rome, April 1970.

[19] F.L. BAUER (ed)
Advanced Course in Software Engineering
Lecture Notes in Mathematics and Economical Systems, 81, Springer Verlag, 1973.

[20] E.W. DIJKSTRA
      Notes on Structured Programming
      Report 241, Technische Hogeschool, Eindhoven, 1969.

[21] Machine Oriented Languages Bulletin
      Published periodically under the auspices of WG2.4 of IFIP.

[22] H.D. MILLS
      Mathematical Foundations for Structured Programming
      Report FSC 72-6012, IBM, 1972.

[23] R.W. FLOYD
      Assigning Meanings to Programs
      Proc. Symp. in App. Math., Vol. 19, AMS, 1967.

[24] M. GRIFFITHS
      Notes from the summer school, Marktoberdorf, Aug., 1975.

[25] J. COURTIN, J. VOIRON
      Introduction à l'algorithmique et aux structures de données
      Traduction de schémas de programme en FORTRAN
      Université de Grenoble, 1975.

[26] W.L. VAN DER POEL, L.A. MAARSSEN (eds)
      Machine Oriented Higher Level Languages
      North Holland, 1974.

[27] C. KAISER
      Quelques problèmes de Parallélisme et leurs solutions par Sémaphore
      ESOPE/A/019, IRIA, Nov. 1971.

ELEMENTE DES ÄRZTLICHEN ERKENNTNISPROZESSES

F. Hartmann, Hannover

I DIAGNOSTIK UND DIAGNOSE

Unter Diagnostik verstehen wir den methodisch geleiteten Weg der ärztlichen Erkenntnis. Jedoch deckt das Wort dia-gnoscein zwei unterschiedliche Ziele:

1. Das Durchunddurch-Erkennen, Durchschauen, mit dem Ziel einer Erklärung des krankhaften Geschehens.

2. Das Auseinander-Kennen, das Unterscheiden (Differential-Diagnose) mit dem Ziel, die krankhaften Erscheinungen eines Kranken einem bekannten Bild, einem Typus von krankhafter Veranstaltung der Natur zuzuordnen; es ist ein Wiedererkennen, pattern recognition.

Die Methode für den ersten Fall ist die der Analyse, der Rückführung der einzelnen Ereignisse, Beschwerden, Befunde, Daten auf ihre Ursachen und Bedingungen. Es wird ein zeitlicher Zusammenhang zwischen einzelnen Ereignissen hergestellt (Pathogenese), auch wenn Gleichzeitiges von zeitlich aufeinander Folgendem unterschieden wird.

Im zweiten Fall ist das Verfahren das Vergleichen. Es ist um so zuverlässiger, je deutlicher das Krankheitsbild bekannt ist. Wenn in einem Fall nach verborgenen Befunden (röntgenologisch, laborchemisch, histologisch) gesucht wird, so dient die Analyse des Falles der bestmöglichen Vervollständigung des Bildes, des Musters mit dem Ziel größtmöglicher Zuverlässigkeit des Vergleichs, der richtigen Zuordnung. Wenn in diesem Zusammenhang von Intuition gesprochen wird, so handelt es sich nicht um eine angeborene Fähigkeit, sondern um ein geschultes Kombinationsvermögen für Beobachtetes, Gehörtes, Gelesenes.

Diagnostizieren ist ein Wechselspiel von Denkprozessen und Handlungen, ein Untersuchungs- und Entscheidungsverfahren. Diagnose ist eine Aussage, daß ein individuelles Geschehen einem allgemeinen Begriff, dem Namen für eine Krankheit zugeordnet, ihm subsumiert werden kann.

Der Begriff der Diagnose ist deswegen so unscharf und mißverständlich, weil er benutzt wird:

1. für das Ergebnis der Suche nach einer Erklärung,
2. für die Aussage, daß eine individuelle Krankheit einem
   Typus, einem Bild, einem anerkannten Muster angehört, mit
   ihm übereinstimmt,
3. für den Namen der Krankheit.

Die beiden Wege des Diagnostizierens münden also in einem Ziel, der Namensgebung.

Viele Gründe haben es verhindert, daß diese Situation kritisch überprüft wird. Diese Gründe sind:

1. Praktisch; die Diagnose dient:
   a) der Benennung und Einordnung beobachteter krankhafter
      Ereignisse,

b) der Begründung für diagnostische Tätigkeiten,
c) der Rechtfertigung von therapeutischen Maßnahmen.

2. Historisch:
a) Krankheiten werden als natürliche Gestalten wie Mineralien, Pflanzen, Tiere, chemische Elemente angesehen; sie sind Parasiten mit einer natürlichen Existenz außerhalb des Kranken; sie haben ihre eigene Naturgeschichte. Sie wachsen, blühen, reifen und verdorren (SYDENHAM). Man spricht von ontologischem Krankheitsbegriff oder substantieller Krankheitsauffassung.

b) Krankheiten haben eine natürliche Ordnung in Klassen, richtige Klassifikation wäre ein treues Abbild der Natur.

c) Die Namen der Krankheiten geben die Natureinheit, die diese Merkmale hat, wieder. Das ideale diagnostische System ist identisch mit dem natürlichen.

3. Wissenschaftlich:
a) Ärzte interpretieren das Stellen einer Diagnose, das Machen eines diagnostischen Urteils (clinical judgment), das Schlußfolgern aus Beobachtungen als Anwendung der induktiven Methode.

b) Ärzte halten den diagnostischen Prozeß für ein dem natur-wissenschaftlichen Experiment analoges Verfahren. Induktive Methode und Gewinnung von Erfahrungen gelten ihnen als Ausweis von Wissenschaftlichkeit.

c) Eine diagnostische Erkenntnis wird mit einer wissenschaft-lichen Erkenntnis gleichgesetzt.

Diese Konstellationen von Bedingungen verhindern es, daß der Begriff der Diagnose in Frage gestellt wird. Man fürchtet die damit verbundene Verunsicherung. Das weist auf verdrängte Ängste um die Wissenschaftlichkeit, Gesichertheit der ärztlichen Verfahren und um das Ansehen in der Öffentlichkeit und in der Scientifique Society hin. Man schämt sich der Merkmale Handeln und Anwenden im theoretischen und tiefenpsychologischen Unterbau ärztlichen Selbstverständnisses. Durch den Sozialisationsprozeß ist der Begriff der Diagnose mit starken Gefühlen des Erfolges, der Selbstbestätigung, des Stolzes und der Selbstrechtfertigung besetzt. Der Zwang zur Standardisierung der Verfahren - um einen verlässlichen ärztlichen Dienst unter variablen Bedingungen zu sichern - führt in der Medizin so zu einer Mythologisierung des Begriffs Diagnose und zu einer Ritualisierung der Verfahren. Deswegen ist es notwendig, Aufgabe und Möglichkeiten der Diagnose auf ihren rationalen Kern zurückzuführen und von Gefühlen zu befreien.

Wenn ärztliche Erkenntnis, die zu einer Aussage, der Diagnose führt, nicht Ergebnis eines induktiven Schlußverfahrens ist, muß die Frage gestellt werden, wie sie in moderne Vorstellungen der Wissenschafts- und Erkenntnistheorie einzuordnen ist.

Karl POPPER hat für die Entwicklung der Wissenschaften ein Schema vorgeschlagen, dem man etwa folgende Form als Flußdiagramm geben kann.

Allgemeiner Forschungsprozess- einzelner Erkenntnisvorgang

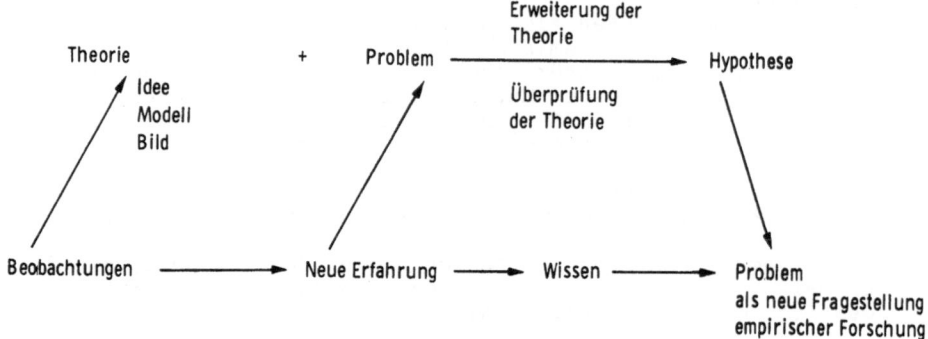

Es soll nun untersucht werden, ob dieses wissenschaftshistorische Modell übertragbar ist auf die Geschichte, die Zeitgestalt der Lösung diagnostischer Probleme im Einzelfall.

Der Arzt geht mit einem Vorwissen, das zum Teil seiner unspezifischen Lebenserfahrung, seinem Studium und seinen bisherigen Berufserfahrungen entstammt, in einen konkreten diagnostischen Prozeß hinein. Zu seiner theoretischen Ausrüstung gehören auch die Krankheitsbilder, die er gelernt und gesehen hat. Eine neue Beobachtung versucht er nun in Übereinstimmung zu bringen mit diesen Bildern, er vergleicht, versucht zur Deckung zu bringen. Er bringt Beobachtung eines Falles und Typus ihm bekannter Bilder in einen problematischen Zusammenhang. Problematisch ist dieser Zusammenhang schon dann, wenn er die diagnostischen Begriffe, die Klassifikation und Namen ebenso für vorläufig hält, wie seine Beobachtungen, denen es an letzter Genauigkeit und Vollständigkeit mangelt. Um das Problem zu lösen, müssen neue Erfahrungswerte eingebracht werden, meist gezielte Untersuchungen. Der Arzt erwartet in der Regel, daß seine Theorien bestätigt werden, seine Bilder und Modelle zu den Beobachtungswirklichkeiten passen. Wenn ihm das nicht gelingt, so zweifelt er zunächst an den Beobachtungen, nicht aber an der Wirklichkeit und Gültigkeit der Bilder und Modelle. Jeder neue Fall kann zu einer Überprüfung oder einer Erweiterung der Theorie Anlaß geben: Aus dem praktischen Problem wird ein wissenschaftliches. Jeder neue Fall, der einer Theorie eingefügt wird, um ein Problem zu lösen, macht die Theorie vorübergehend zu einer Hypothese, d.h. er erweitert die Theorie um ein bisher in ihr noch nicht vorkommendes Element. Jede neue Beobachtung prüft also die Theorie, stellt sie in Frage. Diagnosen sind immer nur Aussagen für einen besonderen Einzelfall. Eine Betrachtung relativ kurzer Zeiträume in der Medizin überzeugt einen schon vom ständigen Wandel der Diagnosen, der Vorläufigkeit, ihrer Namen, Gültigkeiten und Klassifikationen. Dem historisch-kritischen Arzt offenbaren sie ihren Charakter als Konstrukte, die die Wirklichkeit zu simulieren suchen.

Wenn ein Einzelfall nicht in befriedigender Weise mit einem Bild, einem Modell, einer Theorie in Übereinstimmung zu bringen ist, so geht der diagnostische Prozeß vom Vergleichen zum Erklären über. An diesem Übergang müssen Probleme formuliert werden, die die nicht übereinstimmenden Teile der neuen Beobachtung und der bekannten Bilder und Theorien enthalten. Hierher gehört das Verfahren der Ausschlußdiagnose. Dazu werden Probleme formuliert, auf die die Nichtzugehörigkeit als Antwort erwartet wird.

H - O - Schema der deduktiv — nomologischen Erklärung

nach Hempel und Oppenheim (1948)

G_1, G_2	Gesetze, Hypothesen (allgemeine Gültigkeit; empirischer Gehalt)	Explanans
A_1, A_2	Antecedensbedingungen (Randbedingungen nach Popper)	

E	Das zu erklärende Ereignis	Explanandum

Anwendungen : Begriffsbestimmung (Explikation) von Diagnose, Prognose

G_1, G_2 .... + A_1, A_2 .... $\longrightarrow$ E   Deduktion, Prognose

A_1, A_2 .... + E $\longrightarrow$ G_1, G_2 ....   Wissenschaftliche Entdeckung

E   + G_1, G_2 .... $\longrightarrow$ A_1, A_2 ....   Hypothese, Diagnose

Folgerung : Gleiche logische Struktur von Erklärung, Diagnose, Prognose

Im folgenden will ich den Versuch machen, die Diagnose als Formulierung ärztlicher Erkenntnis in die Schematik der Aussage-Logik der modernen Wissenschaftstheorie einzuordnen. Das gilt besonders für das deduktiv-nomologische Modell nach HEMPEL und OPPENHEIM. Dieses verbindet einen empirischen Sachverhalt, der erklärt werden soll (E = Explanandum) und eine allgemeine Aussage (G = Gesetz) mit Hilfe einer Feststellung von Randbedingungen (A = Antecedensbedingungen).

Beispiel:

Erklärt werden soll eine Zuckerausscheidung im Urin und eine Blutzuckersteigerung bei Herrn X. Das ist das Explanandum (E), das zu Erklärende.

Das allgemeine Gesetz, das zur Erklärung herangezogen wird, lautet: Wenn die Zuckerausscheidung im Urin bei hohem Blutzucker auftritt, liegt ein Diabetes mellitus vor.

Um das Explanans, das Erklärungsgefüge aus G + A zu vervollständigen, muß ich die Antecedensbedingung einführen: "Herr X hat einen Diabetes mellitus".

Man erkennt nun, daß eine Diagnose den logischen Schluß aus der Zuordnung eines Explanandums zu einem allgemeinen Gesetz zieht:

$$G + E = A.$$

Eine Diagnose nennt die Antecedensbedingungen. Sie wird zu einer vorläufigen Annahme, wenn ich sie als Bindeglied zwischen einem allgemeinen Gesetz und einem Muster von Symptomen benutze.

Es handelt sich hier um ein rein logisches, also formales Verfahren der Erklärung von Sachverhalten und Sachzusammenhängen, Explanation. Ich benutze, wie die meisten Naturwissenschaftler, den Begriff Erklärung für eine vollständig empirisch durch wiederholte Beobachtung verschiedener Beobachter oder durch Experiment belegbare Aufklärung kausaler Zusammenhänge zwischen den einzelnen Komponenten eines Ereignisses. Das wird aber im deduktiv-nomothetischen Verfahren nicht angestrebt. Es ist nicht kausalanalytisch.

Für die Anwendbarkeit dieses logischen Verfahrens in der praktischen Medizin müssen die einzelnen Komponenten der D-N-Schlußfigur untersucht werden.

1. In der Medizin stehen für die Gesetze die Begründungen für die Einheitlichkeit (Substanz) eines diagnostischen Begriffs. Diesem Begriff liegt eine wenn-dann-Aussage zugrunde. Diese ist in der Regel statistischer Natur, sagt also eine Wahrscheinlichkeit aus. Sie ist gültig innerhalb einer Konvention, eines Systems diagnostischer Begriffe. Erklärungen, die diesen Typ von allgemeiner Aussage benutzen, nennt man auch induktiv-statistische. Ich vermag aber nicht zu erkennen, wie ein Verfahren, in dem eine statistische Wahrscheinlichkeit an die Stelle eines Gesetzes tritt, sich von der Deduktion zur Induktion wandeln soll. Denn Kern des Verfahrens bleibt die Zuordnung, die Subsumption eines Explanandums, eines Ereignisses unter einem allgemeinen Begriff.

2. Das Explanandum, das richtig einzuordnende Ereignis, hat ebenfalls die Form einer Aussage. Diese Aussage ist selbst problematisch; denn die Beobachtungen, Beschwerden und Meßwerte werden vorläufig zusammengefaßt, als ob sie eine Einheit bildeten. Es ist aber möglich, daß ein Kranker 2 oder 3 Krankheiten gleichzeitig hat. Dann gehören die Beobachtungswerte mehreren Krankheiten zu. Das Explanandum besteht in Wirklichkeit in diesem Falle aus mehreren Explananda. Diese Möglichkeit muß immer offengehalten werden.

3. Die Formulierung der Antecedensbedingungen ist eine Aussage über eine Vermutung, eine vorläufige Annahme. Wenn eines oder beide Glieder des Vorsatzes (G, E) problematisch sind, ist auch die Aussage einer Diagnose problematisch. Ist die allgemeine Annahme eine Wahrscheinlichkeitsaussage, so ist auch die Diagnose nur wahrscheinlich. Ist der Aufbau des Explanandums aus seinen empirischen Inhalten vorläufig, so ist es auch die Diagnose.

Die Anwendung des formal-logischen Verfahrens der deduktiv-nomologischen Erklärung nach HEMPEL und OPPENHEIM in der Medizin, in der Aufhellung der Struktur ärztlicher Aussagen über diagnostische Erkenntnisse, ist begrenzt. Ihr Wert liegt in dem Nachweis der gleichen logischen Struktur von Diagnose, Prognose und wissenschaftlicher Erkenntnis. Im Falle der Prognose ist das Explanandum nicht gegeben, sondern es wird gesucht. Es ist das zukünftige, zu erwartende Ereignis. Dieses wird deduziert aus der Übereinstimmung von vorliegenden Antecedensbedingungen mit einem Krankheitsbegriff,für dessen zugehörige Krankheit statistische Wahrscheinlichkeiten zukünftiger Ereignisse bekannt sind. PEIRCE hat den Schritt E + G als Hypothese bezeichnet. DUCASSE hat aber bereits erkannt, daß der gleiche Schritt der Weg seiner diagnostischen Aussage ist. Es überrascht nicht, daß Diagnose und Hypothese die gleiche logische Struktur und Stellung im Erklärungsverfahren haben. Diese Gemeinsamkeit tritt noch deutlicher hervor, wenn man dem Hinweis WIELANDs folgt, daß das Antecedens, die diagnostische Aussage, keinen eigenen empirischen Gehalt hat, der überprüfbar wäre. Die empirische Stütze findet das Antecedens Diagnose im Explanandum. Ich möchte hinzufügen, daß es seine empirische Absicherung aber auch durch die Gesetzesaussage oder die

Wahrscheinlichkeitsaussage erhält. WIELAND schreibt: "Die Richtigkeit einer Diagnose läßt sich also immer nur dadurch bestätigen, daß sie - und unter Voraussetzung des Systems der Krankheitsbegriffe nur sie - die verlangte Erklärung auch wirklich leisten kann". Ich gebe WIELAND darin Recht, wenn er zwischen dem deduktiv-nomologischen oder dem induktiv-statistischen Erklärungsmodell und dem diagnostischen Prozeß nur eine Analogie sieht. Der Versuch dieser Analogie zeigt aber außerdem, daß die diagnostische Aussage immer nur gültig für den einzelnen Fall ist; die wissenschaftliche Aussage dagegen zielt auf allgemeine Gültigkeit. Eine Diagnose ist immer nur die Darstellung eines Beispiels für einen übergeordneten Begriff, im günstigsten Fall ein Gesetz, in der Regel eine Wahrscheinlichkeit. Ein Name, nicht eine wissenschaftliche Erkenntnis, verbindet beide. Für die Formulierung der Diagnose genannten Aussage ist es zweckmäßig, die Form des Problems zu wählen, wenn allgemeine Aussage und Struktur des Explanandums problematisch sind.

Die Aussage von WIELAND "die Diagnose ist keine Erklärung, sondern sie hat eine bestimmte Funktion in einer Erklärung" gilt, wenn man unter Erklärung nur die Reihenfolge:

Diagnostischer Begriff + Diagnose = Erklärung für Symptom-
konstellation

versteht. Das Verfahren ist also nur im Rahmen einer Konvention über gut begründete und allgemein angenommene diagnostische Begriffe möglich. Die Grenzen der Schlüssigkeit der Aussagen ärztlich-diagnostischer Art werden deutlich, wenn man erkennt, daß die wenn-dann-Folge auf mehreren Ebenen wiederkehrt.

G	+	E	$\longrightarrow$	A
<u>Wenn</u> die Bedingungen x, y... vorliegen, <u>dann</u> trifft der Begriff Krankheitsname = N zu.		<u>Wenn</u> alle Beobachtungsdaten zusammengehören, <u>dann</u> liegt ein einheitliches Explanandum vor.		<u>Wenn</u> E mit G zur Deckung zu bringen ist, <u>dann</u> hat dieser Kranke die Krankheit N.

Die Folge G + A $\longrightarrow$ E führt gar nicht zu einer Diagnose. Sie führt auch nicht zu pathogenetischen Aussagen, wenn nicht G außer durch statistische Symptomkonstellationen auch durch Kausalanalysen definiert ist. Eine Erklärung von E im wissenschaftlichen Sinne liegt nur dann vor, wenn festgestellt wird: für den kausalen Zusammenhang der Inhalte des Explanandums gelten auch die pathogenetischen Begründungen für die Einheitlichkeit von G. Eine wissenschaftliche neue Erkenntnis liegt vor, wenn G bisher nur statistisch, als Syndrom definiert war, es aber in einem Einzelfall gelingt, die kausalen Zusammenhänge aufzuklären. Dieser Fall würde sich so darstellen:

$$E \quad + \quad A_{mult.} \quad \longrightarrow \quad G.$$

Es gibt Fälle, in denen die Analyse eines einzigen Falles genügt, z.B. die Entdeckung eines Enzymdefektes oder eines Gendefektes als Ursache von Stoffwechsellücken und zugehörigen Symptomen. In der Regel bedarf es vieler A ($A_{mult.}$), um zu einer statistischen Aussage hoher Allgemeinheit, G, zu kommen.

Die Wahl eines Namens für ein vom Arzt beobachtetes krankhaftes Geschehen, eine Diagnose, ist also weniger eine Erklärung als ein Urteil, eine Beurteilung. Diagnose ist ein handlungstheoretischer Begriff. Er begründet Handlungen und löst sie aus. Diagnosen werden zum

Zweck von Handlungen gestellt. Sie stellen die Ereignisse krankhaften Geschehens für ein zweckmäßiges Handeln zurecht. WIELAND nennt deswegen eine Diagnose eine praktische Aussage.

Wenn die auf Handlungen ausgerichteten Funktionen der Diagnose ihr wesentliches Kennzeichen sind, dann muß die Kritik, die Wahl einer Diagnose zwei Einflußfelder berücksichtigen:

1. Die Bedingungen, unter denen der Arzt erkennt, urteilt, ordnet, Diagnostik veranstaltet.
2. Die Zwecke, die eine Diagnose erfüllen soll.

In beiden Feldern sind die Bedingungen und Zwecke vielfach variabel. Die Wahl hat Ursachen und Folgen. Diagnostische Begriffe, Namen für krankhaftes Geschehen, vermitteln zwischen den Ausgangsbedingungen und den Zwecken in einer Weise, die justitiabel im Sinne von Versicherungen, Gerichten und Verwaltungen, wissenschaftlich begründbar, legitimierend dem Kranken und seiner Mitwelt gegenüber und kommunikabel im System der Gesundheitsdienste sein soll. Wenn die Diagnose eine vermittelnde Aussage in einem so vielgestaltigen Handlungsgefüge ist, muß auch nach einer Aussagepraxis gesucht werden, die der praktischen Aussagefunktion der Diagnose gerecht wird. Diese wird von mir in der Problemorientiertheit ärztlichen Denkens und Handelns gesucht.

Im folgenden sollen die beide Fragen untersucht werden:

1. Wie kommen praktische Aussagen, Diagnosen, zustande?
2. Was sollen die praktischen Aussagen bewirken?

WIELAND bemerkt zu Recht, daß das Stellen einer Diagnose schon selbst eine Handlung ist. Jedoch geht er nach meiner Auffassung zu weit, wenn er daraus einen wesentlichen Unterschied zwischen einer Hypothese und einer Diagnose ableitet. Sein Argument ist, daß eine Hypothese ohne Folgen bleibt, eine Diagnose die praktischen Folgen, z.B. Therapie, immer mit einschließt. Die Beobachtung der Folgen eines praktischen Handelns aufgrund einer Diagnose ist auch immer die Überprüfung der Richtigkeit dieser Diagnose. Aber auch eine Hypothese geht in ihre Überprüfung über, z.B. in ein Experiment. Mit diesem Experiment wird die Hypothese überprüft. Natürlich kann derjenige, der die Hypothese aufgestellt hat, auf ihre Überprüfung verzichten. Genausogut kann und muß - in gewissen Situationen, z.B. der Allgemeinmedizin - der Arzt die Diagnose abwartend offenlassen. Stellt er jedoch eine Diagnose, so ist die praktische Schlußfolgerung unausweichlich. Diese Unterscheidung von der notwendigen Überprüfung einer Hypothese ist aber nur graduell und nicht grundsätzlich. Der Wissenschaftler, der auf die experimentelle Überprüfung einer Hypothese verzichtet, riskiert nur seinen Ruf als Wissenschaftler. Man setzt aber sein Ansehen als Arzt aufs Spiel, wenn man eine Diagnose ohne praktische Folgen läßt. Nur für die Praxis der Schlußfolgerungen, nicht aber für die logische Struktur gilt der von WIELAND gemachte Unterschied zwischen Hypothese und Diagnose. Er stützt diesen Unterschied vor allen Dingen auf das ernst zu nehmende Argument, daß die Handlungsfolgen aus einer Diagnose irreversibel sind; denn der Handlungszwang schließt sich zeitlich unmittelbar an die Entscheidung für eine Diagnose an. Das gilt für das Tun und für das Unterlassen. Die Überprüfung einer Hypothese kann herausgeschoben werden. Die Hypothese kann durch eine andere ersetzt werden, bevor eine Überprüfung stattfindet oder es können mehrere Hypothesen alternativ zur Überprüfung gestellt werde. Das Stadium der Differentialdiagnose ist diesem Stadium der Hypothesenüberprüfung kongruent; denn solange der differentialdiagnostische Prozeß nicht abgeschlossen ist, liegt auch noch keine Diagnose mit Handlungsfolgen vor.

Die folgende Abbildung gibt die Einflußgrößen wieder, die dazu führen, daß das krankhafte Geschehen bei einem Kranken mit einem Namen, einem legitimierten Krankheitsbegriff, benannt wird. Auf der linken Seite sind die Bedingungen aufgeführt, unter denen der Arzt eine diagnostische Aussage erarbeitet. Sie beeinflussen wesentlich die Wahl von Begriffen. Das erkennt man daraus, daß Ärzte unter vergleichbaren Praxisbedingungen einmal viele, ein andermal wenige diagnostische Begriffe verwenden. Frau L. VON FERBER hat gezeigt, daß Allgemeinärzte und Fachärzte für den gleichen krankhaften Sachverhalt nicht nur verschiedene, sondern auch mehr oder weniger Namen benutzen. Da auch der vom Arzt oft geübte diagnostische Prozeß gewisse Gewohnheiten einschleift, wirken die Häufigkeiten, mit denen ein Arzt bestimmte Diagnosen stellt, auf seine Aufmerksamkeit und Erwartung zurück. Das kann dazu führen, daß im Laufe seines Lebens die häufigen Krankheiten immer häufiger und die seltenen Krankheiten immer seltener werden. Das ist bisher bei der Aufstellung von sog. Fälleverteilungsgesetzen in ärztlichen Praxen nicht beachtet worden.

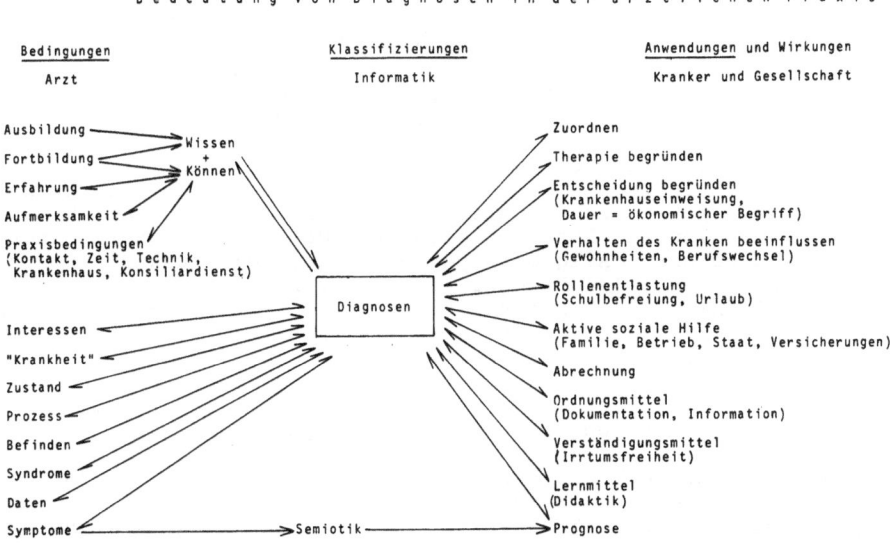

Auf der rechten Seite des Schemas sind die Zwecke aufgeführt, denen Diagnosen dienen, wenn sie einmal gestellt sind. Es ist also das Gefüge von Handlungen, die aus einer Diagnose folgen. Auch hier ist leicht einzusehen, daß die Zwecke, besonders auch die Häufigkeiten, mit denen sie angestrebt werden, auf die Wahl der diagnostischen Begriffe durch den Arzt zurückwirken. Eine Krankheit, an die der Arzt während des diagnostischen Prozesses nicht denkt, kann er auch nicht diagnostizieren. Sein Wissen ist also ein Rahmen oder ein Sieb, das die Wahl diagnostischer Begriffe, seine Aussagefähigkeit für die Beschreibung krankhafter Prozesse auf das ihm Bekannte begrenzt. Dieses Wissen entstammt seiner Ausbildung. Es hängt davon ab, wie beflissen er während seiner Berufstätigkeit das Wissen durch Fortbildung ergänzt,

überprüft oder ersetzt. Schließlich hängt es davon ab, wie er seine
ärztlichen Erfahrungen reflektiert. Einen großen Einfluß auf die Zahl
wählbarer Begriffe üben die organisatorischen und technischen
Praxisbedingungen aus, z.B. welchen persönlichen Kontakt der Arzt mit
seinen Kranken hat, das Vorwissen, das er aus einer gemeinsamen
Lebenswelt mit den Kranken, z.B. als Allgemeinarzt, mitbringt, die
Zeit, die er für einen Kranken aufwenden kann, Zahl, Häufigkeit und
Breite von Laboratoriumsuntersuchungen. So werden in Krankenhäusern und
von Fachärzten mehr und andere Begriffe zur Kennzeichnung krankhaften
Geschehens verwendet als in Allgemeinpraxen. Andererseits differenziert
der Allgemeinarzt ein Krankheitsbild mehr nach den Varianten
individueller Ausprägung. Die Möglichkeit, einen Konsiliarius in
unklaren Fällen zuzuziehen, bestimmt ebenfalls das Begriffsspektrum,
das ein Arzt verwendet. Aus all diesen Bedingungen baut sich für jeden
Arzt eine bestimmte Aufmerksamkeits- und Erwartungshaltung angesichts
seines Krankengutes und den darin verborgenen krankhaften Zuständen und
Verläufen aus.

Die zweite Gruppe von beim Arzt liegenden Bedingungen der Erkennung,
Unterscheidung und Benennung von Krankhaftem beruhen auf
Vorentscheidungen des Arztes darüber, was er unter einer "Einheit
krank" verstehen will. Die einen verstehen unter Krankheit nur die in
Lehrbüchern niedergelegten klassischen Krankheitsbilder. Andere folgen
mehr der Syndromatik häufiger Symptomkonstellationen. Seit eh und je
hat es in der Medizin eine Einstellung gegeben, auch einem Symptom den
Wert einer Krankheit zu geben, besonders, wenn es die den Patienten am
meisten belästigende Beschwerde oder die sein Leben am meisten
bedrohende Veränderung ist. Wenn in diesen Fällen dem Symptom nicht der
Rang einer Diagnose eingeräumt wird, trotzdem aber eine Handlung, z.B.
die Abwehr eines gefährlichen Verlaufes abgeleitet wird, haben wir den
Fall einer Medizin ohne Diagnose vor uns. Die sogenannten
Allgemeinsymptome haben schon immer in der Semiotik an der Diagnose
vorbei zu prognostischen Aussagen geführt; denn die Prognose hängt im
Einzelfall von solchen Allgemeinsymptomen ab, die Auskunft darüber
geben, ob der Patient leicht oder schwer krank ist, ob der Verlauf
günstig, zweifelhaft oder hoffnungslos ist. Die Zuordnung zu einer
Diagnose ist im Einzelfall nur eine statistische Hilfe. Entscheidender
ist die Aussagekraft der Allgemeinsymptome im vorliegenden Fall.
Insofern war schon immer und ist auch heute die Prognose eine Medizin
ohne Diagnose, aber die Vernachlässigung der Einübung der Semiotik hat
leider zu ihrer einseitigen Bindung an die Diagnose geführt.

In der Einstufung dessen, was eine Krankheitseinheit ist, unterscheiden
sich die Ärzte auch in Bezug auf bevorzugte Einstellungen, auf
Krankheitszustände oder Krankheitsprozesse. Die einen sehen das
Wesentliche eines Krankseins im Befinden des Kranken, die anderen in
den Befunden der Laboratorien. Wissenschaftsgeschichtliche Einflüsse
und wissenschaftstheoretische Entscheidungen gehen also in das
Auswahlverhalten des Arztes vielfältig ein. Seine Interessen können
unterschiedlich gerichtet sein auf die Person des Kranken, der sich mit
dem Leiden auseinandersetzt oder auf die meßbaren Ereignisse, die im
oder am Kranken geschehen. All dies würde erkennbar sein, wenn die
Ärzte ihre Beobachtungen und Beurteilungen in einem oder mehreren
Sätzen beschreibend zusammenfaßten. Bringen sie die Bedingungen, die
die Aussage vorbereiteten, aber auf einen Begriff, so deckt dieser die
Hintergründe zu. Es ist dann auch nicht erkennbar, warum ein bestimmter
Arzt einen bestimmten Fall auf diese und nicht auf eine andere Weise
benannte und zuordnete.

Die Herkunft diagnostischer Begriffe im allgemeinen, in dem
Wahlverhalten eines bestimmten Arztes und im Fall eines einzelnen
Kranken aufzuhellen, ist nur bedingt Aufgabe ärztlicher Informatik, die
im Unterschied zur medizinischen Informatik das ärztliche Verhalten mit

einbezieht. Sie ist aber Aufgabe einer Wissenssoziologie der Ärzte und einer Wissenschaftssoziologie der Medizin.

Als praktische Wissenschaft ist die Medizin auch vielfältig in ihr soziales Umfeld verflochten. Ihre Begriffe müssen deswegen praktikabel sein. Diagnosen haben praktische Funktionen. Sie ordnen die Folgen des Krankseins eines Individuums für die mitmenschliche Umgebung. Sie ordnen das kranke Individuum und seine Krankheiten in das System der Medizin ein und sie organisieren und aktivieren die Hilfsmechanismen, die die Medizin und die Gesellschaft bereitstellen. In den Kommunikationsprozeß mit dem Kranken selbst gehen die Funktionen Begründung für weitere diagnostische Schritte und Therapien, Beratung über Lebensweise, Anleitung zum Einhalten therapeutischer Maßnahmen und die Prognose ein. Die Organisation sozialer Hilfe bezieht sich auf die Befreiung von Verpflichtungen sozialer Rollen, Aktivierung von Hilfen in der Familie und anderer Einrichtungen, Auslösung von Versicherungsmaßnahmen, vorübergehende oder dauernde Freistellung von Arbeit. Das Begründen bestimmter Therapien gehört überall dort zur Sozialwirksamkeit einer Diagnose, wo öffentliche Mittel kontrollierbar eingesetzt werden: Krankenhauseinweisung, Kurverschickung, Verordnungen, deren Notwendigkeit und Kostspieligkeit von Prüfungsgremien, z.B. den kassenärztlichen Vereinigungen überprüft werden. Diagnostische Begriffe gelten also auch für Abrechnungsverfahren und haben eine Funktion in der Sicherung des Unterhaltes für den Arzt. Im System Medizin dienen die diagnostischen Begriffe dem Zuordnen des Krankheitsgeschehens in einem allgemein akzeptierten Klassifikationssystem. Dieser Schritt ist notwendig für die Dokumentation und alle Formen der Information. Diagnostische Begriffe sind Verständigungsmittel; da sie unscharf sind, bedarf es einer hohen Redundanz, damit ihr Gebrauch möglichst irrtumsfrei ist. Diese Redundanz wird dadurch erreicht, daß die Nennung eines Begriffs einem zu Informierenden gegenüber bei dem auf diese Weise Informierten ein Gefüge von Aussagen zu diesem Begriff aktiviert oder daß zum Beispiel in Epikrisen, Arztbriefen und Nachrichten an Versicherungen die Diagnose mit zusätzlichen redundanten Aussagen begründet wird. Schließlich werden alle Prognosen, seien sie für den Kranken selbst, seine Angehörigen oder für Versicherungen abgegeben, durch einen diagnostischen Begriff begründet und abgesichert.

Kommen wir von dieser Analyse der Multikonditionalität und Multifungiobilität diagnostischer Begriffe, ihrer Geschichte, ihrem Zustandekommen im Einzelfall und ihrer öffentlichen Wirkung zu ihrer Funktion und Stellung in einer Theorie ärztlicher Erkenntnis- und Urteilsbildung, so erfassen wir das am besten durch das folgende Schema. Es geht von 4 Fragen aus, die dem Arzt in jedem Fall zur Beantwortung gestellt sind. Die Antworten auf diese Fragen bilden die Elemente eines Begründungszusammenhanges. Die Zusammenführung von Erkenntnis und Erklärung nennen wir eine diagnostische Aussage oder Diagnose. Das wird mit einem Namen bezeichnet. Die Beibehaltung dieser Bezeichnung wird im Verlauf der Krankheit durch das Eintreten oder Nichteintreten vorauszusagender Ereignisse ständig kontrolliert. Das ist aber nur dann möglich, wenn die Prognose nicht vollständig abhängig von der Diagnose ist, gewissermaßen eine Funktion der Diagnose. Die Möglichkeit der Überprüfung - Verwerfung oder Bestätigung - der Diagnose durch die Prognose ist nur dann gegeben, wenn die Prognose bestimmende empirische Inhalte hat, die in der Diagnose nicht vorkommen. Das sind die in der Semiotik zusammengefaßten allgemeinen Krankheitszeichen.

Auch das ärztliche Handeln, das sich dem Einzelnen und der Öffentlichkeit gegenüber rechtfertigen und verantworten muß, strebt eine größtmögliche Sicherheit ihrer Urteils- und Entscheidungsverfahren an. Deswegen ist das Schema auf den Begriff des Beweises hin angelegt.

Schema der ärztlichen und Urteilsbildung

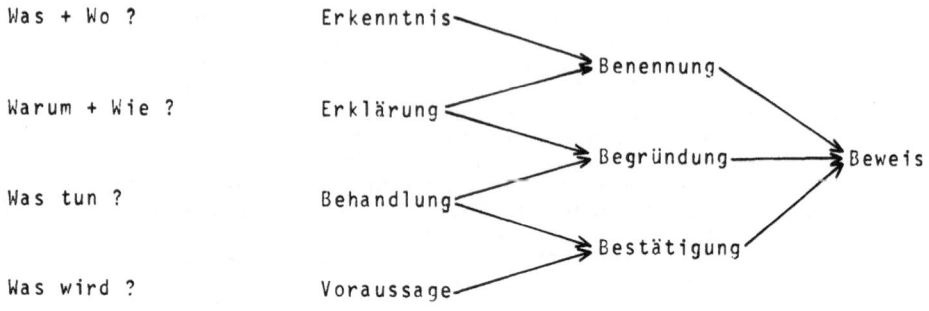

Er wird gebraucht in Analogie zum mathematischen und juristischen Beweis, d.h. als Indizienbeweis vom Typ der Schlußfolgerung wenn-dann. Dadurch, daß die richtige Diagnose, die zutreffend gestellte Prognose und die erfolgreiche Behandlung übereinstimmen, wird bewiesen, daß die 4 gestellten Fragen richtig beantwortet wurden. Das Schema will vor allem zeigen, daß die Diagnose als Beweismaterial nicht ausreicht. In der Theorie erkenntnisgeleiteten ärztlichen Handelns hat sie aber eine bedeutsame Funktion. Wenn eine Erklärung wie unter den Bedingungen der Allgemeinpraxis oder von Notfallsituationen in der Intensivmedizin nicht möglich ist, sollte an die Stelle einer Benennung lediglich eine Beschreibung treten; denn der Beweis für die Richtigkeit des Handelns ist dann nur aus dem Erfolg der Behandlung und aus dem Eintreffen der Vorhersage zu erbringen.

Bei der Bewertung eines für einen Fall benutzten diagnostischen Begriffs als Information muß auch der medizinische Informatiker berücksichtigen:

1. Werden und Wandel der Namen für Krankheiten.
2. Das Wahlverhalten des Arztes.

Wir haben kein System von Naturkonstanten vor uns und keinen systematischen Katalog der Bezeichnungen, der einem Prinzip und Bauplan folgen würde. Jahrhunderte haben mit ihren Beobachtungen auch ihre Deutung, mit ihren Messungen auch ihre Vermutungen und Veranschaulichungen, mit den Erfahrungen auch die Theorien und mit den neutralen Beschreibungen auch ihre Metaphern in die Begriffe hineingelegt und sie zu einem unordentlichen Haufen getürmt. Eine Pyramide wurde es nicht. Von Zeit zu Zeit werden Teile dieses Haufen umgeschichtet. Geschichtlicher Wandel arbeitet an den Inhaltsverzeichnissen unserer klinischen Lehrbücher. Selbst unter der Oberfläche stabiler Begriffe ändern sich die Tatsachen. Beispiele sind Hepatitis und Pneumonie in den letzten 40 Jahren. Und die gleichen Tatsachen müssen sich andere Namen anbequemen. Beispiel: Myodegeneratio cordis --> Myokardfibrose --> congestive Cardiomyopathie. Ein Bewußtsein dieser Unschärfen - Definitionen sollen ja scharfe Grenzen zeigen und Termini sollen das Ende eines Begriffs, seine genaue Reichweite und Gültigkeit angeben - führte in den letzten Jahrzehnten zu deutlichen Unsicherheiten der Benennung und Begriffsbildung. Wo man früher eine neue Beobachtung in den Rang eines "Morbus" erhoben hätte, spricht man heute vorsichtiger und vorläufiger von Syndromen und Syntropien. Nosologie wird zunehmend schwieriger. Kaum jemand beschäftigt sich deswegen mit ihr. Aber es besteht ein Trend, sie zunehmend auf definierte pathogenetische Prozesse zu gründen. Für diese aber fehlt eine ausgearbeitete Begrifflichkeit.

Vielfalt und Wandel kennzeichnet auch die Wahlverhalten des Arztes für die diagnostischen Begriffe, die er verwendet. Der Motive seiner Vorzugs- und Lieblingsdiagnosen ist er sich ebensowenig bewußt wie der objektiven Bedingungen, die seine Möglichkeiten zu erkennen, zu benennen und zu ordnen begrenzen.

Werfen wir aber einen Blick zurück auf die vorwiegend sozialen Funktionen, die die Markierung eines Kranken mit einem Krankheitsbegriff hat, so verwirrt uns nicht nur deren Vielfalt. Es wird uns auch bewußt, welche Rückwirkungen sozialer Wandel, Änderungen im System der Gesundheitsdienste, der Versicherungen, der Arbeitsverhältnisse auf Wahl, Verwendung, Inhalt und sprachliche Form der diagnostischen Begriffe haben.

Der Alltag des Gebrauchs diagnostischer Begriffe stellt uns die Aussage-Praxis relativ stabil dar. Eine medizinische Informatik, die eine inhaltliche und formale Verbesserung dieser Aussagen anstrebt, muß aber aufmerksam sein für die Bewegung und Unruhe. Sie muß die Gründe dafür kennen und die Trends wahrnehmen. Tut sie das nicht, so reproduziert sie und stabilisiert sie nur das, was sie vorfindet. Wissenschaft wäre das nicht mehr. Nach meiner Auffassung sind medizinische Informatik und eine umfassende Theorie der Medizin nicht voneinander zu trennen. Aufgabe einer solchen Theorie ist es, die in den beiden vorstehenden Abbildungen wiedergegebenenen variablen Elemente der Medizin als praktische Wissenschaft zu verbinden mit den stabilen logischen Strukturen, die unser Verstand uns ermöglicht, aber auch vorschreibt.

II PROBLEMOFFENES ÄRZTLICHES VERHALTEN UND MEDIZINISCHE INFORMATIK

Der diagnostische Prozeß ist ein Vorgang der Erkenntnis, des Durchschauens, des einer Sache auf den Grund gehens. Eine Diagnose ist nicht sein eigentliches oder gar sein einziges Ziel. Die Wahl eines passenden diagnostischen Begriffs für einen komplexen krankhaften Vorgang ist ein rein deduktives Verfahren, ein Zuordnen, ein Subsumieren. Es hat keinen Anspruch auf Wissenschaftlichkeit. Es bietet keinen Ansatz für Innovationen. Es wird weder der Lage des Kranken noch der des Arztes, noch der der medizinischen Wissenschaft gerecht. Man wird in Zukunft der Kunst, Probleme formulieren zu können, einen höheren Rang einräumen müssen als der Einübung der Assoziationsfähigkeit im System diagnostischer Klassifikationen. Diese für den praktischen Gebrauch hilfreichen und notwendigen Ordnungen werden ihren Gewinn davon haben.

Es gibt gute Gründe, aus der Enge einer diagnostischen Begriffs-Scholastik immer wieder in die Offenheit von Problemformulierungen auszubrechen: Die Bruchstückhaftigkeit unseres Wissens, die Begrenztheit unseres Könnens, die Unsicherheiten der Vorhersagen, die einmaligen Anteile der Lagen von Kranken und Ärzten, die Lückenhaftigkeit der Verfügbarkeit von Wissen, Können und Organisation im konkreten Fall, die unterschiedlichen Wertigkeiten der Befunde.

Ein problemoffenes ärztliches Verhalten steht nicht unter dem Zwang, das an einem Kranken zu beobachtende und zu messende, von ihm gefühlte und erlebte krankhafte Geschehen auf einen Begriff bringen, es einem einzigen Typus zuordnen zu müssen, wobei das Individuelle, Persönliche des Krankseins und auch die einmalige Gestalt der Krankheit regelmäßig verlorengehen. Denn die Wirklichkeit eines Kranken wird nicht auf ein Problem gebracht, sondern in ein Gefüge, einen Satz von Problembeschreibungen.

Die gleiche komplexe Wirklichkeit wird von verschiedenen methodischen Ansätzen her betrachtet. Aber auch bei gleicher Methodik kann der Gesichtspunkt, die Fragerichtung eine andere sein. Es besteht auch kein Zwang, alle Probleme aufeinander zu beziehen, sie miteinander zu harmonisieren. Das Ganze der Problem-Beschreibungen muß angemessen wiedergeben: Die Lage des Kranken, die Lage des Arztes, den Stand der Erkenntnisse, die Bedingungen der Entscheidungen und Handlungen, die Folgen der Eingriffe, die Gründe für Erwartungen und Vorhersagen.

Die Unvollständigkeit und Inkongruenz des Problem-Gefüges ist selbst ein Problem, d.h. Aufforderung zur Verbesserung von Einsicht und Steigerung der Anstrengung. Ein problemorientiertes ärztliches Verhalten kann in Grenzen das ärztliche Dilemma überwinden, der Sachbezogenheit immer ein Stück Personbezogenheit zu opfern. Es kann das Typische mit dem Individuellen verbinden; es enthält nomothetische und ideographische Aussagen; es stellt Erklären und Verstehen, Messen und Werten gleichrangig nebeneinander.

Problemoffenes ärztliches Verhalten enthält die Eigenschaften angemessen, richtig, genau, gültig, vollständig. Die Aufgabe besteht darin, die Ergebnisse dieser Haltung, die natürlich die Qualität nachvollziehbarer, nachprüfbarer und intersubjektiv annehmbarer Erfahrungen und Aussagen haben müssen, in Information umzusetzen, die der medizinischen Informatik als ein Material dienen können, die über die bisherigen Zuordnungs-Verfahren hinausgehen. Die Anstrengungen der problemoffen arbeitenden Ärzte sind nur gerechtfertigt, wenn die medizinische Informatik aus den Ergebnissen Wege zur Verbesserung der Lage des Kranken und des Arztes in konkreter Lage, zur Steigerung der allgemeinen diagnostischen und therapeutischen Vermögen, zur größeren Genauigkeit der Unterscheidungen und Zuordnungen und schließlich in Aufgabenstellungen für klinische Forschung aufzeigt. Es ist aber auch erkennbar, welchen didaktischen Wert dieses problemorientierte Denken für Ärzte in der Ausbildung hat: Sie lernen, der Unabgeschlossenheit ärztlichen Handelns im Einzelfall und in der medizinischen Wissenschaft gerecht zu werden, auf Überraschungen vorbereitet, für Neues offen zu sein und all dies sich mit einem intellektuellen Handwerkszeug für zweckmäßiges Handeln zurechtzustellen. Mit Recht hat WEED deswegen das Instrument des problem-orientierten Krankenblattes für die Ausbildung zum Arzt entwickelt. Wenn die medizinische Informatik die Ergebnisse richtig nutzt, kommt ihr eine höhere Bedeutung für die Ausprägung und Aufrechterhaltung kritischer und wissenschaftlicher ärztlicher Haltungen zu als bei einer auf Katalogisierung, Klassifizierung, Diskriminierung gerichteten Einstellung, die schließlich in einer maschinellen Kanonisierung einer scholastischen Begriffswelt endet. Die Gefahr dazu ist angesichts der Gegenstandskataloge zur neuen Approbationsordnung (in der Bundesrepublik) groß genug.

Das problemgerichtete Denken in der Medizin wurde von L. L. WEED angestoßen und durch den Vorschlag seines problemorientierten Krankenblattes veranschaulicht. Anlaß und Zweck dazu waren erzieherisch: Das ärztliche Denken sollte diszipliniert werden; die Studenten und jüngeren Ärzte sollten diese Disziplin früh lernen. Diese pädagogische Absicht hat breite Anerkennung, das problem-orientierte Krankenblatt Nachahmung und Verbesserung erfahren. Kritik richtet sich gegen die zeitliche Aufwendigkeit. Die Ansprüche an die medizinische Informatik sind hoch; der Kranke kommt breiter zur Darstellung, das problem-orientierte Krankenblatt könnte und sollte die krankenzentrierte Krankengeschichte der Zukunft werden; denn sein Anlaß und sein Ziel ist eine umfassende Sicht der Probleme des Kranken mit dem Zweck, in einer ebenso umfassenden Behandlung (Comprehensive Care) der Gesamtsituation des Kranken gerecht zu werden. Das kommt besonders in den Veröffentlichungen von F.A.NEELON und G.J.ELLIS ("A syllabus of problem-oriented patient care", 1974) und H.K.WALKER, J.W.HURST und N.F.WOODY ("Applying the problem-oriented system", 1973) zum Ausdruck.

Die erzieherische Absicht des problem-orientierten Krankenblattes wurzelt in Erfahrungen über eine mit der Zahl der Daten zunehmende Ungenauigkeit, Unordnung und Unvollständigkeit in den Krankengeschichten:

1. Alle Probleme der Kranken sollen vorurteilslos erfaßt und aufgelistet werden (Problem-Liste).
2. Alle Daten sollen zu Problemen zusammengefaßt oder solchen zugeordnet werden.
3. Für jedes Problem soll zu Beginn ein Plan für Lösung und Behandlung aufgestellt werden.
4. Die Abhängigkeit der Probleme voneinander soll festgestellt und überprüfbar gemacht werden.
5. Jedes Problem soll im Krankheitsverlauf überprüft werden; nichts soll vergessen oder vernachlässigt werden (Progress-Notes).
6. Die Epikrise, der Arztbrief soll auf alle zu Beginn der registrierten und auf die während des Verlaufes neu hinzugekommenen Probleme eingehen. Damit soll der Arzt sich selbst überprüfen lernen.

Ausweis einer nach diesen Grundsätzen angelegten und geführten Krankengeschichte ist, daß der, der sie liest, die Problemlage und -entwicklung des Kranken, die Denkprozesse des behandelnden Arztes, die Rationalität der diagnostischen und therapeutischen Maßnahmen, die Schlüssigkeit der diagnostischen und prognostischen Aussagen erkennen und nachvollziehen sowie Richtigkeit und Vollständigkeit nachprüfen kann.

Die Verdienste von WEED und derjenigen, die seine Ideen aufgenommen, verwirklicht und verbessert haben, können nicht hoch genug eingeschätzt werden. Jedoch hat die Konzentration auf die praktischen Aspekte zu einer Vernachlässigung der erkenntnistheoretischen Implikationen geführt. Ein Beispiel ist die Definition, die HURST für den Begriff Problem gegeben hat: Ein Problem ist die Ursache, die ärztliches Handeln und diagnostische Maßnahmen veranlaßt. Diese Definition ist operational zutreffend, aber sie enthält nicht die Qualitätsmerkmale, die ein Problem haben muß, wenn es ein Problem genannt werden soll. Eine ähnlich pragmatische Einstellung erkennt man aus den Elementen, aus denen ein problem-orientiertes Krankenblatt zusammengesetzt ist. In zeitlicher Reihenfolge sind diese:

1. Die Datenbasis (Patienten-Profil, Krankengeschichte, Befunde, Laboratoriumsergebnisse).
2. Problem-Formulierung (Titling of Problems).
3. Problem-Liste.
4. Problem-Lösungsplan für alle in der Liste aufgeführten Probleme, gegliedert in diagnostische Maßnahmen, Therapie und Auskunft oder Ausbildung für den Kranken.
5. Fortschrittsbericht (progress notes), gegliedert in Angaben des Patienten (subjektiv), Informationen durch physikalische

Untersuchung oder Laboratoriumsergebnisse (objektiv), Interpretation
der subjektiven und objektiven Daten, Entscheidungen und Pläne
(diagnostisch und therapeutisch), die aus den Daten folgen. Das
dokumentierte Ergebnis ist ein Fluß-Bericht, der sich über den
gesamten diagnostischen und therapeutischen Prozeß erstreckt
(flow-sheets).
6. Entlassungsbericht, Arztbrief oder Epikrise (discharge summary).

Es fehlt bisher eine Definition des Begriffes Problem. Die
amerikanischen Autoren haben einfach den Alltagsgebrauch dieses
Begriffs übernommen. Sie bezeichnen zunächst alles als Problem, was den
Patienten belästigt oder beunruhigt hat: Kopfschmerzen,
Appetitlosigkeit, Beklemmungen in der Brust, leichte Ermüdbarkeit,
usw., also alles, was das Wohlbefinden oder das Gefühl, gesund zu sein,
beeinträchtigt. So liest man in einer Vorschrift für Studenten: "The
problem should be expressing diagnosis provided the diagnostic criteria
are met". Hier ist die Problemformulierung identisch mit einem
diagnostischen Begriff. Wenn das nicht möglich ist, haben auch
Symptome, physikalische Untersuchungsbefunde, Laboratoriumsergebnisse
oder patho- physiologische Syndrome, wie Angina pectoris, die Qualität
eines Problems. Als Beispiele für Probleme im Sozialverhalten werden
angeführt: Depression und wirtschaftlicher Zusammenbruch.
Zusammenfassend bestehen also erhebliche Unklarheiten in der Definition
des Begriffs Problem und in der Art, wie ein Problem sprachlich
dargestellt werden soll. Die amerikanischen Autoren greifen auf die
bekannten diagnostischen Begriffe, wie z.B. Diabetes mellitus oder auf
Befundbeschreibungen, wie Tachykardie, Hypokaliämie usw. zurück. Für
die medizinische Informatik ist diese Unklarheit von großer Bedeutung.
Sie bedarf eines genauer definierten Begriffs von Problem, wenn Problem
etwas anderes sein soll als die bisherigen Diagnosen, Befunde,
Symptome, Labordaten. Für die Dokumentation braucht sie außerdem eine
Entscheidung darüber, ob ein Problem mit einem Namen ausgedrückt werden
soll, oder ob zur Formulierung eines Problems immer ganze Sätze
gehören, in denen mehrere Beschwerden, Befunde und Daten in einen
Zusammenhang alternativer Entscheidungen gebracht werden.

Es ist notwendig, das Konzept und die Praxis problem-orientierten
ärztlichen Denkens und Handelns, für das das problem-orientierte
Krankenblatt das tragende Dokument ist, um folgende Elemente zu
erweitern und zu vertiefen:

1. Definition des Begriffs PROBLEM.
2. Regeln für sprachliche Formulierung von Problemen zum Zwecke
   medizinischer Informatik.
3. Ordnung und Gliederung der Probleme nach Gesichtspunkten, die der
   Lage des Kranken im System seiner umfassenden Betreuung angemessen
   sind.
4. Methode der fortlaufenden Beurteilung der Entwicklung und
   einzelner Probleme sowie der gegenseitigen Abhängigkeiten und
   Beeinflussungen der Probleme im Problem-Gefüge (Flußdiagramme des
   jeweiligen Zustandes der Problem-Liste im Prozeß des
   Krankheitsverlaufs, der Diagnostik, der Therapie und der
   Sozialbeziehungen des Kranken).

1. Definition des Begriffs PROBLEM

Problem ist ein handlungstheoretischer Begriff. So hat Aristoteles in
der "Topik" das "dialektische Problem" definiert als eine "zur
Untersuchung aufgestellte Frage, die entweder auf Tun oder Lassen oder
auch nur auf das Wissen und die Kenntnis der Wahrheit sich bezieht". Er
stellt sich die Erörterung eines Problems vor als einen argumentativ
geführten Dialog, entweder zwischen Wissenschaftlern und dem, was er
die Menge nennt, oder auch zwischen Wissenschaftlern. Ein Problem ist

also nicht einfach eine Frage, sondern die in eine bestimmte Form gebrachte Frage. Die Frageinhalte werden geordnet und zur Beantwortung zurechtgestellt. Die Frageinhalte bekommen eine bestimmte Struktur. Sie werden in ein Gefüge von Beziehungen zueinander gebracht. Das Problem hat also eine innere Ordnung, eine Struktur. Die einzelnen Inhalte der Frage sind nicht problematisch: Beschwerden und Selbstbeobachtungen des Kranken, Befunde und Meßwerte des Arztes. Wenigstens werden diese Daten vorläufig so behandelt, als ob sie unproblematisch wären. Das Problem entsteht dann durch die Art, wie diese Einzeldaten zueinander in Beziehung gesetzt werden. Diese Beziehung ist ein Modell oder eine Hypothese. Sie ist auf vielfache Antworten offen angelegt. Ihr Ergebnis sind Alternativen. Zwischen diesen wird auf Grund neuer Befunde oder Argumente entschieden. Eine Frage wird zwar entscheidbar gemacht, wenn sie die Form eines Problems hat. Aber die Entscheidung muß nicht unbedingt im ersten Schritt erfolgen. Das macht den dialektischen Charakter noch deutlicher. In einer praktischen Wissenschaft wie der Medizin kann dieser Prozeß jedoch nicht unendlich sein. Deswegen zielt die Definition des Aristoteles zuallererst auf die Entscheidung Tun oder Lassen und erst dann auf wahr oder unwahr, richtig oder falsch. Im Tun oder Lassen erkennen wir sofort die ärztliche Kernsituation. Das Grundprinzip aller ärztlichen Entscheidungen "Mehr nützen als schaden" gilt ja sowohl für das eingreifende Handeln wie für das abwartende Unterlassen.

Problemdenken ist Denken in Alternativen. Das erkennt man an den Anlässen, die zur Problematisierung von Tatbeständen oder bisherigen Selbstverständlichkeiten der Zusammenhänge, Erklärungen, usw. führen: Zweifel, Ungenügen, Unsicherheit und Unruhe, wenn ein Wissen sich als Meinung entpuppt, ein vermeintliches Gesetz sich in Regeln mit immer mehr Ausnahmen auflöst, eine anerkannte Theorie eine neue Beobachtung nicht in sich aufnehmen kann oder eine neue Beobachtung zu keiner Theorie paßt, eine Hypothese nicht hält, was sie verspricht, ein geprägtes Krankheitsbild randunscharf wird, eine Therapie aus unerklärlichen Gründen versagt, eine Prognose sich nicht erfüllt. Die Sache ist nicht mehr oder - bei Neuem - noch nicht eindeutig in einem Schritt entscheidbar.

Die Inhalte der in Problemform gebrachten Frage können selbst problematisch sein, z.B. ein Meßwert, der nicht ins Bild paßt und deswegen überprüft wird. Zu den problematischen Inhalten gehören aber auch diagnostische Begriffe. Das bekannte Verfahren der Differentialdiagnose ist eine Problematisierung: Es werden mehrere Diagnosen in der Weise miteinander in Beziehung gesetzt, daß die Hinzufügung von Daten eine Entscheidung möglich macht. Aus dem Vergleich von uns vertrauter Differential-Diagnose und dem uns noch ungewohnten Verfahren der Formulierung und Lösung von Problemen lernen wir drei wichtige Kriterien:

a) Ein Problem enthält mindestens ein "oder".
b) Die Antwort liegt nicht in einer Richtung; sie kann ja oder nein sein.
c) Die Antwort, die Schlußfolgerung, die Entscheidung, kann selbst ein problematisches Urteil sein.

Problematische Urteile sind in der Medizin die Regel. Sie geben nicht vollständige Gewißheit. Sie unterscheiden sich durch Grade der Gewißheit, die auch in einer medizinischen Informatik berücksichtigt werden müssen: Vermutungen (Konjekturen) - Möglichkeiten - Wahrscheinlichkeiten.
Urteile, die nur Möglichkeiten und Wahrscheinlichkeiten aussagen, und Entscheidungen, die daraus abgeleitet werden, sind problematisch. Wird der Anspruch erhoben, mit einem Urteil die Wirklichkeit und Wahrheit wiederzugeben und auszusagen, so spricht man von einem

assertorischen Urteil. Die Selbsttäuschung vieler Ärzte, die
Zuordnung eines diagnostischen Begriffs gäbe die Wirklichkeit eines
Krankheitsbildes wieder und die Klassifikationen diagnostischer
Systeme stünden in Übereinstimmung mit naturgesetzlich festgelegten
natürlichen Systemen, beruht auf solchen assertorischen Urteilen.
Schließlich gibt es noch das apodiktische Urteil, die Behauptung,
die einzige Schlußfolgerung sei die notwendige Antwort und Lösung
des Problems.

Problemoffenes Denken folgt also einer Logik des unabgeschlossenen
Erkenntnis-Prozesses und nicht der Logik vollkommener Erkenntnis
(WILD). Es ist aufbrechendes, aufforderndes, suchendes Denken. Das
Problem ist die abstrakte Form dieses wissenschaftliche Erkenntnis
und Praxis kennzeichnenden Suchverhaltens. Deshalb sprechen wir -
wie Aristoteles - von Unter-Suchung. Wie der Naturwissenschaftler
aus einem Problem einen Entwurf für ein Experiment macht, um zu
einer Lösung zu kommen, so benutzt der Arzt das Problem, - bisher in
der Form der Differential-Diagnose und -Therapie - um zu
diagnostischen und therapeutischen Fragestellungen zu kommen, die
die Sache entscheidbar machen. Auch wenn die ärztliche Handlung
anscheinend abschließenden Charakter hat, so bleibt sie doch als
praktische Folgerung aus einem problematischen Urteil selbst
problematisch. Auch für die wissenschaftliche Medizin gilt die
Aussage Karl POPPERs, daß die wissenschaftliche Erkenntnis von
Problem zu Problem fortschreitet und nicht von Problemlösung zu
Problemlösung. Was in der Medizin als Problemlösung im Einzelfall
erscheint, ist die pragmatische Beendigung eines
Erkenntnisprozesses, ein Problemabbruch. Oder ein Problem erledigt
sich von selbst durch Heilung oder Tod. Vor allem aber dient die
Erziehung zu problemoffenem Denken dazu, die Abweisung, Verdrängung
oder das Vergessen von für den Kranken wichtigen Problemen zu
verhindern oder zumindest zu erschweren.

Bevor die praktischen Möglichkeiten der Verwendung des Begriffs
Problem in der Medizin ausgekundschaftet werden, soll die abstrakte
Form vorgestellt werden, die DESCARTES in den "Regulae"für die
Verfahren der Problemstellung und Problemlösung vorgeschlagen hat:

1. muß in jedem Problem etwas unbekannt sein, sonst würde man es
   nämlich vergeblich stellen,
2. muß eben dieses auf irgendeine Weise bezeichnet sein, sonst wären
   wir nicht darauf festgelegt, eher dies als etwas beliebiges Anderes
   aufzufinden,
3. kann es nur durch etwas Anderes, das bekannt ist, so bezeichnet werden

" ....
Damit aber darüberhinaus das Problem auch vollkommen sei, fordern wir,
daß es vollständig bestimmt werde, so daß nichts gefragt wird, das
einen größeren Umfang hätte als das, was aus dem Gegebenen deduziert
werden kann, z.B.: Jemand stellt an mich die Frage, was man über die
Natur des Magneten ausschließlich aus denjenigen Experimenten
erschließen müsse, die GILBERT versichert, ausgeführt zu haben, mögen
sie nun richtig oder falsch sein".

"Wir verstehen aber unter Problemen alles, wobei wahr und falsch
vorkommen kann. Ihre verschiedenen Arten müssen aufgezählt werden, um
zu bestimmen, was wir bezüglich jeder von ihnen leisten können".
"Wir suchen aber bei unseren Problemen die Sachverhalte aus den Worten
oder die Ursache aus den Wirkungen oder die Wirkungen aus den Ursachen
oder das Ganze, bzw. andere Teile aus den Teilen oder schließlich
Mehreres zugleich aus dem Genannten".

Die Problemstellung muß erkennen lassen "an welchen Zeichen er das
Gesuchte, wenn es etwa unterläuft, erkennen soll". "Obgleich aber
andererseits in jedem Problem etwas unbekannt sein muß, denn sonst
würde das Problem ja zwecklos gestellt, sollte dasselbe doch durch
bestimmte Bedingungen so bezeichnet sein, daß wir in jeder Beziehung
festgelegt sind, eine Sache und nicht eine andere aufzuspüren".
"Man muß sich hüten, engere und mehr Bedingungen zugrunde zu legen als
gegeben sind".

2. Formulierung eines PROBLEMS

Problematisieren ist ein Verfahren, Inhalte für eine sinnvolle Aussage
und eine zweckmäßige Verwertung durch eine Frage aufzuschließen. Das
Verfahren der aufschließenden Frage ist von den Inhalten abgelöst
(GADAMER). Dieses abstrakte Schema muß bestimmte Merkmale haben, wenn
es in allen Wissenschaften vergleichbare Funktionen haben soll.

Die Formulierung eines Problems kann nicht in einem Wort, einem Begriff
bestehen. Hier liegt meine Kritik an der Verwendung des Begriffs
Problem in der anglo-amerikanischen Literatur.

Ein Problem kann nur in ganzen Sätzen formuliert werden. Diese Sätze
sind Protokollsätze eines Denkvorganges, den der Arzt geleistet hat.
Diese Protokollsätze müssen folgende Kriterien erfüllen:

I. Inhaltlich:
a) Sie müssen mehrere Inhalte haben.
b) Die Inhalte müssen miteinander verknüpft sein.
c) Die Verknüpfungsmöglichkeiten müssen mehr als eine sein.
d) Auch wenn die Inhalte mit verschiedenen Methoden, z.B. chemisch,
   psychologisch, gewonnen worden sind, muß die Problemformulierung
   einen leitenden Gesichtspunkt enthalten, der die Verknüpfung
   erlaubt.
e) Die Problemformulierung muß aussagen, an welchem Kriterium die
   Lösung des Problems zu erkennen sein soll.
f) Die Problemformulierung muß die Richtung möglicher oder notwen-
   diger Neuformulierungen anzeigen, wenn sie selbst nicht zu einer
   Entscheidung führt.

II. Formal:
a) Das Motiv dessen, der das Problem aufstellt oder der Anlaß der
   Problematisierung müssen erkennbar sein.
b) Es muß deutlich sein, daß es sich um einen Versuch, ein Untersuchung, ein Denk-Experiment, eine Konstruktion, d.h. ein
   vorläufiges Zurechtstellen von Inhalten, ein Zusammenstellen von
   Tatsachen zueinander oder mit Annahmen handelt.
c) Die Verknüpfungen müssen der Form nach mehrere Lösungen offenlassen, d.h. es muß mindestens ein "oder" enthalten sein; dies
   "oder" kann auch "ja" oder "nein" sein.
d) Die Problemlösung muß Anknüpfungspunkte für neue Problemstellungen
   enthalten.
e) Die Problemstellung muß erkennen lassen, welcher Art das Unbekannte
   ist, nachdem in einem bekannten Zusammenhang gesucht wird.

Das Problematische am Problematisieren ist:
a) daß Motive, Situationen, Interessen, Erwartungen in die Formulierung eingehen,
b) daß an sich Problematisches, wie z.B. Diagnosen als unproblema-
   tischer Inhalt verwendet werden,
c) daß in bestimmten Grenzen die Problem-Stellung die Problem-Lösung
   vorwegnimmt; genauer: Jede Problem-Stellung läßt nur bestimmte
   Problemlösungen zu.

Um diesen Behinderungen durch Vorgaben, Vorurteile und Vorentscheidungen wenigstens teilweise zu entgehen, ist es notwendig, die gleichen Inhalte in verschiedenen Problem-Stellungen miteinander in unterschiedliche Zusammenhänge zu bringen. Diese Aufgabe wird uns bei der Problem-Liste noch einmal begegnen: Die Aussage von Julian HUXLEY "Wer ein Problem definiert, hat es schon halb gelöst" ist also eine in sich problematische, dialektische Aussage, die die Widersprüche und Grenzen des Problematisierens zeigt. Sie verweist die "quaestio perfecta" des DESCARTES ins Reich der idealen Erkenntnis-Verfahren. In ihr sind die Frageinhalte so gewählt und geordnet, daß sich nur eine Lösung ergeben kann, nämlich die richtige.

Ein Problem zu formulieren, ist also eine geistige Leistung. Sie setzt Erfahrung und Beobachtung voraus; denn das Gerüst der als Problem zurechtgestellten Frage sind Tatsachen. Das gesuchte Unbekannte muß klar ausgesprochen sein und mit dem Bekannten in entscheidbare Zusammenhänge gebracht werden können. Das Problem der Problem-Stellung liegt darin, daß der Fragende in dieser geistigen Leistung etwas hinzufügt, etwas mitbringt: Unbewußte Erfahrungen, Erlebnisse, Vorstellungen, Erwartungen, Vergessen, Verdrängen, Nichtwissen, Vorzugswissen, Einschätzungen des Behandelnkönnens gehen in die Formulierung des Problems ein. Diese Formulierung läßt aber besser als ein diagnostischer Begriff die Einflüsse von Bedingungen und Zielen erkennen, die in die Wahl eines Namens für einen krankhaften Vorgang einwirken. Das ist eine Forderung an die Formulierung: Der, der die als Problem aufgestellte Frage nachvollzieht, muß die Motive der so und nicht anders gestellten Frage, die Absicht der Ordnung, der Inhalte erkennen und nachvollziehen können. Es gehört viel intellektuelle Selbstbeherrschung und Aufrichtigkeit dazu, zu vermeiden, daß die Problem-Stellung die Problem-Lösung vollständig vorwegnimmt.

Die gute Problemexposition führt in der klinischen Medizin, in der so häufig Für und Wider gegeneinander stehen, zur Argumentation, zum Austausch von Gründen und Gegengründen, Ansichten und Gegenansichten, Vorteilen und Nachteilen.

Im Verhältnis von Problem zur Diagnose ist das Problem der Diagnose übergeordnet; denn im Erkenntnisprozeß und in der Problemformulierung sind diagnostische Begriffe Teilinhalte, Elemente von Problemen. Andererseits ist ein Problem zusammen mit anderen Problemen Teil und Stadium des diagnostischen Prozesses, wenn dieser als ein Erkenntnisprozeß und ein diagnostisch-therapeutischer Entscheidungs- und Handlungszusammenhang verstanden wird. Schließlich werden auch in Zukunft diagnostische Begriffe als Kurzformeln einer Problem-formulierung oder einer vorläufigen Problemlösung dienen. Aus praktischen Gründen ist nicht zu erwarten, daß die Begriffsapparate von PROBLEM und PATHEM die diagnostischen Begriffe und Klassifikationssysteme vollständig ablösen.

Damit stellt sich die Frage, ob nicht in der Medizin die Definition von Problem flexibler gestaltet und gehandhabt werden muß als das in den Definitionen von DESCARTES gefordert wird. Die Beispiele, die weiter unten folgen, machen die besonderen Aspekte der Verwendung des Begriffs Problem in der Medizin deutlich. Man wird die Diskussion über die zulässigen Formen von Problemformulierungen eröffnen und zu Übereinkünften kommen müssen. Daran müssen die medizinischen Informatiker beteiligt werden; denn die Ergebnisse solcher Konventionen sind gleichzeitig Determinanten von Programmen der Anlage und Auswertung von Daten.

Die folgenden Abweichungen vom abstrakten Problembegriff sind Vorschläge für die Zwecke der Medizin:

1. Die Frageinhalte dürfen z.T. selbst problematisch sein: Anamnestische Angaben, die der Überprüfung bedürfen, Schilderungen von Beschwerden, die durch Nachfragen bestätigt und präzisiert werden müssen, Laboratoriumsbefunde, die wegen Zweifel an der Methodik wiederholt werden müssen, Ergebnisse der körperlichen Untersuchung, die nicht eindeutig sind.

2. Für die Problemliste darf die Problemformulierung auch die Form eines Merksatzes haben, der die Absicht des Arztes dokumentiert, einem bestimmten Zusammenhang nachzuspüren, d.h. es können mehrere Kennzeichen verschiedener Antworten auf die Frage genannt werden.

3. Die Andeutung einer Richtung des Nachdenkens oder diagnostisch-therapeutischen Handelns kann die Stelle der Intention einer bestimmten Antwort auf die Frage einnehmen.

4. Nicht alle Alternativen müssen ausgesagt sein. Die Möglichkeit erwarteter und unerwarteter Ereignisse kann offen bleiben, d.h. es wird eine größere Planlosigkeit als von DESCARTES gefordert, zugelassen.

5. Die Antwort auf die im Problem gestellte Frage kann auch ein problematisches, diagnostisches oder therapeutisches Handeln sein.

6. Ruhende Probleme, die jederzeit wieder aktiv werden können, z.B. Anämie aus Eisenmangel, besonders, wenn der Grund des Eisenmangels nicht gefunden werden konnte.

7. Ereignisse, die einmal ein Problem für den Kranken waren; für seine jetzige Krankheit aber somatisch inaktiv sind, nicht aber für die Verarbeitung der Krankheit, z.B. eine ausgeheilte Gonorrhoe, die Schuldgefühle hinterläßt oder eine Tuberkulose, deren Reaktivierung befürchtet wird.

Weitere Besonderheiten ergeben sich aus der Gliederung und Ordnung der Probleme eines bestimmten Kranken aus den dazu gegebenen Beispielen. Ausgeschlossen aber bleibt der Ersatz einer Problemformulierung durch ein Wort, einen diagnostischen Begriff, das titling of problems.

3. Ordnung und Gliederung der Probleme

WEED, NEELON und ELLIS sowie WALKER, HURST und WOODY haben den größten und fast einzigen Wert auf die Vollständigkeit der Problem-Liste gelegt. Alle Probleme des Kranken sollen protokolliert werden: "The student or physician should list all the patient's problems, past as well as present, social and psychiatric as well as medical" (WEED). WALKER definiert Problem wie folgt: "A problem is defined as anything that requires diagnosis or management or that interferes with the quality of life as perceived by the patient. Thus a problem may or may not be a diagnosis". Aus den Beispielen, die in den drei genannten Monographien mitgeteilt werden, läßt sich keine Systematik der Gliederung der Probleme erkennen. Zwar soll jedes Problem eine Nummer in der Liste haben; aber welcher Gesichtspunkt die Reihenfolge bestimmt, wird nicht gesagt. Jedoch kann man erkennen, daß bei einem "somatischen Fall" die somatischen Probleme, bei einem "psychischen Fall" die psychiatrischen Probleme an der Spitze der Liste stehen. Es sollen medizinische und soziale Probleme, aktive und inaktive, Probleme der Anamnese und der Befunde berücksichtigt werden; ihre Reihenfolge bleibt offenbar beliebig.

Deswegen wird hier ein Vorschlag vorgelegt, der auch nicht ideal ist.
Er erleichtert aber Vollständigkeit der Erfassung aller Probleme und
eine Bewertung im Hinblick darauf, was zuerst getan werden muß.

Problemliste

Programm relevanter Probleme	Problembewertung / Problem für wen? / Zielperson bzw.-gruppe								Pläne für Problemlösungen	Problemgefüge					Problemaktivität					
	Kranker	Arzt	Mitwelt	Staat	Verwaltung	Organisation	Dienstleistung	Wissenschaft		parallel	interdependent mit	konvergiert zu	verschmilzt mit	divergiert von	Erkenntnisstand	Konzentration	Lösungsstand	objekt. Aktivität	Handlungszwang	Reaktion des Kranken
1. Biographisch																				
2. Diagnostisch-symptomatologisch (Arbeitsdiagnosen)																				
3. Prognostisch-semiologisch (Allgemeinsymptome; Hypothesen)																				
4. Pathogenetisch-pathematologisch (Erklärungsmodelle)																				
5. Psychosoziale Dimension (Leidensdruck; Beruf; Familie)																				
6. Individuelle Reaktionsformen (Konstitution; Disposition; Gewohnheiten)																				
7. Therapeutische Modelle (wenn - dann)																				

Die Problem-Liste hat die Form eines Programms mit 7 Gruppen oder
Kategorien von Problemen. In jeder Gruppe kann eine Reihenfolge der
Probleme nach ihrer Bedeutung für das Leiden des Kranken oder für das
Handeln des Arztes gebildet werden, d.h. es wird nicht eine Priorität
gesetzt; sondern es sind bis zu 7 Prioritäten möglich, die gleichwertig
nebeneinander stehen. An der Spitze sollte jeweils das Problem stehen,
das sofortiges Handeln erfordert. Denn mit WEED stimme ich überein, daß
die Problem-Liste Voraussetzung eines Planes für Handeln ist.

Die Beschwerden, Befunde und Labordaten werden nun nicht willkürlich
oder gleichmäßig auf die 7 Kategorien verteilt. Zwar erscheinen in den
Problemformulierungen einer Kategorie verwandte Daten, die mit der
gleichen Methode gewonnen wurden: Befragung, Biographie, Epidemiologie,
physikalische Untersuchung, Bakteriologie, klinische Chemie, usw.

Der vorgelegte Vorschlag zwingt dazu, die Daten verschiedener Quellen,
die Ergebnisse verschiedener Methoden einem Problem unter- und
einzuordnen. Der gleiche Befund kann und muß in verschiedenen
Problemzusammenhängen erscheinen. Er hat nur unterschiedliche
Stellenwerte: einmal lösungsführend, ein andermal lösungshelfend. Die
gleichen Beschwerden, Befunde und Labordaten können in
Problemformulierungen verschiedener Problemkategorien auftreten. Je

häufiger das der Fall ist, um so dichter wird das Problemgefüge eines
Kranken strukturiert.

Aber wer handelt? Mit welchen Zielen wird gehandelt? Die von mir
vorgeschlagene Gliederung der Problem-Liste in 7 Kategorien ermöglicht
eine Verteilung der Aufgaben, eine umfassende Organisation von
gleichzeitigen Handlungen. Deswegen ist das zweite Haupt-Kennzeichen
dieser Problem-Liste die Frage: Für wen ist ein Problem ein Problem?
Wer ist am meisten betroffen und wer kann das Problem am besten lösen:
der Kranke, die Familie, der Arzt, die Schwester, der soziale Dienst,
die Verwaltung, die Versicherung, ein Laboratorium? Oder ist das
Problem Anlaß einer wissenschaftlichen Untersuchung?

Für die Zielpersonen haben die Probleme unterschiedliche Werte und
Bedeutungen; die Reihenfolge der Prioritäten ist für den Kranken und
seinen Arzt oft unterschiedlich. Bei der Hyperthyreose kann für den
Kranken seine Obstipation oder Gewichtszunahme, für den Arzt Ursache
und Schwere, für die Familie der Abbau der Persönlichkeit und für den
Arbeitgeber die Vernachlässigung von Dienstpflichten das Hauptproblem
sein.

Die Frage: "Für wen ist dieses Problem ein Problem?" kann den
Betroffenen meinen, den Kranken, der etwas Bestimmtes befürchtet, z.B.
einen Krebs oder auch den Arzt, der vergeblich nach einem Sitz oder
einer Erklärung der Krankheit sucht. Sie kann aber auch an die Person
gerichtet sein, die am ehesten geeignet ist, ein Problem zu lösen, zu
helfen. Der Plan, der aus der hier vorgeschlagenen gegliederten, nach
Problem-Kategorien geordneten Problem-Liste abgeleitet wird, hat die
Merkmale einer Organisation von Handlungen, Entscheidungen, Hilfen, die
nicht nur den Arzt betreffen; die notwendigen Aufgaben werden
umfassender definiert und verteilt.

4. Dynamik des Einzelproblems und des gesamten Problemgefüges

Daß die Problem-Liste im Laufe der Krankheit eines Patienten sich
verändert, hat WEED bereits berücksichtigt: Probleme können nicht nur
im Anfang aktiv oder inaktiv sein, sie können es auch im Laufe der
Krankheit werden; die Problem-Liste muß dauernd überprüft, ergänzt,
korrigiert werden: "The problem list is added to and updated as new
problems occur and previous ones are resolved".

Die Dynamik des Prozeßgefüges veranschaulicht man am besten durch ein
Fluß-Diagramm der Aktivitäten (Ordinate) der einzelnen Probleme im
Zeitverlauf der Krankheit (Abszisse).

Prozeßgefüge ist das Ganze der bei einem Patienten bestehenden
Probleme. Sie können voneinander unabhängig sein, z.B. kann jemand
einen hohen Blutdruck und eine Anämie haben; sie können einander
bedingen oder einander folgen, wie das Pleuraempyem als Komplikation
der Pneumonie, sie können einander gegenseitig beeinflussen, wie
chronische Bronchitis und Asthma bronchiale, sie können aufeinander
zulaufen, schließlich miteinander verschmelzen wie ein Herzinfarkt und
eine arterielle Verschlußkrankheit, wenn ein Diabetes mellitus
festgestellt worden ist. Sie können sich aber auch aus einem
ursprünglich einheitlich aussehenden Problem differenzieren, wenn z.B.
die Magenbeschwerden einer hypochondrisch gefärbten Depression sich
schließlich als durch ein Magencarcinom bedingt herausstellen. Bei all
diesen verschiedenen Möglichkeiten der Beziehung von Problemen
zueinander wird es vagabundierende Beschwerden, Befunde und Daten
geben, die zu mehreren Problemen passen oder deren Zugehörigkeit in der
Dynamik des Problemgefüges geändert werden müssen. Hauptprobleme können
zu Nebenproblemen werden und umgekehrt. Problemlösungsführende

Beschwerden, Befunde und Daten können problemlösungshelfend oder
irrelevant werden und umgekehrt.

AKTIVITÄT

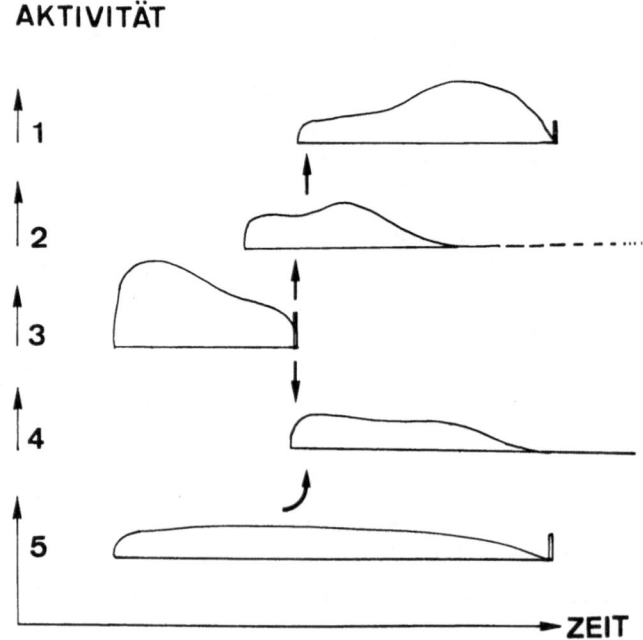

VERLAUFSDIAGRAMM DER PROBLEME

Aber auch der Begriff der Problem-Aktivität fordert die Frage heraus,
an welchem Maßstab (Ordinate) die Aktivitäten gemessen werden sollen.
Es kann sich um Bezugspersonen handeln: Was ängstigt, belästigt,
behindert den Kranken am meisten und beeinflußt sein Verhalten? Was
beschäftigt den Arzt am eindringlichsten, worauf konzentriert er sein
Denken und organisiert er sein Handeln? Es kann sich um die Krankheit
handeln: Was bedroht den Kranken am meisten, was zwingt zu welchen
sofortigen Eingriffen? Wie ist der Stand des objektiven
Krankheitsverlaufes (Fieber, Infiltrationen in der Lunge, Urinbefund,
usw.)? Und schließlich kann die Problem-Aktivität sich auf den Stand
der Erkenntnisse, auch auf die Präzision der Problemformulierung oder
auf den Stand der Lösung - diagnostisch und therapeutisch - beziehen.

Beispiele

1. Sind die von Herrn X angegebenen nächtlichen Anfälle von Atemnot
durch einen Bronchialspasmus oder durch ein Herzversagen oder durch
Angstträume bedingt?

Der Patient würde die Lage anders problematisieren, z.B.: Kann ich in einem solchen Anfall ersticken?

Die Problemformulierung für den Arzt führt nicht zu einer Anwort im ersten Schritt, sondern nur zur Formulierung differenzierter Teilprobleme. Die Inhalte dieser Teilprobleme könnten z.B. anamnestische Angaben sein.

Die Kurzformen, Asthma, nächtliche Dyspnoe, decken die Problemlage und die notwendigen Planungen zu; sie entfalten sie nicht.

2. Ist die klinisch und röntgenologisch bei Frau Y nachgewiesene Insuffizienz des linken Herzens Ursache oder Folge der ebenfalls nachgewiesenen Insuffizienz der Mitralklappe?

Die übliche Kurzform relative oder absolute Mitralinsuffizienz macht dem Studenten, der die Lage entscheiden lernen soll, den von ihm geforderten Denkprozeß nicht deutlich.

Für den Kranken ist dies überhaupt kein Problem.

Betrachtet man die Lage vom Standpunkt der Problem-Aktivität aus, so ist für Kranken und Arzt das therapeutische Problem der Herzinsuffizienz am aktivsten.

Herzinsuffizienz aber ist keine Problemformulierung: Diese muß vielmehr so geartet sein, daß sich ein der individuellen Lage des Kranken angepaßter, umfassender und differenzierter Behandlungs- und Pflegeplan daraus ableiten läßt.

Den bedeutsamen Unterschied zwischen dem diagnostischen Begriff Herzinsuffizienz und seiner Problematisierung erkennt man, wenn man den Versuch macht, das Problem einmal aus der Lage, den Beschwerden, den Beobachtungen des Kranken zu entwerfen und mit dem Ergebnis eine arztgerechte, handlungsanweisende Formulierung vergleicht.

3. 30-jähriger Mann mit einem diabetischen Vater und einem seit 17 Jahren bekannten Diabetes mellitus, dessen Insulinbedarf steigt; er sucht den Arzt auf wegen Verschlechterung des Sehvermögens und plötzlich auftretender Wadenschmerzen bei schnellem Gehen.

Diese Problemformulierung ist für Studenten besonders lehrwirksam. Sie verbindet eine Problemlage des Kranken, die der Anlaß zu einem Arztbesuch ist, mit einem Problemgefüge, aus dem heraus sich pathophysiologische, prognostische, erbbiologische und therapeutische Probleme und deren Lösungen entwickeln lassen.

Der Satz hat nicht die Form einer Frage; er enthält kein "oder". Es ist offen für verschiedene und verschiedenartige Antworten.

4. Gehbeschwerden bei Hallux valgus.

Es kann sein, daß der Patient das Problem selbst so stellt oder daß es das Ergebnis der Kombination von Beschwerden mit einem ersten Befund durch den Arzt ist. Als Frage behandelt zielt die Problemformulierung auf "ja"oder "nein". Um diese Frage beantworten zu können, muß ein diagnostisches Problem formuliert werden, das Antworten auf die Frage Gicht, chronische Polyarthritis, arterielle Verschlußkrankheit, usw. formuliert. Für den Arzt als Zielperson folgt ein diagnostisches Programm aus der Problemformulierung. Hauptprobleme für den Kranken bleiben seine Beschwerden und die Frage, wie diese zu beseitigen sind; er hat ein subjektives und ein prognostisches Problem.

5. 30-jährige Frau, Mutter eines Schul- und eines Kleinkindes mit einem blutenden Ulcus duodeni.

Diese Problemformulierung macht den Protokollsatz dadurch als eine Verknüpfung von Problemen erkennbar, daß die Schwierigkeit, die er zur Lösung aufstellt, unmittelbar vor Augen steht: Die Frau ist gleichzeitig zu Hause unabkömmlich, wenn nicht soziale Hilfen organisiert werden; sie muß gleichzeitig in ein Krankenhaus. Der Satz deutet eine Konfliktlage (Alter, Kinder) als Bedingung der Erkrankung und die Möglichkeit einer Operation an. Die Hauptprobleme, die zuerst gelöst werden müssen, liegen für die Kranke und für den Arzt auf verschiedenen Ebenen.

6. 45-jähriger, starker Raucher mit einem unstillbaren Husten seit einem Jahr und einem kupferfarbenen Auswurf seit 6 Wochen.

Diese Problemformulierung bündelt die Informationen: Raucher, Husten, Auswurf, Farbe, Zeiten so, daß eine Ja-Nein-Antwort als Lösung gesucht wird.

7. Seit 6 Monaten Fieber ohne Schüttelfröste, das bei Behandlung durch den Hausarzt auf Corticosteroide, nicht aber auf Antibiotica ansprach.

In der Problemformulierung wird ein einengend definierter Fiebertyp - ohne Schüttelfrost, seit 6 Monaten - in Verbindung gesetzt zu einer bereits vorliegenden therapeutischen Erfahrung. Die Einzelinhalte bleiben in sich problematisch. Trotzdem kann die Lösung in der Kombination zweier Probleme gesucht werden. Für den Kranken mag das nicht abklingen wollende Fieber das aktivste Problem sein; für den Arzt, der die Lage in diese Formulierung bringt, ist es das nicht.

Zusammenfassend läßt sich sagen, daß in einem richtig formulierten Problem der Arzt sich selbst eine definierte Aufgabe stellt. Mit den anglo-amerikanischen Autoren stimme ich darin überein, daß die häufig gemachte Anmerkung "Ausschluß von ....." keine Problemstellung ist; denn sie läßt nicht erkennen, welche Inhalte mit welchen Methoden in dem Problem zusammengefaßt werden sollen und welche Kennzeichen die angestrebte Lösung haben soll. In der Regel haben die in der Medizin gestellten Probleme nicht die grammatische Form einer Frage, aber die Lösung eines gut formulierten Problems in der Form eines aus der Problemstellung ableitbaren Plans für Handlungen, ist äquivalent mit der Anwort auf eine in Problemform gestellte Frage. Es ist auch kein systematischer Unterschied zwischen einer wissenschaftlichen und einer klinischen Problemformulierung zu erkennen.

III PATHEM

Diagnosen erfüllen ihre Funktionen schlecht oder gar nicht. Sie geben nicht die Information, die sie zu geben versprechen. Sie sind Bezeichnung, aber nicht Beschreibung oder Erklärung. Der Grund ist: die Wirklichkeit, die sie wiedergeben und ordnen sollen, ist sehr komplex. Die diagnostischen Begriffe, die ein Arzt für die Kennzeichnung und Einordnung eines krankhaften Geschehens verwendet, geben wieder:

1. Die Beschwerden, Beobachtungen und Befunde.
2. Die Bedingungen, unter denen die Diagnostik verlief.
3. Die Zwecke, denen die Diagnose dient.
4. Die Theorie, mit der der krankhafte Prozeß erklärt werden soll.
5. Die Struktur des Klassifikations-Systems, das der Arzt verwendet und dem der diagnostische Begriff entnommen wird.

Was der praktizierende Arzt heute dem medizinischen Informatiker liefert, ist ein Gemisch von Worten, Begriffen, Tatsachen, Vermutungen, Hypothesen, Schlußfolgerungen und Absichten. Demgemäß haben die Informationen unterschiedliche Qualitäten und Wertigkeiten: Genauigkeit, Verläßlichkeit, Gültigkeit, Bedeutung.

Um diese Situation zu verbessern, gehen wir auf die elementaren ersten Schritte des ärztlichen Erkenntnisprozesses zurück:

1. Sammlung erster Wahrnehmungen, Eindrücke, Untersuchungsergebnisse und einzelner Laboratoriumsdaten.

2. Primitive Unterordnung unter einfache, allgemein anerkannte Standard- Begriffe. Diese reduzieren, selektieren, evaluieren und kondensieren bereits die einzelnen Fakten.

Ein zweites Verfahren ist primär synthetisch: das Erkennen von Gesamtheiten, Bildern und Verläufen von Krankheiten; "Klinischer Blick" und "pattern recognition". Es ist das Hineinsehen oder Herauslesen von "Gestalten" (Eidos), ein idiographisches Verhalten der empiristischen Heilkunde.

Theoretisch besteht ein Krankheitsprozeß aus kleinsten Gliedern einer Ereigniskette. Das Ideal praktischer, wissenschaftlich begründeter Medizin wäre, jeden Schritt zu kennen und zu messen. Wir nennen ein solches Elementarereignis in einer pathogenetischen Kette ein Pathem. Es besteht mindestens aus einem Ereignis und einem Folgeereignis. Die Beziehung kann linear, aber auch eine Wechselwirkung sein. Es sind auch Konvergenzen verschiedener Bedingungen auf ein gemeinsames Folgeereignis und Divergenzen von Folgeereignissen aus einem vorhergehenden Ereignis möglich. Ein Beispiel für linear: Hypalbuminämie $\longrightarrow$ Ödem; für Wechselwirkung: Schmerz $\longrightarrow$ Muskelspannung $\longrightarrow$ Schmerz. Hat ein Folgeereignis mehrere Bedingungen, ohne die es nicht zustandekommen würde, gehören alle notwendigen Bedingungen zu dem Pathem. Beispiel: Kalium + Veränderung der Wasserstoffionenkonzentration + Freisetzung von Prostaglandin E $\longrightarrow$ Schmerz. Das gleiche gilt umgekehrt, wenn ein Ereignis mehrere Folgeereignisse nach sich zieht. Der Begriff des Pathems ist anwendbar auf alle mit der Erfahrung zu ermittelnden Tatsachen; er ordnet Phänomene, ohne auf einen theoretischen Zusammenhang angewiesen zu sein. Er ist anwendbar auf physikalische, chemische, biologische, psychische und psychosoziale Vorgänge und auch auf die Übergänge dieser methodisch bedingten Bereiche ineinander. Er bleibt aber abhängig von den Meßbedingungen und tatsächlichen Beobachtungen. Aber er erlaubt - im Unterschied zur Diagnose - keine Aussage über etwas, das nicht beobachtet oder gemessen wurde.

Eine pathogenetische Kette besteht also aus zahlreichen Pathemata. Je nachdem, ob diese nur das Minimum von zwei oder aber mehr durch Daten belegbare Ereignisse enthalten, wird man Pathemata 1., 2., 3. etc. Ordnung unterscheiden können. Viele Pathemata werden bei vielen Krankheiten vorkommen, so die aus der allgemeinen Pathologie bekannten. Aber sie haben nicht immer den gleichen Stellenwert. Man wird also essentielle von accidentellen Pathemata - so wie früher bei den Krankheitszeichen - unterscheiden können: Ein Pathem, daß bei einer Krankheit essentiell ist, wie z.B. der Eisenmangel bei hypochromer Anämie, ist bei einer anderen accidentell, wie der Eisenmangel beim Carcinom.

Eine andere Gliederung der Pathemata ist die in Leit- oder Haupt-Pathemata und in Neben-Pathemata.

Wichtig ist, die Beschwerden der Kranken, Befunde und Labordaten auf Pathemata zurückzubeziehen; denn Beschwerden (Complaints), Krankheitszeichen (Symptoms) und Befunde (Signs) sind Epiphänomene von Pathemata. Eine begründete Therapie muß nachweisen können, in welches Pathem sie auf welche Weise eingreift.

Die Pathogenese ist die zeitliche Ordnung der Patheme

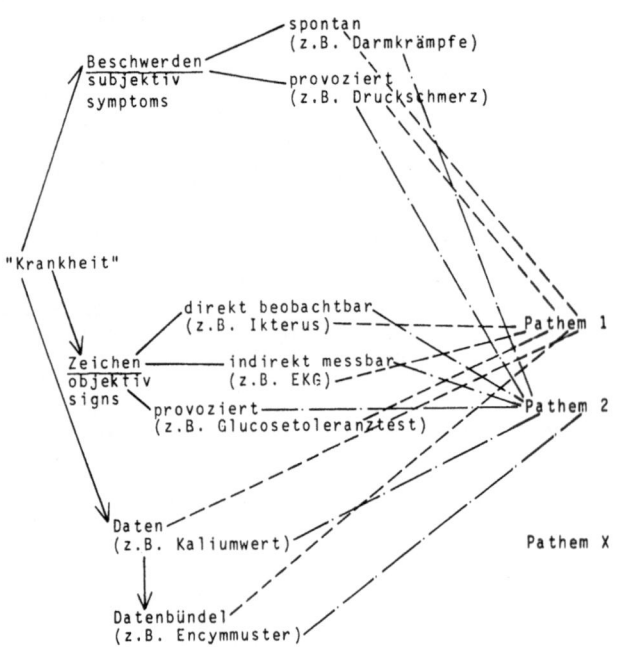

Die bisherigen diagnostischen Begriffe sind ein recht unsystematischer nominalistischer Überbau über der natürlichen Ordnung der Pathemata. Nicht die Krankheiten - wie SYNDENHAM meinte - sind die natürlichen Gestalten des Krankhaften, sondern die Pathemata.

Der Zusammenhang des bisherigen Krankheits-Begriffs mit dem Pathem-Begriff ergibt sich aus dem obigen Schema.

Die Pathogenese ist die zeitliche Ordnung der Patheme. Das zeigt die folgende Abbildung.

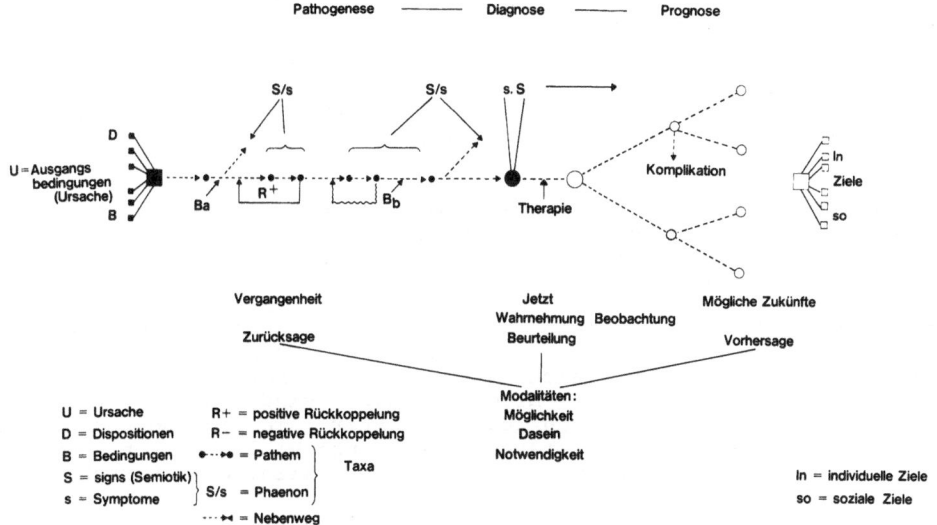

Wenn der analytische Prozeß der ärztlichen Erkenntnis einsetzt, sind ein Teil der Pathemata nicht mehr wirksam. Sie müssen in alternativen Modellen rekonstruiert werden. Allen noch nachweisbaren Veränderungen liegen aber noch wirksame Pathemata zugrunde. Entscheidend wichtig wird aber die pathemgeleitete - und nicht mehr nur phänomenologische - Beobachtung des Verlaufes der Krankheit. Auch der gezielte therapeutische Eingriff in Haupt- und Neben-Pathemata ist eine Erkenntnis- und Entscheidungsquelle. Nur hat das "ex juvantibus" nicht mehr eine Diagnose zum Ziel, sondern Elementarprozesse, ist also näher an der Wirklichkeit des krankhaften Geschehens ausgerichtet. Im günstigsten und erstrebenswerten Fall ist dies das Primär-Pathem, die erste Ursache und ihre erste Wirkung oder die Konstellation der ersten ungünstigen Bedingungen mit dem Schritt zur ersten krankhaften Störung. Diese Beschreibung des Pathembegriffs macht deutlich, daß er auf eine verstärkte und vertiefte klinische Forschung zur Gewinnung zuverlässigerer und relevanterer Daten zielt. Er verschiebt das Schwergewicht des diagnostischen Prozesses, der in der Vergangenheit auf einem Gleichgewicht induktiver und deduktiver Schritte beruhte, zugunsten der induktiven Methodik. Das Pathem ist ein Versuch, das Subjektive und Zufällige aus der ärztlichen Erkenntnis und Entscheidung noch mehr zu eliminieren als bisher. Die Daten für die Informatik sollen härter werden. Sie sollen aber übersichtlich, logisch und durch Experiment und Beobachtung begründet so geordnet sein, daß die Informatik sie zu höheren Ordnungen des Verständnisses - der Erklärung der Entscheidung für therapeutische Eingriffe und der Vorhersage verarbeiten kann.

Die Gliederung der Pathogenese in Pathemata erlaubt es der medizinischen Informatik auch, die Ergebnisse ihrer logischen Verknüpfungen in Modellen, ihre Vergleiche mit der Auswertung bekannter Pathem-Konstellationen oder Therapiefolgen und mit theoretischen Konstrukten von Pathogenese als Problem, als diagnostischen oder Forschungsauftrag oder auch als Anregung zu einem Behandlungsversuch an den Arzt zurückzugeben. Selbstverständlich können die Ergebnisse dieser Ordnungsvorgänge auch den bekannten Diagnosen zugeordnet werden. Aber es wird auch zu einer Qualitätsprüfung dieser Diagnosen und ihrer Klassifikationen kommen. Einige werden dabei bestätigt, andere verworfen werden.

Das Beispiel des Pathems zeigt wieder einmal, daß eine genauere Messung und Kenntnis von Vorgängen die Reduktion von Komplexität erfordert. Wenn man das Ganze des menschlichen Krankseins mit diesem Instrument beschreiben oder bestenfalls erklären will, müssen Pathemata mit physikalischen, chemischen, biologischen, psychologischen, und sozialpsychologischen Methoden gleichwertig nebeneinander gestellt werden. Außerdem müssen sie Elemente der Verknüpfung enthalten. Insofern sind sie zugleich natürlich, aber angesichts des Gesamtzusammenhangs, dessen Elemente sie sind, auch künstlich, Konstrukte unserer methodischen Zugriffe. Aber sie sind besser als die Diagnosen geeignet, eine angemessene Zahl und Vielfalt von Problemen für den einzelnen Kranken und für die klinische Forschung zu formulieren.

Die Wortbildung PATHEM ist in Analogie zu den Begriffen PHONEM und LEXEM gewählt worden. In der Linguistik heißt die kleinste Zahl von Buchstaben, die in eine Folge gebracht, einen Sinn ergibt, der verstanden werden kann, ein LEXEM. Der kürzest mögliche Laut oder eine Klangfolge, die eine zuverlässige und genaue Information in der sprachlichen Kommunikation vermittelt, heißt PHONEM. Entsprechend ist das PATHEM die kleinste denkbare Einheit eines pathogenetischen Prozesses, der für das Zustandekommen dieses Prozesses notwendig ist, der eine in sich geschlossene Einheit darstellt, die ein Kettenglied in verschiedenen pathogenetischen Prozessen sein kann, die quantitativ beschreibbar und experimentell reproduzierbar ist.

DECISION MAKING METHODS IN MEDICINE

F. GREMY et M. GOLDBERG (PARIS)

I - MEDICINE AND DECISION MAKING

I.1. MEDICAL ACTION

Medicine is a discipline of judgment and action. At each moment of his professional life, the physician must suggest decisions and actions to his patient. In order to do this, he must gather some pertinent information and extract in the most logical and the surest way arguments allowing him to achieve his objectives.

Medical action can be summarized in the following way. From his patient, the physician extracts a certain information I_1, made up of : a) "Clinical data" collected by the physician himself by inquiry and examination of the patient (motives of the consultation, story of the disease, signs of functionnal and organic disorders, ...) ; b) "paraclinical data" (biochemical tests, bioelectrical signals, radiological pictures ...) provided by special apparatus, calling for extra costs and demanded by the doctor.

In addition he must master the current medical knowledge concerning pathology, physiology, therapeutics and so on, in other words an I_2 information. He must compare both kinds of information to elaborate a decision that will lead to an action.

This procedure : collection + knowledge $\longrightarrow$ decision is often cyclical : it must be separated in partial problems which must be solved one after the other. For instance, a first step can be gathering signs to form a syndrome ; the next step is to link this syndrome to a disease by searching associated signs and syndromes. In other words, this procedure leading to diagnosis is made of a variable number of cycles, each of them being composed of collecting information and comparing it to a certain knowledge : this comparison often suggests the search of new information and so on up to the final decision. Medical action still often implies a written record of the major signs and decisions. This "medical record" may serve several objectives : it may be progress notes that the physician can consult and update each time he sees his patient or a similar one ; it may also be the systematical collection of information gathered for research. In this last case, a statistical analysis of a sufficient number of records may improve medical knowledge. Let us call I_3 and I_4 the information streams converging towards medical archives. The following diagram summarizes the procedures we have just described.

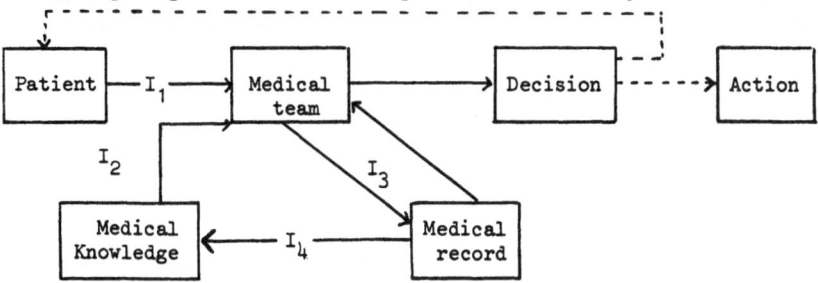

I.2. DIFFICULTIES IN MEDICAL PRACTICE

Medical practice is becoming more and more difficult. This is owing to the constantly increasing amount of possible information - 3000 diseases and syndromes were identified in the beginning of the century : they are now about 30 000 ; the number of marketed drugs - that everyone finds excessive - is close to 8 000 in France and its increase is about 300 a year ; the number of tests one can ask for, is also constantly increasing and one must know the limits and signification of each of them.

This increase of knowledge is often confusing or even destressing for the physician to whom a huge effort of memorization is asked. But it is a well known fact that the human can only manage simultaneously a very small number of different information. This means that an excessive number of information confuses more than it helps.

In addition to his human responsability, we must not underestimate the doctor's economical power : he often commands great expenses (for instance certain frequent radiological examinations can cost more than 750 dollars).

I.3. AID TO DECISION TAKEN IN A LARGE MEANING

Considering these difficulties, it seems justified to use computer sciences methods and technics to help the physician in his action. As a matter of fact, the computer has been used in several points of the previous diagram :

- aid for collecting information : for instance by the mean of self questionnaires ;
- help for access to medical knowledge ; this is the field of certain data banks (for instance drugs or enzymes data banks) and of documentation systems such as MEDLARS and now MEDLINE or the french SABIR ;
- aid for medical records management.

Since all the physician's activities lead to decisions, all these kinds of systems that are made to facilitate these activities may be considered as aid to decision.

I.4. AID TO DECISION IN A RESTRICTIVE MEANING

But alongside this outside aid, informatics can help the decision procedures themselves, in other words, the specific intellectual activity by which the physician compares the information gathered from the patient to his own knowledge and builds his judgments and choices. In this case one can speak of help for decision in a restrictive meaning.

Usually, one divides the medical activity in three distinct parts : 1) diagnosis, which is classing the patient in one or more pre-established categories of pathology ; 2) prognosis, which is foreseeing the patient's near and distant future ; 3) therapeutics, which is the choice of the most appropriate treatments.

Evidently, each of these parts implies a decision. However, we will mostly consider the diagnosis problem ; which is sufficiently representative of the decision procedures. Morever, we will exclude the automatical analysis of paraclinical tests (such as EKG, radiological pictures ...) since too many technical explanations would be necessary.

This paper will therefore mostly concern the aid to diagnosis when all the information involved in the procedure are already interpreted ; for instance, we will consider that an EKG is normal or abnormal without reference to the way this result is obtained.

Note : Alongside patient oriented medicine, there is another field where one must take decision and act, which is public health (population-oriented). We will only consider here the individual practice problems, decision in population oriented medicine being considered elsewhere ("Information ssystems in Public Health").

II - "NATURAL" DIAGNOSIS METHODS

II.1. GLOBAL AND SEQUENTIAL DIAGNOSIS

Two major mechanisms are more or less unconsciously used : global diagnosis and sequential diagnosis.

Global diagnosis is similar to "pattern reco ition". In a crowd, we recognize an individual among many others without having to analyze separately the form of his face, the colour of his eyes, his hair-do, etc ... All these information are almost instantaneously combined by our brain. In the same way, a dermatologist recognizes at first sight an eczema without having to make a preliminary analysis of the lesion. In each case, it is the global comparison of all the characteristics of a known disease which leads to diagnosis.

Sequential diagnosis is mostly used when one symptom is largely predominant. Each step of the reasonning is composed of a question to which there are two or more answers, determining the choice of the next question. This sequential procedure is in fact far from being strictly linear ; the symptoms are not gathered separately but by groups ; the ordering in which they are inserted in the reasonning is fairly random ; there are often recurrences, the discovery of new symptoms leading to a new interpretation of the previously known symptoms.

II.2. COMPLEXITY OF THE PROCEDURE OF DIAGNOSIS

Practically, it is impossible to foresee the proportion in which each of these diagnosis procedures is used. This depends on many factors ; the psychological profile of the physician, his more or less synthetic intellectual training. These factors can lead to the preferential use of one of the two methods. Different patients having the same disease may, depending on the major symptoms, induce the developpement of one of these procedures. In addition, one can change of method at any time depending on the previous results : the first examination of the patient may incite to a first synthetic step ; then recognition of a predominant symptom, the need to ask for paramedical tests in a correct order may bring to the use of a sequential procedure ; finally, to operate the synthesis of the collected informations, one may recur to a global procedure ... Furthermore, the physician often takes into account considerations of "a priori" frequencies ; in the case of an acute angina, the very rare dipheteria is now one of the last diagnosis evoked.

Other factors can also influence the choice of the methods : the trained physician is naturally more apt to use a global procedure ; but for the needs of teaching he may however submit himself to the slower ways of the analytic methods.

Finally, it seems quite unrealistic to propose a general procedure of diagnosis. That procedure varies considering men and circumstances. Therefore, the automatization of diagnosis cannot choose to follow exactly the "natural" procedures ; it must build its own methods and the choice of these cannot come from their degree of similarity with the natural diagnosis, but from their efficiency.

II.3. MAJOR DIFFICULTIES OF DIAGNOSIS

Dr. F.T. de DOMBAL (LEEDS, U.K.) made an excellent analysis on a series of
600 patients who presented an acute abdominal pain, of the major causes of
errors in diagnosis [12] . He found 4 main reasons :

- the bad quality of the clinical examinations(omitted signs or uncorrect
  interpretation). This led him to suggest a very vigourous method for inquiry
  and examination ;
- the excessive importance the physicians give to typical aspects of diseases.
  Usually, they tend too often to reason by similarity and don't take suffi-
  sant account of the real frequency of symptoms in different diseases ;
- ignorance of certain rare diagnoses ;
- human thought's difficulty to manage simultaneously many information.

If the first cause decreases in the same way the performances of a computer
and of a trained brain, the three others show the computer's superiority :
under the condition that one has provided correct data, the computer's performance is not affected by a large amount of information. Its performances do
not decrease when this amount increases, while contrary is true for physicians.

The man capabilities of managing simultaneously different information were
more precisely studied by the mean of a specific experiment : two groups of
individuals - doctors and not doctors - had to recognize figures of an increasing complexity (composed of an increasing number of distinct elements
that must be simultaneously identified). Each figure represents a diagnosis.
The goal of the experiment was to measure the diagnosis procedure's efficiency connected with the number of elements to be taken into account simultaneously. The results are given by the following curve :

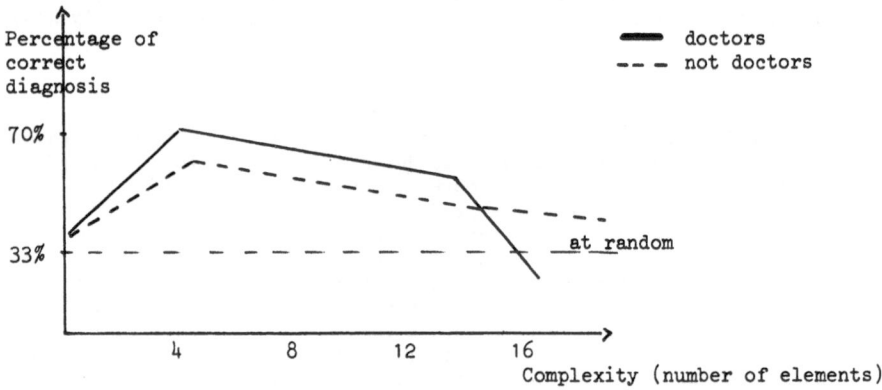

It clearly stands out that man's behaviour is like a limited capacity channel and, morever, this capacity is poorly extensible, as shown by the little
difference between trained people - the doctors - and the others. By opposition, the behaviour of a computer is independant of the complexity. It is
one of the major reasons of its utilisation in diagnosis procedures [9].

III. METHODS USING A COMPUTER

We will find here the same distinction between sequential and global methods.

III.1. ANALYTIC SEQUENTIAL METHODS

All these methods proceed by means of the sequential acquisition of the elements of information : after each new acquisition of decision is made concerning the next action to be taken. The application of such methods implies a logical modelisation of the decision-making process   ; this model can be represented by means of a graph, which is often a tree-like one since it is the simplest kind to construct.

The major tools used to read the graph are boolean algebra, theory of probability and theory decision.

III.1.1. Boolean (or Logical) Methods [3, 10, 20]

Boolean algebra is the algebra of variables that can take only two values. It can be applied particularly well to logical formalisation because a simple proposition can only be true or false : a patient has or does not have a disease D ; he or she has or does not have the symptom S.

One can object that symptoms may be present in more than two ways only. The patient's weight may be normal, or it may have gone up or gone down, for instance, or it may exist an infinite number of states in certain cases – for example, in biochemical dosages. But, it is always possible by breaking them down in a suitable manner to put symptoms into binary classes.

Three fundamental operations can be made on boolean variables :

- complementation of a variable : the complementary of a variable S is a new variable $\bar{S}$. It is linked to the first by the following rule :

if S is true, $\bar{S}$ is false $S = T \Longleftrightarrow \bar{S} = F$

if S is false, $\bar{S}$ is true $S = F \Longleftrightarrow \bar{S} = T$

Thus, if S is a present symptom, $\bar{S}$ will represent the lack of symptom.

- the logical sum of two variables S_1, S_2 is a third variable :

$\Sigma = S_1 + S_2$. Σ is true if at least one of the two variables S_1 or S_2 is true. Elsewhere, it is false. The logical sum corresponds to the "inclusive or" logical operation which is often expressed as "and/or" in medical literature. The logical sum can be stated as follows in the table below :

S_1	S_2	$S_1 + S_2$
F	F	F
F	T	T
T	F	T
T	T	T

Let us take for instance the measles (M) : two specific symptoms – a particular skin rash (R) and "Koplik's spots" or the buccal mucosa (K) – may be

present at the same time or separately. This may be expressed in the following way :

$$M = R + K$$

- the <u>logical product</u> of two variables S_1 ans S_2 is a new variable :

$$\Pi = S_1 \times S_2$$

Π is true only when S_1 and S_2 are true simultaneously, and false in other
cases. The logical product corresponds to the logical operation :"AND" :

S_1	S_2	$S_1 \times S_2$
F	F	F
F	T	F
T	F	F
T	T	T

In medicine, a frequent application of this is the definition of a syndrome. The nephrotic syndrome (N) is the association of proteinuria (pro-
tein in urine : P) and hypoproteinemia (diminution of the proteins in
blood : h) which may be formulated : $N = P \times h$.

It is clear that $S + \bar{S} = T$ and $S \times \bar{S} = F$

Boolean algebra use three basic operations in a systematic way by develop-
ping techniques adapted to binary computation, in order to solve complex
logical problems.

Among the relations created by logical algebra, one is particularly useful :
the relation of implication symbolized by " ————> ".
S ————> D means : if S is true, <u>then</u> D is true. Expressed in another
form : $S = T \Longrightarrow D = T$.

For instance, there is in neurology a very important sign called
Babinski's reflex (B) : when it is found, one can be sure that the patient
has what is called "pyramidal syndrome" (Py) but it expressly excludes poliomyelitis (Po). This can be stated as follows :

$$B \longrightarrow Py \qquad ; \qquad B \longrightarrow \bar{\bar{Po}}$$

A simplistic example will show how these notions may be applied in medical
diagnosis. Let us state the problem as follows :

We want to know if a patient has cirrhosis (C) ; four signs are defined :
each of them may be found when cirrhosis exists - but may also be found
in conjunction with other diseases. These symptoms are : hepatomegaly
(increase of the liver's size : H), splenomegaly (increase of the spleen's
size : S), ascites (accumulation of fluid in the peritoneal cavity : A),
spider angioma (tumours derived from blood vessels and having a particular
appearance : Sa). In addition, we want to distinguish between two kinds of
cirrhosis : atrophic cirrhosis (AC) and hypertrophic cirrhosis (HC).

The first step will be the symptomatical description of diseases. Let us
admit that medical knowledge will lead us to express this as follows :

$$HC = H \times S \times (A + Sa) \qquad ; \qquad AC = S \times A \times Sa$$

and it becomes clear that :

$$C = \left[H \times S \times (A + Sa) \right] \quad + \quad \left[S \times A \times Sa \right]$$

In the next step these relations may be represented in a binary form by means of a table where 1 indicates that a sign or a disease exists and 0 that it is missing.

	H	1	1	1	0	1	1	0	0
Symptoms	S	1	1	1	1	0	1	1	1
	A	1	1	0	1	1	0	0	1
	Sa	1	0	1	1	1	0	1	0
	C	1	1	1	1	0	0	0	0
Diseases	HC	1	1	1	0	0	0	0	0
	AC	0	0	0	1	0	0	0	0

Each row describes a possible combination of signs and the compatible diagnoses. In the left part of the table are the combinations corresponding to the previously defined diseases (C, HC, AC) ; in the right part, the combinations of symptoms which are not related to cirrhosis.

The final step will consist in programming a computer in order to sort the present signs and to check them against this table.

In fact, the number of signs and combinations is much greater, but the combined power of boolean algebra and computers make the computation of very complex problems possible.

One of the advantages of boolean methods is that they proceed in much the same way as the natural sequential method. On the other hand, they don't take into account the notion of frequency : the result of a computation is only the name of one - or more - possible diseases but it gives no estimation of probability.

Another point is the difficulty of purely logical formalisation of medical knowledge in false and true terms : in most cases, the physician would prefer to say that the symptom S is exceptional in the disease D, rather than S is never possible in D. In other words, the physician very often uses, more or less explicitly, the notion of frequency. The fact that logical methods neglect this reality is their major flaw.

III.1.2. Methods using the Theory of Probability [5, 6, 7, 8, 11, 14, 16, 21, 22, 29]

In opposition to logical methods, they take into account the frequency of the diseases and the frequency of signs in diseases. These methods are based on BAYES' theorem : it is used to compute the disease D_i's probability when a symptom - or syndrome - S has been looked for and given the result S_j, i.e. $P(D_i/S_j)$. It presupposes that the "prior" probability of D_i $(P(D_i))$ and the probability of finding S_j when D_i exists $(P(S_j/D_i))$ are known. Bayes' theorem links these probabilities in the following way :

$$P(D_i/S_j) = \frac{1}{K} \; P(D_i) \; P(S_j/D_i)$$

where K is a constant chosen in such a way that $\sum_i P(D_i/S_j) = 1$

One can clearly see that the BAYES' theorem implies :

- exhaustivity and exclusiveness of the list of all possible diseases D_i ;
- previous knowledge of all the $P(D_i)$ and $P(S_j/D_i)$ as mentioned above.

It is clear that probabilistic methods don't "make" a diagnosis ; but they give a "posterior" probability - that may equal zero - to each possible diagnosis. The physician must choose from a list of diagnoses in order of decreasing probability but he must know that in "particular cases" the accurate diagnosis is not always the most probable.

Probabilistic methods are especially well adapted when diagnosis's procedure is a step by step one. The BAYES' theorem may be used in iterative way : at each step, new signs are collected and the posterior probability of the previous step becomes the prior probability of the present step. The D_i diagnosis's probability, during the collection of symptoms evolves as follows :

$$P\ (D_i) \longrightarrow P(D_i/S_{1j}) \longrightarrow P(D_i/S_{1j} \text{ and } S_{2k}) \longrightarrow \text{ etc } \ldots\ldots$$

D_i's prior probability

$S_{1j}(S_{2k})$ is the modality j (k) of the result of test 1 (2).

In fact there are some theoretical and practical difficulties in using BAYES' theorem :

- the first is the exclusiveness and exhaustivity of the diagnosis ; in real cases, D_1 and D_2 may be present simultaneously for one patient : the solution is to consider that there are not 2 but 3 diagnoses : D_1, D_2 and $D_1 \times D_2$.

   As for the exhaustivity of the list, it can always be guaranteed by introcing the item "other diagnoses". This is obviously reasonable only if these other diagnoses represent only doubtful possibility, that is, with low prior probability. This is the case with acute abdominal pain syndrome which de Dombal has studied. He noted that out of 300 cases observed in the Leeds Hospital system, 96 % of the acute abdominal pain syndromes were represented by 7 diagnoses ; the "other diagnoses" rubric, representing only 4 % of the cases, was sufficient to make the list of possibilities exhaustive [8] .

- determining the prior probability of various diseases $P(D_i)$ isn't always simple ; it depends to a great extent on the limitations of the consultation : geographical location, season, speciality of the department involved, the doctor's reputation ... Estimating it isn't easy and requires statistics that have been correctly organized and brought up to date. To give an example, the round shapes on X-rays of the thorax studied by J. Lellouch and A. Alperovitch [1] were considered to be of tubercular origin 9 % or 34 % of the time, according to what hospital department the patient came from. Furthermore, there are some cases in which the different possibilities have prior probabilities that vary greatly. The least likely ones run the risk of having a heavy handicap to overcome and never showing up after a reasonable number of investigations. That is why one can suggest to adopt Laplace's hypothesis, that is, all possibilities having equal prior probability.

- the $P(S_j/D_i)$ probabilities are themselves not very well known in most cases. Correct statistics are rare. Some authors think that even a very approximative estimation by doctors, based on their experience, is sufficient. But de Dombal seems to believe otherwise : in his bayesian algorithm applied to the diagnosis of acute abdominal pains, he first introduced the probability supplied to him by trained clinicians, and then the frequencies provided by the statistical analysis of a series of 600 cases : the proportion of correct diagnoses given by the computer was 82 % in the first case and

91 % in the second (N.B. : the clinicians' diagnoses were correct for 79 % of the cases) [8] .

- the iterative use of Bayes theorem doesn't imply, as it is often argued, the stochastic independance of the symptoms and signs sequentially collected.

Indeed, when one writes

$$P(D_j/S_{1i} \text{ and } S_{2k}) = \frac{1}{K} P(D_j) P(S_{1i} \text{ and } S_{2k}/D_j)$$

One must evaluate $P(S_{1i} \text{ and } S_{2k}/D_j)$, that is

$$P(S_{1i} \text{ and } S_{2k}/D_j) = \frac{1}{K} P(S_{1i}/D_j).P(S_{2k}/S_{1i} \text{and } D_j)$$

and more generally, one must know the sequence :

$$P(S_{1i}/D_j), \ P(S_{2k}/S_{1i} \text{ and } D_j), \ P(S_{31}/S_{1i} \text{ and } S_{2k} \text{ and } D_j) \ \ldots$$

That means, the probability of the results of the nth test in diagnosis D_j, knowing the results of tests number 1, 2, ... , n - 1.

Practically, it is impossible to know so many parameters. It is why the assumption of stochastic independence is so often made. That means for instance, that

$$P(S_{1i} \text{ and } S_{2k}/D_j) = P(S_{1i}/D_j).P(S_{2k}/D_j)$$

Much research has been made in order to get rid, at least partly, of this too strict assumption [15 bis, 20 bis].

In the case, very important when a clinical investigation is concerned, when all the symptoms are of the boolean nature (S and $\bar{S}$), the final formula can be written :

$$P(D_j/ \Sigma) = \frac{1}{K} P(D_j) \prod_{k \in I} P(S_k/D_j) \prod_{k \in \bar{I}} P(\bar{S}_l/D_j)$$

I   set of symptoms and signs being present
$\bar{I}$ set of the symptoms and signs being absent
Σ corresponding clinical profile.

One sees that bayesian method takes into account as well the absent as the present symptoms and signs. This is one of the main reasons of its power. Now, it happens that several symptoms reveal the same illness in a different way. The idea here is to regroup (by means of a boolean fonction, for example) the symptoms correlated into syndromes, such that the latter are independant of one another.

Even if such precautions are taken, the probabilistic independance of symptoms or syndromes is far from being proved in practice. Although such a theoretical difficulty would appear to be prohibitive, in practice it apparently has not harmed a certain number of programs.

- finally, it has been objected that a list of diagnoses in decreasing order of probability is of no interest. The most probable diagnosis is not necessarily the most interesting or most useful one ; thus given a list of the following type :

        . simple indigestion : 65 %
        . appendicitis   : 20 %

It would perhaps be unwise to be satisfied with the diagnosis of indiges-

tion and not to operate. A mistake in diagnosis can have serious consequences or less serious ones depending on whether Diagnosis A has been
opted for, when it should have been Diagnosis B or vice versa.

This entails completing the program by introducing the cost of diagnostic
mistakes. Let C_{ij} be the cost of accepting Diagnosis D_i when the correct
diagnosis is D_j. If $p_1 \ldots p_n$ are the posterior probabilities of these
different diagnoses, the average cost of the decision D_j is

$$C_j = \sum_{i=1}^{n} p_i \, C_{ij}$$

The average cost of all possible decisions may be calculated in this way
and the one whose cost is least is chosen. It is only if all the C_{ij} are
equal that the best choice is the most probable one.

Theory of information

In an iterative process like the bayesian one described above, it is important to try to determine from out of all the signs that can be collected those
that can lead the most quickly to the diagnosis.

The theory of information makes it possible to arrive at this result by allowing us to select the one which will provide the most information.

Let us then consider, at a given stage i, diagnostic uncertainty. The latter
can be expressed, after examination i and before examination i+1, as

$$H = - \sum_j p_j \log p_j$$

where p_j are the posterior probabilities of the diagnoses D_j.

Now let us consider a new examination S that it has been decided to recur to
at a stage i+1. Let us suppose it is binary, that is, that it can give a
"positive" or "negative" result. If it is positive, the posterior probabilities
of the diagnosis will become p'_j. The uncertainty will be :

$$H' = - \sum_j p'_j \log p'_j$$

and the gain in information will be given as $G' = H - H'$.
If it is negative, the posterior probability will be p''_j, the uncertainty will
be H'', and the gain of information $G'' = H - H''$. We can then calculate the
expectancy of gain in information, which is merely the mean of gains in information weighed by the prior probabilities of examination S having a positive
or negative result : $G = \pi_+ \, G' + \pi_- \, G''$

This calculation can be done again for all possible examinations and the one
having the best gain in information will be chosen.

The combination of Bayes' theorem with the theory of information gives rise
to the "theory of questionnaires".

But it is clear that the information supplied by an examination is not the
only criterion used in choosing it. In fact in some cases, it may be preferable to choose examinations which, taken individually, supply less information
but which, altogether, cost less in financial terms. One may and should take
into account factors connected with the patients' confort and safety. If this
is done, it may turn out to be very difficult to choose between several strategies and to define an objective criterion for choosing. The choice of the
best decision resides in considering one numerical variable that has to be

optimized : it is easy, in theory at least, to find the strategy that maximizes the amount of information provided by each examination and minimizes the number of examinations to be done, or the one that, without taking into account the number of examinations, minimizes the overall financial cost of the latter, or again the strategy that minimizes the risk-to-life for the patient (all one needs to know is the risk each individual examination brings to light). It is more difficult if the patient's discomfort is to be taken into account because it is subjective, it cannot be quantified and at best, can only be expressed in qualitative terms. It is even more difficult if all the factors are to be taken into account at once because it would then be necessary to weigh them and express them in terms of a single numerical variable which would express the overall cost to be minimized (or the utility to be maximized). The attempt to find the numerical functions of several quantitative or qualitative variables is one of the problems of and obstacles to formalizing diagnostical decisions.

III.1.3. Theory of Decision [1, 13, 27, 28]

The methods described up to this point are applicable to diagnostic decision-making or occasionally to prognosis decision-making that is, they are applicable to essentially static situations : a decision is made on the basis of the examination of a patient at a given moment (even if the examination lasts several days, during which the necessary investigations will be pursued in sequential fashion). But in Lusted'opinion, a purely diagnostic decision is no more than the product of academic activity, very often futile if not followed up by the therapeutic decision, that is, an action that can change the "natural" course of the illness. To achieve the latter, the dynamic process of the disease must be got at, and the previous methods, which do not take into account the temporal progress of the disease, are inadequate [19] .

The more complex model of the theory of decision must be called into play. It presupposes that a model of the evolution of the illness will have been constructed taking into account the various actions that can be put into practice. The latter model is a tree-like graph on which the nodes are alternately decision nodes (the arrows going out from them represent the various decisions concerning possible action that a doctor can make) and nodes of nature's responses to these same decisions (the arrows that go out from them, each one having been assigned a probability, represent the possibilities that can occur).

For each possibility, the decision-maker must be able to answer by one and only one of the possible decisions,and so forth. This diagram, which represents an interaction between the decision-maker and nature, gives a broad overview and is characteristic of "decision trees". Each path leading from the top of the tree to one of its outer branches represents a possible strategy. In order to be able to make a rational choice among these paths, each one of them must be assigned an "overall cost" - or a "utility" which is none other than the "overall cost" with the opposite sign. This utility must, in general, depend on the "cost" of all actions taken on the path under consideration (the term "cost" being used in the manner discussed above) and above all on the patients' condition at the end of the path. The path that should be chosen will be the one that gives, in term of expectancy, the maximal utility or the minimal cost.

It can be objected that it is very difficult to compute with the same unity costs that vary widely as financial costs, the costs of suffering, discomfort, risk-to-life and impairment of functioning, etc ... It can be answered that the doctor who makes a choice between two or among several strategies implicitly sets up a relationship of order between them by weighing in his own way the different elements that enter into "the cost". Determining the costs, which is difficult but possible, results in making such choices more easily to be replicated.

III.2. GLOBAL METHODS [15, 23, 25]

They are essentially based on multivariate statistical analysis techniques : what differentiates them above all from sequential analytical methods is the fact that they make it possible to examine the data "innocently" by not seeking in any way to imitate or even to be inspired by the "natural" medical procedure. In fact they require of the doctor no special effort to elaborate an algorithm : all he or she has to do is provide the exact information.

Another difference between global methods and sequential ones is that the former usually allow for a choice among only a small number of decisions. This is one of the reasons why most of these global methods are used particularly in stages prior to the diagnosis properly speaking ; they make it possible basically to study the different criteria that come into play in the diagnosis.

III.2.1. The Variables

All the methods which will be described depart from the collection of data from patients. These data can be of several kinds : they can be either qualitative (the sex, the existence of a pain are boolean variables ; to possess caucasian, mongoloid or negro features is a variable with 3 values), or quantitative (number of cg of glucose per liter of blood, systolic blood pressure ...). At the boarder between qualitative and quantitative data, there are variables which may be called semi-quantitative : there are not the result of a measure and as such are qualitative ; but their values can be ranked in a definite order, aspect which make them close to numbers (degree of a jaundice, response to a serological test ...).

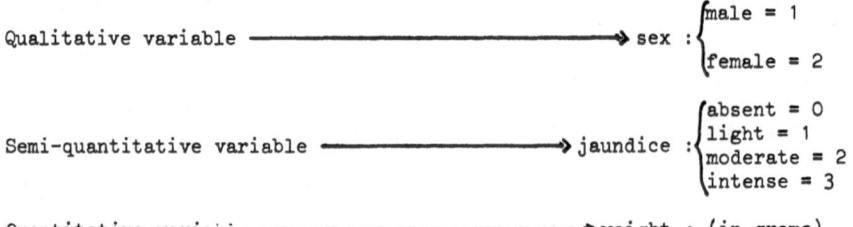

Qualitative variable ⟶ sex : $\begin{cases} male = 1 \\ female = 2 \end{cases}$

Semi-quantitative variable ⟶ jaundice : $\begin{cases} absent = 0 \\ light = 1 \\ moderate = 2 \\ intense = 3 \end{cases}$

Quantitative variable ⟶ weight : (in grams)

It is always possible to transform a quantitative variable into a semi-quantitative one (by dividing the range into several distinct domains), and a semi-quantitative into one or several boolean qualitative variables.Doing so, one looses information, but this transformation is often most useful for some kind of analysis. Obviously, to go in the reverse direction from qualitative to quantitative description of a same data is logically impossible and then forbidden.

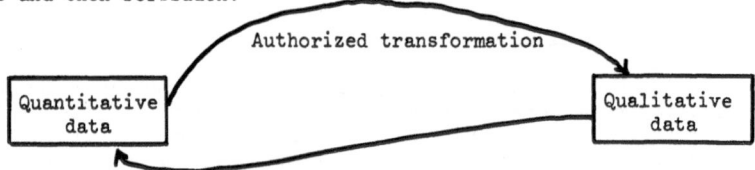

Authorized transformation

| Quantitative data | | Qualitative data |

Forbidden transformation

The matrix of the data

Finally one collects p variables from n patients. They can be presented on a matrix of n rows and p columns. Two important points must be pointed out : a) it is necessary to have $n > p$; b) the matrix must be full : empty places resulting from the missing data can make the analysis difficult if there are few of them, and impossible if they are numerous.

		Sex			Jaundice		Weight		
n patients									
child n°231		1			2		2250		

(n patients, p variables)

III.2.3. Multivariate methods

In multivariate analysis, instead of examining the variable one by one as is done in classical univariate statistical methods, one considers as a whole, at the same time, **all** the variables collected on a patient. Some geometrical considerations can help to understand the general principles of the analytical methods.

This matrix can be represented geometrically by a cloud of n points in a space of p dimensions, called R^p. The following figures gives a graph of a cloud in a space of 3 dimensions, the largest one that can be graphically represented. Each point represents a patient.

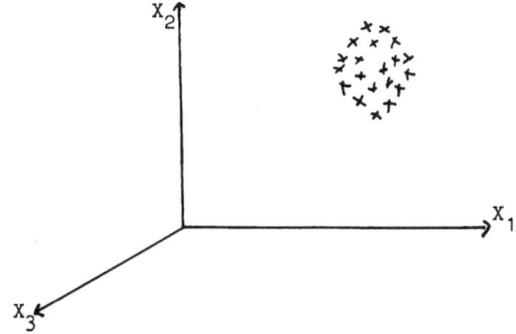

The methods can be divided into two groups : the purely descriptive methods ; the decisionnal methods.

III.2.3.1. The descriptive methods

These methods are used to describe the shape of the cloud, and to examine whether it can be divided into several distinct subclouds.

The method used to analyse the shape of the cloud is called <u>factorial analysis</u>.

Let us consider two possible situations.

1) The cloud can be almost spheric, that means that it has about the same size in every directions. This shape can be interpreted by the fact that there is no correlation between variables.

2) In fact, in practical cases, the variables collected on a patient are always correlated and often strongly. That means that the information collected is redundant. That also implies that the cloud has not the same dimension in every direction and that it is (more or less) contained in a subspace of R^p. It can be described with an excellent approximation by q variables only ($q < p$)

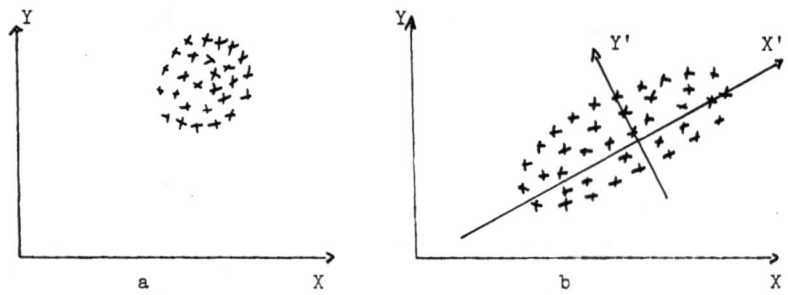

The figure gives an example of what can happen in the case of p = 2 dimensions. Instead of having a circular cloud (a), one can have a very long cloud (b). This suggests strongly to change the axes, and to consider <u>new variables</u> X' and Y'. In fact, the variable X' will be nearly sufficient to describe the cloud : the more elongated the cloud, the better the reduction to the simple variable X'. The new axes are called <u>factorial axes</u>, and the new variables which give the coordinates of the points on the factorial axes are called <u>factors</u>. So one can say, that is the case b, the factor X' is sufficient to give a good approximation of the cloud.

Let us now return to the R^p space. One finds the factorial axes in the same way : the first one is chosen along the direction of maximal elongation of the cloud (and the abscisse on this axe is the first factor) ; the next one is perpendicular to the first, and runs the direction of the next maximal elongation and so on ...

Finally we have succeeded in changing the system of axes in the R^p space, Most of time, it appears that a few axes and the corresponding factors are sufficient to describe the cloud. Falling from p original variables to a very few factors (3 or 4), we have obtained a <u>substantial data reduction</u>. An important feature is that the few new variables, which can be calculated from numerous mutually correlated variables, are mutually uncorrelated.

It is possible to consider the planes built on the first and second factorial axes, on first and third, on second and third ... and project the clouds on these planes, called <u>factorial planes</u>. Doing that, one can observe the possible clustering of the points (i.e. the patients) : this can suggest a classification of the patients.

A special kind of factorial analysis, called "<u>analyse factorielle des correspondances</u>" (A. F. C.) due to the french mathematician J.P. BENZECRI

[4] , is particularly interesting, because by a mathematical procedure which is beyond the scope of this paper, it allows to project on the factorial planes, not only the patients, but also the variables. The interpretation of the graph obtained is the following : two patients very much alike project close to each other ; two variables highly correlated project also close to each other : if a patient is particularly well explained by a variable, both are neighbors on the graph.

Another kind of description methods is the classification methods. If the examination of factorial graphs suggest clustering of patients (and/or of variables in the case of A. F. C.), factorial analysis methods do not build classes. Classification methods allow to define the classes (or clusters) into which one can put every patient of the sample. First, one must choose an index of similarity and compute it for all the $\frac{n(n-1)}{2}$ couples of patients.

Afterwards a rather simple kind of algorithm gives a hierarchical classification of the individuals of the sample. Unfortunately, the result of the algorithm - i.e. the proposed classification - depends the most often on the choice of the similarity coefficient, and of the algorithm of clustering.

III.2.3.2. The decisionnal methods

Some other multivariate methods are used to describe the sample in such a way that it provides a way of making a decision for new patient (that means that it does not belong to the sample), and so it can be used for diagnosis. In this case, one of the variables, let say Y, plays a special role. The problem is how to explain and to predict the value of this particular variable from all others, let say X_1, X_2, ... , X_p. Two cases must be separated :

a) Y is a qualitative variable : for instance the type of a jaundice, mechanical or not ; or else the issue of a disease : death or survival. Each value of variable Y represents a predefined class of patients. The kind of analysis is called discriminant analysis. From the other variables, for instance symptoms, physical or biological signs, can be predicted the type of jaundice, or the death of the patient.
b) Y is a quantitative variable : for instance the duration of survival. This method is then a regression analysis method.

We shall here envisage only linear discriminant and regression analysis.

Linear discriminant analysis. In order to explain this method let us consider first that Y is a boolean variable (two predefined classes) and that there are only two explaining variables X_1 and X_2.

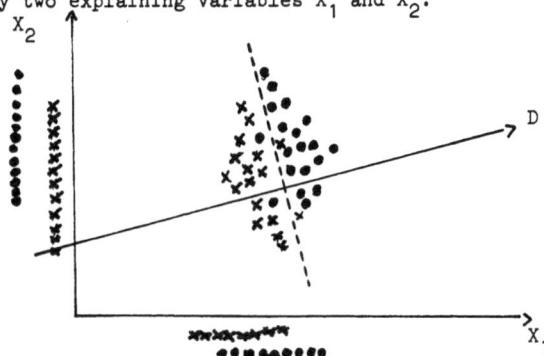

It is obvious on the graph that none of the X_1, or X_2 is able alone to provide a good separation between the two classes. But if we change the axes
and consider the D axis,it is obvious that a new variable (which can be
expressed linearly from both X_1 and X_2 : $D = a_0 + a_1X_1 + a_2X_2$) will lead
to a much better discrimination.

If there are p explaining variables $(X_1 \ldots X_p)$, one can proceed on similar
lines, and find from the <u>sample</u> the best linear discriminant function :

$$D = a_0 + a_1X_1 + \ldots + a_pX_p$$

Now, if we have a new patient, for which we know the explaining variables
$X_1, \ldots X_p$, it is possible to compute for him the value of D and then
to <u>predict</u> for him the value of Y, that means to which class he should be
allocated.

So, one may say that discriminant analysis proceeds in two steps.

1) a descriptive step : from a <u>training</u> sample of patients for which <u>all</u>
   variables are known (the explaining ones,and the explained Y), one can
   determine the discriminant function (that is compute the coefficients
   $a_0, a_1 \ldots a_p$)

2) a decisionnal step : for a <u>new</u> patient, for which Y is unknown, one
   compute the discriminant function, and according the value obtained
   decide to which class he belongs.

One extremely important point is that, when determining the discriminant
function, it is possible to proceed <u>stepwise</u> : first, one extracts, among
all the X_i, the most discriminating, then the second most discriminating
one, and so on ... It appears, in nearly all the cases, that one can
reach the <u>best linear discrimination</u>, using only a restricted subset for
all the X_i (let us say 5 to 7). Then 5 to 7 X_i are sufficient for the best
possible linear decision ; the others are of a poor informationnel value
for the decision. This aspect can be of course of a great interest, both
theoretical and practical.

<u>Linear regression analysis</u>. Here the explained variable is quantitative. One
tries to find the <u>best</u> linear function that explains Y.

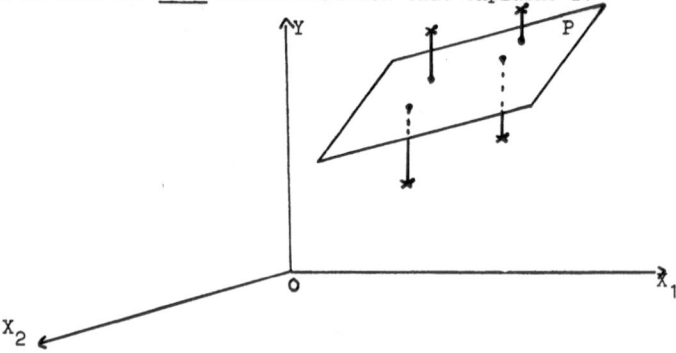

The figure shows an example when p = 2 (X_1 and X_2). The idea, underlying
the mathematical procedure, is that each observed value Y can be written

$$Y = \underbrace{b_0 + b_1X_1 + b_2X_2}_{\text{plane P}} + e$$

wheree is the vertical distance, along the OY direction, from the observed points to the plane P. One must find b_0, b_1, b_2 in such a way that e_s are as small as possible (in fact, one imposes the condition to minimize the sum of the e_s^2). The plane found is the best linear approximation of the cloud.

So it appears that as well as for discriminant analysis, there are two steps in regression analysis, descriptive and decisionnal.

1) from a <u>training</u> sample (Y known) one derives the best linear function

$$Y = b_0 + b_1 X_1 + \ldots\ldots\ldots + b_p X_p$$

2) for a new patient (Y unknown), one computes the linear function and predicts the value of Y.

It is possible to select the best subset of explaining variables by a stepwise procedure.

III.2.4. Conclusion

An important point to rise is the fact that all the signs, symptoms, results of tests we collect on patient are highly redundant, and that probably a small subset is sufficient to make the correct decisions. This idea, that should have a great practical impact, deserves our reflexion and can be the ground for future research.

Methods Aid to	Factorial analysis	Classification	Discrimination	Multiple Regression
Nosology Classification Epidemiology	+++	++		
Diagnosis	+		++	
Prognosis	+		++	++

Global Methods and Their Medical Application Field

IV. EVALUATION OF THE QUALITY OF A DECISION-MAKING PROCESS

The decision to use or not to use an informational system of aid-to-diagnosis can only be made by taking into account a certain number of criteria, the essential one being the evaluation of its efficiency. We are going to demonstrate how it is possible to make such an evaluation.

As an example, let us take a sample of 150 subjects about whom we <u>know</u> that the correct diagnosis is d for 70 of them (d = cardiac infarction, for example) and d̄ (no cardiac infarction) for 80. Let us call δ and δ̄ the decisions proposed by the decision-making process.

An <u>ideal</u> decision-making process would make no mistakes, that is, the results could be expressed as follows

Correct decision, that is, <u>Correct diagnosis</u>

	d	$\bar{d}$
proposed decision δ	70	0
that is, the		
chosen diagnosis $\bar{\delta}$	0	80
	70	80

In most cases, it doesn't work like this and efficiency in making the correct diagnosis gives results of the following type :

Correct diagnosis

	d	$\bar{d}$
proposed δ	63_{TP}	12_{FP}
diagnosis $\bar{\delta}$	7_{FN}	68_{TN}

The two boxes that were empty before aren't any longer : 7 cases of illness d were not diagnosed as such ; these are the cases that were mistakenly declared negative, in other words, the <u>False Negatives</u> (FN); diagnosis d was attributed to 12 patients who do not have the illness : the <u>False Positives</u> (FP). This leaves only 63 True Positives (TP) and 68 True Negatives (TN).

How should this performance be evaluated ? One idea consists in computing the <u>proportion of correctly classified subjects</u>, that is the relation :

$$\frac{TP + TN}{TP + FN + FP + TN} = \frac{63 + 68}{150} = 0.87$$

and that is what is often done. But let us take the following example :

	d	$\bar{d}$			d	$\bar{d}$
δ	70_{TP}	19_{FP}		δ	51	0
$\bar{\delta}$	0_{FN}	61_{TN}		$\bar{\delta}$	19	80
	70	80			70	80

which corresponds to two extreme situations :
- <u>all the cases of infarction</u> were detected (no false negatives)
- <u>all the chosen diagnoses of infarction</u> are correct (no false positives)

yet both have the same ratio of correctly classified subjects as the previous ones.

table (= 0.87)

Since calculating the ratio of correctly classified subjects is inadequate, a diagnostic process is often characterized by <u>two</u> parameters that must be considered <u>simultaneously</u>.

- sensitivity - Sy - or the proportion of subjects suffering from d to whom this diagnosis was in fact attributed. It equals

$$\frac{TP}{TP + FN}$$

that is, respectively

$$\frac{63}{70} = 0.90 \; ; \; \frac{70}{70} = 1.0 \; \text{and} \; \frac{51}{70} = 0.73$$

In terms of probability, sensitivity can be expressed Proba (δ/d). The sensitivity of a diagnostic process expresses the ability of the latter to detect <u>illness d when it exists</u> (and to make decision δ when the correct decision is D)

- specificity - Sp - equals $\frac{TN}{TN + FP}$. It is the proportion of subjects who do not have illness d and for whom this diagnosis was effectively eliminated.

It equals respectively $\frac{68}{80} = 0.85 \; ; \; \frac{61}{80} = 0.76 \; ; \; \frac{80}{80} = 1$, in the three cases envisaged above. In terms of probability, specificity is none other than Proba $(\bar{\delta}/\bar{d})$. Specificity expresses the aptitude of a process to eliminate illness d when it doesn't exist.

It is more or less obvious that these two qualities are somewhat contradictory. If we wish to detect all cases of infarction, we will have to make the criteria of selection less exacting. But if we increase sensitivity in this way, we also increase the chances of applying this diagnosis incorrectly, that is we decrease <u>specificity</u>. Inversely, if we choose to use only very stringent criteria, all the cases detected will in fact be cases of infarction but the diagnostic net will not catch all the cases of <u>real</u> infarction. Depending on the case, very good sensitivity or very good specificity will be stressed in making the decision. For example, in a systematic detection of diabetes, the aim is to have as high sensitivity as possible, even if it entails detecting in view of further exploration of subjects who are not in fact diabetics. Inversely, in research work on a given illness, it is preferable to count only subjects who definitely have the illness, that is achieve <u>excellent specificity</u>. Work done on an individual whose diagnosis was uncertain, would lack scientific value and would therefore be a waste.

Comments

These two parameters "sensitivity" and "specificity" characterize a decision-making process perfectly. The latter is in effect represented by 2x2 table for which the total of the two columns are fixed, that is with two degrees of freedom. The proportion of correctly classified or the proportion of success :

$$Su = \frac{TN + TP}{TN + FN + TP + FP}$$

is only the average of sensitivity and specificity weighed by the sizes d and $\bar{d}$.

Indeed : $$Sy \times \frac{TP + FN}{TP + FN + TN + FP} + Sp \times \frac{TN + FP}{TP + FN + TN + FP} = Su$$

It is obvious that sensitivity and specificity are strictly symmetrical: sensitivity for decision d is the equivalent of specificity for $\bar{d}$, and vice versa.

Still, there is most often asymmetry with respect to the practical consequences of the two alternative decisions : to diagnose an infarction or reject this diagnosis ; to operate or not.

Some authors also introduce the concept of reliability which expresses the degree of confidence one can have in a process. This concept in fact takes in two parameters :

- on the one hand, the reliability of a decision chosen δ is the probability that this decision is the correct one, that is, Prob (d/δ). It can be estimated by :

$$R_\delta = \frac{TP}{TP + FP} \quad \text{or} \quad \frac{63}{63 + 12} = 0.84$$

in our example above.

- on the other hand, there is the reliability of $\bar{\delta}$, which is Prob$(\bar{d}/\bar{\delta})$. It

equals : $R_{\bar{\delta}} = \frac{TN}{TN + FN} = \frac{68}{7 + 68} = 0.91$

Of course, these two parameters are linked to the first two by virtue of Bayes'theorem. For example :

$$R_\delta = \frac{prob\ (d)\ .Sy}{prob(d)\ .\ Sy + prob\ \bar{d}(1 - Sp)} \quad \text{with} \quad prob\ (d) = \frac{70}{150} = 0.467$$

and $prob(\bar{d}) = \frac{80}{112} = 0.84$ which gives $R_\delta = \frac{0.467 \times 0.9}{0.467 \times 0.9 + 0.533(1-0.85)} = 0.84$

and similarly

$$R_{\bar{\delta}} = \frac{prob\ (\bar{d})\ .\ Sp}{prob(\bar{d})\ .\ Sp + prob\ (d)\ .\ (1 - Sy)}$$

The case of K alternative decisions (K > 2)

Let us imagine that the decisions are mutually exclusive and exhaustive. In this case, the results of the decision-making process can be given in a square table K x K

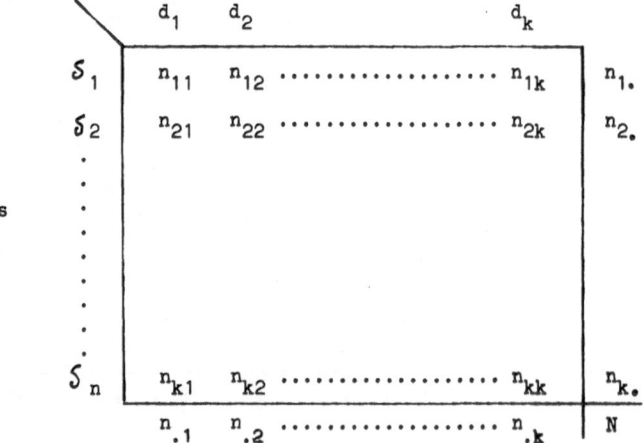

correct decisions

	d_1	d_2	d_k	
δ_1	n_{11}	n_{12} .... n_{1k}		$n_{1.}$
δ_2	n_{21}	n_{22} .... n_{2k}		$n_{2.}$
Decisions proposed δ_n	n_{k1}	n_{k2} .... n_{kk}		$n_{k.}$
	$n_{.1}$	$n_{.2}$ .... $n_{.k}$		N

n_1, n_2 ... are the sum of the sizes of lines 1, 2, ... That is, of the sizes of each of the decisions proposed δ_1, δ_2 ....

$n_{.1}$, $n_{.2}$, ... are similarly, the sizes of the columns that correspond to d_1, d_2, ...

This table possesses $K(K - 1)$ degrees of freedom, the total K sizes of each column are given, and for each column an arbitrary number K-1 sizes can be established.

There would therefore have to be $K(K-1)$ relations.

In practice a smaller number of parameters will be satisfactory, for example :

- the proportion of correctly classified subjects $(n_{11} + n_{22} + \ldots + n_{kk})$ / N
- the sensitivity of each decision

$$\text{prob} \left(\delta_i / d_i \right) = \frac{n_{ii}}{n_{.i}}$$

- the reliability of each decision $\text{prob} \left(d_i / \delta_i \right) = \frac{n_{ii}}{n_{i.}}$

V. MEDICAL EXAMPLES

V.1. AID TO NEUROLOGICAL DIAGNOSIS USING A BAYESIAN METHOD

This work has been realized by our department (R. SALAMON) and the department of Neurology (Prof. C. DEROUESNE) in the CHU Pitié-Salpétrière (PARIS) and in collaboration with the department of Neurology of Hotel-Dieu Hospital (Prof. SAMSON, Rouen).

In this work, several original points can be noted :

a) the application field : the authors chose a very wide field, the whole pathology of the nervous system, and they take into account a great deal of symptoms - especially clinical ones -

b) the aim of the system : in fact, aid to diagnosis in neurology has only a limited practical interest ; therefore, for the authors, the system is considered essentially as a teaching tool for medical students, and more precisely as an aid to determine the content of teaching.

Two major difficulties exist :

- semiology is a vast and complicated field : it is often based on statistical considerations - more or less explicit - and rarely on physiopathological facts (only a few symptoms are directly linked to precise nervous system lesions).
- diagnosis is quite difficult to make precisely due to the fact that neurological diagnoses are divided into etiological (diagnosis of the cause) and topographical (diagnosis of localization) ones.

The authors wanted to simplify these problems by focusing on therapeutical acts.

This was done in the following way :

- the selected diagnoses lead to a single way of medical strategy (annex 1). This is why the different diagnoses implying the same therapeutical attitude were gathered. For instance, heredodegenerescence, amyotrophic lateral sclerosis and PICK-HERZHEIMER disease have been gathered in a single category called "degenerative diseases" ; only Parkinson's disease is differentiated because it requires a special treatment.

- only a few neurological signs have been selected and they were greatly
simplified (annex 2). The authors think - and the purpose of this work is
to prove it - that students are perfectly capable of discriminating a
given "operational" neurological diagnosis by using a very simple semiology.

c) Selection of   prior   probabilities

For pedagogical reasons, the authors have chosen an equiprobable reparti-
tion of diseases to initiate the process.

The aim of this choice is to compute diagnoses,with a bayesian method,
using only the results of the patient's clinical examination : in fact
it seems to be dangerous if the students mix up information coming from
patients and much wider considerations, resulting from prior frequencies
of diseases.

Obviously, coming at the end of the process, relative frequencies of possible diagnoses must be given to students, and they have to take them into
consideration.

d) Evaluation of $P(S_j/D_i)$ conditional probabilities

These probabilities, as mentioned above, are very difficult to estimate.
Most of the time, we have a choice between methods:

- this evaluation can be made by analysing a great number of medical
records ;
- or it can be obtained from the physician in an empirical way.

The first choice - the best one, when it is possible - was here ruled out :
its would require too many records because 31 diagnoses and close to 150
symptoms are used.

Since the purpose of computer-aided diagnosis is an objective evaluation of
the probabilities related to every diagnosis, choosing the second method
would have been really dangerous as the computation would be based on subjective and biased data.

The authors chose an intermediate method, which can be summarized as follows :

1 - the neurologist estimates the different probabilities he wants to express
by a mark from 0 to 5 ; these different "weights" relative to each symptom are vague enough to be reasonably estimated by a neurologist (annex 3)

2 - afterwards, from a little sample of patients with a known diagnosis, a
probability, P(x), is attributed to each weight by using the formula :

$$P(x) = \frac{N(x)}{N_{max}(x)}$$

where :

. $N(x)$ is the number of symptoms having the weight x in the patients'
sample ;
. $N_{max}(x)$ is the maximum number of symptoms having the weight x that
sample's patients could have (annex 4)

3 - Finally, these P(x) probabilities are weighted by the real frequencies
computed from the patients with known diagnoses each time new patients'
records come in (annex 5). Finally, the probability used in the bayesian
process is the following one :

$$P(S_j D_i) = \frac{K\ P(x) + N_i\ f(S_j/D_i)}{N_i + K}$$

where :

. $f(S_j/D_i)$ is the real frequence of S_j in D_i, computed from N_i patients
having the diagnosis D_i that are recorded in the system ;

. K is a constant which corresponds to the number of patients'records
in the system, to which is given the same value as the neurologist's evaluation. After several trials, the value K = 10
was chosen (annex 6)

As the sample increases constantly, this"self-training"method gives more and
more new "objective" probabilities.

e) management of the patients' records

One of the consequences of the self-training method is the necessity to
manage the patient's record. A very large amount of information concerning
the patients is kept in the records - more than is needed for the aid-to-
diagnosis program. A management system was created which allows mainly for
sorts on various keys and display   of the records.

This system made it possible to use the same patient   sample for another
neurologist, with different symptoms and diagnoses.

f) the "useful diagnosis"

The result of the bayesian process is the vector of the most probable diagnoses. But very often the medical action remains difficult to decide, if
several possible diagnoses lead to different strategies (strategy here
means the actions to be taken following the discovery of the diagnosis :
prognosis, non-standard para-clinical tests, treatment). The authors have
therefore made a distinction between the "useful diagnosis", which implies
a specific strategy, and the "descriptive diagnosis" which has the higher
probability : these two diagnoses   are not always the same, and it is very
very important to give both.

The useful diagnosis is computed according to :

- its probability,
- the utility of taking it into account if it is not the
right one.

A "matrix of utilities" has been built, in which the generic term $U(i,j)$
measures the utility of treating the diagnosis i if the right one is j.

The selected useful diagnosis is the one for which the utility expectancy:
$U(i) = \sum_j P(D_j)\ U(i,j)$ is maximal (annex 7 and 7bis).

This method seems to have provided good results on a sample of 277 patients. But the matrix of utilities, which has been initially defined em-
pirically has to be adjusted by a precise analysis of the results which
is in progress now.

Current Results

At the present time, this method gives   rather good results (annex 8).
But it is important not to stop at the global results : it is quite interesting to analyse the results for each diagnosis and to extract three

basic notions for each of them, as mentioned above :

- its sensitivity,
- its specificity,
- its reliability.

This study is now in progress : it is based on an analysis of a so-called "matrix of coincidences" which is established by the computer (annex 9). The generic term of the matrix, $M(i,j)$, is :

the number of times when the patients having D_i have been classified as D_j by the computer. For instance :

$$\frac{\sum_{j \neq i} M(i,j)}{\sum_j M(i,j)}$$ is the percentage of errors by default for the diagnosis D_i

and

$$\frac{\sum_{i \neq j} M(i,j)}{\sum_i M(i,j)}$$ is the percentage of errors by excess for the diagnosis D_j

V.2. THEORY OF DECISION APPLIED TO THE TREATMENT OF CARDIAC INFARCTION

We are concerned with work done by D. Teather, P.A. Emerson and S.A. Handley [28] on the following problem : one of the major complications connected with cardiac infarction is deep vein thrombosis (DVT) that is, the formation of blood clot in a vein which can migrate and provoke pulmonary embolism (obstruction of blood vessels leading to the lungs) the consequences of which can be fatal. In order to ward off DVT, patients with CI can be given a drug called heparin which thins the blood and therefore theoretically prevents clotting. But the problem with this treatment is that it, too, can cause fatal complications by provoking hemorrhages that are the result of the lack of clotting the treatment causes. So we see that the decision to give preventive treatment to patients isn't so simple.

The authors then formalized the decision-making process in the following manner :

(see next page)

where :
   h : probability of hemorhage by heparin
   e : probability of pulmonary embolus complicating untreated DVT
   t : probability of pulmonary embolus complicating treated DVT
   x : probability of DVT developing

443

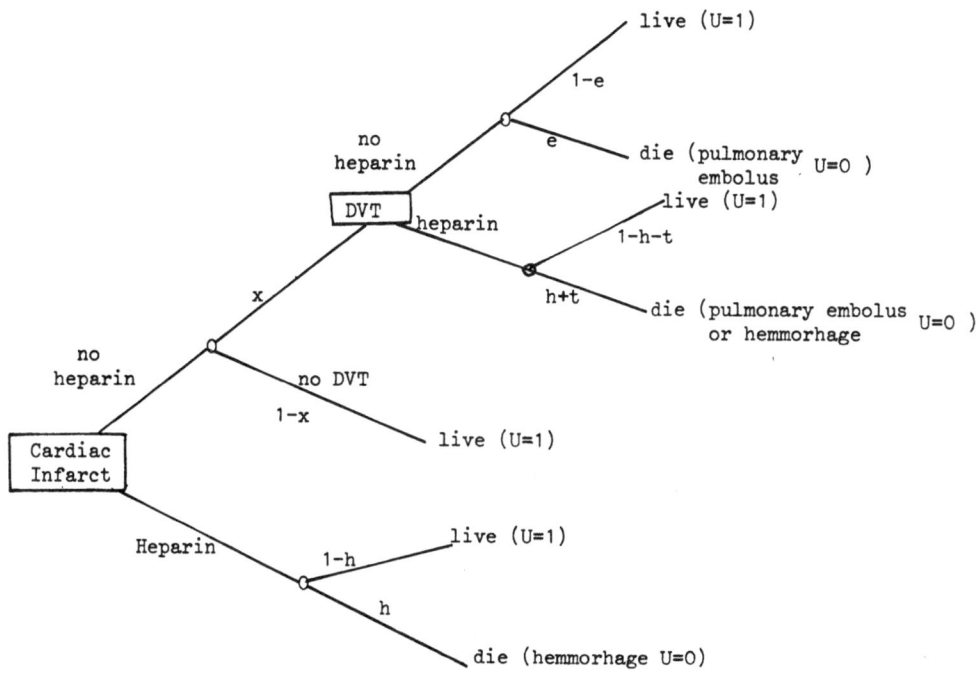

As the terminal states considered were death or survival; tne financial cost
of heparin as well as the various non-fatal disadvantages of heparin treatment and of DVT .can be disregarded and then utility 1 can be assigned to
survival and 0 to death.

Suppose we are at node DVT : if heparin treatment is begun, the expected
utility equals 1(1 - h - t) + 0(h + t) = 1 - h - t. If heparin treatment
isn't begun, the expected utility will be 1-e. At this stage heparin is
begun if 1 - h - t $>$ 1 - e, that is, if e $>$ h + t.

A cursory glance at the litterature and experience of all cardiologists leads
us to believe that it is always this way : the recognized cases of DVT are
always treated.

Suppose we are at the first node now : if heparin is given starting from
this stage, the utility is h ; if no heparin treatment is given, the utility
is (1 - x) + x(1 - h - t).

Heparin treatment must be decided upon as soon as the patient is admitted if :

$1 - h > (1 - x) + x(1 - h - t)$, that is, if x $> \dfrac{h}{h + t}$

Thus in order for a useful decision to be made, x , h and t must be known.
On the basis of their own personal experience and of that written up in the
litterature, the authors were able to estimate the probabilities for different categories of patients (age, medical history, habits, etc ...). They
arrived in this way at the following decision-making process algorithm :

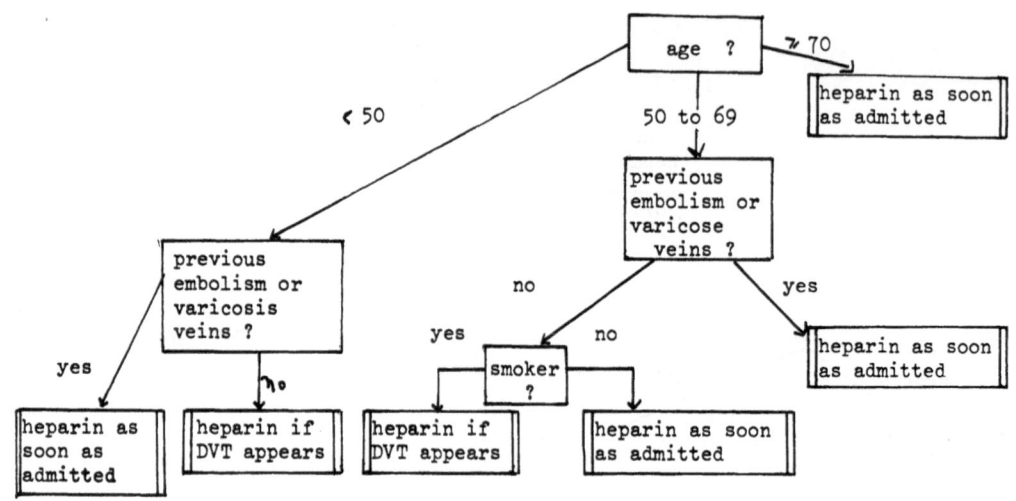

V.3. DIAGNOSIS OF TYPE OF JAUNDICE BY DISCRIMINANT ANALYSIS

The objective of the work we did in our department [25] was to solve the following problem : two types of jaundice can be distinguished according to their cause : (1) medical jaundices most commonly of infection origin and (2) mechanical jaundices caused by compression of the gall ducts. When a patient is suffering from a jaundice, it is important to classify it in one of these two categories, for the treatment will vary greatly (medical in one case, surgical in the other). A rather large number of clinical labora-tory tests are currently available to this end. The training sample was made up of 137 patients (44 medical and 93 mechanical jaundices) ; 84 tests (clinical signs and laboratory tests) were conducted for each subject. A discriminant analysis done on this sample made it possible to establish a simple discriminant function allowing for the classification of new patients in one of the two groups with a success ratio of 80 %. It is interesting to note that in this function, only 6 signs out of 84 are used since they suffi-ce to obtain the best discrimination possible: a useful reduction of data was thus accomplished. Furthermore, it happens that of these 6 signs, 5 are easi-ly collected clinical signs and the sixth is a very banal inexpensive labo-ratory test.

As a conclusion, it is possible to stress some very important points :

a) first, one must remind that the methods described here should not be conside-red as decision-making tool ; they are only an aid to medical decision. The responsability of decision remains to the medical staff.

b) another crucial question is the practical use of such tools. It must be recog-nized that most of the experiments described in the scientific litterature are prototypes. Very few are used on a routine basis.

The reason for this is the fact that they concern mainly very narrow and specia-lized fields of medicine, where the number of possible decisions is usually limi-ted. Very highly specialized staff do not feel the need of using a system in which they resent as a heavy burden and which, according to their opinion, does not work

better than themselves; (this opinion may be wrong : when the computer program
uses the true probabilities, it delivers better results than the best specialist
- see de DOMBAL -).

If the present state of practical applications is not rewarding, what can be
predict about the future ? It seems to us that at least, two direction may be
concerned by the implementation of aid to decision tools. First the extension
to broader domaines of medicine : trials like application to a whole discipline
(like described above for neurology) should be encouraged. Second, the chances
of such help to decision systems appears to be great for mass health screening
where one of the most difficult problems is the lack of qualified physicians.

c) Now, even if the routine applications were to remain negligible, we do think that
these efforts will be very fruitful. The interest of these methods stays elsewhere
than previously expected. The collision between two ways of thinking - medical
and informatical - contributes very significantly to the improvement of the former.

Doctors have at their disposal very broad knowledge, continuously increasing,
but due to the lack of method, do not know how to use it. Very often, and even
with the best, their way of solving problems is erratic ; they hide their uneasi-
ness by requesting a large amount of laboratory tests, often superfluous, sometimes detrimental ; they lack of strict intellectual frames, of strong logical
models. Data processing method and especially those we are concerned with in this
paper, forces the doctors to build and/or to adopt such frames and models.

That may have its first consequence in medical education : for training both of
students and of teachers. These informatical tools can provide the latter objective arguments to decide whether a strategy is better or not than another, which
symptom is useful, and in which order they must be searched.

Giving the doctors better intellectual tools, they will improve the quality of
their practice. One may also notice that, being indirect, the improvement does
not necessarily imply the use of computer by the doctor in his daily practice.

d) Allowing a better use of the doctor's mind, the aid-to-decision system can do a
lot for allowing a better use of the patient's or the community's money. Indeed,
as it has been pointed out, a general result of these methods is to show which
sign, symptom and/or test is useful. They reveal that the correct decision can
be reached with restricted amount of them. Very often, it is possible to avoid
the use of the most expensive, or at least, to require them only when strictly
necessary.

446

VI. REFERENCES

1. Alperovitch, A., Gold, A., Lellouch, J.
   L'aide de l'Ordinateur dans le Diagnostic des Images Rondes Intra-thora-
   ciques
   Presse Méd. 1971, 79, n° 4, 137

2. Barker, J.P., Bishop, J.M.
   Computer Analysis of Symptoms Patterns as a Method of Screening Patients at
   Special Risk of Hypothyroïdism
   Brit. J. Prev. Soc. Med. 1970, 24, n° 4, 193

3. Begon, F., Tremolières, R., Sultan, C.
   Présentation et Illustration d'un Modèle Logique du Diagnostic à Propos
   d'un Exemple Hématologique
   Journées d'Informatique Médicale   Toulouse 1972   IRIA éd.

4. Benzecri, J.P.
   L'Analyse des Données - Tome 2 : l'analyse des correspondances
   Dunod - Paris 1973

5. Billewicz, W.Z., Chapman, R.S., Crooks, J., Day, M.E., Gossage, J.,
   Wayne, S.E., Young, J.A.
   Statistical Methods Applied to the Diagnosis of Hypothyroïdism
   Quart. J. Med. 1969, 38, n° 150, 255

6. Bishop, C.R., Warner, A.R.
   A Mathematical Approach to Medical Diagnosis : Application to Polycythemic
   States Utilizing Clinical Finding with Values Continuously Distributed
   Computers and Biomedical Research 2, 486-493 (1969)

7. Burbank, F.
   A Computer Diagnostic System for the Diagnosis of Prolonged Undifferencia-
   ting Liver Disease
   Amer. J. Med., 1969, 46, n° 3, 401

8. de Dombal, Leaper, D.I., Staniland, I.R., Mc Cann, A.P., Horrocks, J.C.
   Computer-Aided Diagnosis of Acute Abdominal Pain
   Brit. Med. J., 1972, 2, n° 5804, 9

9. de Dombal,F.T., Horrocks, J., Staniland, J.R., Guillou, P.J.
   Pattern Recognition : a Comparison of the Performance of Clinicians and
   Non-Clinicians with a note on the Performance of a Computer-Based System
   Meth. Inform. Med. 11 (1972) 32-37

10. Fries,J.F.
    Experience Counting in Sequential Computer Diagnosis
    Arch. Inter. Med. vol 127, Oct. 1970

11. Fragu, P., Patois, E., Huber, C., Lellouch, J.
    Original Approach of the Hyperthyroïdism Diagnosis with Computer
    Medinfo 1974, pp. 559-564. North-Holland Ed.

12. Gill, P.W., Leaper, D.J., Guillou, P.J., Staniland, J.R., Horrocks, J.C.
    de Dombal, F.T.
    Observer Variations in Clinical Diagnosis - A Computer-Aided Assessment of
    its Magnitude and Importance in 552 patients with Abdominal Pain
    Meth. Inform. Med. vol 12, n° 2 (April 1973), pp. 108-113

13. Gorry, G.A., Kassirer, J.P., Essig, A., Schwartz, W.B.
Decision Analysis as the Basis for Computer-Aided Management of Acute Renal
Failures
Amer. J. Med. vol 55 (October 1973)

14. Hadley, T.P., Geer, D.E., Bleich, H.L., Freedberg, I.M.
The Use of Digital Computers in Dermatologic Diagnosis : Computer-Aided
Diagnosis of Febrile Illness With Eruption
Journal of Investigative Dermatology, 62 : 467-471, 1974

15. Hall, P., Hallen, B., Selander, H.
Linear Discriminatory Analysis : a Patient Classifying Method for Research
and Production Control
Meth. Inform. Med. vol 10, n° 2 (April 1971), pp. 96-102

15 bis. Huber, C., Lellouch, J.
Estimation dans les Tableaux de Contingence à un Grand Nombre d'Entrées
Int. Stat. Rev. Vol. 42, n° 2, 1974, pp. 193-203

16. Knill-Jones, R.P., Stern, R.B., Girmes, D.H., Maxwell, J.D., Thompson, R.P.H.,
Williams, R.
Use of Sequential Bayesian Model in Diagnosis of Jaundice by Computer
Brit. Med. J., 1973, 1, 530-533

17. Lebart, L., Fenelon, J.P.
Statistiques et Informatique Appliquées
Dunod - Paris 1973

18. Lodwick, G.S., Haun, C.S., Smith, W.E., Keller, R.F., Robertson, E.D.
Computer Diagnosis of Primary Bone Tumors : a Preliminary Report
Radiology, 1963, 80, n° 2, 273

19. Lusted, L.B.
Introduction to Medical Decision Making
C. Thomas Ed. Springfield Illinois

20. Namba, H., Kamac, M., Hizikuri, F., Takayama, J., Miyawaki, K., Nakamura, K.,
Nakamura, M
Diagnosis of Congenital Heart Diseases with an Electronic Computer
Med. J. Osaka Univ., 1965, 16, n° 1-2

20 bis. Norusis, M., Jaquez, J.A.
Symptom non Independance in Mathematical Models for Diagnosis
Computer and Biomedical Research, vol. 8, n° 2, April 1975, p. 156-172

21. Oddie, T.H., Hales, I.B., Stiel, J.N., Reeve, T.S., Hooper, M., Boyd, C.M.,
Fisher, D.A.,
Prospective Trial of Computer Program for the Diagnosis of Thyroid Disorders
J.C.E. and M. 1974, vol 38, n° 5, 876-882

22. Overall, J.E., Kan, M., Williams, C.M.
Conditional Probability Program for Diagnosis of Thyroid Function
J. Amer. Med. Ass. 1963, 183, 307

23. Pipberger, H.V., Klingeman, J.D., Cosma, J.
Computer Evaluation of Statistical Properties of Clinical Information in the
Differential Diagnosis of Chest Pain
Meth. Inform. Med., 1968, 7, n° 2, 79

24. Romeder, J.M.
    Méthodes et Programmes d'Analyse dDiscriminante
    Dunod – Paris, 1973

25. Romeder, J.M., Hecht, Y., Guille, C., Garçon, C.
    Diagnostic des Ictères Cholostatiques
    Rev. Med. Chir. Malad. Foie, 46, 159-170 – 1971

26. Taylor, T.R., Aitchinson, J., Mc Girr, E.M.
    Doctors as Decision-Makers : a Computer-Assisted Study of Diagnosis as a
    Cognitive Skill
    Brit. Med. J., 3, 1971, 39-40

27. Taylor, T.R., Shields, S., Black, R.
    Study of Cost-Conscious Computer-Assisted Diagnosis in Thyroid Diseases
    Lancet, July 8, 1972, 79-83

28. Teather, D., Emerson, P.A., Handley, A.J.
    Decision Theory Applied to the Treatment of Deep Vein Thrombosis
    Meth. Inform. Med. vol. 13, n° 2, 1974

29. Warner, H.R., Toronto, A.F., Veasy, L.G., Stephenson, R.
    A Mathematical Approach to Medical Diagnosis – Application to Congenital
    Heart Diseases
    J. Amer. Med. Ass. 1961, 177, n° 1, 77

(Annex 1)

D I A G N O S T I C

1 TUMEUR SUS-TENTORIELLE BENIGNE

2 TUMEUR SUS-TENTORIELLE MALIGNE

3 TUMEUR SOUS-TENTORIELLE BENIGNE

4 TUMEUR SOUS-TENTORIELLE MALIGNE

5 COMPRESSION MEDULLAIRE

6 ACCIDENT ISCHEMIQUE CEREBRAL D'ORIGINE CARDIAQUE

7 ACCIDENT ISCHEMIQUE CEREBRAL D'ORIGINE ATHEROSCLEREUSE

8 ACCIDENT ISCHEMIQUE CEREBRAL DE TYPE LACUNAIRE

9 ACCIDENT ISCHEMIQUE MEDULLAIRE

10 HEMORRAGIE CEREBRALE LIEE A L'HYPERTENSION ARTERIELLE

11 HEMORRAGIE CEREBRALE LIEE A UN ANEVRYSME ARTERIEL

12 HEMORRAGIE CEREBRALE LIEE A UN ANEVRYSME ARTERIO-VEINEUX

13 MALADIE DE PARKINSON

14 AUTRES AFFECTIONS DEGENERATIVES

   (SLA, PICK, ALZHEIMER, HEREDO-DEGENERESCENCE)

15 MALFORMATION DE LA CHARNIERE CERVICO-CRANIENNE ET SYRINGOMYELIE

16 AFFECTIONS METABOLIQUES HEREDITAIRES : WILSON, LEUCODYSTROPHIE...

17 AFFECTIONS METABOLIQUES ACQUISES

18 AFFECTIONS PARANEOPLASIQUES

19 S.E.P.

20 AFFECTIONS VIRALES OU APPARENTEES (LESS, CREUTZFELDT-JACOB)

21 ABCES CEREBRAL

22 AFFECTIONS A PYOGENES EN DEHORS DE L'ABCES

23 AFFECTIONS TOXIQUES

24 DETERMINATION D'UNE MALADIE GENERALE

25 AFFECTIONS MYCOSIQUES OU PARASITAIRES

26 TUBERCULOSE CEREBRO-MENINGEE

27 SYPHILIS DU SYSTEME NERVEUX

28 AFFECTIONS TRAUMATIQUES : HEMATOMES INTRA-CRANIENS

29 AFFECTIONS TRAUMATIQUES (EN DEHORS DES HEMATOMES INTRA-CRANIENS)

30 AFFECTIONS PSYCHIATRIQUES

31 AUTRES (EPILEPSIE PRIMAIRE, ...)

(annex 2)

E X A M E N   N E U R O L O G I Q U E

1 DEFICIT HEMIPLEGIQUE

2 DEFICIT PARAPLEGIQUE

3 DEFICIT LOCALISE A LA FACE

4 DEFICIT SENSITIF EN DESSOUS DE LA FACE

5 DEFICIT SENSITIF DE LA FACE

6 SIGNES PERIPHERIQUES (REFLEXES ABOLIS, ATROPHIE, FASCICULATIONS)

7 DEFICIT VISUEL MONOCULAIRE

8 DEFICIT VISUEL BINOCULAIRE

9 DIPLOPIE OU STRABISME

10 NYSTAGMUS

11 SURDITE UNILATERALE

12 TROUBLES MODERES DE LA VIGILANCE

13 TROUBLES DU COMPORTEMENT EN L'ABSENCE DE TROUBLES DE LA VIGILANCE

14 AUTRES

15 SIGNES RACHIDIENS

16 TROUBLES MOTEURS NON DEFICITAIRES

17 TREMBLEMENTS

18 MOUVEMENTS ANORMAUX

19 TROUBLES DE LA DEGLUTITION

20 TROUBLES DU LANGAGE OU DE LA PAROLE

21 TROUBLES DE LA MARCHE OU DE L'EQUILIBRE

22 TROUBLES DE L'OLFACTION

23 TROUBLES DE L'HUMEUR

24 TROUBLES SPHINCTERIENS

25 TROUBLES DE LA MEMOIRE

26 DIMINUTION MAJEURE DES FONCTIONS INTELLECTUELLES

27 SIGNES EVOQUANT H T I C

28 COMA

(annex 3)

NOTES ATTRIBUEES PAR LE NEUROLOGUE

	① TUMEUR SUS-TENTORIELLE BENIGNE	② TUMEUR SUS-TENTORIELLE MALIGNE	③ TUMEUR SOUS-TENTORIELLE BENIGNE	④ TUMEUR SOUS-TENTORIELLE MALIGNE
⑫ DEFICIT HEMIPLEGIQUE FRUSTE	2	2	1_A	1_B
⑬ DEFICIT HEMIPLEGIQUE MASSIF	1_A	1_B	1_A	1_A

(annex 4)

FREQUENCES ASSOCIEES AUX

NOTES ATTRIBUEES PAR LE NEUROLOGUE

Fréquence

0	0,014	TROUVE	24	FOIS	SUR	1 748
1A	0,038	TROUVE	747	FOIS	SUR	19 677
1B	0,116	TROUVE	1 114	FOIS	SUR	9 620
2	0,312	TROUVE	1 064	FOIS	SUR	3 408
3	0,495	TROUVE	635	FOIS	SUR	1 283
4	0,674	TROUVE	437	FOIS	SUR	645
5	0,990	TROUVE	0	FOIS	SUR	0

(annex 5)

FREQUENCES REELLES

	① TUMEUR SUS-TENTORIELLE BENIGNE 15 malades	② TUMEUR SUS-TENTORIELLE MALIGNE 27 malades	③ TUMEUR SOUS-TENTORIELLE BENIGNE 26 malades	④ TUMEUR SOUS-TENTORIELLE MALIGNE 16 malades
⑫ DEFICIT HEMIPLEGIQUE FRUSTE	26 %	37 %	7 %	25 %
⑬ DEFICIT HEMIPLEGIQUE MASSIF	6 %	8 %	0 %	0 %

(annex 6)

FREQUENCES PONDEREES

UTILISEES DANS LE PROCESSUS BAYESIEN

	① TUMEUR SUS-TENTORIELLE BENIGNE	② TUMEUR SUS-TENTORIELLE MALIGNE	③ TUMEUR SOUS-TENTORIELLE BENIGNE	④ TUMEUR SOUS-TENTORIELLE MALIGNE
⑫ DEFICIT HEMIPLEGIQUE FRUSTE	28 %	35 %	6 %	16 %
⑬ DEFICIT HEMIPLEGIQUE MASSIF	5 %	9 %	1 %	1 %

(annex 7)

Dossier n°   Nom :

DIAGNOSTIC   CLINIQUE : MENINGITE CARCINOMATEUSE

DIAGNOSTIC APRES EXAMENS COMPLEMENTAIRES : IDEM

DIAGNOSTIC ANATOMO-PATHOLOGIQUE : MENINGITE CARCINOMATEUSE

INFILTRATION MENINGEE DIFFUSE (ADENO K DU POUMON)

DIAGNOSTICS CALCULES :

Probabilité :

    0,939   pour TUMEUR SOUS-TENTORIELLE MALIGNE

    0,024   pour TUMEUR SOUS-TENTORIELLE BENIGNE

    0,023   pour TUMEUR SUS-TENTORIELLE BENIGNE

    0,005   pour HEMORRAGIE CEREBRALE LIEE A UN ANEVRYSME
                    ARTERIO-VEINEUX

    0,003   pour ABCES CEREBRAL

DIAGNOSTIC UTILE :

    9,79   pour TUMEUR SOUS-TENTORIELLE MALIGNE

(annex 7 bis)

Dossier n°   Nom :

DIAGNOSTIC   CLINIQUE : ?

DIAGNOSTIC APRES EXAMENS COMPLEMENTAIRES : METASTASES CEREBRALES.

DIAGNOSTIC ANATOMO-PATHOLOGIQUE : LACUNE DANS LES NOYAUX LENTICULAIRES
ET LE THALAMUS, SURTOUT A DROITE

DIAGNOSTICS CALCULES :

Probabilité :

    0,366   pour ACCIDENT ISCHEMIQUE CEREBRAL DE TYPE LACUNAIRE

    0,344   pour AFFECTIONS METABOLIQUES ACQUISES

    0,122   pour ACCIDENT ISCHEMIQUE CEREBRAL D'ORIGINE ATHEROSCLEREUSE

    0,082   pour AFFECTIONS TRAUMATIQUES : HEMATOMES INTRA-CRANIENS

    0,035   pour AFFECTIONS VIRALES OU APPARENTEES
                       (LESS, CREUTZFELDT-JACOB)

DIAGNOSTIC UTILE :

    8,32   pour AFFECTIONS METABOLIQUES ACQUISES

(annex 8)

POURCENTAGE DE DIAGNOSTICS EXACTS PAR POSITION

DIAGNOSTIC	TOTAL	POSITION				
		1	2	3	4	5
1	15	93	6	0	0	0
2	27	70	14	0	7	3
3	26	88	7	3	0	0
4	16	68	18	0	0	6
5	13	100	0	0	0	0
6	23	91	8	0	0	0
7	30	73	16	3	0	0
8	17	70	17	5	0	5
9	8	100	0	0	0	0
10	18	83	5	11	0	0
11	15	100	0	0	0	0
12	6	66	16	16	0	0
13	13	92	7	0	0	0
14	13	84	15	0	0	0
15	1	100	0	0	0	0
16	0	*	*	*	*	*
17	8	87	12	0	0	0
18	0	*	*	*	*	*
19	22	100	0	0	0	0
20	2	100	0	0	0	0
21	1	100	0	0	0	0
22	0	*	*	*	*	*
23	1	0	100	0	0	0
24	1	0	0	100	0	0
25	0	*	*	*	*	*
26	0	*	*	*	*	*
27	0	*	*	*	*	*
28	1	100	0	0	0	0
29	0	*	*	*	*	*
30	0	*	*	*	*	*
31	0	*	*	*	*	*

(annex 8 bis)

R E S U L T A T S

84 % DE DIAGNOSTICS CORRECTS EN PREMIERE POSITION

94 % DE DIAGNOSTICS CORRECTS SUR LES 2 PREMIERES POSITIONS

96 % DE DIAGNOSTICS CORRECTS SUR LES 3 PREMIERES POSITIONS

97 % DE DIAGNOSTICS CORRECTS SUR LES 4 PREMIERES POSITIONS

98 % DE DIAGNOSTICS CORRECTS SUR LES 5 POSITIONS

(annex 9)

MATRICE DE COINCIDENCES

Diagnostics calculés

diagnostics présentés	1	2	3	4	5	6	7	8	9	10	11	12	13	14	15
1	14	0	0	0	0	0	0	0	0	0	1	0	0	0	0
2	3	19	0	0	0	0	1	0	0	0	0	1	0	0	1
3	1	0	23	1	0	0	0	0	0	0	0	0	0	0	0
4	0	0	1	11	0	0	0	0	0	0	0	1	0	0	0
5	0	0	0	0	13	0	0	0	0	0	0	0	0	0	0
6	0	0	0	0	0	21	0	0	0	1	0	0	0	0	0
7	0	1	0	0	0	2	22	2	0	0	1	0	0	1	0
8	0	0	0	0	0	1	1	12	0	0	0	0	0	0	0
9	0	0	0	0	0	0	0	0	8	0	0	0	0	0	0
10	0	0	0	0	0	1	0	0	0	15	2	0	0	0	0
11	0	0	0	0	0	0	0	0	0	0	15	0	0	0	0
12	0	0	0	0	0	0	0	0	0	0	2	4	0	0	0
13	0	0	0	0	0	0	0	0	0	0	0	0	12	0	0
14	0	0	0	0	0	0	0	0	0	0	0	0	1	11	0
15	0	0	0	00	0	0	0	0	0	0	0	0	0	0	1

COMPUTER ASSISTED
MEDICAL HISTORY

J.R. MOEHR, HANNOVER

1. The Medical History

1.1 INTRODUCTION

The medical history, as well as the process by which it is obtained is
often termed 'anamnesis'. This expression is derived from the Greek
word for 'recollection', 'remembrance'. In medicine, this term is
applied to the recollection of past events and sensations related to a
physician by a patient for purposes of medical care.

Although patient-physician communication is a two way process even in
history 'taking', the term denotes mainly one aspect of doctor -
patient communication, in which the information flow is predominantly
directed from the patient to the physician. Aspects of information
being transmitted predominantly from the physician to the patient, e.g.
patient education, are not covered by the term.

Since direct communication between patient and physician is not in
every instance feasible, the meaning is extended to those occasions
where persons such as a child's mother or the physician's aides become
active in the process of communication. Also, the term applies to the
process of eliciting information, as well as to the document which
results as a by-product of this process.

There are two major subjects that history taking deals with

- the history of the disease
- the history of the diseased.

HARTMANN (c.f. e.g. 49, 50) has repeatedly pointed out, that during
hippocratic times medical records were essentially histories of
diseased persons and that under the influence of the natural sciences
during the eighteenth and nineteenth century they became histories of
'a disease'. Today, both aspects are considered to be equally
important.

The process of anamnesis or 'history taking' as such is part of the
treatment process which includes diagnostic and therapeutic activities.
It starts with the first patient-physician contact and is only
temporarily terminated with the end of a particular treatment episode.
If the patient consults his physician again, the anamnestic process is
continued. If a new physician is consulted during the treatment
episode, he may often and above all initiate the anamnestic process
anew for himself.

It has to be emphasized that history taking necessitates active
involvement of the patient as well as of the physician. It is an
essentially humane process for which abilities for

- talking
- listening and
- thinking

are essential prerequisites (50). Much information, however, is also non-verbally conveyed by the patient's posture and gestures as well as his reactions to the questions.

1.2 REVIEW OF PURPOSE, CONTENTS, MEANS AND STYLES

1.2.1 TRADITIONAL PURPOSE

Medical care was traditionally delivered in a process that involved a single patient and his physician and was primarily directed at treating sickness. History taking in this situation served the purpose of

- providing the basis for treatment decisions, and
- generating a documentation of this process.

The accomplishment of this purpose is closely related to two other major functions of the history

- establishing and consolidating the patient-physician relation

and

- serving a cathartic function by providing the patient with an opportunity to verbalize and maybe rationalize his worries.

Also history taking is part of a continuous process of enforcement and correction of the physician's professional experience and it therefore serves

- the promotion of professional experience.

In order to provide the basis for the physician's treatment decisions, history taking should specifically aim at:

1 Disclosing speedily and economically an accurate and objective picture of the patient, including an account of
   - his symptoms
   - his personality, in particular his perception of and attitude towards his illness
   - his environment, in particular its sources of worries and resources for care.
2 Revealing risks for the patient as posed by
   - allergies and idiosyncrasies
   - previous treatment
   - previous or concurrent dise.ase

As a by-product, there should result a documentation of the history including the measures taken with regard to symptoms and risks and in consideration of personality and environment. The resulting document should

- serve as a basis for communication between physicians in that it provides guidance through the physician's reasoning and

      consequent actions
- serve as a justification of the physician's actions and
- allow interindividual evaluation for scientific and
  teaching purposes.

In this latter sense, the document should make the experience gained by an individual physician

- more objective and
- communicable to others

Achievement of the goals of history taking in sick care depends to a great extent on a relaxed, confident attitude of the patient towards his physician since a timid, cunning or distrusting patient may consciously withhold or distort information. Establishment and consolidation of a favourable doctor-patient relationship are therefore also frequently named among the general goals of history taking.

As far as history taking is concerned, there is so far little known about the actual information requirements. The statements concerning the purpose and contents of anamnestic interrogation are usually of a normative kind, based on conjectural medical concepts and influenced by didactic considerations. They state the respective author's opinion on what <u>should be</u>.

Positive statements on what <u>is</u> are rare, and further insight based on empirical investigation is only slowly gained. In particular, we owe significant contributions to advances in medical sociology (139). These investigations show that the way in which the physician communicates information to the patient about his illness may determine the patient-physician relation even to a greater extent than the way in which he elicits information from him. Providing the patient with information (patient education) also affects the history taking process in another way. A patient may only communicate correctly what was told to him correctly and understandably during earlier encounters.

The same results pertain to our views of the cathartic function of history taking. The therapeutic effect attributed to the relief caused by verbalization and rationalization of worries and anxieties may be equaled or even surpassed by the relief of anxiety concerning diagnosis, prognosis and planned therapy that is caused by propper information of the patient.

In summary, the primary purpose of history taking in sick care of the individual is to provide a documented basis for treatment decisions. A favourable effect on the patient-physician relation is closely related to this purpose. A therapeutic effect may be attributed to the entire communicative process, i.e. to the communication of information from patient to physician as well as inversely from physician to patient. Through documentation, the gained information may be communicated for the purpose of individual patient care as well as for other purposes, e.g. promotion of medical science.

1.2.2 PURPOSE IN RESPONSE TO PRESENT DAY REQUIREMENTS

In our industrial societies, the responsibilities of medicine have considerably been extended beyond the scope of individual sick care.

Diagnostic achievements have made it possible to recognize disease states at ever earlier stages. Sometimes, this requires diagnostic techniques which are very costly in terms of money, skilled man power or patient discomfort. Their application therefore requires thorough and reliable prior diagnosis in order to determine whether these measures are indicated. Therapeutic achievements on the other hand make the effort worthwhile. Frequently yet, therapeutic results are not such as to completely restore health but rather to create a state that needs continuous attention. Medical care as a whole may therefore start earlier and continue longer for a given individual.

A number of factors contribute to the fact that more individuals are asking for medical attention. One is that the financial consequences no longer have to be borne by the individual. Others lie in the fact that medicine provides the legitimation for obtaining a number of social benefits. Finally, life in contemporary industrialized societies seems to lead to a number of states perceived as disease even without organic derangement. These contribute further to an increase in the demand for medical attention.

Apart from these factors stimulating the demand for medical services beyond that of conventional sick care on the part of the consumer, there is increasing awareness within the medical society itself that further progress may not lie `entirely within the scope of individualized care but rather in the care for collectives. This collective health care is primarily directed to prevention and early recognition of disease. This is achieved through identification of factors that constitute risks and of persons subject to such risks.

All these factors contribute to a widened spectrum of purposes for the medical history. These now include

- screening for early sick
- surveillance for chronically ill as well as
- providing a basis for health care decisions
  which might concern an individual or a collective.

Concurrent with this extension of the purpose of history taking is a need for better understanding of the validity of anamnestic data. This has the effect that anamnestic information is increasingly subject to scientific investigations and contributes as such to the improvement of medical science.

1.2.3 CONTENTS

Virtually every account of

- observable facts
- sensations or
- emotions

that may pertain to the patient's condition may be relevant within the purposes of a history. It will therefore be worth being considered and documented. The volume of the document, the time and skill that is needed for its preparation are largely determined by the number of different purposes a history has to serve, and by the complexity of these purposes. Histories serving only as a reminder for the physician himself will be much more economical than if they have to be meaningful for others as well. Disciplines with a small choice of standard problems may rely on a set of few standard questions. This is frequently the case in surgical disciplines. Others have more complicated histories. Examples of the latter are internal medicine with its claim for encompassing responsibility of the patient or the psychiatric disciplines in which the diagnostic armamentarium includes little besides history taking.

These differences are appropriately reflected in the schemes for standard history that various disciplines have produced. These schemes usually assume an encounter with a previously unknown patient and are mostly devised for use in the hospital care setting.

The elements of a general standard history have repeatedly been characterized - mainly from the point of view of internal medicine (21, 31, 37, 41, 49, 50, 95). As stated above, it should cover a history of the diseased as well as of the disease.

The history of the diseased encompasses

- family history
- patient history
- review of systems
- social history

The family history includes

- hereditary diseases, e.g. bleeding troubles, diabetes
- diseases of particular frequency in the family
- causes and age at death of the patient's relatives.

It is necessarily limited by the patient's memory, unless other sources of information are referred to. Usually, one recommends that ascending, collateral and descending family be covered.

The patient's own history contains an account of his development in health and disease, including

- development during
  = infancy
  = puberty
  = adult age
  = climatic period
  = old age
- habits (drinking, smoking)
- diets
- previous
  = diseases
  = periods of hospitalization
  = operations
  = periodic and chronic medication
  = vaccination
- allergies and risk facts
- sexual habits
- in women
  = menstrual cycle
  = pregnancies

The review of systems is an account of sensations and troubles concerning the organic systems for

- sensation
- digestion
- respiration
- circulation
- locomotion

- secretion
- generation (59).

Views differ a little whether these subjects should be covered according to their functional or topographic relations. Some claim that questioning is more meaningful for the patient if questions are posed according to topographic regions while the resultant documentation is thought to be medically more meaningful if presented according to functional relations.

The social history covers aspects of the patient's

- professional life
- leisure life
- family life
- education.

Particularly the aspects of medical relevance like occupational hazards (noise, dust, toxic agents) and social stress should be covered.

The history of the disease includes

- chief complaint
- supposed causes
- previous circumstances
- course and development with
    = prodromata, the symptoms preceeding the outbreak of disease
    = initial symptoms
    = alteration of troubles
    = actions taken
- an account of the present state of the disease.

Standard history schemes for other disciplines than internal medicine may place more detailed emphasis on certain parts while neglecting others. The outline given is therefore rather encompassing. In many instances limited subsets of the indicated spectrum will be considered sufficient. Still, however, these recommendations are again of a normative kind, based to a large extent on convention and fitted to convenience while often little is known about the spectrum of information that is really needed. History schemes often contain sections on childhood diseases or family history that are considered of little relevance by the physician obtaining the history and are then notoriously halfheartedly - if at all - completed. The advances in automatic support of history acquisition begin to shed some light on questions concerning the real need of information.

Also the rigorously systematic approach does not fit certain situations of patient care. In the primary care setting of the family physician, for instance, the typical patient-physician contact extends over years. Each consultation adds facts to an account of a witnessed patient history in the propper sense of the word. At the occasion of the next encounter these will be part of the patient's history - whether it was a note on the physician's action or on a sensation the patient recorded. For this setting, BRAUN (7) suggested that the physician asks the following set of standard questions:

"Why have you come - did you call me ? "
"What is the cause ? "
"What do you guess it is ? "
"What worries you ? "

Another occasion, where only a minimal history can be obtained is the
emergency encounter with a previously unknown patient. FASSL (31)
suggests in this situation to record and consider:

- previous information
- first impression
- reason for consultation
  (Why have you come, did you call me?)
- chief complaint(s)
  - Spontaneous complaints, worries, troubles
- causes
  (What happened, how did it come about?)
- measures previously taken
- risk facts
  (allergy, diabetes, bleeding troubles, chronic medication)
- identification
  (name, age, profession)

At the other end of these suggestions for a minimal history are
unlimited possibilities for extension of the scope of a history. As
long as there remains doubt or unresolved problems, the history may
have to be widened by addition of more subjects or deepening through
inclusion of more details. Thus, a previously neglected family history
may be added or it may be completed to the extent of consulting other
hospital records of family members or interviewing them personally. The
reason for such extensions may reach from patient care over legal
justification to scientific purposes.

1.2.4 MEANS AND STYLES

The primary, most appropriate and most effective means for obtaining a
patient's history is that of direct verbal communication between
patient and physician. Anamnesis has therefore been called the foremost
diagnostic instrument of the physician caring for humans (H.H.BERG
quoted according to 49). In the process, the physician has the entire
spectrum of styles of human dialogue available to him (Fig. 1.2.4-1;
after (49)).

The typical form is that of an anamnestic conversation (49, 61): A few
neutral opening remarks should put the patient at ease and convince him
of getting attention so that he loses his inhibitions. He should be
encouraged to start his account where he senses his troubles. During
this phase of spontaneous subjective account, the physician should
assume the role of a rather passive and permissive listener. The
establishment of an affective relation between patient and physician
has been indicated as the purpose of this phase.

Thereupon the physician should assume a more leading role to get a more
objective picture by asking for details, and validating the items
offered by the patient. Finally, the account should be completed by
asking questions on subjects the patient did not think of by himself.

It is a matter of the physician's skill and expertise, not to arrive at
false conclusions through suggestive channeling of the patient's
spontaneous account, and yet to obtain information, the patient may not
have been consciously aware of himself.

This may necessitate easing and resolving the patient's fear - e.g. of
serious or dishonouring disease - or disrupting a wall of artificial

constructs the patient has built around himself. Depending on occasion and purpose the physician may have to assume a dominantly leading role in a forceful interrogation, he may have to provoke emotional engagement of the patient or guide him through an objective interview. The ultimate refinement of these techniques of free anamnesis will still depend largely upon the physician's individual talents, his experience, and techniques.

```
                                 scope of styles for

                       free anamnesis     structured
                                          history
dispute                                   acquisition
                            T             device
discussion                  |
                            |
dialogue                    |
                            |
talk                        |
                            |
anamnestic conversation     |
_____         |
                            |
exploration                 |             T
                            |             |
interview                   |             |
                            |             |
inquiery                    |             |
                            |             |
interrogation               |             |
                            |             |
```

Figure 1.2.4-1

Scope of styles for free anamnesis and structured techniques.

In a number of ways one tries to support history taking since one cannot expect these qualities in their optimal representation from every physician, and since there are situations, which do not favour their exercise. Minimal means for support consist of forms, which in general offer a structure for documentation of the medical history much as the one outlined above. They serve simultaneously as a reminder of its contents.

These forms are usually of the open format type and structured for being completed by the physician during or after the encounter with a previously unknown patient. Somewhat less frequently they are of the closed format type, offering only a limited choice of answers. They may in this case also be completed by the patient himself. Since the document may serve other functions than the orientating interview, by which it is completed, it may have a sequence and structure differing from that of the interview.

The use of such aids is mainly advisable in situations characterized by
- serious time constraints
- need for comparable data provided by examiners
  of varying skill
- teaching purposes
- scientific purposes.

An example of a history form in a research- and teaching environment is the history form devised for use at the Medical School Hannover (Fig. 1.2.4-2). Similar devices exist in many medical schools and teaching hospitals.

If - as in the example - they are of the open format type, they contain spaces for all parts of the history that are considered standard for the particular institution.

The first page of the form used at the Medical School Hannover contains space for

- identification data
- a brief summary of the history
- working diagnoses.

Second is a description of the patient's chief complaint and present illness, followed by a scheme for a review of systems.

Two more pages give an outline of previous diseases, operations and treatment, habits, genital, social and family history.

Figure 1.2.4.-3 gives an example of a more concise history scheme used in outpatient clinics of the surgical department.

The variations in forms used and ways of administration suggest that there are wide varieties in emphasis placed upon and significance attributed to anamnestic findings. The question arises whether there might be a "too much" on one side or a "too little" on the other.

Evidently, the value of a history may only be judged by its contribution to the goals one attempts to achieve, by the contribution to the management of the patient's problems, or to the improvement of individual or general knowledge.

Effective management of the patient's problems may be achieved through a few skillfully posed questions and correctly interpreted answers. This is the typical situation in primary care, in the family physician's office. During hospital rounds it may be easily demonstrated that a brief interrogation by an experienced clinician may completely reverse the picture derived from an extensive elaboration prepared by a junior staff member. It is this potential for correction by few experienced physicians, which warrants the widely used practice, that the least experienced physicians in a hospital acquire the bulk of initial histories.

ANAMNESE der jetzigen Krankheit

Die Hauptbeschwerde Dauer Stärke Art und Ort Beziehung zu Funktionen	
Bisheriger Krankheitsverlauf und Begleitbeschwerden Benutzen Sie die System-übersicht (S. 3) als Gedächtnisstütze Im Rahmen des chronologischen Krankheitsverlaufs werden die Begleitbeschwerden dargestellt, die mit der Hauptbeschwerde zusammenhängen. Bei Rezidiven und chron. Verläufen mit dem ersten Krankheitsereignis beginnen. Bisherige Behandlung der jetzigen Krankheit erwähnen.	

Figure 1.2.4-2.1

Example of a free format history documentation form. The figure shows the second page of the form used at the Medical School Hannover. It contains spaces for chief complaint and a summary of the history of the current diseases.

SYSTEM-ÜBERSICHT

Hier sind Beschwerden und Besonderheiten als **Gedächtnisstütze** nach Organsystemen geordnet. Sie werden entsprechend den Angaben des **durchkreuzt** und im Krankheitsverlauf (S. 2) erläutert.

Bemerkungen

Allgemein-Beschwerden:					
Appetitmangel	Übelkeit	Erbrechen	Durchfall	Verstopfung	Gew.Veränd./Z.
übermäß. Durst	Nykturie	Polyurie	Anurie	Potenzstörungen	Schwäche
Schwindel	Gleichgewichts-Störungen		Ohnmacht	Bewußtlosigkeit	Angst
Erregbarkeit	Unruhe	Kopfschmerzen	geschw. Füße	geschw. Beine	geschw. Gesicht
Herzklopfen	Krämpfe	Lähmungen	Schweißausbr.	Veränderung der Hautfarbe	
Veränderung d. Körperbehaarg.		Fieber	Schüttelfrost	Einschlafstör.	Durchschlafstör.

Kopf:	Schmerzen	Haarausfall			

Augen:					
verminderte Sehfähigkeit		Flimmern	schwarze Fleck.	Doppelbilder	Nahbrille
Fernbrille	vermehrter Tränenfluß		Druckgefühl	Brennen	Schmerzen

Ohren:	Hörstörung	Ohrensausen	Absonderung	Schmerzen	

Nase:	Behinderung der Nasenatmung	Störung des Geruchssinns		Nasenbluten	Absonderungen

Mund:	Zahnfleischblut.	Zungenbrennen	kein Geschmack	Zahnschmerzen	

Rachen:	Halsschmerzen	Schluckbeschw.	Heiserkeit		

Hals:	Schwellungen	Knoten am Hals	Nackenschmerz.	eingeschränkte Beweglichkeit	

Brustkorb:	Schwellungen	Knoten in der Achselhöhle		Verändrg. d. Bruste/Brustwarzen	

Atmung, Herz, Kreislauf:					
kurzatmig (Ruhe, Anstrengung)		nächtliche Dyspnoe		Todesangst	Husten
Auswurf (weiß, gelb, rot)		Brustschmerzen	Nachtschweiß	unregelmäßiger Herzschlag	
plötzliches Herzrasen					

Verdauungstrakt:					
Schluckbeschw.	Aufstoßen	Sodbrennen	Oberbauchbeschwerden		Völlegefühl
Bauchschmerzen (erläutern)		Blähungen	zunehmender Bauchumfang		Unvertr. f. Fett
Kaffee	Gewürze	Obst;	Übelkeit	Erbrechen: .... x / 24 h	
Änderung d. übl. Verdauung		Stuhlgang m. ziehd. Schmerzen		Brennen	Stuhl schwarz
schleimig	blutig	unverdaute Speisen		Würmer	

Urogenitalsystem:					
Harnstottern	Startschwierigk.	Tröpfeln	Schmerzen	Brennen beim Wasserlassen	
Urin nicht halten können		Nierenschmerz.	Urin dunkel	blutig	schaumig
trübe	Steine	Schmerzen	Blutung beim/nach Geschl.-Verk.		

Hämatopoet. und Lymphsystem:					
Verletzungsblutung » 5 Min.		ungewöhnliche blaue Flecken	schlechte Wundheilung		
Knoten in der Achselhöhle		i. d. Leiste			

Extremitäten, Muskel- und Skelettsystem:					
Schmerzen in Gelenken		Schmerzen in den Gliedern		im Rücken	Beweg.Einschr.
Mißempfindung	Kältegefühl	Schmerzen beim Gehen		in Ruhe	

Neurolog., psychiatr., psycholog.:					
Ungeklärte Traurigkeit		Grübeln	„Nervenzusammenbrüche"		Gedächtnisstör.
Konzentrationsstörungen		Halflosigkeit	Taubheit	Kribbeln	Schmerzen
Gangstörungen	Sprechstörungen	Lähmungen			

Endokrin:	Auffallend viel Urin		Empfindlichkeit gegen Wärme	gegen Kälte	Hitzewallungen

Sonst. Beschwerden und Erläuterungen

Fehlerhaftes Ankreuzen bitte durch Nachziehen des Kästchens korrigieren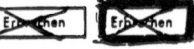

Figure 1.2.4-2.2

Example of free format history documentation form. The system review section lists coarse classes of complaints for guidance of the examiner, who may add more detailed comments on previous page.

PAT.-AKTE.

10

Medizinische Hochschule Hannover

Chirurgische Klinik
und Poliklinik

Hausarzt Tel. Aufnahmearzt

Zuständig: Prof. Dr. H.G. Borst Tel. Prof. Dr. R. Pichlmayr Tel.

Vorgeschichte:

Beschwerden:

Diagnose:

Therapie:

Therapie - Vorschlag:

Befund:

Diagnostik:

1. Durchschrift für die Krankenakte bestimmt

/262-02/75

Figure 1.2.4-3

Example of free format documentation form including a small history section, as used in the surgical outpatient clinics of the Medical School Hannover.

1.3 CRITIQUE

History taking offers a virtually unlimited source of information for treating a case as well as for gaining insight into human disease and ill-being. This may be used by the experienced to his advantage. For the unexperienced and less skilled, however, it may constitute risks with the result that the produced histories fall short of expectations or are misleading.

Principally, histories may suffer three types of shortcomings:

- errors of omission
- errors of commission
- poor documentation

Errors of omission are a lack in completeness considering the goals that are to be achieved, whereas errors of commission designate inadequate consequences drawn from correct primary information or the stimulation of incorrect utterances. In this category also fall incorrect semantic interpretations of statements by the patient in his own language. Both kinds of errors are closely related in the process of history taking, since a complete data base is a prerequisite for correct interpretation and since correct interpretation on the other hand is a prerequisite for meaningful completion of an incomplete data base. The process of history taking in the conventional form is therefore highly redundant and characterized by extensive crosschecking and crossvalidation.

Causes for shortcomings have to be sought on the side of

- the patient or
- the physician or
- their relation.

1.3.1 CAUSES OF ERRORS - THE PATIENT

There are several reasons for errors of omission or commission that may be attributable to the patient:

- incomplete memory
- modified memory
- resistance to communication.

The gradual onset of disease may get lost in a patient's other preoccupations. His account may be strongly influenced by his own interpretation, by his idea of the significance of his symptoms, of their meaning and by his endeavour to explain to himself what he is experiencing. He may report other laymen's and even other physician's incorrect or misunderstood interpretations.

REISSNER (106) and HARTUNG (51) pointed out that the process of history taking has a training effect for the patient. A first interview may cause the patient to think things over, to talk certain problems over with his family. This may improve the yield of subsequent interviews.

FAHRENBERG (29) discerns several tendencies for systematic distortion of answers through the patient, such as the tendency

- to present oneself in a socially desirable way
- to respond by yes without much reflection
- to prefer unconspicious neutral answers
- to choose extreme answers which may
  represent either
    = aggravation or
    = dissimulation.

Beyond that the patient may vehemently resent the physician's intrusion into what he considers his private sphere and therefore withhold, guard or distort information. This is enhanced if there is a danger of resulting disadvantages in style of life or social status.

While these effects may be encountered in all instances of history taking, a special situation may arise in social or legal medicine, when the role of the patient changes from that of a person asking for professional help to that of a consumer claiming his right for social services or compensation. In these cases a strong determination to present a false picture may be encountered.

1.3.2 CAUSES OF ERRORS - THE PHYSICIAN

These circumstances necessitate subjective involvement of the physician in the anamnestic process. His role is to validate the responses offered by the patient for

- completeness,
- correctness and
- value

in the context of the persued goals (31).

In this sense, the physician's subjectivity is an essential ingredient of an effective history taking process. Yet it may just as well constitute a source of errors on the physician's side.

- Limited perspective, e.g. to the scope of a
  medical subspecialty
- preoccupation with the proof of an early suspicion
- strong expectations
- lack of attention
- lack of knowledge and experience

may be causes for errors of omission as well as of commission.

Reasons are variations in individual doctor's disposition as well as differences in qualification between different examiners. Of great influence is a lack of time causing insufficient exposure during patient-physician contact and favouring the deficiencies just enumerated through exhaustion of the physician.

An initial history in internal medicine will take anywhere from fractions of an hour to several hours if prepared in a hospital setting, by the average house officer. In the primary care setting the total time available for an encounter rarely exceeds a few minutes (6, 34, 47, 79, 102).

These tremendous differences have several reasons:
- The problems dealt with in primary care are of lesser
  complexity than in a hospital. Only a small fraction
  (around 5 percent) of the cases treated will reach the hospital.
- Histories in the primary care setting are not of the all inclusive
  systematic type but aim at special problem management.
- The documentation serves primarily as a reminder for the physician
  himself.
- History data are almost exclusively used for patient care
  purposes.

Typically, physician's errors are detectable and correctable because
they pertain to facts and findings that may be reproduced. Whenever a
patient is treated by several physicians simultaneously, there are
chances for correction of errors, - much less so in the primary care
setting where a 1 : 1 relation between patient and physician is more
characteristic. Still however, in this instance a corrective effect may
be attributed to the length of exposure. The greatest need for
corrective and supportive measures exists therefore in situations
characterized by brief singular encounters between patients and
individual physicians. This situation prevails for

- practicing specialists
- health "check up" environments
- emergency clinics,
just to name a few examples.

For matters of completeness it should be pointed out that the
physician's responsibility is not limited to the objective aspects of
pathology. He is confronted with human illness and suffering. To
prevent or to treat disease requires understanding interpretation to an
extent that may elude objective reproducibility and therefore the
detection and correction of errors.

1.3.3 CAUSES OF ERRORS - THE PATIENT PHYSICIAN RELATION

The outlined deficiencies on the patient's as well as the physician's
side are complemented by deficiencies in their relation, but certainly
they may also affect their relation.

- Lack or lessening of care
- obstinacy
- aggressiveness
- strangeness
- shame

are obstacles to effective communication (49) favoured by

- lack of time
- language or semantic problems
- sociocultural differences.

The time constraints characterizing the physician's situation have been
mentioned above. The language problems may be an absolute obstacle to
history taking, especially in recent years where "horizontal migration"
crossing language borders has increased manifold. The problems that
physicians in industrialized nations have to deal with in treating
foreign workers are analogous to those of the physicians in the
workers' home countries in treating tourists.

But even within a common mother language problems posed by the differences between professional and laymen's language, received or stard language and dialect, jargon or slang may be severe (33, 63, 130). Words have different meanings at different language levels. For example, the German word for gout (Gicht) is often used popularly to denote any kinds of diseases of the rheumatic family. Again, the physician may use such differences to his advantage. He may open the dialogue in slang to initiate the spontaneous account and thereafter lead the objectivating interview over to the level of the received standard language (49).

1.3.4 POOR DOCUMENTATION

Even though the history had been successfully obtained, the resulting documentation may be poor. It may pose
- problems of legibility,
- intelligibility and
- completeness.

The problems of legibility resulting from doctor's notoriously poor handwriting have frequently been documented and illustrated in this context. They are a nuisance if several physicians care for a given patient and they may render scientific evaluation of the document impossible. However, they may be solved by typing out the notes.

The problems of intelligibility are far more complicated. The structures of standard histories exemplified above yield a frame work within which one may search for specific information or within which such information may be added to a given history. They allow a certain control over completeness of the initial data base. However, they still may not trace the physician's reasoning in the treatment of a given case. They afford no measure for assessing the completeness with respect to findings obtained later in the course of treatment. In this respect WEED's (134) concept of problem oriented documentation constitutes a considerable advance. According to WEED's suggestions, a physician is required to

1 obtain and document a complete, defined data base,
2 identify all of a patient's problems, describe and list identified by numbers
3 work out a plan of action for each problem
4 document follow up notes by indexing each further action and finding by number of the problem it relates to.

This procedure does not only allow to keep track of the reasons underlying the actions taken, but it also allows control of completeness of the follow-up history. The conventional use of a structure just for the initial data base often leads to neglecting to document the more important findings that are produced later in the course of treatment.

Still however, completeness of a record with regard to patient care purposes may be different from what is considered completeness in the scientific sense. This is a cause for frequent deficiencies with respect to the scientific value of patient histories prepared in a busy patient care environment. MELLNER et al. found that particularly senior physicians tend to be negligent about the potential scientific value of a history document (71, 72).

Almost invariably, negative findings are omitted from documentation, making it thus difficult or impossible to decide whether they actually were negative or just not asked.

While the health care delivery systems function on the whole rather well and therefore seem to cope with the various shortcomings of history taking, the effects may be serious in individual cases. Impressive case histories have been reported in the literature. They range from successful attempts of suicide because of failure to discover a suicidal inclination (8) over serious misjudgements concerving causes of chronic disability (116) to accounts of "serious errors in 40 - 50 percent" of reviewed records (73). GOEPEL (39) found 15 cases of severe disease in a sample of more than 800 patients who were submitted to a systematic examination in his general practice. BERNER and HAEHN (2, 3) found that 8 out of 112 patients that completed our experimental history questionnaire had to be referred to specialists solely on behalf of information acquired by this device.

Interesting quantitative data are given by COCHRANE et.al. (17) who compared the results of several physicians obtained by brief interrogations (average time 5 minutes per man) of coal miners. For symptoms such as cough and sputum highly significant differences in positive answers were found between the various observers. The percentages for positive answers for cough ranged from 23.4 to 40.3, those for sputum from 13.0 to 41.9 in the 5 observes, despite of the fact that the interviewed population samples were not significantly different.

These findings stress the importance of efforts to improve quality, effectiveness and consistency of history taking. They are conceivable as

- improving the teaching of history taking
- motivating physicians to devote their time and skills to history taking
- devising supportive techniques.

Only the latter kind will be treated in the following discussion.

2. SUPPORTIVE TECHNIQUES

2.1 GENERAL PURPOSE

The use of a form for a standard history or a checklist for use by the physician is the simplest form of technical support. These approaches will however not be considered in the following unless computer processing of the acquired data is involved. Positively speaking the following discussion will therefore be restricted to questionnaire techniques used for history acquisition directly from the patient, or through another intermediary than a physician with or without computer processing.

So far only one description of a computer system could be found which is designed specifically to support the recording of histories acquired by a physician (40).

Questionnaire techniques are widely employed in the medical field mainly for

- surveys in epidemiology
- testing in the psychological disciplines of medicine
- specialized scientific investigations
- screening in prevention and early recognition of disease
- surveilling the course of disease
- providing a data base in individual sick care.

The following discussion will focus on the latter aspects, the support of preventive and curative care directed at somatic diseases.

The principal objectives of supportive techniques in this context are improvements with respect to

- standardization
- quality of documentation
- expense of physician time
- foreign language problems
- enhancement of science from interindividual evaluation.

2.1.1 IMPROVEMENT OF STANDARDIZATION

Three different levels of standardization may be discerned. At the first level, standardization may be viewed as an attempt to increase the number of constants in the history taking process so that more homogeneous and comparable results are obtained, even if the various shortcomings cannot be entirely eliminated. Apart from covering positive and negative responses to a standard set of questions, standardization pertains to aspects that influence patient performance:

- layout, environment
- language chosen
- time requirements.

A system standardized to this extent will be more uniform. To the patient it will be more evenly appealing or appalling, - both to an extent that can be reckonned with.

Least amenable to standardization may be the patient's characteristics. Wide variations in

- intelligence
- medical knowledge
- interest in one's illness
- language characteristics
- familiarity with technical devices
- ability to handle such technical devices
- patience
- degree of impairment by disease

will have to be taken into account and possibly compensated. In this respect, the homogeneity of the population that is using a particular device is of importance.

The second level of standardization then insures that essential characteristics of the instrument can be accounted for. If, for instance, the purpose of the instrument is primarily diagnostic classification, the accuracy of diagnostic classification achieved by use of the instrument may be specified. An instrument standardized to this extent will yield results which are predictable with respect to the investigated characteristics, although it may not yet meet independently defined requirements.

Even though predictable, the results may still be considered inadequate. Correction of such deficiencies then constitutes the third level of standardization. It means that the instrument meets defined requirements.

The distinction seems important since high expectations are sometimes attached to instruments which in fact are barely meeting requirements of first level standardization.

2.1.2 OTHER OBJECTIVES

It is assumed that providing the physician with a standard data base in history findings will serve as a primer and a backup in special problem management. Reduction of the error of omission through provision of a more complete data base may indirectly reduce the error of commission.

As far as scientific evaluation is concerned it should be pointed out, that the objectives aiming at improving individually oriented patient care are in some contrast to those aiming at improving the scientific value of medical history data. The questionnaire is not per se a research tool, even though it still requires a lot of research to become a useful tool in medical care.

In order to be useful in medical care the value of each question and the entire questionnaire should be known with respect to given objectives. As long as this is not the case, routine application will be a waste of time, effort and money. Until so far, it is sufficient to test the instrument on samples of respondents. Thereafter, during routine application, further insights into the value of history data acquired by the instrument will be restricted to relating these findings with other data, e. g. from laboratory procedures.

If data acquisition is the dominant purpose already in conventional history taking, this is even more true for supporting devices. So far at least attempts to integrate e.g. aspects of patient education with history acquisition are not known to us.

2.2 OUTLINE OF APPROACHES TO SOLUTION

The fact that it is not possible to simply ask a patient to write down his medical history, because he lacks the knowledge of what would be important, has led to the development of questionnaire techniques which are employed to channel the patient's attention appropriately.

The principle is not new. HARTMANN (110) points out that mailed questionnaires were used already in the 17th century by Theophraste Renaudot, a physician in Paris.

However, there seem to exist no direct links relating this work to contemporary endeavours in this field.

The early development of medical questionnaires, which was taken up in the late thirties (35) and resulted in the development of such devices as the Cornell Medical Index Health Questionnaire (CMI) in the late fourties (8), was influenced to a great extent by the development of measuring devices in psychology and epidemiology. The advent of computers, which became available in the late fifties in the medical field, has definitely stimulated the developments in this area just as much as the growing awareness of a change in the goals and responsibilities of medicine.

So far, three stages of development may be identified:

1 checklist approach
2 simulation of patient-physician dialogue through logic branching
3 complex acquisition and presentation techniques.

2.3 FIRST STAGE OF DEVELOPMENT: CHECKLIST APPROACH

The lack of technical alternatives and perhaps the influence of psychometric instruments had the effect, that at first paper and pencil forms were developed which the patient could complete where he wanted, at home as well as in bed on the ward. The completed questionnaire served simultaneously as a documentation of its results.

Typically, the patient gets a list of printed questions each presented with a choice of answers of the yes/no or true/false type. It is estimated that 90 percent of the adult population are capable of completing such a list of questions (30), which usually requires to mark the intended answer (as opposed to crossing out the wrong answer). The completed form may then be read by the physician by scanning the answers.

A typical example is the CORNELL MEDICAL INDEX HEALTH QUESTIONNAIRE (CMI, 8) (figures 2.3-1 and 2.3-2). It consists of a list of 195 questions, presented in two columns on four pages. Associated with each question are the yes/no choices of answers which may be specified by encircling the intended response.

The questionnaire is combined with a "diagnostic sheet" that enables the physician to summarize concisely his conclusions drawn from the completed questionnaire.

The CMI has gained wide acceptance in a number of different institutions and is still in use in the original form. As a matter of fact, it may be used more widely in daily routine than any other single history taking device. Extensive testing has demonstrated its value in screening situations (9, 10, 11, 12, 13, 14, 26, 27, 28). Impressing case reports demonstrating the superiority of the information acquired with the aid of the CMI over the histories acquired in clinical routine were given by BRODMAN in the initial publications describing the approach (8, 9).

It is particularly important that BRODMAN showed clearly that while the CMI histories were invariably more complete with respect to coverage of general symptoms, physician's histories were more complete with respect to details pertaining to a given patient's problems.

Since then, numerous questionnaires of similar structure have been developed, often relying heavily on the CMI in format as well as content. The clear structure, ease of use and effectiveness of these questionnaires have won them many friends. It is considered particularly useful that the physician may go over the answers with the patient and add personal comments to an otherwise satisfactory document.

Their wide spread use and extensive application in routine practice is also a prerequisite which made it possible to test some of these devices thoroughly (e.g. 1, 16, 60, 107, 108, 113, 136).

Nevertheless, a physician's history will frequently have to be more comprehensive, more detailed and be focussed more appropriately at the patient's specific problems. This need together with the availibility of technological advances lead to further developments.

Patient _____ History Number _____

Interpreter of CMI _____ Date _____

THIS IS A SPECIMEN COPY

DIAGNOSTIC SHEET

THE CORNELL MEDICAL INDEX-HEALTH QUESTIONNAIRE

Underline the organ systems about which the CMI reveals symptoms requiring diagnostic investigation. Add your tentative diagnoses.

If the symptoms about an organ system appear to be associated with an emotional disturbance, add the diagnosis "emotional."

Letters in the left hand column refer to sections on the CMI.

A Eyes or ears

B Respiratory system

C Cardiovascular system

D Teeth

D Gastrointestinal, liver and gall bladder

E Musculoskeletal system

F Skin

G Nervous system

H Genital system

H Urinary tract

Other

From the evidence on the CMI, underline the severity of the patient's emotional disturbance:

(1) Not significant   (2) Mild   (3) Moderate   (4) Severe

The CMI reveals evidence of an emotional disturbance, in complaints referring to the body (yes answers scattered over the first three pages) or those referring to moods and feelings (yes answers on the last page).

The number, distribution, and clinical importance of the yes responses indicate the severity of an emotional disturbance.

The following numbered questions on the CMI refer to histories of specific diseases:

20 Hay Fever	90 Epilepsy	130 Goiter
21 Asthma	100 Hernia (in men)	131 Tumor or Cancer
26 Tuberculosis	107 Kidney or Bladder Disease	133 Underweight
28 Hypertension	124 Scarlet Fever	134 Overweight
39 Heart Disease	125 Rheumatic Fever	135 Varicose Veins
56 Stomach Ulcers	126 Malaria	136 Major Operation
61 Hemorrhoids	127 Anemia	137 Major Injury
63 Liver or Gall Bladder Disease	128 Venereal Disease	168 Nervous Breakdown
87 Paralysis	129 Diabetes	170 Mental Hospitalization

Figure 2.3-1

The Cornell Medical Index Health Questionnaire Diagnostic Sheet (9).

THIS IS A SPECIMEN COPY

History Number_____

(MEN)

CORNELL MEDICAL INDEX

HEALTH QUESTIONNAIRE

Date_____

| Print Your Name | Your Home Address |

How Old Are You?_____ Circle If You Are . . Single, Married, Widowed, Separated, Divorced.

Circle the Highest Year You Reached In School | 1 2 3 4 5 6 7 8 | | 1 2 3 4 | | 1 2 3 4 | What Is Your Occupation?_____
Elementary School   High   College

Directions: This questionnaire is for **MEN ONLY.**

If you can answer **YES** to the question asked, put a circle around the (Yes)

If you have to answer **NO** to the question asked, put a circle around the (No)

Answer all questions. If you are not sure, guess.

A

1. Do you need glasses to read? .... Yes No
2. Do you need glasses to see things at a distance? ...... Yes No
3. Has your eyesight often blacked out completely? ...... Yes No
4. Do your eyes continually blink or water? ... Yes No
5. Do you often have bad pains in your eyes? .. Yes No
6. Are your eyes often red or inflamed? ...... Yes No
7. Are you hard of hearing? ...... Yes No
8. Have you ever had a bad running ear? ...... Yes No
9. Do you have constant noises in your ears? ..... Yes No

B

10. Do you have to clear your throat frequently? Yes No
11. Do you often feel a choking lump in your throat? ...... Yes No
12. Are you often troubled with bad spells of sneezing? ...... Yes No
13. Is your nose continually stuffed up? .... Yes No
14. Do you suffer from a constantly running nose? ...... Yes No
15. Have you at times had bad nose bleeds? ...... Yes No
16. Do you often catch severe colds? .... Yes No
17. Do you frequently suffer from heavy chest colds? ...... Yes No
18. When you catch a cold, do you always have to go to bed? ...... Yes No
19. Do frequent colds keep you miserable all winter? ...... Yes No

20. Do you get hay fever? ...... Yes No
21. Do you suffer from asthma? ...... Yes No
22. Are you troubled by constant coughing? ...... Yes No
23. Have you ever coughed up blood? ...... Yes No
24. Do you sometimes have severe soaking sweats at night? ...... Yes No
25. Have you ever had a chronic chest condition? Yes No
26. Have you ever had T.B. (Tuberculosis) ? ...... Yes No
27. Did you ever live with anyone who had T.B.? Yes No

C

28. Has a doctor ever said your blood pressure was too *high?* ...... Yes No
29. Has a doctor ever said your blood pressure was too *low?* ...... Yes No
30. Do you have pains in the heart or chest? ...... Yes No
31. Are you often bothered by thumping of the heart? ...... Yes No
32. Does your heart often race like mad? ...... Yes No
33. Do you often have difficulty in breathing? ...... Yes No
34. Do you get out of breath long before anyone else? ...... Yes No
35. Do you sometimes get out of breath just sitting still? ...... Yes No
36. Are your ankles often badly swollen? ...... Yes No
37. Do cold hands or feet trouble you even in hot weather? ...... Yes No
38. Do you suffer from frequent cramps in your legs? ...... Yes No
39. Has a doctor ever said you had heart trouble? Yes No
40. Does heart trouble run in your family? ...... Yes No

OPEN TO NEXT PAGE

Cornell University Medical College
1300 York Avenue, New York 21, N. Y.

Figure 2.3-2

The Cornell Medical Index Health Questionnaire. First page with 40 out of 195 questions (8).

2.4 SECOND STAGE DEVELOPMENTS: DETERMINISTIC SIMULATION OF PATIENT - PHYSICIAN DIALOGUE

2.4.1 BASIC CONCEPT AND CONSEQUENT TECHNICAL REQUIREMENTS

The work of BRODMAN had shown that

- self-administered history acquisition was able to provide useful

information of the general type
- physician acquired histories were superior in detail.

It was logical therefore to attempt to obtain more detail with self-administered devices.

An example might illustrate the problem:

There are three questions in the CMI, which may refer to gastroduodenal ulcers:

54 Do you suffer from constant stomach trouble?

55 Does Stomach trouble run in your family?

56 Has a Doctor ever said you had stomach ulcers?

To find out whether positive answers to any of these three questions really refer to a gastric ulcer one might want to ask, whether the trouble increases in the spring and autumn season, whether the pains get worse at night and whether eating and or antacids are of help. In order to get this kind of detail, one would either have to increase the number of questions asked or else use very complicated questions like

"Do you suffer from stomach trouble that gets worse at night and better from eating or taking antiacids"

Volume and phrasing would soon become prohibitive.

A solution to the problem was expected from simulating the logical conduct of an anamnestic interview, in which the physician is supposed to ask for detail only when previous information seems to make questioning worthwhile in this direction. The concept was based on the assumption that the physician's questioning process follows a logic path, according to medical concepts of disease. Consequently, it was thought to suffice to transmit this medical logic to the computer, and have the computer react deterministically according to the rules derived from medical model concepts.

The development of such

- programmed interviews

had as prerequisites the employ of essentially three types of extensions of the previously used techniques:

- extended choice of reply options
- questionnaire branching, and
- condensed presentation of results.

These extensions can be used to varying extent either singly or in combination.

Although, the basic ideas at this stage of development were thoroughly influenced by computer technology and computers were widely and extensively applied in these approaches, their use is not mandatory for achieving the stated goals.

2.4.1.1 REPLY OPTIONS

Even though the simple reply options of the YES/NO type are supposed to be manageable by patients with below average intelligence (29) they may present problems to patients of average or higher intelligence.

This kind of patients may find it difficult to decide between yes or no, because they simply are not sure enough of either or because they might prefer to respond by an answer like "yes - sometimes".

This lead frequently to an extension of answer choices to

- don't know.

This option still contains ambiguity because it might either pertain to the question or to what the question asks for. The patient might not understand the question or not know the answer. Realizing this lead to offer the two options

- don't know and
- don't understand.

A fifth option has also been suggested (104, 124), but apparently is rarely used. It is

- rather don't want to answer.

These five answer options are the maximum suggested for standard type questions in questionnaires using paper and pencil as recording media. If different devices, such as computer terminals are used, a few more options may become necessary for controlling the sequence of questions and the recording of answers. The most common are:

- backward branch (previous question)
- branch to last answered question
- branch to specified question
- forward branch (next question)
- transmit response
- erase response
- display explanation.

Thus, a total of some 12 options results, which of course need not all be used. For instance, the option "forward branch" might be used instead of the "don't know", "don't understand" and "rather not answer" option.

The two to twelve options represent a standard set of multiple choice answers. Multiple choice techniques are extensively used for detailed answering of more complex questions. For instance, they may be used to specify for a given complaint such characteristics as

- location
- duration
- time of occurence
- accompanying circumstances
- causes
- intensity
- quality

```
- quantity
- previous actions taken.
```

Multiple choice questions may be of the exclusive or inclusive type, depending on whether just one or several options may be specified simultaneously.

The answer options given above would represent an exclusive choice of answer options. Examples of exclusive questions would be

```
    Are you
        - A man
        - A Woman

    Which type of school did you attend at last
        - Elementary School
        - Highschool
        - College
        - Other
```

An inclusive multiple choice question would be

```
    Have you ever been treated for
        - Heart trouble
        - High blood pressure
        - Diabetes
```

Here, either none or any to all of the options offered may apply in a given patient.

Numerical entries were frequently found desirable as an additional answer option in questionnaires based on paper and pencil medium as well as on terminal devices. Usually numerical entries are found to be handled sufficiently well by untrained users for specifying such items as age, number of children or current date. The precision of memory for other items such as onset of a disease, date of an operation or time of earlier hospitalization , seems not to justify more extensive recording of numerical answers (55). This applies likewise to their use in recording such items as average number of cigarettes smoked. Here not only the imprecision of the question and the patient's memory but also his unwillingness to supply the correct information make it preferrable to use an exclusive multiple choice question instead for obtaining approximate specifications. (See also example below).

Despite the fact that it is usually strongly recommended that the physician records pertinent answers as given by the patient, the option to have the patient complete the questionnaire by filling in answers in free text is abandoned. It increases the burden for the patient (8) and makes the result less accurate and less comparable if it can be obtained at all. One might think of using such techniques for recording the patient's spontaneous phrasing. However the reluctance of most patients to write at all, and the use of "written" instead of spontaneous language precludes the use of such techniques even for this purpose. Free text answers are therefore restricted to such items as patient's name and chief complaint or reason for consultation. These few items may even be added to a completed history by trained personnel.

In own experience the option to specify a chief complaint or reason for referral was used by roughly 25 percent (see section 4.2) of patients, a finding which corresponds to those of MELLNER (71). MAYNE (76) and GIERE (58) obtained handwritten responses to these questions from more

than 50 (70) to more than 90 (58) percent. This may be due to the fact
that their experiments were conducted in a private outpatient clinic
environment with a greater proportion of upper middle class worried
well patients in their clientele.

2.4.1.2 BRANCHING

Branching means that the sequence of questions may be altered depending
on the answers obtained. It is the essential characteristic of the
second stage of developments.

Branching is frequently used in connection with multiple choice answer
techniques for eliciting details on summarily recorded findings. A
typical example would be

A
    Do you have children?
        - Yes
        - No
    If no, continue at B

A 1
    How many children do you have?
        - 1
        - 2 or 3
        - More than 3

B
    Where do you live?
        - City
        - Suburb
        - Town
        - Village or Country
        - Other

For design and evaluation of acquisition devices it is important to
distinguish between

    - simple and
    - complex

branching (15). Simple branching denotes branching that is determined
by the answer to the current question and does not require mathematical
operations to be performed, while complex branching involves at least
an answer to a previous question.

If paper and pencil based techniques are employed, the simple branching
can usually be controlled sufficiently well by the patient. Since
questions are usually phrased in such a way that a negative answer
implies a state which is not pathologic or not otherwise worthy of
further elaboration, a branching instruction may be attached to a
negative answer as in the example given above. In a printed
questionnaire, the patient may nevertheless read the questions that he
is supposed to skip and if the branching question was answered wrongly,
he may still respond to the questions at the lower level correctly.
This possibility is lost if branching is accomplished automatically,
since the skipped questions remain hidden. Since the patient's answers
may be incorrect faulty branching will result. One of the major
objectives of third stage developments is to eliminate this shortcoming
of the deterministic branching technique used in the second stage.

The distinction between simple and complex branching is noteworthy for automatic devices because simple branching may be achieved mechanically without computer Complex branching on the other hand requires even in its most primitive form that answers pertinent to later branching decisions be stored for later action upon them. The acquisition device will therefore to some extent have to incorporate programmable logic. The essentials of automatic branching for this type of automated history acquisition systems have comprehensively been summarized by BUDD et.al. (15). The basic operations consist of

- displaying a question
- recording the response
- analysis of the response
- execution of a branching instruction.

Questionnaires invariably are constructed in such a way that each question is presented only once. They are not reentrant. Nevertheless, the same text may be presented in different medical context. For instance, it may be necessary several times to find out whether a given symptom is observed on the right, the left or both sides of the body. In this instance the same phrases could be reused several times.

Such a questionnaire could then correspond to a directed graph. The questions would be represented by nodes which are interconnected by lines. Branches along these lines are possible only in one direction which is indicated by an arrow head.

A node would then consist of

1) a node identifier
2) a text identifier
3) two or more answer options with
4) associated branch instructions.

Figure 2.4.1.2-1 gives an example. Here node identifiers are represented by uppercase letters, text identifiers by numbers and answer options by lower case letters. The branch instruction represented by a Greek letter would be of the type "If at A the answer to text 1 is b go to B".

As illustrated in figure 2.4.1.2-1 branch instructions may result in skipping a sequence of questions or in parallel sequences of questions.

Skips may be nested and several parallel sequences may be used. Care has to be taken however, that no circles result which would trap the respondent in a portion of the questionnaire.

If complex branching is used, several characteristics may be identified which relate to the design of the acquisition device (15). These are:

- the number of questions which may be reached from the current question
- the number of answers which must be stored to determine the branching actions
- the type of mathematical operations which have to be performed on the given answers in order to determine the ensuing question.

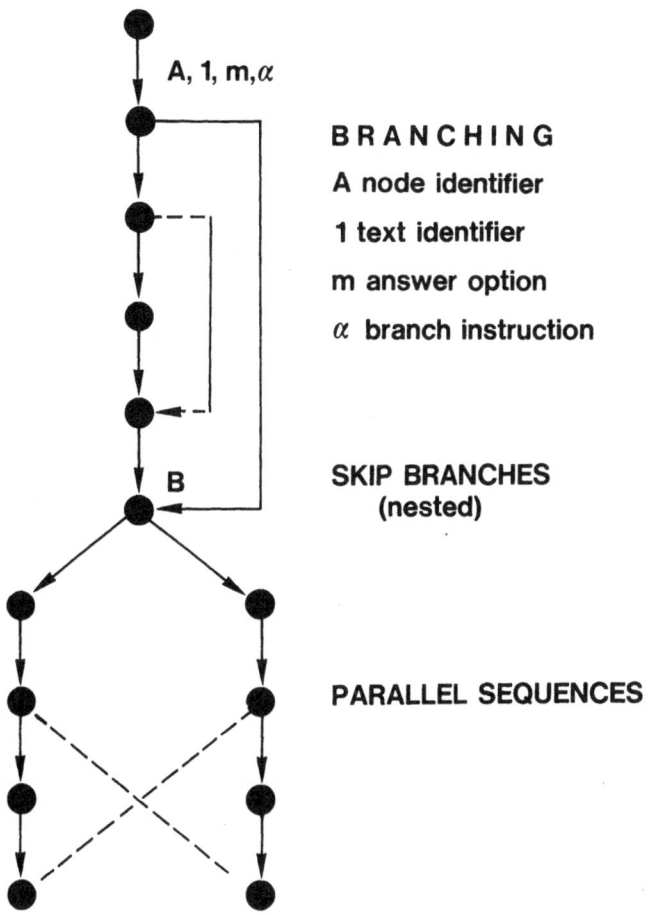

A, 1, m, α

BRANCHING

A node identifier

1 text identifier

m answer option

α branch instruction

SKIP BRANCHES
(nested)

PARALLEL SEQUENCES

Figure 2.4.1.2-1

Directed graph representing a branching questionnaire.

For the design of acquisition devices it is crucial to realize that the storage of answers for the purpose of complex branching is of different type than the recording of answers for later evaluation or presentation to the physician. While for this latter purpose it might suffice to add code to an output stream, it is necessary for branching purposes, to store answer code as well as the addresses of possible target questions in a retrievable form.

2.4.1.3 CONDENSED PRESENTATION OF RESULTS

The extension of questionnaires to the gathering of greater detail requires condensed presentation of the acquired data, just as it required the employ of branching techniques in acquisition.

This is achieved by extracting and editing techniques. Extraction denotes that only relevant parts of the acquired data are presented (usually represented by positive answers). In the simplest way this may mean that the answer referring to some kind of derangement or to a subsystem of the organism is presented. A listing of the remainder of answers may be supplied in addition for optional reference.

The editing functions start with the presentation of simply rephrased sentences which read better than the combination of question and answer. The answers given to several distinct questions may be rearranged into a single phrase. In this case the 1 : 1 correspondence between question and report text frequently has to be replaced by more complex logical relations. This leads then to fully programmable text editing systems (101).

Invariably hardcopies of the acquired data are produced, which may be added to the patient's conventional record. The display of acquired data on terminals does only then constitute an advantage, when the displays are available, where the information is needed. Usually it is yet safer and more universally applicable, if hardcopies are made available that may accompany the patient on his route through different units or institutions.

2.4.2 SURVEY OF SYSTEM PROPOSALS

The variety of technical alternatives at the second stage of development lead to a still proliferating number of alternative systems. Hardly any combination of acquisition and presentation techniques seems to have been spared.

A number of portable acquisition devices, that the patient may use where he deems it is appropriate, have been developed. They share with the first stage developments a significant operational advantage which makes it possible that these systems have often been validated more thoroughly than stationary ones. COLLEN (19) introduced in the early sixties a simple procedure which required the patient to sort questions printed on punched cards into boxes according to whether the intended answer was affirmation or denial.

These cards were fed into a computer to produce a printed record. Besides its remarkable simplicity, the approach is noteworthy for the fact that questions may be presented in random order.

Wide acceptance was gained by mark sense forms and cards for interfacing with the patient, (2, 58, 66, 67, 69, 77) but we are not aware of the use of optical character reading devices in this context. MAYNE et.al. (67) realized some kind of complex branching with paper and pencil devices by using questionnaires printed by computer on mark sense sheets. These were individualized for the patient on the basis of a previously completed questionnaire.

An interesting variety of a computer independent portable system was described by KANNER (57). It offered the advantages of covering a broad spectrum of questions and producing a compact type written summary at low cost through use of a text editing typewriter. Of course the acquired data may be transcribed to machine readable devices for computer processing.

Stationary devices used for data acquisition range from standard typewriter terminals over CRT-terminals to special purpose devices including multimedial approaches. The basic response options may be realized using a numerical keyboard including few special keys e.g. for signs, decimal point and a "shift" key. A full typewriter keyboard may confuse patients and should therefore be reduced by masking out unused keys or replaced by a special purpose keyboard. Function buttons are a common feature on special purpose devices.

Apart from their superiority in speed and noiselessness CRT-terminals are usually preferred to other stationary devices for the possibility of employing light pen techniques which eliminate the necessity to translate an intended answer into a key board response. This advantage lead even to the development of special purpose recording screens (68). Pictures stored on media like projection slides, film strips or microfilm may be projected onto such a screen. They can be used to illustrate a question or instead of a question. The answer is then given by pointing to an appropriate area on the screen.

SIMMONS and MILLER (119, 120) combined the display of written question with graphic illustrations automatically projected onto a screen and the playoff of spoken text stored on a tape recorder.

Such special purpose devices may again operate independently of a computer, as exemplified by the SADE Programmed Film System introduced by CDC (15). In this system all displayed information as well as data controlling the display sequence was stored on 16 mm film. Answers were registered by means of 12 function buttons and either recorded on punched paper tape or transmitted to a computer. This system even allowed the display of motion picture scenes during the interview.

Along the same general line are attempts to use graphic displays to support history acquisition (25, 56, 90, 118).

In a different kind of attempt, SLACK (125) tried to extend the acquisiton of data during interview beyond the actual responses chosen by the patient. He monitored heart rate and response latency (time lag between display of a question and the recording of the answer) and used these data in conjunction with the patient's responses to route the sequence of displayed questions. Elevation of heart rate and response latency would result in skipping of certain questions or the display of explanatory or reassuring frames of text.

Despite of the great variety in alternatives for stationary systems, few seem to have proven useful enough to justify routine application, which on the other hand is a prerequisite for meaningful validation. The system of SLACK (121, 122, 123), which initially involved dedicated use of a LINC Computer, and another dedicated commercial system, described by HAESSLER (25, 46), probably have to be named first in this context.

Within the Medical System Hannover (MSH; 104, 105), an experimental system for support of medical history acquisition has been developed and evaluated. In the following this system will be described and the obtained results and consequences discussed.

3. THE EXPERIMENTAL MSH AUTOMATED HISTORY

3.1 THE CARRIER SYSTEM

Our experimentation with impersonal history acquistion was based upon a program system developed by IBM specifically for application in medicine: the Clinical Decision Support System (CDSS).

The system can be considered an early prototype of a data directed interactive system. It was developed from 1964 on according to a concept outlined by MOORE (80, 81, 82, 83, 84, 85, 86). Its chief underlying idea is that it should be possible to delegate complex medical decisions to a computer by subdividing them into modular components and to transfer these 'decision modules' to the computer.

This concept has been tested in our institution in a different context (76, 97, 98). It was found to be unsatisfactorily realized in CDSS, it has, however, some interesting characteristics which are dealt with in section 5.6.1.

Other features of CDSS motivated us to use it as supporting system for computer supported history acquisition. These were:

- data directed program control
- an appropriate set of basic functions
- availability

The program system consists of close to 50 programs supplied in four program packages written in PL/1 with a few routines written in Assembler language:

- presystem programs
- system build programs
- system operate programs offline
- system operate programs online.

Originally conceived to be operated in batch mode, the system was later modified for online operation under DOS (Disk Operating System) as supervisor, using MISP (Medical Information System Programs) as teleprocessing executive. This version was installed in 1970 at the Medical School Hannover. Versions executable under OS as supervisor were provided by IBM in 1971 for the presystem, system build and system operate offline programs for better integration into the Medical System Hannover (MSH) which is based upon OS (Operating System) as supervisor and BEST (Baylor Executive System for Teleprocessing) as teleprocessing executive (104). Adaption of the online system operate programs to the OS/BEST environment of the Medical System Hannover (MSH) was accomplished by REICHERTZ.

The program packages have the following functions:

- Presystem programs:

    The presystem programs serve to manipulate the user provided control data (see below). With their aid the control data is loaded on files, various data sets are interrelated and control listings produced. Central to this package is an editor program which serves to correct and modify the data base in the batch mode.

- System build programs:

   The system build programs employ the user provided data base to
   generate the data sets needed for system operation, such as a
   text file, an area where patient data may be stored and various
   pointer tables interrelating the data sets.

- System operate programs:

   These use the data sets generated by the system build programs
   and the commands provided by the user either in the form of
   descriptive data or as commands in the propper sense to
   accomplish the system functions which are
   = acquisition
   = storage
   = presentation and
   = interpretation of medical data.

The rationale underlying CDSS was to supply the user with a system that
he would be able to control without using a formal programming
language.

This was realized by providing a system which accepts two kinds of
data:

- control data
- descriptive data.

The control data appear to the user as 'medical experience', written
down in a fairly informal way and fed into the computer. The system
uses this data to generate data sets that are referred to during
operation. Descriptive data on the other hand are data describing a
particular case by supplying data, e.g. concerning the medical history,
physical examination, lab results etc. Both kinds of data control the
system's action.

In this manner, the user is able to program the system to his
particular application using a very limited set of commands, which do
hardly resemble commands. In particular he is able to control:

- the kind and amount of medical data to be handled by the system
- the type of device used for data acquisition
- the editing of text used in data acquisition or
  presentation
- the branching logic of data acquisition dialogues
- the logic for medical interpretation of data (using decision
  modules)
- calculations to be performed on numerical data entered.

For this purpose, the user initially had to provide only three kinds of
data:

- node hierarchy
- questionnaires and
- decision modules.

Special coding forms are provided for all user supplied control
information. As the system evolved into an online system, some other
sets of control data were developed for such functions as execution of
numerical calculations, use of special data entry devices etc.

The 'node hierarchy' represents the core of the system concept. It consists of a list of identifiers called 'nodes' that may be hierarchically structured. At least two levels of hierarchy are required, but as much as 10 may be used. (The hierarchy serves mainly for controlling 'spreading' of answers to nodes at other levels in the hierarchy than the answer was obtained for. It is also useful in editing and generating of reports). Associated with each identifier is a medical text that serves to give it a semantic content. This text is provided by the system with a unique identification number, which the user programing the system must refer to. Apart from the text the user has to supply some additional information:

A 'node type' determines whether it is a

- decisional node or a
- descriptive node.

The value of decisional nodes is determined by the system on the basis of a threshold logic, that is provided by the user in the form of decision modules. The value of descriptive nodes is entered as part of the descriptive data entered during system operation. Descriptive nodes may further be subdivided into

- text nodes
- numerical nodes and
- boolean nodes,

depending on the type of values that a particular node may be given. Each node may be identified as 'single' or 'multiple', depending on whether multiple results may replace each other or have to be stored separately. This information is crucial, because the computerized patient record consists essentially of a fixed length image of the node hierarchy in which each node of the hierarchy is represented with a certain amount of storage according to its type. In addition an overflow area is provided. Depending on the type of node either the value given to the node or a pointer to the location of the data in the overflow area are stored in this 'node status vector'. In this fashion storage of varying amounts of text or of multiple values is accomplished.

A few additional control data of lesser importance have to be supplied, but are not necessary for understanding the basic function of the node hierarchy which consists in linking all functions of the system for a given patient together. Also it has to be emphasized that the node hierarchy is just what is supplied by the user 'programming' the system and is not as such represented in the system. During system generation it is processed to generate the various data sets used during system operation.

The questionnaire input provided by the user is a list of question texts. Each question text has to be associated with at least 1 hierarchy node.

Of particular interest in the context of history acquisition is the control over data acquisition and -presentation. A great variety of data entry devices may be used. The best support however is given to the use of

- mark sense forms and
- terminals.

The mark sense forms and frame sequences for either mode of data entry
are generated by the system on the basis of questionnaire data provided
by the user. For this purpose the user has to specify

- the wording for texts
- the response options
- branching controls
- a few editing controls.

Two kinds of text are required:

- question text and
- report text.

The report text is the text provided with the node hierarchy. The
differentiation is necessary if the report text is to be concentrated
and condensed. It opens the possibility of adapting to the patient's
needs to the extent of using a foreign language as questionnaire text.

Response options available differ only slightly for online and offline
data acquisition. Basically they consists of:

- yes
- no
- don't know (online)
- don't understand (online)
- multiple choice inclusive
- multiple choice exclusive
- numerical entry
- text entry

For offline text entry one has to resort to punch cards or analogous
devices.

The option to control branching with the questionnaire control data
requires to construct the questionnaire also in hierarchical form. It
may however differ from that of the node hierarchy. In order to achieve
branching one has to specify

- the level of the questionnaire hierarchy that the branch has to
  skip to
- the identifier of the hierarchy node that controls
  the branch
- the value or values of that node that will cause skipping the
  questions at lower hierachical levels.

In this fashion only 'skip' type branches may be realized. On mark
sense forms this is achieved by generating a printed instruction to the
user to skip questions and continue at a specified question. The
instruction may read

    If no skip to next A

telling the user that if he just answered 'no' he may skip to a
question marked 'A'.

During online system operation the skipping is, of course, done
automatically without being noticeable to the user. Here the need for
parallel sequences also arises. These cannot be realized through use of
questionnaire control data. Instead it is necessary to load part of the

questionnaire on a particular point on the controlling data set and specify in the questionnaire control data a branch to this point. Inconsistencies in the system design such as this arise from the fact that CDSS was originally conceived as offline system and only later converted to an online system.

During the development of the program system some other features were added to the system which all require the user to specify his control information in a less convenient fashion than for node hierarchy, questionnaire and decision modules. The most important in this context is the patient summary description feature (PSD) that puts the programming user into the position to control

- selection
- context
- kind and
- sequence

of data to be included in an so called 'patient summary', the printed report generated for data presentation.

The presentation is largely independent of the structure of the hierarchy, and entirely independent of the kind of input and its manner of acquisition. Therefore it is possible, e. g. to combine the presentation of laboratory test results with physical examination findings and history data.

The specifications supplied by the 'programmer' include again the identifier for the hierarchy node and the condition, under which it is to be included in the report. It may be reported unconditionally or conditionally depending on the value it has. This value may have been supplied by the user entering descriptive data or derived by the system on the basis of the decision module logic. Also text belonging to a node, its value or both may be presented. Part of the text may be suppressed if it is identical for adjacently presented nodes. The presented text may be concatenated or listed in tabular form. Also the presentation may include text constants that were only once supplied to the system as part of the control information but are not part of user entered descriptive data or system generated decisional data. Several PSDs may be made available to suit varying needs of information by the user. The same data may therefore be presented in a variety of formats and contexts, depending on the PSD chosen.

3.2 CONTENTS AND GENERAL CHARACTERISTICS

The own initial work was directed at implementing a computer assisted dialogue under CDSS. This work was based on existing questionnaires which had been obtained from the following workers and institutions:

M.F. Collen	Kaiser Permanente Medical Group	Oakland, Calif.
H. Deicher	Medizinische Hoch-schule Hannover	Hannover
W. Giere	Deutsche KLinik fuer Diagnostik	Wiesbaden
P. Hall	Karolinska Sjukhuset	Stockholm

H.R. Thompson   Duke University   Durham, N.C.

W.V. Slack   Beth Israel Hospital   Boston, Mass.

L.L. Weed   University of Vermont Burlington, Vmt.

The first result was an extensively branching questionnaire comprising some 1700 questions. It could be used in its entirety or partially and was equipped with a training section that was meant to familiarize the user with the response options. After completing any chosen questionnaire the respondent was branched to a section elliciting some answers concerning the attitudes towards various aspects of the interview. In summary then the following choices werde made available:

A   Comprehensive Questionnaire
B   Short version
C   Social history
D   Training section
E   Attitude section.

The questions were displayed to the respondent via an IBM 2740 or SIEMENS 8151 terminal and consisted mainly of 1 to 8 questions, or an introductory question and several answer options for multiple choice answers. Also free text or numeric entries were used. Free text entries were only expected from clerical personnel to be added to the answers given by the patient. Numerical entries were demanded on a few occasions from the patient himself.

A mask was constructed for the SIEMENS 8151 terminal that covered the typewriter keyboard of the terminal and converted it into a special purpose keyboard with conspicious indication of the various buttons' functions.

Branching used in these questionnaires was predominantly of the simple type. A few answers such as the respondent's sex were refered to repetitively during the interview. Only very limited use was made of the complex branching capability provided by the CDSS decision modules. It was used only for prohibiting access to real patient histories, i.e. for insuring confidentiality of the data. The reason was that all functions considered necessary at the time could be accomplished using the simple branching technique and the feature provided for construction of parallel questionnaire sequences. Also during different experiments conducted parallel to the described investigations it turned out that due to the fact that essential features of CDSS were designed for batch operation, an effective linkage of the decision calculation feature with online dialogue processing was not achievable (76, 97, 98).

Initial tests of patient performance with the online dialogue showed that a paper and pencil medium would be superior to it at this stage of development because it is easier available to the patient who may fill in the answers where and when he likes.

Therefore a mark sense form was developed which was identical in content to the short questionnaire supplied online. This in turn was tailored to resemble closely the questionnaire used in the outpatient departments of the Hannover Medical School which was developed by DEICHER and RUGE.

The development of the offline questionnaire included 3 succesive stages

- Version I
- Version II
- Version III.

The initial version was tested on 20 patients and found to be too complicated because it contained too many different response options and branches (figure 3.2-1). The response options were then mostly converted from exclusive or inclusive multiple choices to explicit yes/no answer options. Most of the branches were eliminated. The resulting version II was tested on more than 150 patients on the acute care wards of the Department of Internal Medicine. The test showed shortcomings of a number of questions which were worked over in cooperation with internists. The resulting version III (figure 3.2-2) was then tested on close to 600 patients. Until it was introduced, a total of 262 patients had completed version II in a manner that made evaluation possible. Version III could be evaluated for 526 patients.

Version II comprised 417 questions presented on 26 pages, Version III included 444 questions on 29 pages. In the third version between 318 and 415 questions had to be answered by a patient, depending on whether a man took the shortest route or a woman the longest through the branchings (Table 3.2-1).

Table 3.2-1

Questionnaire Characteristics
- Number of Questions -

| | Number of Questions to be Answered | | | | total |
| | by men | | by women | | Number of |
	maximum	minimum	maximum	minimum	Questions
Version III	406	318	415	312	444
Version II	384	328	404	331	417

The questionnaire contains the following sections:

- identification
- review of systems and present symptoms
- accidents, operations
- prior diseases
- family diseases
- drugs
- allergy
- habits
- social
- assessment of questionnaire.

Table 3.2-2

Characteristics of Questionnaire
- Contents -

	Maximum Number of Questions	
	Version II	Version III
Identification, sex, length of stay	7	7
Systems review and present symptoms		
head, eyes, ear, nose and throat	32	29
cough, respiratory system	12	12
heart, circulatory system	32	23
digestive tract	33	36
urinary tract	13	12
male genital tract	12+3	12+3
female genital tract	32+3	28+3
musculo skelettal system	15	13
general symptoms	3	3
endocrinology	16	15
skin and appendages	15	15
neurology	16	15
Accidents and operations	24	24
Prior diseases	36	36
Family diseases	40	40
Drugs	27	27
Allergy	8	9
Habits		
drinking	1	22
smoking	1	17
Social	32	39
Assessment of Questionnaire	7	7

498

```
JA NEIN
         A. HATTEN SIE JEMALS HARTE KNOTEN
           * IN DER MUNDHOEHLE?
(    )     * IN DER ZUNGE?
(    )     * IN DEN LIPPEN?
(    )

         A. HABEN SIE SCHON EINMAL FOLGENDE VERAENDERUNGEN AM HALS, UNTER DEN
            ACHSELHOEHLEN ODER IN DER LEISTENGEGEND TASTEN KOENNEN?
           * KNOTIGE VERAENDERUNGEN?
(    )     * DRUESENSCHWELLUNGEN?
(    )

         A. HATTEN SIE INNERHALB DER VERGANGENEN 6 MONATE EIN BRENNEN AUF DER
(    )      ZUNGE?
         A. HABEN SIE BESCHWERDEN BEIM SCHLUCKEN?
(    )
         A. HABEN SIE MANCHMAL EIN KLOSSGEFUEHL IM HALS?
(    )
         A. MUESSEN SIE OFT HUSTEN?
(    )      BEI NEIN WEITER BEI A.
         B. BITTE TEILEN SIE UNS GENAUERES UEBER IHREN HUSTEN MIT.
           * HABEN SIE SEIT LAENGER ALS 4 WOCHEN HUSTEN?
(    )     * HABEN SIE AUSWURF BEIM HUSTEN?
(    )     * PFEIFT ODER BRUMMT ES BEIM HUSTEN IM BRUSTKORB?
(    )

         A. LEIDEN SIE UNTER ATEMNOT ODER KURZATMIGKEIT?
(    )      BEI NEIN WEITER BEI A.
         B. WIE OFT HABEN SIE ATEMNOT?
           * NUR ZEITWEISE?
  /        * HAEUFIG?
/  /

         B. WOBEI HABEN SIE ATEMNOT?
           * HABEN SIE NUR ATEMNOT, WENN SIE SCHNELL GEHEN (WENIGER ALS 100
/  /         METER) ODER TREPPENSTEIGEN?
           * HABEN SIE SCHON ATEMNOT, WENN SIE NORMAL GEHEN (WENIGER ALS 100
/  /         METER)?




22.06.72    28 FORMULAR NR.00001                          SEITE   04
```

Figure 3.2-1

MSH Automated History Questionnaire, Version I. The form is generated on a line printer. Extensive use of various answer options, represented by different types of brackets in answer column.

JA NEIN

B. WOBEI HABEN SIE ATEMNOT?

(:::: ::::) C. NUR WENN SIE SCHNELL GEHEN (WENIGER ALS 100 METER) ODER TREPPEN
STEIGEN?

(:::: ::::) C. ODER SCHON WENN SIE NORMAL GEHEN (WENIGER ALS 100 METER)?

(:::: ::::) C. ODER HABEN SIE SOGAR ATEMNOT, WENN SIE LANGSAM GEHEN?

(:::: ::::) C. HABEN SIE NUR ATEMNOT, WENN SIE GANZ FLACH LIEGEN?

(:::: ::::) C. WACHEN SIE NACHTS MANCHMAL DURCH ATEMNOT AUF?
BEI NEIN WEITER BEI A.

(:::: ::::) * IST DIE ATEMNOT, DIE NACHTS BEI IHNEN AUFTRITT, SO STARK, DASS SIE
ENGEGEFUEHL UND TODESANGST EMPFINDEN?

A. DIE FOLGENDEN FRAGEN BETREFFEN HERZ UND KREISLAUF

(:::: ::::) B. HABEN SIE HERZSCHMERZEN (SCHMERZEN UNTER DEM BRUSTBEIN)?
BEI NEIN WEITER BEI B.

C. WANN ODER WODURCH WERDEN IHRER MEINUNG NACH DIE HERZSCHMERZEN
(SCHMERZEN UNTER DEM BRUSTBEIN) AUSGELOEST?

(:::: ::::) * NUR IN RUHE, WENN SIE SICH NICHT BESCHAEFTIGEN?

(:::: ::::) * DURCH ESSEN ODER SONSTIGES SCHLUCKEN?

(:::: ::::) * DURCH ERREGUNG (FREUDE, KUMMER, AERGER, USW.)?

(:::: ::::) * DURCH SCHWERE KOERPERLICHE BELASTUNG Z.B. LAUFEN?

(:::: ::::) * DURCH LEICHTE KOERPERLICHE BELASTUNG (BERGAUFGEHEN,
TREPPENSTEIGEN)?

B. HAT EIN ARZT EINE DER FOLGENDEN HERZERKRANKUNGEN BEI IHNEN
FESTGESTELLT?

(:::: ::::) * EINEN ANGEBORENEN HERZFEHLER?

(:::: ::::) * EINEN HERZINFARKT?

(:::: ::::) * EINEN KLAPPENFEHLER?

(:::: ::::) * 'RHEUMATISCHES FIEBER'?

(:::: ::::) * ANDERE HERZERKRANKUNGEN ALS ANGEGEBEN?

15.10.73   20 FORMULAR NR.00005   SEITE   04

Figure 3.2-2

MSH Automated History Questionnaire, Version III. Exclusive use of
explicit yes/no answer options. Questions have also been rephrased.

GEBRAUCHSHINWEISE
▪▫▪▫▪▫▪▫▪▫▪▫▪▫▪▫

1.) Blaetter voneinander trennen. Nicht knicken, koennen sonst vom Computer nicht gelesen werden!

2.) NUR DEN BEIGEGEBENEN BLEISTIFT VERWENDEN!

3.) Die Antworten werden angestrichen, nicht angekreuzt. Auf den Markierungsboegen selbst darf nichts geschrieben werden.

4.) Ein Strich links bedeutet "Ja" als Antwort, ein Strich rechts bedeutet "Nein". Oben in jeder Seite sind die Spalten entsprechend mit "Ja" und "Nein" bezeichnet (s. Pfeil).

5.) Die Strichmarkierungen koennen nur gelesen werden, wenn sie in den Klammern und zwischen den roten Linien liegen.

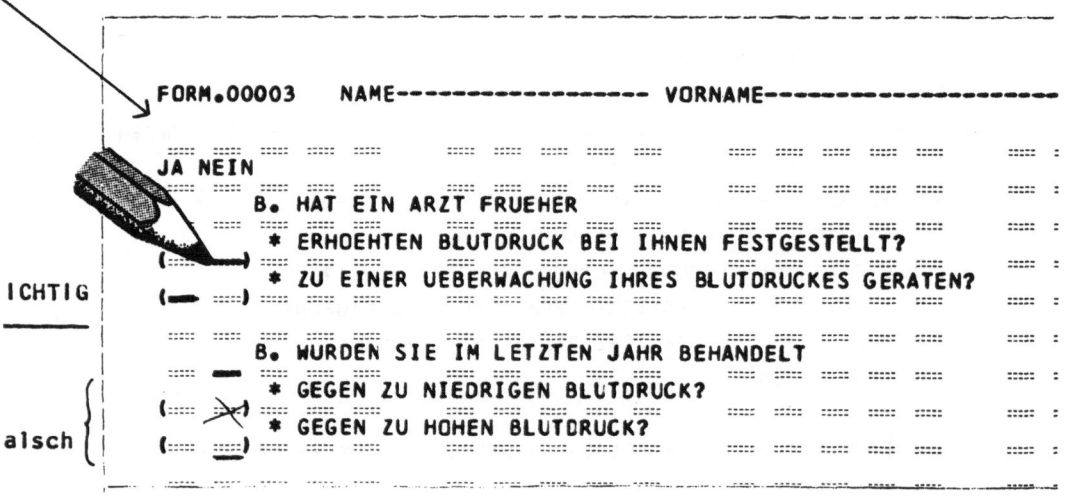

6.) Wenn Sie einen falschen Strich gemacht haben, streichen Sie ihn bitte durch und machen Sie einen Pfeil an den Rand. Machen Sie dazu einen Strich an die richtige Stelle.

Figure 3.2-3

Sample page of printed instructions for completing the questionnaire.

```
KURZANAMNESE
******************************************************************
FI█████████████F, 21B
******************************************************************
I-ZAHL 2207471810
GESCHLECHT MAENNLICH
ALTER 25


PAT. BEFINDET SICH IN STATIONAERER BEHANDLUNG, SEIT ABGER. 0 WOCHE


HAUPTBESCHWERDEN BZW. AUFNAHMEGRUND:
----------------------------------------
SCHMERZEN IN HUEFT- UND, SCHULTERGELENKEN




SYSTEMUEBERSICHT
------------------------------------------------------------------




GASTRC- INTESTINALTRAKT:
------------------------------------------



VCM ARZT FESTGESTELLT, LEBERVERGROESSERUNG

NIERE UND HARNWEGE:
------------------------------------------
HARNDRANG HAEUFIGER IN DEN VERG. 3 MON.

BEWEGUNGSAPPARAT:
------------------------------------------
GELENKSCHMERZEN, INNERH. DER VERG. 6 MON.
GELENKVERSTEIFUNG (BEWEGUNGSEINSCHRAENKUNG), MORGENSTEIFIGKEIT

PSYCHIATRISCHE ANAMNESE:
------------------------------------------
NERVOESE UNRUHE INNERHALB DER VERGANGENEN WOCHEN

MEDIKAMENTEN ANAMNESE
------------------------------------------
ANTIBIOTIKA
VITAMINE (MEHR ALS 3 X WOECHENTLICH)
SCHMERZSTILLENDE MITTEL (TAEGL. MEHR ALS 4 TABL. AN MEHR ALS 3 TAG
    PRO WOCHE)
ANTIRHEUMATICA
```

Figure 3.2-4

Sample page of history report generated on the basis of a completed
questionnaire. Chief complaint / reason for referral was indicated
in free text and entered via terminal. Other findings are a result
of compiled and translated positive answers.

The review of systems is organized according to systems in a roughly topographical order, as represented in table 3.2-2. From the same table it is evident that the difference in total number of questions between the second and third version is due mainly to an extension of the section on drinking and smoking habits.

The other sections were rather affected in a qualitative than an quantitative sense by the conversion from version II to version III.

The questionnaire forms were distributed on the wards by medical documentation assistants to all newly admitted patients that seemed to be able to complete the form. The patient was given a few minutes of introduction into the handling of the form. The assistant filled in the identification number and demonstrated thereby how to mark the positions. In particular the patient was asked, not to try to erase wrong markings, but to cross them out and indicate the mistake by an arrow on the edge of the form.

Along with the demonstration the patient received a printed form (figure 3.2-1) of four pages explaining the purpose of the procedure and providing an illustration and description of how to fill out the form. On the second page the patient was asked to note his chief complaint, his reason for consulting a physician and, if he liked, to add additional comments for the physician. This version of the form was the third, the preceeding ones being less illustrative and more lengthy).

The patients were asked to complete the form within two days. Actually it took most of them longer due to the extensive diagnostic and therapeutic activities that characterize the first days of a hospital stay. The completed forms were collected by the assistant who then scanned them thoroughly, corrected and documented errors. Because the computer generated mark sense forms were not reliable enough, they were first trial read and if errors occurred these were corrected before reading the mark sense forms again and printing the summary which was then distributed to the wards. During the processing procedure some additional data were entered via terminal. These included the patient's name, the ward number, and the chief complaint and reason for consultation if the patient had indicated them.

In an independent experiment the histories were distributed to the patients consulting a general practitioner in a rural community on three days. The patients were introduced in a simular manner as in the hospital to the use of the mark sense forms (Version III) and provided with the printed instructions and an addressed envelope for returning the questionnaire. 112 out of 117 distributed questionnaires were returned within three months (96 percent return rate). 20 to 30 patients had to be reminded on the phone to return their forms.

Only one standard patient summary was used for generating the printout supplied to the physician (figure 3.2-2). It contained the patient's identification data, and, chief complaint and reason for consultation if indicated by the patient. This was followed by a condensed listing of the patient's positive responses ordered roughly in the same sequence in which they had been obtained through the questionnaire. Brief headings separated each paragraph pertaining to a given system. Answers to the social history part and evaluation of the questionnaire were not included since they had been selected mainly as reference data for evaluation of the form.

All available information concerning the evaluation of history acquisition devices pertains to first and second stage developments. Specifically

- patient acceptance
- physician acceptance
- medical validity of the acquired data

have been examined. As far as acceptance by patients and physicians are concerned it has to be differentiated between the assessment of indicators of

- subjective attitude and
- objective performance.

4. EVALUATION OF THE MSH AUTOMATED HISTORY AND
OTHER FIRST AND SECOND STAGE DEVELOPMENTS

4.1 SUBJECTIVE PATIENT ACCEPTANCE

The subjective attitude of the patients concerning

- general attitude towards being questioned in this fashion, and
- intelligibility of questions
- the number of questions
- the effort required for completing the questionnaire
- preference of this type of questioning over a physician conducted
  interview

was asked from the patients.

The questions concerning patient attitude were not changed during conversion from version II to version III. These data were supplied by the approximatly 76 percent of patients who were able to complete the questionnaire successfully. As shown in the next section the rate of refusals to cooperate was in the range of 2.1 percent in the hospital. As outlined above the rate of loss was 5 out 117 in the experiment conducted in general practice. These figures were lower than originally expected.

General attitude

The question and answer options aimed at disclosing the general attitude could be translated as:

What is your attitude towards introducing your physician to your history in this fashion.

- I like it
- I neither like or dislike it
- I don't like it at all.

The answers chosen by the patients are summarized in table 4.1-1.

Table 4.1-1

Patient Attitude Towards Questionnaire

Attitude	Department of Medicine Version II Patients		Gen. Practice Version III Patients		Version III Patients		Total Patients	
	number	%	number	%	number	%	number	%
positive	128	48.9	270	51.3	56	50.0	454	50.4
neutral	79	30.2	151	28.7	27	24.1	257	28.6
negative	16	6.1	32	6.1	1	0.9	49	5.4
no response	39	14.9	73	13.9	28	25.0	140	15.6
total	262	100.0	526	100.0	112	100.0	900	100.0

Very uniformly approximately 50 percent of the patients chose the positive response option, 24 to 30 percent decided on the neutral response and six percent of the patients sampled in the hospital preferred the negative response. In the hospital around 14 percent of patients did not answer, in general practice the answer was not given by 25 percent.

If one assumes that all withheld answers are negative responses the total of negative response still hardly exeeds 25 percent, less than half of the positive responses.

The intelligibility of the question phrasing was elicited using the following question and response options (translated):

Did you consider the questions

- all well to understand
- largely understandable with some exceptions
- predominatly obscure and hard to understand.

The responses are summarized in table 4.1-2. The two favourable response options were obtained from close to 90 percent of the respondents only around 7 to 11 percent did not answer. Again striking uniformity in all three samples was obtained. Apparently the great effort invested in converting the questions contained in version II to those of version III had no effect upon the patients' attitude concerning the clarity of the questions. Also one can hardly expect a much better result.

The following phrasing (translated) was used in order to assess the inpact of the number of questions on the patient.

Did you think the number of questions was

- much too large
- somewhat too large
- just right
- too small.

Table 4.1-2

Patient's Assessment of Intelligibility of Questions

Intelligi-bility of questions	Department of Medicine Version II Patients		Version III Patients		Gen. Practice Version III Patients		Total Patients	
	number	%	number	%	number	%	number	%
good	122	46.6	249	47.3	58	51.8	429	47.7
predomi-nantly good	111	42.4	207	39.4	45	40.2	363	40.3
predomi-nantly poor	6	2.3	12	2.3	1	0.9	19	2.1
no res-ponse	23	8.8	58	11.0	8	7.1	89	9.9
total	262	100.0	526	100.0	112	100.0	900	100.0

Table 4.1-3

Patient Attitude Towards Number of Questions

Number of questions	Department of Medicine Version II Patients		Version III Patients		Gen. Practice Version III Patients		Total Patients	
	number	%	number	%	number	%	number	%
much too large	30	11.5	56	10.6	9	8.0	95	10.6
somewhat too large	73	27.9	128	24.3	32	28.6	233	25.9
just right	106	40.5	227	43.2	56	50.0	389	43.2
too small	11	4.2	21	4.0	1	0.9	33	3.7
no response	42	16.0	94	17.9	14	12.5	150	16.7
total	262	100.0	526	100.0	112	100.0	900	100.0

In this case, favourable responses were chosen by approximately 70 percent of the population completing the questionnaire. Fifteen percent left the question unanswered (Table 4.1-3). Around 10 percent considered the number of questions much too large, close to 4 percent considered them too small. It is possible that this question supported a 'central tendency' towards indifferent answers since it is not made explicit enough in the phrasing whether the patient should judge the number of questions by the load of work it represented or by the amount of information he was enabled to deliver through use of the questions. A patient might feel he was not able to disclose information that he regards as essential and may still feel that the number of questions was too large.

The next question was posed in order to assess the subjective effort it took the patient to complete the questionnaire. The phrasing was approximately.

Did you feel answering the questions represented

     - no effort at all?
     - some effort?
     - a great effort?

Table 4.1-4
Patient's Assessment of Effort Required for Completion of Questionnaire

effort	Department of Medicine Version II Patients		Version III Patients		Gen. Practice Version III Patients		Total Patients	
	number	%	number	%	number	%	number	%
none	112	42.7	217	41.3	38	33.9	367	40.8
some	79	30.2	158	30.0	40	35.7	277	30.8
large	15	5.7	25	4.8	2	1.8	42	4.7
no response	56	21.4	126	14.0	32	28.6	214	23.8
total	262	100.0	526	100.0	112	100.0	900	100.0

Again 70 percent of the patients completing the questionnaire gave favourable responses, 14 percent did not answer the question (Table 4.1-4). Close to 5 percent of the respondents chose the option indicating great effort. In this case, again unfavourable responses are less frequent and withheld answers more frequent in the sample obtained in general practice than in the hospital samples, the sums representing very constant fractions of the respective samples (Version II: 27.1 percent, Version III, hospital 28,8 percent, Version III, general practice: 28,5 percent). Adding these two response options for this question may be very justified, since the question represented one of the last in a rather lengthy questionnaire and patients not arriving at the end of it might very well have tended to choose the unfavourable response option. This could indicate that a questionnaire of this length (in the range of 300 to 500 questions) may be close to exceeding the tolerance of a significant number of patients.

The patient's opinion concerning the lack of essential questions is exemplified in table 4.1-5. The question could be translated:

    Do you feel that facts which are important for the doctor have not been asked?

It was answered in a simple yes/no fashion. The responses seem to confirm, just as the responses concerning the effort of answering the questionnaire, that in fact a central tendency played a role in the responses concerning the number of questions. Up to 45 percent of the patients indicated that they felt that essential information was not picked up by the questionnaire. Up to 50 percent of a sample did not answer the question. Interestingly, this was the general practice population. This could indicate that many did not feel competent to answer the question.

Table 4.1-5
Patient Responses Concerning Completeness of Spectrum of Questions

Essential questions are missing	Department of Medicine Version II Patients		Version III Patients		Gen. Practice Version III Patients		Total Patients	
	number	%	number	%	number	%	number	%
yes	57	21.8	236	44.9	16	14.3	309	34.3
no	125	47.7	104	19.8	37	33.0	266	29.6
no response	80	30.5	186	35.4	59	52.7	325	36.1
total	262	100.0	526	100.0	112	100.0	900	100.0

Table 4.1-6
Patient Responses Concerning Preference of Physician or Questionnaire for Supplying their History

Patient prefers to respond	Department of Medicine Version II Patients		Version III Patients		Gen. Practice Version III Patients		Total Patients	
	number	%	number	%	number	%	number	%
directly to physician	165	63.0	312	59.3	55	49.1	532	59.1
through questionnaire	48	18.3	108	20.5	25	22.3	181	20.1
no response	49	18.7	106	20.2	32	28.6	187	20.8
total	262	100.0	526	100.0	112	100.0	900	100.0-

Finally the patients were asked whether they actually preferred the
questionnaire to a physician conducted interview (Table 4.1-6). The
question could be translated as

How would you prefer to supply the answers to these questions?

- directly to the physician
- through the questionnaire

An overall fraction of 20 percent indicated preference of the
questionnaire, the same fraction left the question unanswered. A slight
(statistically unsignificant) increase of preference of the
questionnaire may be noted from version II over version III in the
hospital to the sample answering the questionnaire in general practice.
This was paralleled by a decline in preference of the physician, but
also by an increase in the fraction of unanswered questions.

In summary then the general attitude of the patients is very favourable
and very homogeneous. The effort in answering the questionnaire
bordered what the population was willing to tolerate and the content of
the questionnaire evoked the greatest criticism.

Particulary the homogeneity of the results is striking if one considers
the differences in the tested populations: On one side, a
predominantely urbane population, severely ill, being treated in a huge
acute care installation that is sometimes criticized for impersonality
of care it renders. On the other side a rural population, consulting
its local physician, completing the questionnaire at home, sometimes
with extensive help from family members. This uniformity of response
suggest that it reflects a 'true' attitude in that influences from the
environment, e.g. positive reactions towards the person distributing
the questionnaire or a negative reaction as consequence of a
discouraging comment from the part of the personnel on the wards -
which sometimes were reported - did not systematically influence the
overall response pattern. This is particularly confirmed by the results
obtained in general practice where a very positive attitude towards the
questionnaire existed, unlike the situation on the wards where positive
and negative attitude might have cancelled out each other.

Comparison of the responses among each other, however, leaves some
doubt whether the responses are 'true' in the sense that they reflect
what a questionnaire designer might think they should reflect.
Comparison of the answers concerning number of questions, the effort
required for answering them, and the missing of essential questions
indicated already that the wording of the questions might have
influenced considerably the results obtained.

No correlation of the attitudinal response patterns to age and sex of
the respondents was found in our material.

A number of studies included an assessment of patient's attitudes (2,
24, 44, 58, 75, 120, 122, 139). The recording required prior completion
of an interview. Quite uniformly patients indicated a positive general
attitude including sometimes such factors as curiosity, being thrilled
by the new approach, and feeling at ease and confident with the device
and its thoroughness (24, 42, 58, 120, 139).

Favourable answers were usually given by more than 80 percent of the
patients. Interestingly a substantial fraction varying between 20 and
40 percent even indicated some preference of the impersonal interview

over that conducted by the physician (3, 42, 77, 117, 122). Such
patients indicated that they felt it was easier to confess problems of
the private sphere to the computer.

Also many patients indicated that they felt that the automatic
interview was more thorough, allowed them to identify their problems
adequately and completely (24). Percentages of positive answers ranged
from 50 percent (139) to more than 80 percent (42, 58, 120).

Likewise the number of questions presented (3, 77, 117), the time it
took to answer them (24, 143) and the overall effort that the procedure
required (3, 58, 77, 117, 122) were overwhelmingly judged tolerable.
Even the latter aspect seems remarkable since average times for
completion of an automated history lie often in the order of 1/2 hour
to more than one hour (76, 121). Extremes in our experiment
approximated 3 hours for completion of the history.

In our experiment more than 90 percent of the patients judged the
questions understandable (77, 117). This finding is in good accordance
with findings of KANZLER et.al. (58). In both instances question
printed on mark sense forms were used. According to SIMMONS and MILLER
(120) who took particular care in question design, 35 percent of
patients reported difficulty with some questions using a paper and
pencil questionnaire, whereas even 53 percent of the patients using the
terminal reported some difficulties in understanding (120).

Technical difficulties with the use of various terminals were reported
for a fraction ranging from less than 5 (120, 122) to less than 20 (65)
percent of patients. Difficulties with the use of mark sense forms were
only perceived and noted by 2 percent in the study of the German Clinic
for Diagnostics (58).

4.2 OBJECTIVE PATIENT PERFORMANCE - TECHNICAL ASPECTS.

An interesting observation was made by MELLNER (69) who found that
branching errors occured in 24 percent of the histories in the sense
that screening questions were answered negatively and at least one of
the questions that should have been skipped were answered positively.

Consequently rates of errors may be greater than would be judged from
the patient's own perception of difficulties. The positive attitude of
patients, however, is a factor which justifies further work to
eliminate the existing problems.

Our assessment of patient performance is based upon

- recording reasons for not completing the questionnaire
- analysis of error statistics
- personal discussion with the patients.

During a period of the last ten months of trial application of version
III (Oct. '73 through July '74) the errors made by the patients in
completing the questionnaires and reasons for not completing the
questionnaire were registered for a total of 516 patients in our
experiment. 395 of these completed the questionnaire successfully.
Reasons for not completing the questionnaire are summarized in table
4.2-1 and illustrated in figure 4.2-1.

Table 4.2-1

Completion of Questionnaires by 516 Acutely
Ill Patients on Internal Medicine Wards.

	Patients number	%
Successfully completed	395	76.5
Disability due to disease	78	15.2
Discharged before completion	20	3.9
Lack of German / reading knowledge	12	2.3
Completion refused	11	2.1
Total	516	100.0

COMPLETION OF QUESTIONNAIRES BY AN ACUTELY ILL PATIENT POPULATION

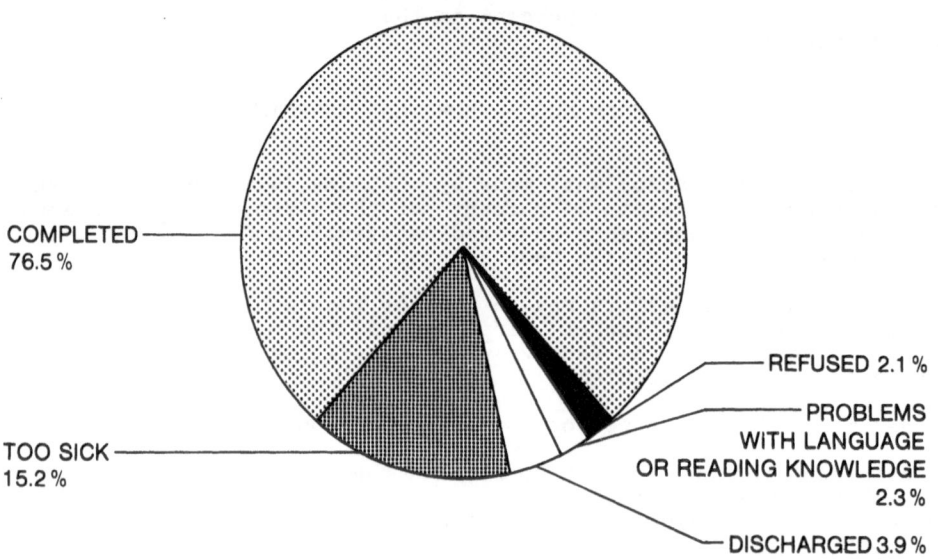

Figure 4.2-1

Completion of questionnaire by 516 patients on internal medicine wards.
Refusal rates are low, most patients are able and willing to complete
questionnaire.

Only a very small fraction (2.1 percent) of patients refused to cooperate. Another similarly small fraction was unable to complete the questionnaire for reasons of being discharged from the ward too early or lack of reading knowledge or language problems. 15.2 percent of the patients admitted to the wards where the experiment was conducted were too sick to complete the questionnaire. Thus quite exactly three quarters of the tested population were able to complete the questionnaire. The data recorded for this remaining sample included

- the utilization of assistance for the completion
- the frequency of
    = indications of errors provided by the patient (arrows)
    = bad markings
    = marking 'yes' in wrong line
    = marking 'no' in wrong line

As detailed in table 4.2-2, close to 80 percent of the patients indicated that they had completed the questionnaire without further help. Only 9 percent said they had been helped, the rest did not answer or were not questioned. For the following results refer to tables 4.2-3 to 4.2-6.

The possibility of marking erroneous responses by an arrow to initiate correction through the assistant was employed by 40 percent of patients 1 to 5 times. Only 2.5 percent used it more often. The remainder did not use the option.

Bad markings that would not have been read by the computer and required correction were noted for 30 percent of the patients, half of these making less than 10 errors of this kind. Again 30 percent of patients marked 'yes' responses in a wrong line. This error was made by only 6 percent of the patients more than 5 times since 'yes' answers constituted the minority of given answers. The same kind of mistake occured for at least one 'no' answer in close to 50 percent of patients, 20 percent making more than 10 errors of this kind. Depending on the type of error, some 50 to 70 percent of the forms were completed correctly.

The use of a more convenient form will certainly contribute to eliminate these types of errors. The fact that with the use of such an unwieldly form the error rate remained within tolerable limits, has to be considered even more promising.

This may have been due to the fact that a demonstration of the use of the questionnaires was given as well as to the manner in which this demonstration was given.

During correction of the forms it was noted that the rate of errors increased towards the end of the questionnaire. In the section on drugs only positive answers were to be registered. In spite of this, a great number of patients recorded also no responses. Great problems posed the specification of numbers, which required that the digits were marked off vertically, the highest counting digits first. 35 percent of the patients made at least one error, which seems remarkably high since the maximum of numbers to be provided was 20, the minimum only three.

These results make it strongly recommendable to use exclusive type multiple choice options, covering the range of possible numbers appropriately, instead of demanding from the patient to supply exact figures.

512

In addition our data compare well with international experience. Concerning patient attitude MAYNE et al (64) registered only 2 refusals in 905 patients at the Mayo Clinic. However, he does not state how many patients were not offered the questionnaire.

In a similar environment characterized by a predominance of upper middle class patients, using also a mark sense type questionnaire KANZLER et.al. (36) noted no refusals in approximately 28000 processed histories. YARNALL et.al. (138) witnessed no refusals in 99 patients that were offered the SEARLE MEDIDATA AUTOMATED HISTORY TAKER, a computer controlled special purpose terminal.

Table 4.2-2
Completion of Questionnaires

	Patients Number	%
alone	304	77.0
with help	35	8.9
unknown	56	14.1
total	395	100.0

Table 4.2-3
Number of Arrows Indicating Wrong Markings (Maximum 22)

Number of arrows	Patients Number	%
0	227	57.5
1 - 5	139	40.0
> 5	29	2.5

Table 4.2-4
Number of Insufficient Markings (Maximum 30)

Number of markings	Patients Number	%
0	277	70.1
1 - 5	47	11.9
6 - 10	20	5.1
11 - 15	18	4.5
> 15	33	8.4

Table 4.2-5
Positive Responses Marked in Wrong Row
(Intended Answer Would not Have Been
Reported to the Physician)
(Maximum 15)

Number of markings	Patients	
	Number	%
0	275	69.6
1 - 5	97	29.6
6 - 10	18	4.6
> 10	5	1.3

Table 4.2-6
Negative Responses Marked in Wrong Row
(Maximum 65)

Number of markings	Patients	
	Number	%
0	209	52.9
1 - 10	109	27.6
11 - 20	44	11.1
> 20	33	8.4

The overall conclusions to be drawn from these results are that the answer options should be as explicit and unmistakable as possible and as uniform as possible, if they are not to confuse a significant number of patients. It is particularly noteworthy that the printed instructions for completion of the questionnaire appeared to have been hardly ever read. This means that the questionnaire itself would have to be illustrative and selfexplanatory. The lack of attention to the instruction form had as a consequence that the space provided for specifying chief complaint, reason for physician consultation, and for written comments was utilized by only 155 out of 599 patients (25,9 percent).

4.3. OBJECTIVE PATIENT PERFORMANCE - RESPONSE PATTERN

We did not attempt to determine test retest reliability since the length of the processing procedure, shortness of average length of stay, and the effort required from the patient for completion inevitably would have resulted in a selection of patients differing from that of the other test population. A trial conducted with well respondents resulted in a return rate of 50 percent only.

Instead we set out to assess summarily the reliability of our
instrument from an analysis of the response pattern. In particular, the
patterns of

  - missing answers and
  - 'yes' answers

were analyzed.

During demonstration of the questionnaire technique, patients were told
to leave out answers entirely, if they felt unable to decide between a
'yes' and a 'no' response option. A missing answer may therefore have
the following meanings:

  - don't know
  - don't understand the question
  - don't want to answer
  - I am exhausted and cannot continue to complete the form.

Table 4.3-1 shows the distribution of system review questions that were
presented to all patients, regardless of branches taken, according to
frequency of missing answers. The mean fraction of missing answers for
this group of questions was 16.8 +/- 6.1 percent. In more than 30
percent of questions more than 20 percent of the patients felt unable
or did not want to answer.

Table 4.3-1
Distribution of System Review Questions according to Frequencies of
Missing Responses. (Versions II - 262 Patients)

Missing Answers	Questions	
%	number	%
< 4.9	1	0.8
5 - 9.9	16	13.1
10 -19.9	64	52.5
20 -29.9	38	31.1
>30.0	3	2.5
	122	100

Figure 4.3-1 (following page)

Pattern of total number of responses ('yes' or 'no' answers) to
questionnaire (version III, 189 respondents).
The figure illustrates the frequency of total number of responses to
each question of the questionnaire, which is represented by a
horizontal bar. First question upper left hand corner, last one lower
right hand corner. The length of the bars corresponds to the percentage
of total responses relative to the number of respondents. The dashed
vertical line corresponds to 90 percent. Branching questions are
indicated by a dash to the left. Abbreviations indicate various
sections of questionnaire (see below). It is conspicuous that questions
offered to all respondents achieve a total response rate in the order
of 90 percent with considerably smaller rates for some questions. On
the right hand side, response rates exact are lower, in part because

patients were allowed to be less scrutinizing, for instance for family
history (FA), in part because only 'yes' answers could be given, e. g.
for the drug section (MED), in part because exclusive or multiple
choice response options were employed, for instance in the social
history section (SA), and female genital history section.

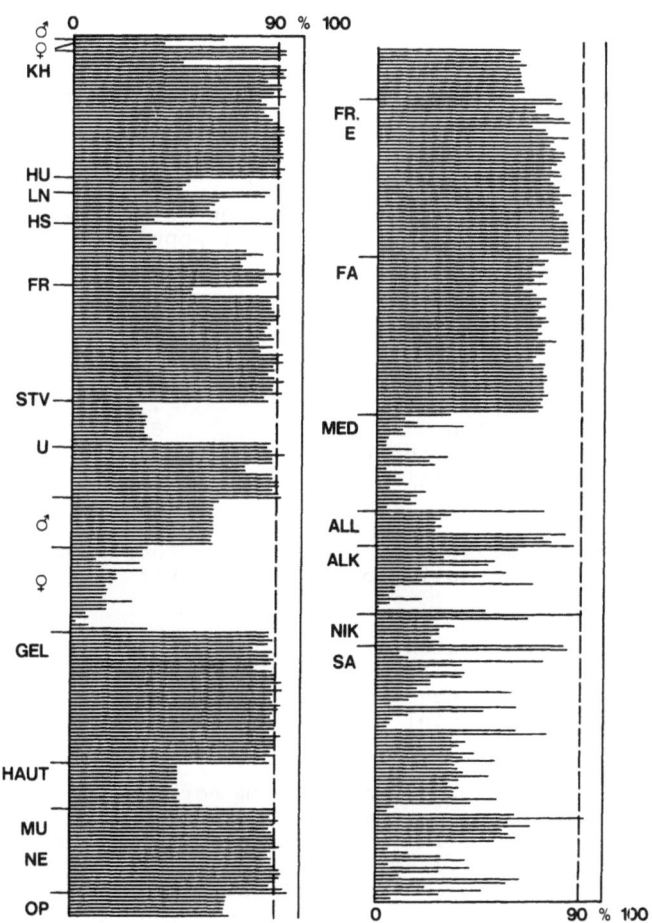

Abbreviations used:
KH: head and neck; HU: cough; LN: shortness of breath; HS: heart
complaints; FR: heart frequency and rhythm; STV: bowel habits; U:
urinary tract, followed by male and female genital history. GEL:
joints; HAUT: skin; MU: musculo-skelettal system; NE: neurologic
section; OP: operations; FRE: earlier diseases; FA: family history;
MED: drugs; ALL: allergies; ALK: alcohol; NIK: nicotine; SA: social
history.

No correlation was found between the number of missing answers and position of a question in the questionnaire sequence, although the assistants correcting the form noted that the rate of errors increased towards the end. This makes it unlikely that a significant number of patients completed only part of the questionnaire with diligence. Instead, a very uniform pattern was obtained for the fraction of patients which answered a given question either by 'yes' or by 'no'. The figure shows that for the 'yes'-'no' choice answers a response rate close to 90 percent was obtained, corresponding to a rate of missing responses somewhat above 10 percent.

Of course, total response rates are much lower in the drug section, where patients were asked explicitely to answer only if they were positive that they had taken the drug in question. Likewise, for exclusive multiple choice questions, the response rates are low, due to the questioning technique.

If one looks at questions with low frequencies of missing responses, it becomes apparent that they usually aim at popular complaints, or facts which apply to most patients to some extent and are familiar to them, such as:

Contents	Missing Answers	
	Version II	Version III
Pains in the heart or chest	8.0	9.1
Shortness of breath	4.2	./.
History of smoking	6.5	10.6
Feeling of lump in the throat	7.3	5.5
Swallowing difficulties	6.9	3.8

High frequencies of missing responses are found for questions which apply only to a small fraction of patients like:

Contents	Missing Answers	
	Version II	Version III
Having a college degree	61.8	46.6
Going still to school	31.7	56.1

Also it becomes evident that, apart from not knowing an answer or not understanding a question because it is expressed in unfamiliar terms or scientific jargon, increasing rates of missing answers seem to reflect slight degrees of inaccuracy or haziness in expression. Missing responses (or analogous answer options) may therefore serve as a rather sensitive indicator of a feeling of uncertainty, inadequacy or shame in a given population of respondents. Typical examples are:

Contents	Missing Answers	
	Version II	Version III
Have items been missed that are important for the doctor ?	30.5	35.4
'Allergy'	26.7	31.7
Treatment for alcoholism	---	55.5

Table 4.3-2
Distribution of System Review Questions According to Frequencies

of Positive Responses

(Version II - 262 Patients)

Yes Answers	Questions	
%	number	%
< 0.9	7	5.7
1 - 4.9	21	17.2
5 - 9.9	31	25.4
10 - 19.9	31	25.4
20 - 29.9	18	14.8 |
30 - 39.9	10	8.2 > 26.3
40 - 49.9	4	3.3 |
> 50.0	0	0.0
	122	100.0

The frequencies of 'yes'-answers are also important, since positive answers implied pathologic findings in our questionnaire. Table 4.3-2 summarizes the distribution of questions among categories of 'yes'-answer frequencies. It is obvious that 26.3 percent of the questions were answered positively by more than one fifth of the patients. This means that roughly a quarter of the findings in the systems review section was presented at least in every fifth patient, sometimes more close to every other patient. This may of course be due to the patient mix that completes the questionnaire or the degree of specialization of the wards, where the questionnaire was tested. Predominance of these kinds of factors is likely to be responsible for the high frequencies of 'yes'-answers obtained for the following questions:

Contents	Frequency of 'yes'-answers (percent)	
	Version II	Version III
wear glasses	45.8	58.1
weight loss exceeding 5 pounds	41.2	43.7

For a different type of question however, the phrasing may strongly influence the frequency of 'yes'-answers one obtains. There are questions aiming at symptoms which anyone may have, but which may also constitute part of a disease pattern, particularly if they exceed a certain limit of severity or frequency or if they change in character.

This type of influence was strongly suggested when we obtained even higher frequencies of 'yes'-answers from a group of medical students for some questions than we had obtained from the acutely ill patients (fig. 4.3-2). Of course, sensitization of the students towards symptoms due to their training and absence of more important troubles contribute to their sensations and symptoms. The findings demonstrate that it is sometimes more unlikely for the frequency of 'yes'-answers to be related to the actual presence or absence of a symptom in a population of respondents than to what the question means to this population.

Examples of such questions are:

Contents	Frequency of 'yes'-answers (percent)	
	Version II	Version III
headaches	31.3	27.7
dizziness	30.9	32.9
changes of appetite	33.6	35.1

Of course, it is also possible that the question misses facts or sensations that are actually present. Our experiment conducted in general practices (see below) and international experience suggests, however, that this is by far the smaller problem. We therefore did not try to persue this possibility.

Instead, we examined the questions with high frequencies of 'yes'-answers and of missing answers. If a correction seemed justified, we tried to alter the wording accordingly. This modification lead from Version II to Version III. In cooperation with physicians who had used the questionnaire, we reworded the questions, with particular attention to

- specifying circumstances of the asked facts or sensations precisely
- using concrete and realistic expressions
- eliminating complicated phrasing consisting of explanations, 'and'/'or'/'not' constructions, and the like.

45 questions of the systems review section were altered. 30 of these were presented to all patients. In 19 of these, a decrease in 'yes'-response frequency, in 24, a decrease in the frequency of misssing responses was hoped to result.

When the answers obtained for version II are actually compared to those obtained for version III, a decrease in 'yes'-answer frequency that was significant with $p < 0.05$ was obtained for 10 questions. For 7 questions the difference in 'yes' answer frequency was not significant, and in 2 instances a significant increase was observed. Likewise a significant decrease in missing response rates was obtained for 17 questions, while 7 showed no significant alteration in either direction. For none of the 30 questions a significant increase in missing response rate was observed (Table 4.3-3).

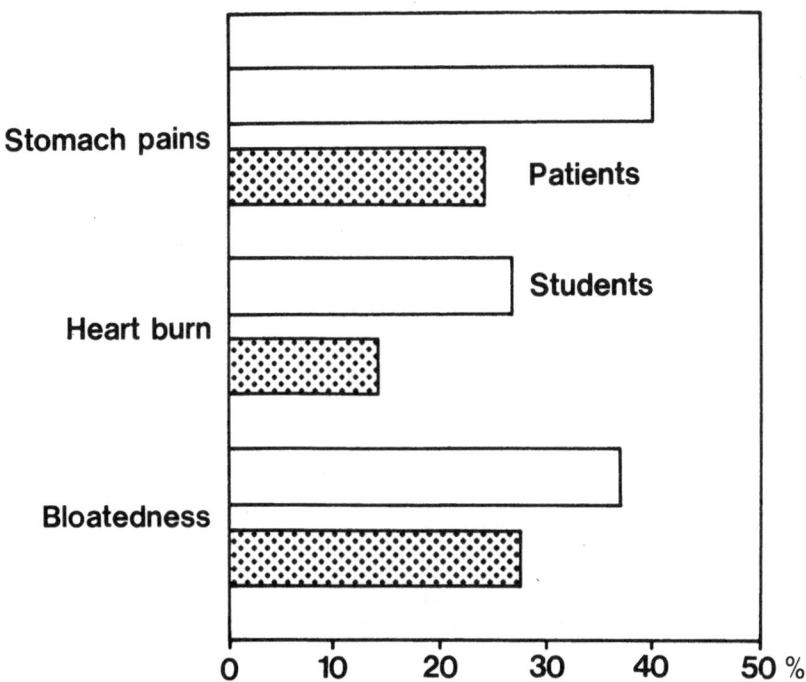

Figure 4.3-2

Frequency of 'yes'-answers obtained from acutely ill patients and students to three questions concerning pains in the stomach, heart burn and bloatedness.

Table 4.3-3
Response Pattern of Version II (262 answers per question) and Version III (526 answers per question) were compared.

	Missing Responses		'yes' Answers	
	Questions		Questions	
	number	%	number	%
Decrease significant	17	70.8	10	52.6
p < 0.05				
not significant	4	16.7	4	21.1
Increase significant	0	0	2	10.5
p < 0.05				
not significant	3	12.5	3	15.8
Total	24	100.0	19	100.0

Table 4.3-4
Examples of Alterations of Questions Resulting in <u>Decrease</u> of
'Yes'-Responses.
Questions are left untranslated for better assessment of differences.

ENo	VNo	Text	YR %	CS
1	II	Troepfelt der Urin nach dem Wasserlassen nach?	21.4	15.8*
	III	Geht nach dem Wasserlassen noch Harn ab?	11.8	
2	II	Haben Sie Schmerzen oder andere Beschwerden im Ruecken?	34.0	17.9
	III	Sind Sie in Ihrer Beweglichkeit im Ruecken durch Schmerzen behindert?	22.6	
3	II	Hatten Sie innerhalb der vergangenen Monate nachts Schweissausbruch?	48.5	43.3
	III	Leiden Sie nachts unter Schweissaus- bruechen, so dass Sie sich abtrocknen oder das Bettzeug wechseln muessen?	28.1	
4		Welche der folgenden Beschwerden, die nur einige Minuten anhielten, sind schon einmal bei Ihnen aufgetreten?		
	II	- Unvermoegen, bekannte Personen oder Dinge mit dem richtigen Namen bzw. der richtigen Bezeichnung zu benennen	11.5	33.1*
	III	- Unvermoegen, bekannte Gegenstaende (z.B. Tisch) richtig zu benennen	2.1	
5		Haben Sie oder andere Personen jemals beobachtet,		
	II	- dass Ihre Haut (besonders Lippen und Fingerspitzen) eine blaeuliche Verfaerbung aufweist (ausser bei starker Kaelte)	12.6	9.8*
	III	- dass Sie auch in Waerme blaeuliche Lippen und Finger haben (Blausucht)	6.8	

* Simultaneously significant decrease in missing reponses
was noted.

ENo = Example Number
VNo = Version Number
YR = Yes Reponses
CS = Chi Square

Table 4.3-5
    Examples of Alterations of Questions Resulting in
              Increase of 'Yes'-Responses.
Questions are left untranslated for better assessment of differences.

ENo	VNo	Text	YR %	CS
	II	Haben Sie unabhaengig von Erkaeltungen Beschwerden beim Luftholen durch die	11.1	
6		Nase?		12.1
	III	Koennen Sie (ohne Erkaeltung) nicht mehr ungehindert durch die Nase atmen?	21.1	
	II	Kommt es vor, dass Sie zwar Harndrang haben, aber erst nach einiger Zeit Wasser	13.7	
7		lassen koennen?		11.1*
	III	Koennen Sie trotz Harndrang meist erst nach einiger Zeit Wasser lassen?	24.3	

* Simultaneously significant decrease in missing responses was noted.

ENo = Example Number
VNo = Version Number
YR = Yes Responses
CS = Chi Square

Tables 4.3-4 through 4.3-6 give examples of questions the rephrasing of
which resulted in significant alterations of the response pattern.
Examples 1,2,3,4,11 and 12 demonstrate the effect of illustrative,
clear, determined language. The contrary is exemplified by example
number 7. (In this case it is not clear whether it refers to voiding
problems arising from adverse circumstances or from anatomical
abnormalities.)

The effect of the elimination of complex structuring of questions,
elimination of interspersed explanations, and the use of "and", "or",
"not" constructions is illustrated by examples 4,5,8,9. Again example 6
demonstrates that the effect is reversible.

In summary then, it appears that the frequencies of 'missing' and 'yes'
responses characterize essential properties of the questions.
Frequencies of missing responses for questions offering a choice
between a 'yes' - and a 'no' - response seem to be sensitive, but
probably rather unspecific indicators of a number of factors reducing
the value of a question as such. Frequencies of 'yes' responses - just
as frequencies of 'no' responses which we disregarded for the reasons
outlined above - may be of use if the frequency of the symptom they
imply or deny is known or if its magnitude can be reasonably well
assumed.

These indices could therefore serve as alternatives for other measures
of the overall quality of a question such as test retest reliability.
Finally, our data demonstrate that the quality of questions presented
to a given population is amenable to correction. An adaptive process of
optimization may therefore be based on these measures.

Table 4.3-6
Examples of Alterations of Questions Resulting in <u>Decrease</u> of Missing
Responses.
Questions are left untranslated for better assessment of differences.

ENo	VNo	Text	MR %	CS
8	II	Konnten Sie einmal fuer einige Zeit (Minuten oder laenger) nicht sehen?	27.9	
				42.3
	III	Konnten Sie einmal fuer einige Minuten oder laenger ueberhaupt nichts sehen?	9.9	
9	II	Haben Sie unabhaengig von Erkaeltungen Halsschmerzen?	16.4	
				41.3
	III	Haben Sie Halsschmerzen (unabhaengig von Erkael-tungen)?	3.4	
10	II	Haben oder hatten Sie jemals ein Taubheitsgefuehl in be-stimmten Koeperpartien?	21	
				20.8
	III	Leiden Sie in bestimmten Koerperpartien oder Gliedern unter Taubheitsgefuehl?	9.3	
11	II	Haben Sie kleine Geschwuere, die seit laengerer Zeit be-stehen		
		- in der Mundhoehle?	19.1	35.7
		- an den Lippen?	18.7	
	III	Haben Sie schmerzlose Ge-schwuere (offene Stellen), die seit laengerer Zeit bestehen		
		- in der Mundhoehle?	5.5	
12		- an den Lippen?	6.7	32.8

ENo = Example Number
VNo = Version Number
MR = Missing responses
CS = Chi square

4.4 SUBJECTIVE PHYSICIAN ACCEPTANCE

During the testing phase, it became evident from discussions with the physicians receiving the summaries that the computer-generated histories were not very enthusiastically received. Criticism focused mainly on two features

- the delay of its availibility
- the fact that a patient's problems were not readily apparent from the listing of complaints.

The delay between admission of a patient and the availability of the history printout was due to the fact that

- forms were distributed only after admission
- the experimental situation demanded extensive error checking and
- the supporting system also required much attention and a lengthy input procedure.

It is evident that a more reliable supporting system processing histories that are distributed in advance so that results are available on admission will obviate this problem.

The need for more intelligible presentation of data concerns a problem that is not as easily solved and which much of our attention is devoted to. It calls for appropriate selection of items to be gathered by the system and suitably emphasized, and for differentiated display of results.

An inquiry conducted after Version II and Version III which had each been tested for more than half a year, served more to document the current state of physician attitude towards the instrument than for a detailed analysis of its features.

The inquiry was conducted anonymously. The form was mailed to 96 physicians and returned by 78 (86 percent). 20 of these stated that they had been treating patients on the wards where the trial was conducted during the period of the trial. 5 of these, (3 faculty members, 2 consulting physicians) were not familiar with the form, 15 (2 faculty members, 13 house officers) could state their opinion regarding the forms. Results are summarized in table 4.4-1.

They reflect a rather reserved attitude in all considered aspects, which included

- taking notice of the supplied data
- usefulness of the data
- number of questions
- lack of essential facts
- presence of inessential facts.

It has to be borne in mind, though, that internists are diligent history takers and proud of their histories and might therefore especially resent an artifical element in this process. The observation that the physician who expressed that the data reported were entirely useles was the same who stated that he had never read a report, illustrates this attitude. He may have been the kind of physician who very justly repeats above all the history, if he is consulted by a colleague. Although internists in a teaching hospital may be least in need of a technical aid in history taking, it was necessary to test the instrument in internal medicine wards, since they are less specialized than other departments. Therefore, it was possible to cover a broad spectrum of diagnoses during the test.

Table 4.4-1
Summary of Responses of 15 Physicians to an Inquiry Concerning the Computer-Generated History

	No.	%
When you received history printouts, did you		
- disregard them?	1	7
- read them a few times?	7	47
- read them occasionally?	5	35
- read them regularly?	2	13
Did you regard the data		
- entirely useless?	1	7
- predominantly useless?	4	27
- occasionally useful?	8	53
- predominantly useful?	2	13
Do you think the number of questions is		
- too large?	8	53
- just right?	5	35
- too small?	0	0
- no response	2	13
Have essential facts been missed?		
- yes	2	13
- no	5	35
- don't know	1	8
- no response	6	40
Are superfluous questions included?		
- yes	4	27
- no	3	20
- don't know	2	13
- no response	6	40

A survey of the literature concerning physician acceptance shows that in contrast to the positive results for the Cornell Medical Index Health Questionnaire, the attitude towards second stage developments is less positive and less uniform, quite in accordance with our results.

OSHER (96) polled physicians' opinions prior to the introduction of a system and obtained from 58 to 84 percent favourable responses on various questions (table 4.4-2). At this stage, physicians may of course not be aware of what is meant by an automatically produced history; still the confident enthusiasm reflected in these figures seems promising.

Table 4.4-2
If a computer-processed history taken by a technician
was placed on the chart within 12 hours would you
(OSHER (96))

	Yes	No
Use it?	53 (84%)	10
Cut down your dictation?	32 (84%)	10
Consider it a significant improvement in patient care?	46 (73%)	23
Consider it a physician convenience and time saver?	51 (84%)	11

Results on physician's attitudes after introduction of the history
acquisition systems vary rather widely from a predominance of
favourable responses (24, 46) over more neutral attitudes (42, 58) to
rather reserved statements (117).

The positive results were obtained in medical (46) and pediatric
clinics (24) using the SEARLE MEDIDATA History Acquisition System and
reported by the designer of this commercially available system. In the
medical clinic, the survey included 35 physicians, more than 7 of whom
felt that the provided history helped to approach the patient history
and saved time. The estimates for time savings were in the order of
less than 30 minutes for about 60 percent of the physicians. 31 percent
felt that information was provided that probably would not have been
obtained otherwise and 34 percent did not think that more or different
information should be included in the profile. GROSSMAN et al. (42)
asked 21 physicians treating 103 patients, some of whom were provided
with automated histories, to appraise their own effectiveness
concerning

- their rapport with the patient
- their understanding of the patient's problems
- the usefulness of historical information
- the effectiveness of obtaining it
- the sufficiency of available time
- the effectiveness of the use of the available time.

They found no difference, whether the physicians were provided with the
history data base or not.

GIERE's group (58) obtained between 23 and 6 positive responses from 21
internists diagnosing 100 cases in an outpatient clinic on questions
concerning

(pos. responses in
percent)

- rapport with the patient   (43)
- quick recognition of important problems   (35)
- saving of time   (50)
- their opinion on whether information had been   (36)
  obtained that would have been missed otherwise.

The authors do not state whether this survey was conducted in the
beginning or after some time of routine application of the

questionnaire. MAYNE (70) supplied data that show that this might be important. In his study, initially 4 out of 27 physicians had a favourable attitude towards the experiment, whereas later only one used it regularly, 16 referred to it to some extent, 3 used it rarely and 8, never.

MAYNE's as well as our data point out deficiencies of history acquisition devices, which we felt had to be given serious consideration, and which prompted much of the research which will be outlined below.

4.5 MEDICAL UTILITY

The experiment conducted in a general practitioner's office (2, 3) allowed to compare the acquired data with the physician's knowledge and with his documentation.

The physician, upon receiving the printed summaries, checked off the items known to him. An independent investigator searched the physician's documentation independently for the items reported in the summary. If important findings were reported by the history that were not subjectively known to the physician nor apparent from his documentation, the patient was asked to present himself again, and the items were checked during an examination. A total of 60 patients were controlled.

Each of the 112 histories reported from 5 to 85 items (mean 34.4, SD 19.8). Between 0 and 39 (mean 12.6, SD 9.4) were apparent from the physician's documentation, and had also been checked off as subjectively known. 0 to 32 (mean 11.2, SD 7.7) were neither apparent from the documentation nor checked off as known and for 0 to 30 (mean 11.4, SD 7.9) there was disagreement between subjective knowledge and documentation. In only two instances, there were more items apparent from the physician's documentation than checked off as known.

Overall, some 4000 positive answers were reported in the 112 histories. 63.4 percent of these were considered known by the physician, the remainder unknown (neither apparent from history nor documentation). Approximately one third of these were rechecked. 63 percent of the reckecked items proved positive, 37 percent negative. (Figure 4.5-1, bottom marginals in table 4.5-1). If these relations are extrapolated to all of the approximately 1400 items unknown to the physician, then 23 percent the positive findings gathered by the questionnaire would have to be considered as gained data. Thirteen percent would be false positives. The overall probability of correct positive findings of the questionnaire would then be .87. (Figure 4.5-2).

A view at the data listed in a similar fashion for the various subsections of the questionnaire, in table 4.5-1, and figures 4.5-3 and 4.5-4, sheds some light on the question, whether the gain in data can be considered again in information.

The data are presented in descending order of the frequency with which unknown items were rechecked, assuming that the extent to which they were controlled represents a measure of the value attached to them. Even though this holds only very approximately true, even for this physician, it becomes immediately apparent that the notoriously neglected parts of the history

- habits
- past diseases
- family diseases

all appear at the bottom of the tables and graphs. The length of the bars in the graphs corresponds to the number of positive findings contained in each of the history subsections. It shows that some of these less interesting parts were extensively covered in the questionnaire. This is due to the fact that many of these items did not correspond to pathologic states, as in the case of the items of the systems review section. They were therefore reported more frequently.

It also is apparent from figure 4.5-3 that in the more important parts of the questionnaire (upper end of the graph) the fraction of unknown items among the positives reported is relatively small, indicating that the physician knows a lot, if he wants to. Exceptions are drinking and smoking habits which appear at the bottom of the graph and yet have only small unknown fractions. The habits are well known in a rural community, and the drugs are, in this single physician community prescribed by the physician himself.

Figure 4.5-4 contains the same figures, with the ratio of correct positive findings to false positive findings extrapolated to all unknown findings.

The estimate of the probability of correct positive findings is an equivalent of 'sensitivity'. It is evident from the figure that the so defined sensitivity of the various sections of the questionnaire is in the order of above 70 for most parts. A problematic area is male genital history which contains only few items pertaining to rather severe, rare diseases. The sensitivity of 10 sections lies in the range from .7 to .9, for 6 sections it exceeds .9. These are the musculo-skelettal part, the endocrinology section, general symptoms, female genital history and smoking and drinking habits. These are the areas where the answers of the patient are most reliable.

The figure also shows that in the upper part containing the vital organ systems, which are in the focus of the physician's attention, the fraction of new data out of all positives picked up by the history, is in the range of 20 to 25 percent. In the middle section, it rises above 30 percent for some categories (e.g. endocrinology, general symptoms, head, eye, ear, nose and throat, female genital tract). Exceptions are again smoking and drinking habits and drugs, but also the skin and allergy sections. For past diseases the fraction exceeds 50 percent. For family diseases it might be even larger but was considered so unimportant that it has not been checked. This means that, although an overall gain in data of 23 percent was observed (figure 4.5-2), this gain may be as low as 7 percent for the more interesting sections concerning vital organ systems, and exceeds 50 percent for the less interesting areas of the questionnaire.

Still the overall gain in the range of 20 percent in the family physician's setting seems promising. The sensitivity figures reported show that in a setting, where no prior information exists about the patient, a rather large amount of correct data may be acquired with the questionnaire.

Table 4.5-1
Medical Utility of Various Sections of Questionnaire in General
Practice. The Sections are Listed in Decreasing Order of Frequency with
which Unknown Items were Rechecked.

	a	b	c	d	e
Respiratory tract	180	17	30	21	70
Urinary tract	127	53	47	22	47
Neurology	130	38	33	20	61
Male Genital tract	13	5	4	0	0
Musculo-skelettal sys.	256	58	45	38	84
Cardiovascular syst.	454	143	103	64	62
Digestive tract	315	111	72	35	49
Endocrinology	132	53	31	24	77
General symptoms	27	12	7	6	86
Head, eye, ear, nose					
and throat	365	148	83	56	68
Drugs	225	43	23	10	44
Skin and appendages	44	21	9	4	44
Allergy	104	44	15	6	40
Female genital tract	264	93	28	23	82
Smoking habits	102	22	6	6	100
Drinking habits	327	37	6	6	100
Prior diseases and					
Accidents	636	359	35	26	74
Family history	312	197	1	0	0
Total	4017	1455	578	367	63

a = Number of positive findings reported
b = Number of items in a unknown to the physician
c = Number of items rechecked by physician
d = Number of items found positive upon check
e = Items positive in % of items rechecked

More data on the utility of automatically obtained history data are
provided by MELLNER (48, 71, 72) and MAYNE (70).

MELLNER allowed the physicians to cancel affirmative statements given
by patients, if they judged them irrelevant. He found that physicians
cancelled from 6.3 to 45 percent of the answers in a questionnaire
divided into two sections, containing

- questions on heredity and previous state of health
and
- questions on present state of health and present symptoms

respectively. Questions cancelled in the previous state of health
sections ranged from 5.4 to 29 percent. In the present state of health
section, they ranged from 7 to 65 percent. Although on the average an
about three times larger fraction of answers (31 percent as opposed to
10 percent) was cancelled in the present state of health section, this
tendency did not apply uniformly to all physicians.

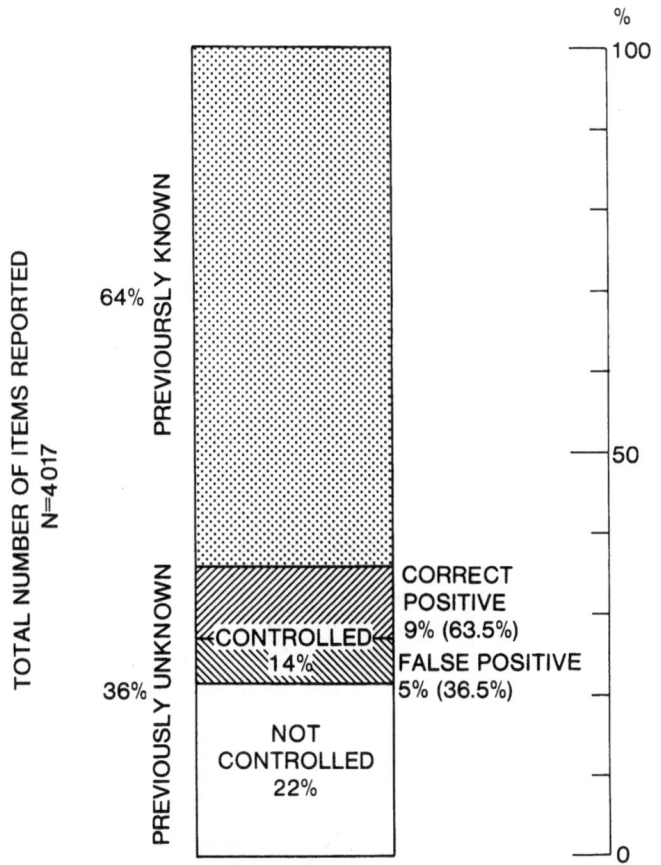

Figure 4.5-1

Questionnaire utility in general practice.

36 percent of more than 4,000 reported items were not previously known.
Out of those controlled (14 percent of total), 63.5 percent were found
correct positive (9 percent of total).

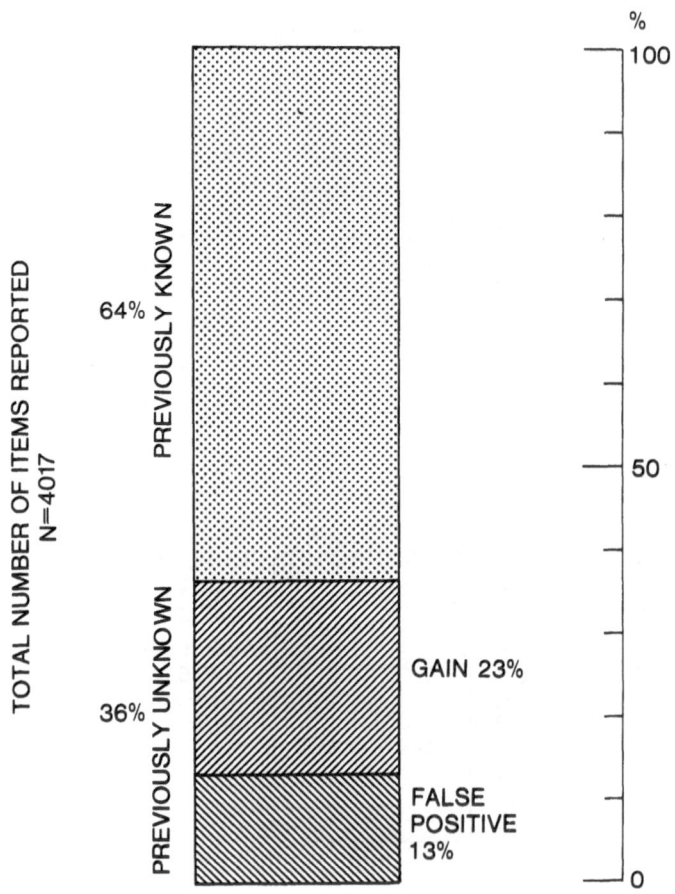

Figure 4.5-2

Questionnaire utility in general practice.

Same data as in figure 4.5-1, however, the relation of correct positives and false positives has been extended to all unknown findings. Under this assumption, the questionnaire would represent gain in data in the range of 20 percent of positive findings in a setting of continuous care.

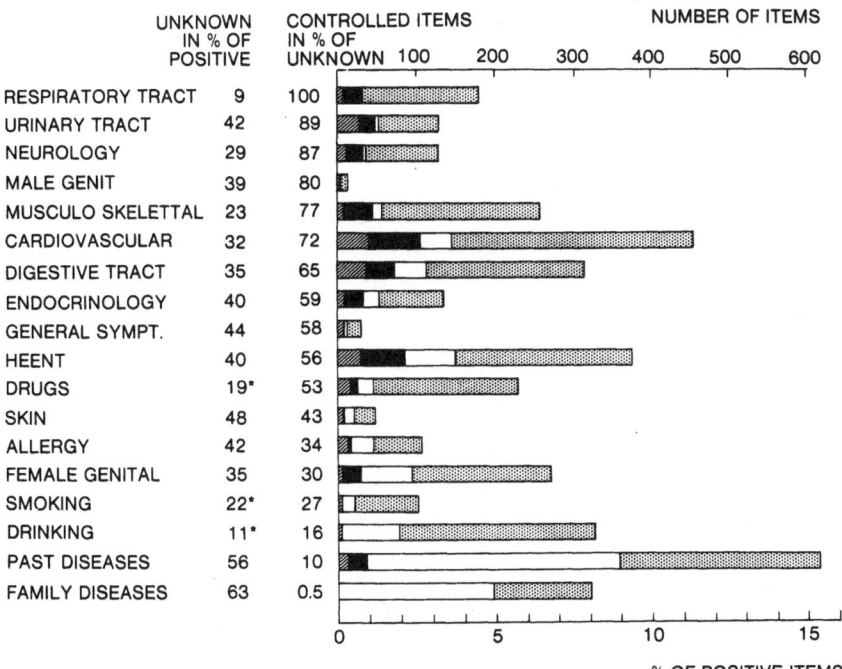

	UNKNOWN IN % OF POSITIVE	CONTROLLED ITEMS IN % OF UNKNOWN		
RESPIRATORY TRACT	9	100		
URINARY TRACT	42	89		
NEUROLOGY	29	87		
MALE GENIT	39	80		
MUSCULO SKELETTAL	23	77		
CARDIOVASCULAR	32	72		
DIGESTIVE TRACT	35	65		
ENDOCRINOLOGY	40	59		
GENERAL SYMPT.	44	58		
HEENT	40	56		
DRUGS	19*	53		
SKIN	48	43		
ALLERGY	42	34		
FEMALE GENITAL	35	30		
SMOKING	22*	27		
DRINKING	11*	16		
PAST DISEASES	56	10		
FAMILY DISEASES	63	0.5		

Figure 4.5-3

Questionnaire utility in general practice.

The reported items have been broken down according to various sections of the questionnaire and ranked in the order of decreasing frequency with which unknown items were controlled. Vital systems appear on top, past history and family diseases at bottom of the list.

The length of the bars corresponds to the number (upper scale) and percentage (lower scale) of positive items. The dotted area represents previously known items, crosshatched area, false positives, black area, true positives and blank area, uncontrolled unknown items.

These differences were attributed to differences in

- attitude towards history taking
- clinical experience
- understanding of the purpose of the history.

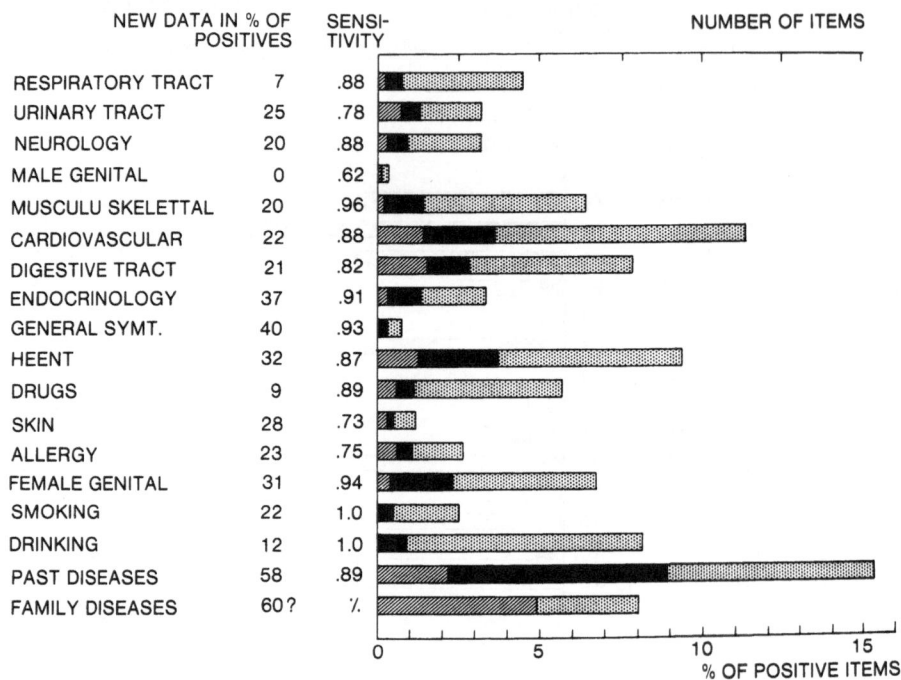

NEW DATA IN % OF POSITIVES		SENSI-TIVITY	NUMBER OF ITEMS
RESPIRATORY TRACT	7	.88	
URINARY TRACT	25	.78	
NEUROLOGY	20	.88	
MALE GENITAL	0	.62	
MUSCULU SKELETTAL	20	.96	
CARDIOVASCULAR	22	.88	
DIGESTIVE TRACT	21	.82	
ENDOCRINOLOGY	37	.91	
GENERAL SYMT.	40	.93	
HEENT	32	.87	
DRUGS	9	.89	
SKIN	28	.73	
ALLERGY	23	.75	
FEMALE GENITAL	31	.94	
SMOKING	22	1.0	
DRINKING	12	1.0	
PAST DISEASES	58	.89	
FAMILY DISEASES	60?	./.	

% OF POSITIVE ITEMS

Figure 4.5-4

Questionnaire utility in general practice

Same data as in figure 4.5-3, however, ratio of true positives and false positives has been extended to all previously unknown items. 'Sensitivity' refers to the probability of true positives in all positive items, 'new data in percent of positives' to the fraction of positive items that was not previously known. In a setting of continuous medical care like a general practice this latter figure would determine medical utility of the questionnaire. During the first encounter of a patient, the 'sensitivity' figures would apply.

Especially the latter aspect was demonstrated by the fact that the more experienced physicians tended to cancel more data than their junior colleagues. It was felt that the junior staff members might have been more aware of the history as a document serving research purposes, whereas the senior staff used it primarily for patient care purposes.

MAYNE (70) found that in 148 out of 300 completed questionnaires there occured at least 1 "wrong" answer, the maximum being 23. Only 21 summaries omitted 1 or more items that in the physician's opinion should have been presented.

MAYNE then set out to study the utility of the acquired data as a basis for patient care decisions. Eleven physicians were asked for 49 cases to arrive at a number of decisions, first on the basis of the summary data from the automated history, then again after completing the examination of the patient. The decisions included:

	(percent agreement)
(1) to judge the urgency of the patient's need of care	(86)
(2) to decide whether the indicated problems were primarily "organic" or "functional"	(59)
(3) to decide whether management of the indicated problems could be handled by one internist or whether several specialists were needed	(65)
(4) to estimate the amount of time that would be needed for the first consultation	(55)
(5) to assign the patient to appropriate sub-specialties	(61)
(6) to request the appropriate laboratory tests	

The agreement was best for the urgency of the medical care. In 5 of 7 misclassified cases the urgency of the need for care was underestimated, in 2 it was overestimated. The agreement was least for the laboratory procedures. All tests for which the results are given in MAYNE's paper, were more frequently cancelled when they had been ordered on the basis of the history data, or requested when the physician had failed to do so than there was an agreement in both instances. The decisions concerning the organic or functional nature of the patient's problems, its complexity, the time needed by a physician for his initial medical consultation and assignment of the patient to an appropriate medical specialty were correct only in 59, 65, 55 and 61 percent of the 49 cases respectively.

The available evidence can be summarized to the effect that even though the data given by the patient may be to a considerable degree 'correct' in that they reflected what the patient intended to report, they may still frequently be considered irrelevant by the physician. It is the quality rather than the quantity of the data that determines the value of the acquisition system. The quality is reflected to some extent by attitudinal surveys. These, however, tend to be rather favourable particularly in the beginning of experimentation with such systems. Where objective data are available for the utility of data acquired by second stage developments, they reveal that the quality of the data is not yet satisfactory.

It is necessary therefore

1) to attribute much greater care to tailoring the medical contents of a questionnaire to the physician's needs
2) to improve the presentation of the acquired data
3) to test the operational value of the offered instruments thoroughly.

5.1 GENERAL EMPHASIS

The experiments described so far pointed out that a fair degree of first level standardization had been attained by our medical history questionnaire and the other second stage devices. The responses were quite uniform with respect to completeness and response pattern. Also the possibility of effecting defined changes in the response pattern through alteration of questions had been demonstrated. However, an inadequate fit of the questionnaire to the physician's need of information and the patient's ability to provide this information had been demonstrated.

Counter measures require to determine both, the physician's need of information and the patient's ability to provide it, and to adjust the instrument in a manner that it serves to transmit this needed information. At least, one should be able to characterize the instrument's performance with respect to transmittal of this information, i.e. attain the second level of standardization. Optimally it should be adjusted to meet specific requirements, which then would constitute what was characterized as third level standardization. The following discussion will summarize principal conceptual prerequisites and experiments pertinent to an achievement of these goals. The conceptual prerequisites concern basic medical and methodological concepts, the prevailing understanding of which seems to have obstructed progress in this field so far.

5.2 OUTLINE FOR DEVELOPMENT OF HISTORY SYSTEMS.

So far, there have been very few descriptions of strategies for medical history questionnaire design. FASSL (31) proposed a rigorously complete attempt at documenting each of a number of leading symptoms with respect to all essential attributes, such as causes, occurrence in time and location, precipitating factors, quantity, quality and the like. He concludes in his analysis, which was not only concerned with the aspects of documentation of the medical history, but also with supporting the art of history-taking through a reproducible, communicable and therefore teachable scientific approach, that this degree of completeness was not achievable in an impersonal interview by automated history acquisition techniques. If then we have to apply automated techniques in a much more restricted sense, the need for an efficient strategy for selecting appropriate contents for a medical history becomes even more imperative.

GRUND-KREHL (45) selected questions from existing questionnaires according to their relevance for a spectrum of frequent diseases, as judged by physicians. The preceeding discussion should have made it clear that this approach suffers the disadvantage of a closed system, limited by the set of questions taken into consideration. Also the judgement of physicians concerning the relevance of questions may be misleading. A physician's judgement of the practical value of a question is based on concepts of the relevance of the symptoms the question is supposed to aim at. Our own experience - as far as outlined up to this point and in particular as summarized in chapter 4 - shows that frequently the assumption is not justified that a symptom is picked up by a question in the desired manner. We suggested and are currently applying a different approach (78) which is based upon a simplified signal transmission model of a history acquisition system (figure 5.2-1).

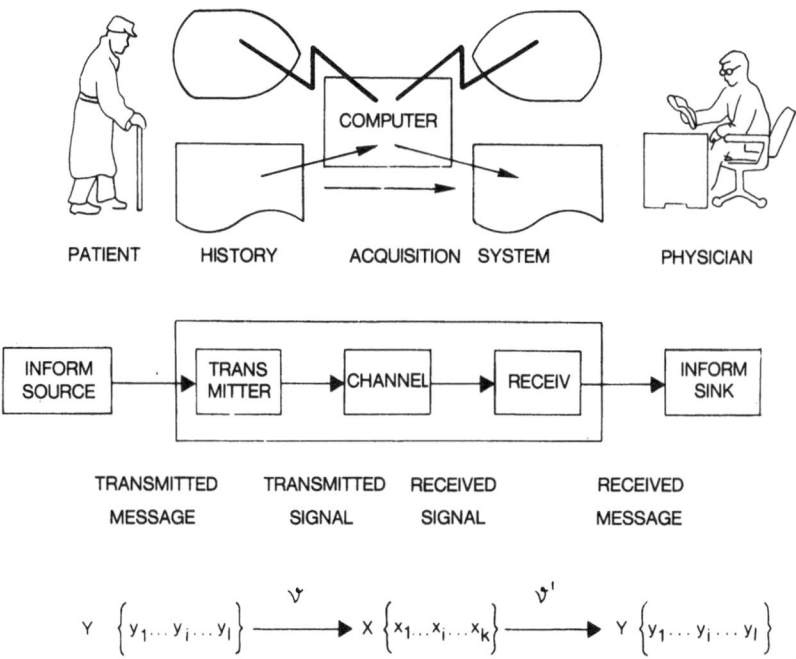

Figure 5.2-1

Model of a history acquisition system based on a signal transmission
concept. The information contained in the patient has to be transformed
into messages processed by the system through application of an
encoding procedure. An inverse procedure is needed for presentation of
the acquired message to the physician.

A history acquisition system is supposed to transmit information from
the patient to the physician, so that the physician is in the position
to carry out decisions concerning this patient.

The model depicts the patient as the information source, and the
physician as information sink. The purpose of this model is to show
that the information contained in the patient and needed by the
physician undergoes a transformation in the process of conversion to
data which is entered into the system. The encoding procedure is a
complex function the result of which is influenced by characteristics
of the environment, such as

    - setting
    - questionnaire
    - each question
    - acquisition device

and characteristics of the patient's personality, such as

- intelligence
- technical ability
- perception of disease
- impairment by disease with respect to physical, intellectual and emotional characteristics
- type of disease combination
- medical knowledge.

These parameters influence the transcription of the information 'contained in' the patient into the messages picked up by the history acquisition device. To the extent that this encoding process is controlled, an inverse process may be applied to decode the messages for presentation to the physician.

The model should further illustrate some consequences for the design of questionnaires. In order to arrive economically at a suitably tailored instrument, it is preferrable to base its contents on a catalogue of decisions, a physician has to face, not on a catalogue of symptoms a patient may have. The latter is infinite, while the former will yield a valid frame of reference, which reflects the information needed by the physician, if adequately defined.

Consequently, the following steps for design and implementation of a history acquisition system are proposed.

1) Definition of circumstantial requirements
   - physician population to be serviced
   - patient population providing the input
   - environment
   - available hardware and software.
2) Definition of a range of relevance in the form of a list of appropriately defined decisions (e.g. problems, risks, diagnoses) reflecting the information needed by the physician.
3) Selection of items in order to arrive at the decisions specified under 2 (questions, tests, tasks).
4) Union of items and adaption to chosen supporting device.
5) Preroutine test. Possibly modification of item collection and repetition of steps 3 to 5.
6) Routine application, preferably with adaption to optimal performance.

In defining the circumstantial requirements on the side of the physician, the considerations have to include such factors as

- medical objectives
- medical methods
- time constraints for availibility of results
- location where results are needed.

Among medical objectives the choice between prevention, screening and early recognition, cure, scientific or teaching requirements, detection of presence of problems or verification of absence of problems are noteworthy. Location and time constraints for availability of results will influence the choice among available acquisition, processing and presentation devices. Medical methods used will finally influence the choice of content of the history. An environment characterized by intensive diagnostic techniques will have different requirements than a

primarily therapeutic setting, such as surgical disciplines, or
radiotherapy. A setting characterized by special problem management
such as most private offices will need a screening history with broad
range of relevance, whereas the afore mentioned examples would require
special problem histories.

From the preceding discussion it should be apparent, to what extent
characteristics of the patient population will have to be considered.
Essential personality features have been mentioned above; of course
other characteristics are also important. Examples are language, the
fact of whether the patients are expected to decide themselves that
they need medical advice, or whether the examination is compulsory, as
in some environments of industrial medicine.

Also important are characteristics of the setting where the instrument
is to be used, - the presence of aides, helping or onlooking family
members or fellow patients; the environment where the questionnaire is
to be completed - home, waiting room or other patient care facility.

These will determine whether all questions are presented at once or
selections made, whether online techniques may be used or one has to
resort to portable devices. The latter choice being of course also
influenced by the alternatives presented by available hardware and
software.

This consideration of circumstantial requirements should be followed by
a definition of the information needed by the physician in the form of
a 'range of relevance' for the instrument. This could be done by
listing the decisions one wants to arrive at with the aid of the
questionnaire. Decisions concerning diagnostic classification are but
one example. The discussion presented in the preceding paragraph should
have shown that even in this case the choice of the items for inclusion
in the list should be carefully considered. Existing diagnostic indices
are not equivalent and very likely the situation, where the
questionnaire is to be applied calls for a specific list with
specifically defined items. However, decisions concerning the
application of costly diagnostic or therapeutic procedures, or
concerning the credibility of the obtained answers (e.g. indicators of
'neuroticism') are other examples of items that could be included in
such a list.

The range of relevance provides a frame of reference, within which the
instrument may be assessed. Once it is defined, it can be considered to
represent the information which the testing instrument is to pick up.
The process of definition is comparable to a process of discretization
by which the continuous, variable and infinite information source that
the patient represents is transformed so that it can be considered as
finite, discrete and in some cases even constant.

If thereafter test items or questions are selected, only those have to
be included, which are considered likely to contribute to the spectrum
of decisions which constitute the range of relevance. In contrast to
the symptom oriented approach, which was characteristic for most
previous endeavours in this field, the problem oriented approach makes
it easier to decide upon the inclusion of a particular item, and should
help to arrive at a close match between the problems a physician has to
solve and the information that is gathered by the history
questionnaire.

In terms of information science concepts, the list of items resulting
from this process can be considered as an alphabet of symbols, each of
which has considerable semantic content. The patient's answer to this

list represents a message containing the information that is to be transmitted to the physician.

The question whether patients are actually able to provide this remains, however, open and must be tested. Initially one can only hope to arrive at a close to optimal set of questions by observing the criteria which characterize good questions. These have been discussed before. Thereafter it is the purpose of preroutine testing and adaption during routine application to assess the quality of questions in order to attain second, and, if possible, third level standardization.

Determination of the validity of the questionnaire for the range of relevance in a representative sample population results in attaining the second level of standardization. It allows to specify the probability of a correctly positive and a correctly negative decision for each item in the range of relevance. The value of the questionnaire becomes known. If the results are unsatisfactory for certain elements within the frame of reference, one may attempt to alter the questionnaire by changing, eliminating or adding questions. If then, finally, certain minimal requirements are met by the questionnaire for all elements of the frame of reference, the third level of standardization has been achieved.

A prerequisite for determination of validity is that the questionnaire has been answered by a representative sample of respondents, and that the decisions defined as range of relevance have been arrived at by methods considered to yield 'true' results. These have to be adequately recorded for each respondent. In this manner, a feedback loop can be established which is a prerequisite for adaption and correction. The data obtained by the instrument are a result of the complex processes of encoding outlined above. The relation of this data to decision outcomes obtained by independent means can be considered to account for the encoding processes summarily in as much as preroutine test conditions are comparable to the conditions of routine application.

Therefore the results of statistical evaluation may be used to derive the information defined as range of relevance and to present the acquired data accordingly. Certainly the definition of the range of relevance will not match exactly and exhaustively the decisions to be arrived at in a given case. It should be defined in a way which serves to prompt the attention of the physician. Hence we do not mean to suggest that the derived decisions constitute the only data to be presented. In combination with a listing of the acquired data which initiated the decisions, the transparency of the decisions as well as the intelligibility of the acquired data should be improved however.

Finally the statistics obtained during validity testing may be used to optimize question selection and question sequencing during interactive data acquisition. Contrary to the deterministic approaches characterizing second stage developments, the question selection may now be based upon measures of the actual performance of a given population using a defined question catalogue. Errors due to differences in the intentions of a questionnaire designer and the understanding of a respondent population may thereby be identified and corrected.

The suggested approach has two essential prerequisites:

1 a reconsideration of the concepts of medical information,
2 the employment of formal methods of validation.

Both aspects will be outlined in the following. The applicability of the principles is not restricted to history acquisition systems, but is generally relevant to computer assistance in documentation and information derivation in medicine.

5.3 SYSTEM VALIDATION

5.3.1 REVIEW OF SOME RELEVANT APPROACHES

While the evaluation experiments reviewed before (section 4.5) provide insight into the practical usefulness of data acquired by impersonal questionnaires, their results do usually apply to rather specialized experimental situations only. In order to develop standardized anamnestic instruments which yield predictable and comparable results at minimal expense, more formal approaches with broader applicability are required.

Only few studies are available wherein the assessment of reliability of general medical questionnaires is reported. COLLEN (22) provided an extensive assessment of test retest reliability of a questionnaire comprising some 200 questions. The results were used to identify inappropriate questions for correction. As outlined in section 5.4, the methods for determination of reliability suffer a number of drawbacks. Among others they require a considerable effort on the side of the respondent and/or the investigator. Depending on the device to be assessed this may preclude effective application of these methods. In our own experiments which are described in detail in chapter 4, we had to refrain from assessing test retest reliability after we obtained return rates in the range of 50 percent only during a pilot experiment. As described above, however, we were able to control gross deficiences of questions in a similar manner as was achieved by COLLEN's group on the basis of reliability estimates by analyzing response patterns - in particular of 'yes' answers and missing answers. At the same time we avoided the drawbacks of methods for determining measures of reliability (see below, section 5.4).

A typical example of standardization is the way which was persued in the development of the so-called "HHM Beschwerdeliste" (153) (HHM list of complaints. HHM standing for "Hamburg, Heidelberg, Munich", the places where the list was predominantly developed and tested). This list contained the most frequent complaints presented in general practice. In most tested versions the questionnaire contained between 60 and 70 complaints, characterized by very short texts, not even complete phrases. In the final versions, these could be answered either in a yes/no fashion or by checking off one of four degrees of applicability (strongly - moderately - slightly - not at all).

Standardization and testing of this instrument was carried out by a group around v. ZERSSEN (153) according to the principles outlined for classical psychological test construction (69). The tests were carried out mainly in the environment of internal medicine (66) and psychiatry (1, 121).

Using particularly factor analytic methods the various authors found support for simply using an overall score arrived at by counting the number of positive answers obtained by administration of the list of complaints. This overall score discriminated only vaguely between twelve diagnostic categories used in internal medicine. This small number of diagnostic classes was investigated more closely because only for them a sufficiently large number of patients (from 12 to 65 out of a total of 760) could be found in each category (66). On the other hand, this overall score correlated closely with other tests of "neuroticism" which are usually quite similar in structure to such a list of complaints. (66, 153). The overall score also discriminated well between "healthy" individuals and psychiatric patients (153). A number of factors considered to be consistent with major psychopathologic traits could be extracted. Use of the list and the total number of positive answers as overall score is recommended for assessing summarily the overall course of disease. In order to facilitate repeated administrations, the list was divided into two parts which produced identical results with respect to the overall score if used in parallel (153). Even though the practical usefulness especially of the recommendation to use the overall score for assessing a degree of illness seems questionable, the investigation clearly points out that in fact not only organic disease but to a large extent psychologic attitude towards illness influences response patterns.

This kind of overall information may not be particularly useful in medical practice, if direct contact between patient and physician is possible, because it may be arrived at with less expense. Very likely it has to be accounted for however, before complaints can be interpreted as evidence of organic disease. So far, no existing medical history device seems to account for the influence of subjective aspects of illness upon the answers obtained. An incorporation of the principle into a history acquisition instrument might therefore be useful.

A different approach in relating testoutcomes (e. g. answers to a history questionnaire) to external criteria (e. g. medical diagnoses) has been described by PIPBERGER et al (107). The authors tried to identify test outcomes that would serve as optimal descriptors and/or discriminators of disease. Close to 500 tests - 429 questions answered in the yes/no fashion and 69 numerical descriptors such as laboratory tests - were analyzed with respect to their value in the differential diagnosis of chest pain. In a first step, those tests with sufficiently high rates of incidence were identified. Then their discriminative power was determined on the basis of Chi square tests. Finally, discriminant function analysis was used for identifying those charateristics that resulted in satisfactory discrimination of the diseases under consideration. This could be achieved on the basis of less than 10 out of the initial 498 symptoms. Though indicating a valid methodologic approach as to the statistical techniques, the study suffers the drawback that it was conducted using a sample of respondents which consisted exclusively of patients with a common leading symptom - chest pain. This restricts general applicability of its results to this particular differential diagnostic situation. The resultant set of "best symptoms" may not apply for a differentiation of the discerned diagnostic categories in an unselected population. An interesting observation on the side of these results was, that anamnestic information was of greater value than outcomes of laboratory tests and physical examinations. The approach is one of a number of alternative approaches of automatic classification and numerical taxonomy, a complete review of which is beyond the scope of this presentation.

The commonest type of approach is based upon the concepts of reliability and validity. Reliability describes the consistency of obtaining a given test outcome. Validity describes the relation of this test outcome to what is attempted to be measured. This is usually represented by an external criterion. These approaches have become commonly applied in epidemiology, social medicine and psychiatric disciplines.

The commonest application concerns again highly specialized questionnaires, e.g. for diagnosing arteriosclerotic heart disease (6, 46, 112, 113) peptic ulcer and rheumatoid arthritis or "low back trouble" (145). Although such widely applied screening instruments as the chest pain questionnaire developed by ROSE (112, 113) resulted from this type of work, the usefullness of its results for the construction of more encompassing questionnaires is limited because there is no way of guaranteeing that the reliability and validity measures of items of such specialized questionnaires do still apply if a new questionnaire is compiled by uniting several such specialized questionnaires.

The main reason is that the validity of a test item is strongly influenced not only by the definition of these qualities, but also by the spectrum of qualities that are included in the frame of relevance that a test is designed for.

An encompassing outline of the assessment of validity on the basis of statistics derived from two by two contingency tables (see below, section 5.4.3) was given by YOUNG (149). Practical application by the same author, however, was restricted to a comparison of answers obtained by aid of a questionnaire to those resulting from personal interview (151). As detailed below (section 5.4.2), this can only be considered a test of validity and not of reliability if the questions aim at detecting no other condition than what is reported in the answer. This is usually not the case for such parts as a systems review section in a general questionnaire. These aim at the detection of underlying causes of complaints. For their assessment a single question is usually not a sufficient test, and the measures derived from two by two tables do not suffice. Based on a method proposed by NEYMANN (99), COLLEN's group outlined an extension of this approach, which is applicable not only to an individual question, but also to sets of questions (20,21,118). In the demonstration example given by COLLEN (20, 21), the sets of questions were defined in accordance with physician's judgement, i.e. according to medical disease concepts, and not on the basis of objective measures of their value as in the approach described by PIPBERGER (107). Measures of validity were obtained by analyzing response patterns obtained in diseased persons and in nondiseased persons. These were related to documented diagnostic classifications. In a later publication, formal strategies for arriving at optimal test sequences on the basis of test outcomes in a large population sample were described but apparently not extensively applied (39). This approach was based on an algorithm proposed by STERLING, POLLACK et.al. (134, 135). Our own approach which will be outlined below relies essentially on these cited papers.

5.3.2 BASIC CONCEPTS

Although the determination of validity is an essential step to arrive at standardized instruments, this technique has been applied only to a limited extent so far, and its applicability was questioned categorically (c.f. e. g. 15). The reasons for this seem to be rooted in difficulties with the basic methodological and medical concepts which determine the application of these techniques. Following the outline of concepts of medical information given above, the concepts of reliability and validity will be discussed in the following, since their relation to the concepts of information is relevant for the methodological alternatives for solution.

Reliability attempts to assess the consistency with which a given test yields a certain outcome.

Validity, on the contrary, attempts to assess the consistency with which a test reflects what it is supposed to measure.

If we are concerned with questionnaires, the test may be a single question or a set of several questions. The answers obtained for these questions constitute the test outcomes. Measures of reliability should reflect the consistency of these outcomes. Measures of validity, on the other hand, should reflect the relation of these test outcomes to the quality the questionnaire is designed to measure. Usually in medical questionnaires, test outcome and quality that is to be determined are not identical.

Reliability - the consistency of a test outcome - may be assessed in different ways. The most important ones are: comparison of the outcomes of the test produced by repeated test application - test retest method - and comparison of the outcome of one test with the outcome of another test - parallel test method.

In questionnaire design, test retest reliability is frequently determined by repeated application of the questionnaire. If, alternatively, the answers obtained by an impersonal questionnaire are compared to those obtained by a personal interview or to documented results of routine anamnesis, these methods have to be regarded as determination of parallel test reliability. Only in those instances where the test is designed to gather no other information than that reported in the answer, this method could be considered an assessment of validity. This situation is typical for the section referring to previous diseases and operations. The fact that a given trauma occurred is the essential quality to be detected. In the systems review section, on the other hand, the questions for various symptoms usually aim at the detection of some underlying derangement. Not the pain as such, but its consequences for the doctor's decisions are important.

In assessing reliability one usually has to cope with two different sources of error:

1 differences between compared tests,
2 change of the state of nature.

Only if the test with unknown reliability is compared to a standardized test, the result can be expected to reflect the reliability of the test. Personal interviews and results of routine documentation can hardly be regarded as standardized test. Differences between the applied methods may then account for the fact that determined measures of reliability do not reflect the high reliability of the test under assay.

The state of nature may change due to various reasons, the most important ones being
      - natural course of events
      - influence of test instrument.
The symptoms referred to in a questionnaire may change. The results of determination of reliability will then again be unduly poor.

On the other hand, the test application may raise memories or cause the respondent to consult sources of information, because he was in doubt about the answer. Again poor measures of reliability will result, which in this instance are justified. Quite likely, however, the opposite effect plays an important role and contributes to unduly good measures of reliability. The respondent may repeat a choice between answers, because he remembers the answer given the first time. Therefore the choice of method for determination of reliability and interpretation of results have to be considered carefully.

Reliability constitutes a limiting value for validity. Even though being highly reliable, a test may still have poor validity. Validity then is the essential characteristic of a test.

For the determination of validity, it is important to note that validity is not only a function of possible test outcomes and the spectrum of qualities one attempts to measure, but also of characteristics of the population of respondents and the environment in which the test is applied. Measures of validity are only applicable to defined populations of respondents in an environment with defined characteristics.

It is therefore not justified to compile a questionnaire from questions with determined validity, and to expect that these still apply. A diagnostic questionnaire designed for the differential diagnosis of a small group of diseases may lose its validity, if other diseases are included in the consideration. It has to be postulated therefore to determine the validity of a questionnaire test against the entire spectrum of qualities that it is to detect. If this is not possible, the spectrum that was considered in the assessment should be explicitely stated. Characteristics of population and environment should be kept as constant as possible.

5.3.3 SOME METHODS FOR STATISTICAL ASSESSMENT

The measures most commonly used for determination of reliability as well as validity can be derived from two by two contingency tables (fig. 5.3.3-1). In this manner they are applicable to binary data only.

Figure 5.3.3-1

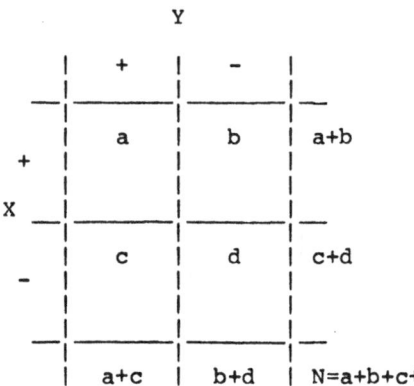

Two by two table for determination of measures of reliability and validity.

The upper case letters X and Y stand for characteristics which may have two states designated by + and -. The lower case letters stand for frequencies with which each one of the four possible states (X+Y+, X+Y-, X-Y+, X-Y-) are observed in a given sample.

If applied to determine test retest reliability, X may be used to represent the answer obtained at the first test (first presentation), Y that obtained at retest (second presentation).

Figure 5.3.3-2

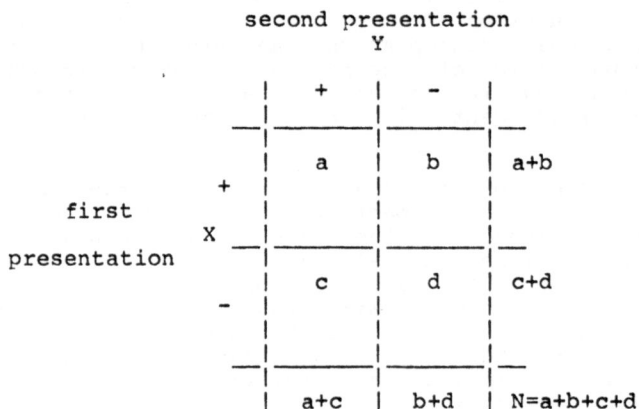

Two by two table for determination of measures of reliability by test retest method.

Figure 5.3.3-3

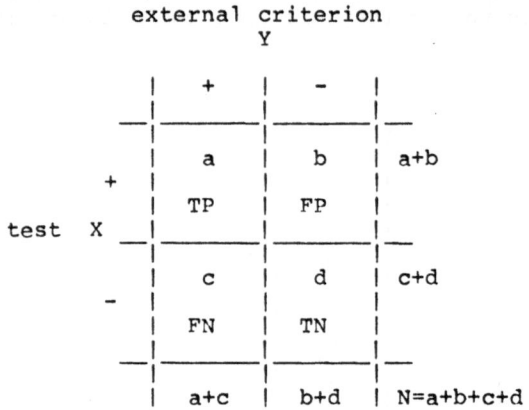

Two by two table for determination of measures of validity

TP true positives
FP false positives
FN false negatives
TN true negatives

The reliability may then be represented separately for the 'yes' and the 'no' responses obtained at the first presentation, by ratios of unchanged answers to total answers of each type:

$$R+=a/(a+b)$$

$$R-=d/(c+d)$$

For determining validity, test results are compared to some external criterion which is assumed to represent the true outcome better than the test. Applying the two by two table we would use X to denote the test and Y to denote the external criterion.

In this case, 'a' denotes the number of cases for which test and external criterion are positive, i.e. the number of true positives (TP). 'b' stands for the number of cases where the test was positive but the criterion negative, i.e. the number of false positives (FP). In similar fashion, 'c' denotes the number of false negatives (FN) and 'd' the number of true negatives (TN). The marginals stand for the number of total positive tests (a+b), total negative tests (c+d), total positives (a+c) or total negatives (b+d), as indicated by the external criterion. The grand total N is given by a+b+c+d. The most commonly used indicators of validity are

sensitivity   a/(a+c)
and
specificity   d/(b+d).

Sensitivity thus stands for the fraction of correctly positive test results obtained in all cases for which the external criterion was positive. It corresponds to the probability of correctly diagnosing a positive case through application of the test. Its complement to 1 corresponds to the probability of not diagnosing the truly positive cases, i.e. the false negatives. This fraction corresponds to the 'error of first kind' or 'Type 1 error'(91, 92).

Specificity stands for the fraction of correctly negative test results in all cases which are negative according to the external criterion. It corresponds to the probability of correctly rejecting a case as negative. Its complement to 1 corresponds to the probability of not diagnosing truly negative cases, i.e. the false positives, an error which was called the 'error of second kind' or 'Type 2 error' by NEYMAN (91, 92).

A total of eight ratios may be calculated from the cell frequencies and corresponding marginals. YOUNG (140) has recently provided an encompassing discussion of their meaning. He also provided measures of variance for these ratios, which had previously been indicated by YOUDEN (138).

The measures termed positive and negative accuracy by YOUNG (140) (accuracy(+)=a/(a+b), accuracy(-)=d/(c+d)) have been called positive or negative predictive values (129, 138). The positive predictive value corresponds to the probability that the criterion is positive, if the applied test is positive, the probability with which a positive test corresponds to a positive diagnosis.

designation	index	variance
sensitivity	a/(a+c)	ac/(a+c)**3
specificity	d/(b+d)	bd/(b+d)**3
accuracy(+)	a/(a+b)	ab/(a+b)**3
accuracy(-)	d/(c+d)	cd/(c+d)**3
apparent error(+)	b/(a+b)	ab/(a+b)**3
apparent error(-)	c/(c+d)	cd/(c+d)**3
true error(+)	c/(a+c)	ac/(a+c)**3
true error(-)	b/(b+d)	bd/(b+d)**3

These measures are also related to the so called 'likelihood ratio' L which in the notation used here would correspond to

L=(a/(a+c))/(b/(b+d)).

It is thus the ratio of the probability of a positive test result in a population with a positive external criterion and the probability of a positive test result in a population with a negative criterion (18, 91, 92) or the probability of a correct positive test divided by the probability for a false positive test.

Also the measures termed 'accuracy' by YOUNG correspond to the measures given above for the assessment of reliability.

In every case two different values are given for the assessment of one essential aspect of reliability and validity. Every index represents an estimate for conditional probabilities.

Likewise, estimates of the unconditional probabilities, e. g. of test outcomes or outcomes of the external criterion may be derived from the marginals.

Each of the ratios varies from 0 to 1. Any two making up a pair determining one aspect of validity or reliability therefore opens up a two dimensional space in which the values for a given test are represented by a single point. It is hard to decide on some kind of threshold from which on a given combination may be called valid enough (figure 5.3.3-4).

There have been a number of attempts therefore to arrive at a single value that adequately represents the aspects of both measurements making up such a pair (5, 20, 36, 43, 44, 87, 88, 138). The main disadvantage of any one of them is that they do not solve the problem of providing a valid criterion for deciding whether a given medical test suits its requirements. The value 'J' proposed by YOUDEN (138) corresponds to the sum of sensitivity and specificity minus 1. All values of sensitivity and specificity that would result in a line parallel to the negative diagonal in figure 5-4 would result in identical 'J' values. (The line plotted in figure 5-4 corresponds to a 'J' value of .2). Other proposed values are only applicable to binary data, i.e. two by two tables (5, 20, 44, 87). These disadvantages are

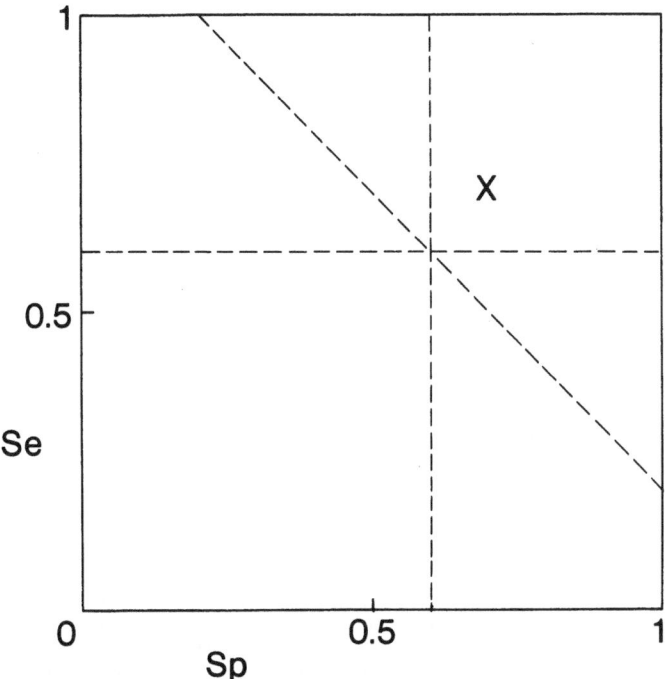

Figure 5.3.3-4

Sensitivity - specificity graph.
The sensitivity/specificity values for a binary test are represented bv
a point (x). Dashed lines represent different possibilities for setting
threshold values for minimal sensitivity and/or specificity. The line
parallel to the negative diagonal corresponds to a 'J' value of .2 (J =
sensitivity + specificity - 1).

not shared by a measure suggested by STERLING et al (127, 128) for what
these authors call 'robot data screening'. This measure 'I' is based on
the concepts of information theory and may serve for comparing
sensitivity and specificity values derived from a two by two table,
although its application is not limited to two by two tables. It is
also related to the Chi square value and therefore may be used as a
statistical test.

This measure 'I' can be figured as the difference in bit between the
entropy of an information source Y with k outcomes and the conditional
entropy of this information source Y, if a test X with l outcomes has
been applied.

$$I(X) = H(Y) - H(Y/X)$$

Since the entropy is a function of the probabilities of the various outcomes of the information source Y,

$$H(Y) = -\sum_{i=1}^{k} p_{i.} \, log_2 \, p_{i.} \qquad \left| \quad \sum_{i=1}^{k} p_{i.} = 1, \; 1 < i < k \right.$$

and conditional entropy a function of these probabilities and the probabilities for the joint outcomes of the test and the dependent variable (information source),

$$H(Y/X) = -\sum_{j=1}^{l} p_{.j} \sum_{i=1}^{k} \frac{p_{ij}}{p_{.j}} \, log_2 \, \frac{p_{ij}}{p_{.j}} \qquad \left| \quad \sum_{j=1}^{l} p_{.j} = \sum_{j=1}^{l} \sum_{i=1}^{k} p_{ij} = 1, \; 1 < j < l \right.$$

the measure 'I' may be derived from the probabilities for which estimates may be derived from a contingency table. 'I' may be estimated from

$$\hat{I}(X) = \frac{1}{N} \sum_{i=1}^{k} \sum_{j=1}^{l} n_{ij} \, log_e \, \frac{n_{ij} N}{n_{.j} n_{i.}} \qquad \left| \quad \sum_{i=1}^{k} \sum_{j=1}^{l} n_{ij} = N \right.$$

Since 2*N*I(X) approximates a Chi square distribution for large N with (k-1)*(l-1) degrees of freedom, this measure constitutes an index of the probability that an improvement of the entropy criterion as large as the one observed could have resulted from an independent variable, which actually produces no improvement (38, 127, 128).

It is particularly illustrative to demonstrate the relation between the measure 'I' and the measures for sensitivity and specificity (in this case regarded as measures of conditional probabilities) for the two by two table, i. e. for k=l=2.

The entropy of an information source with two outcomes is represented by the well-known curve (figure 5.3.3-5) with a maximum of 1 bit for p(Y+)=p(Y-)=0.5 and a minimum of 0 bit for p(Y+) or p(Y-)=1. A similar curve is obtained for the conditional entropy H (Y|X). It is identical with H(Y), if p (X+|Y+) + p (X-|Y-)=1, i.e. if the sum of sensitivity and specificity adds up to 1. This is the case, if test and external criterion (information source) are statistically independent. For all other cases, the curve of the conditional entropy is lower than that of the unconditional entropy. If sensitivity and specificity = 1, it remains on the abscissa. In figure 5.3.3-5, values for sensitivity and specificity of .9 have been assumed. The resulting curve is symmetric to a vertical middle line in the graph. If the values of sensitivity and specificity differ from each other, an asymmetric curve results.

The relation between the measure for sensitivity and specificity and 'I' becomes intuitively clear, if a presentation analogous to that of figure 5.3.3-3 is used. In figures 5.3.3-6 to 5.3.3-8, isoinformation curves for constant values of 'I' have been plotted in the area opened up by sensitivity (p(Y+|X+) and specificity (p(Y-|X-)). Three graphs for differing values of p(Y+) are given, since 'I' depends also on the apriori probabilities, as is also evident from figure 5.3.3-5. In figure 5.3.3-6, an apriori probability of .5 is assumed. The resulting isoinformation curves are symmetric to the positive diagonal. Ten curves have been determined, .1 bit apart. The last one coincides with p(Y+|X+)=p(Y-|X-)=1 and consists of only one point. For other apriori probabilities (figures 5.3.3-7 and 5.3.3-8), the curves obtained are no

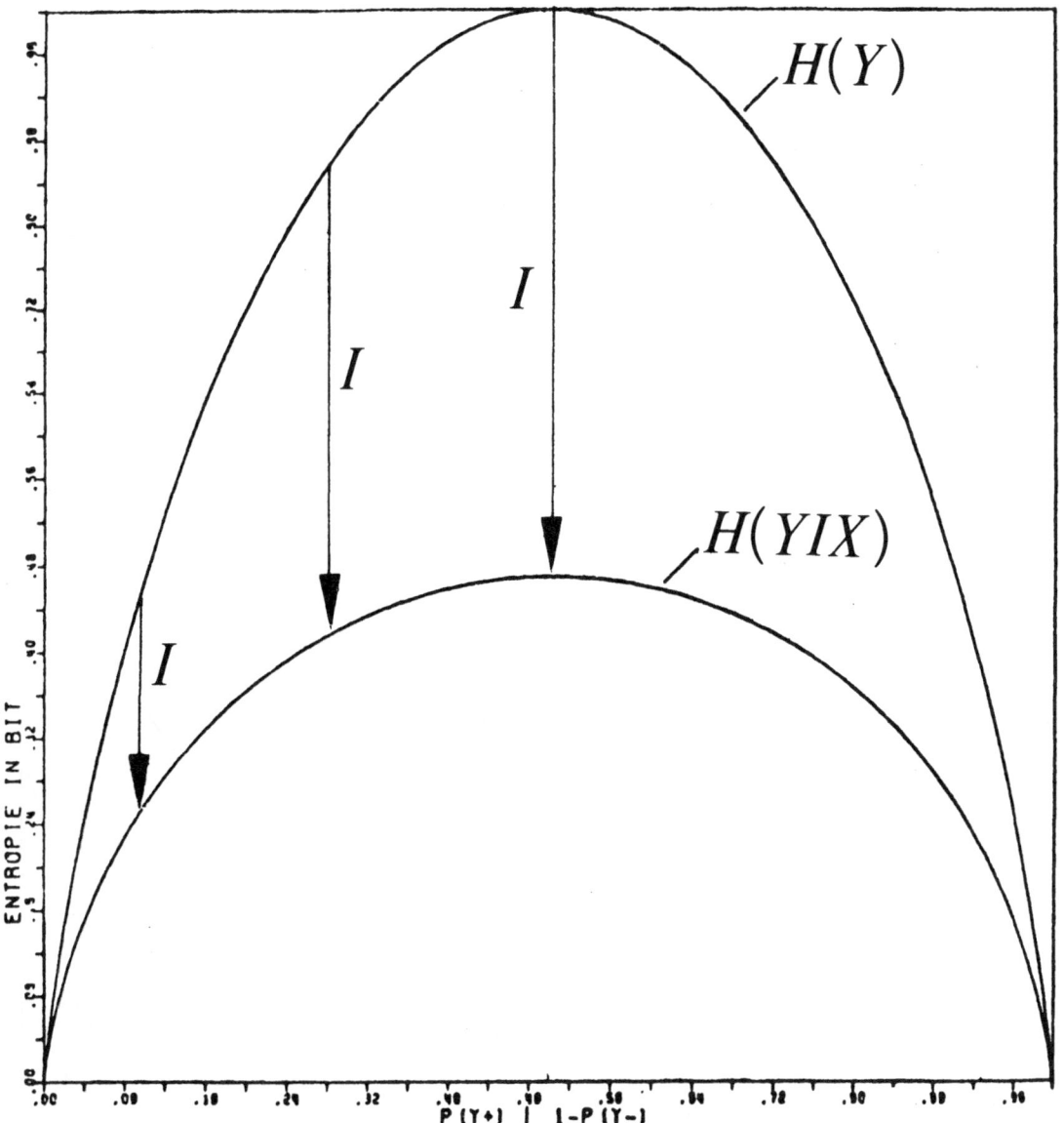

Figure 5.3.3-5

Relation between entropy H(Y), conditional entropy H(Y|X) and "information content I" II : I = H(Y) - H(Y|X). For details refer to text.

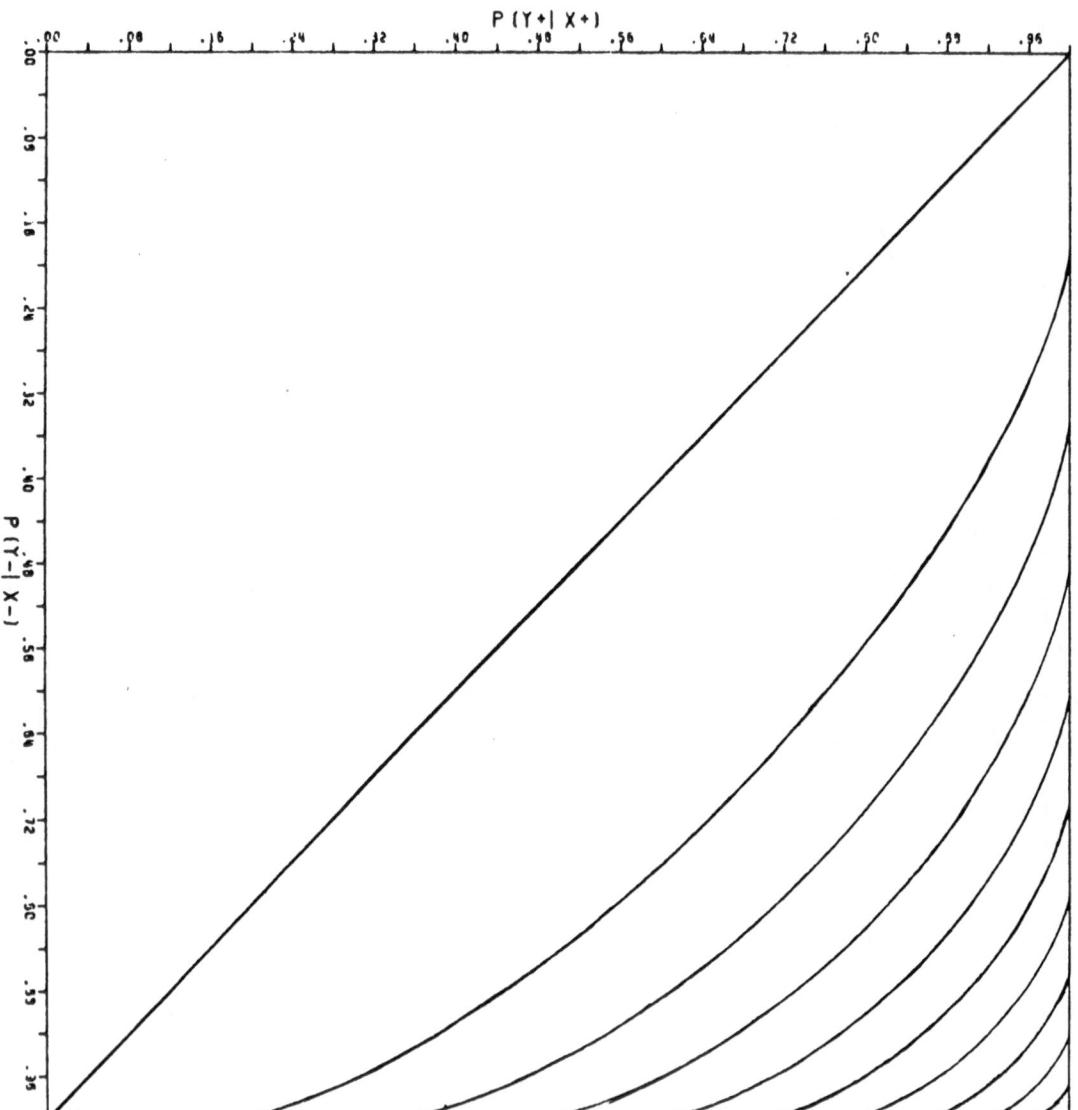

Figure 5.3.3-6

Isoinformation curves.
A sensitivity - specificity graph analogous to figure 5.3.3-4. The
curves represent values of sensitivity and specificity which correspond
to identical information content. The negative diagonal corresponds to
I values of 0 bit. The other isoinformation curves are .1 bit apart.
The last of 10 curves coincides with sensitivity = specificity = 1.
Curves are symmetric to positive diagonal, because an apriori
probability p(Y+) of .5 has been assumed. Curves in the lower half of
the graph have been omitted in this and the following figures.

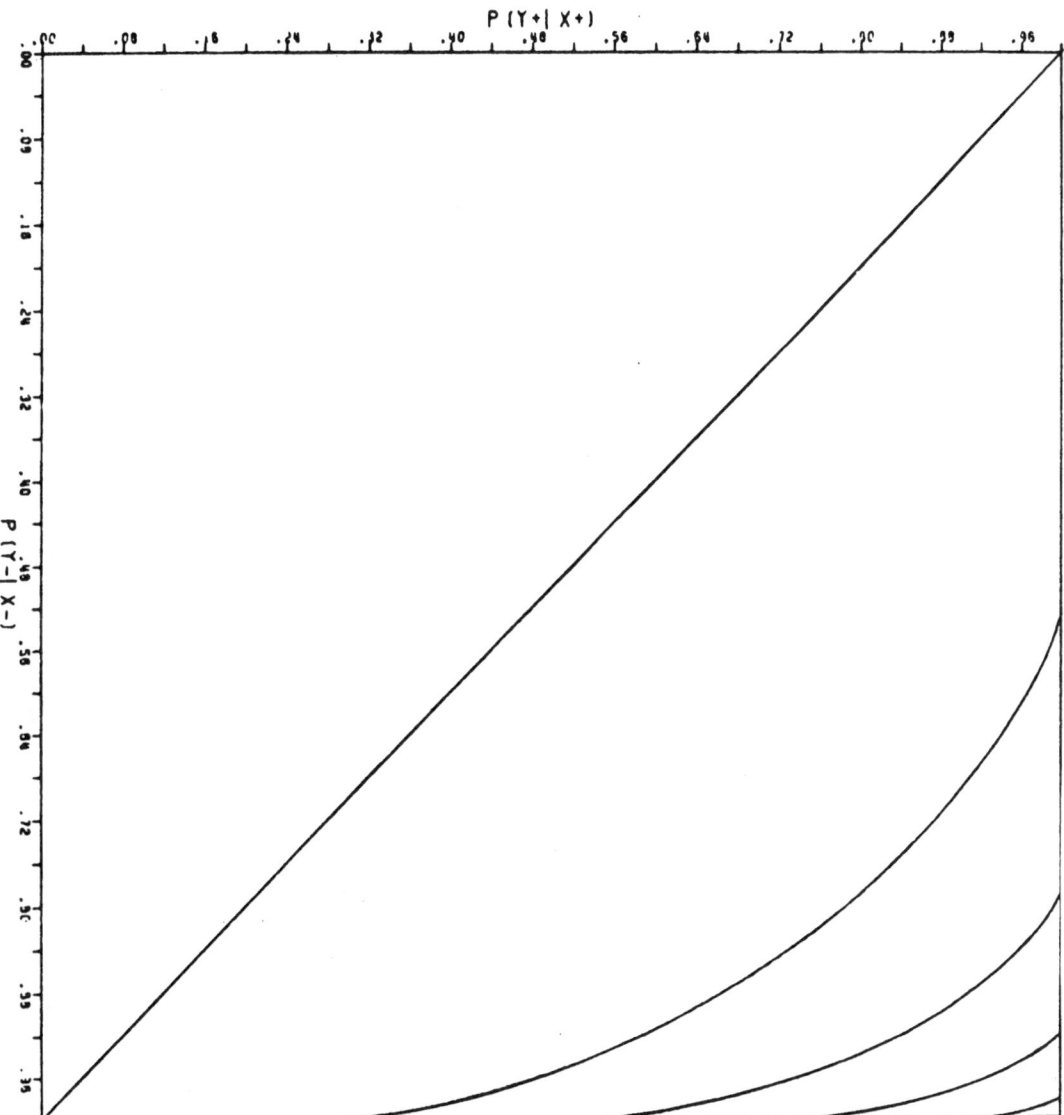

Figure 5.3.3-7

Isoinformation curves.
Analogous presentation to figure 5.3.3-6. However, a value of .1 has been assumed for the apriori probability p(Y+). Curves are no longer symmetric. High specificity at the expense of sensitivity would yield higher 'information content' ('I'). Curves are again .1 bit apart. Maximal values barely exceed .4 bit.

P (Y+) = .90

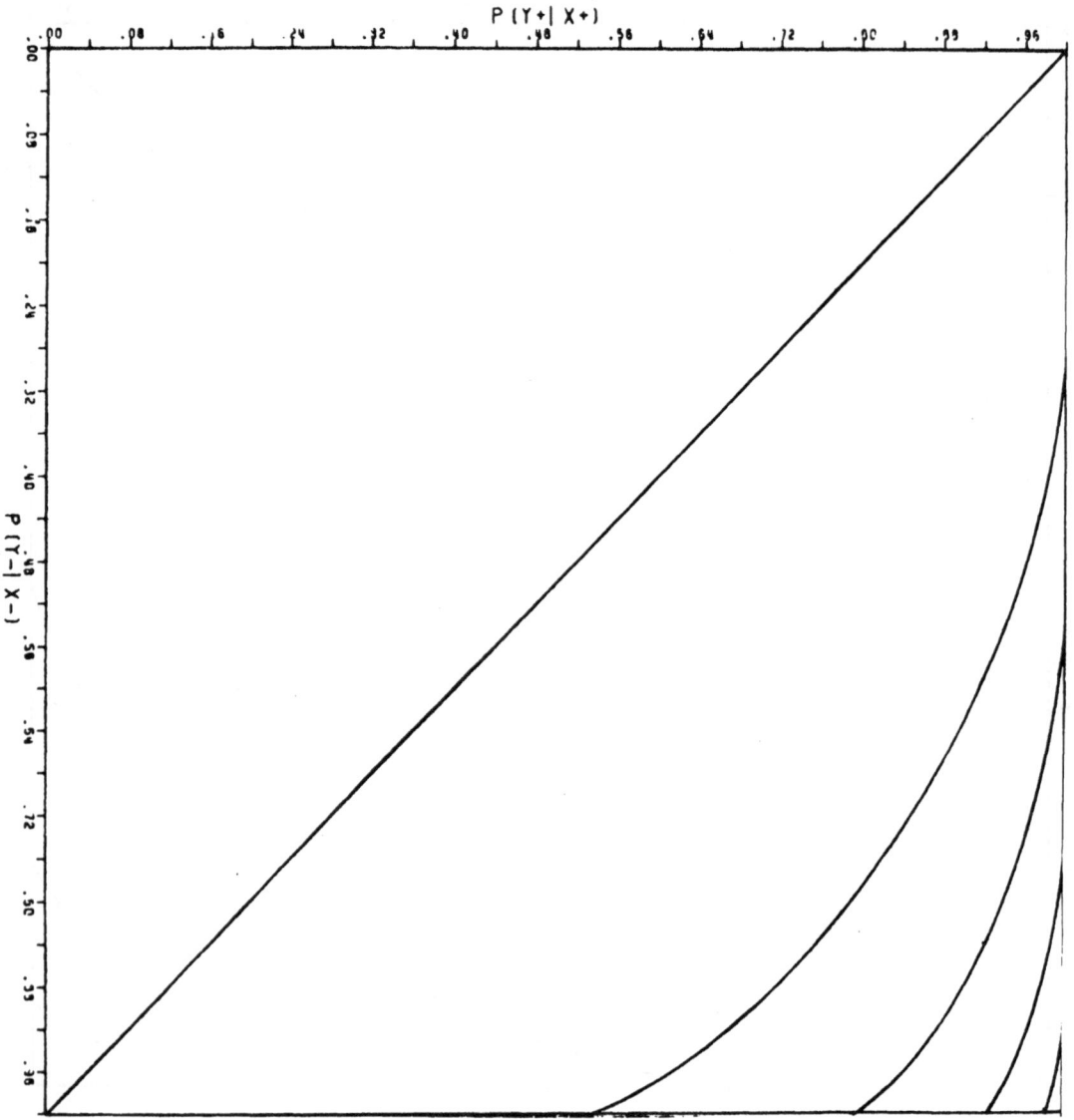

Figure 5.3.3-8

Isoinformation curves
An apriori probability p(Y+) of .9 has been assumed. The asymmetry of
the resulting picture is inverse to that of figure 5.3.3-7.

longer symmetric to the positive diagonal. Corresponding with the smaller values of H(Y) for extreme values of p(Y+) are the smaller values that the measure 'I' may attain, as exemplified by the smaller number of curves which again are plotted with intervals of .1 bit. The maximum information gain that may be obtained in the illustrated cases barely exceeds .4 bit.

It is also evident that for low values of p(Y+), i. e. low prevalence rates of the positive outcomes of the external criterion (information source), a combination of a high specificity value with one of a low sensitivity is preferable to the inverse ratio.

In order to make values determined for different apriori probabilities comparable, the use of an uncertainty coefficient 'U' has been suggested (93).

$$U = (H(Y) - H(Y|X)) / H(Y)$$

It relativates the decrease in uncertainty or gain in information 'I' to the maximal values that these measures may attain for any given apriori probability. 'U' varies between 0 and 1, while 'I' may theoretically attain infinitely large values, if applied to scalar variables.

'U' constitutes thus a single measure, which may be used for determination of the validity interrelating tests and criteria with multiple discrete outcomes.

Determination of this measure for each item of a questionnaire and each decision defined in the range of relevance makes it possible to identify those items which singly contribute most to the reduction in uncertainty concerning each individual decision. Assuming that those questionnaire items which singly contribute most are also likely to contribute most if used in combination, it becomes possible to base each decision contained in the frame of relevance on an appropriate subset of the questionnaire.

Definition of such a subset is desirable, since computation of the validity measures for a questionnaire with several hundred items exceeds computational feasibility. Consider a composite test of n items. If there are i classes of items, each with m (i) outcomes (1 < i < 1), and n' (i) items in each class, the entire test will have

$$SUM(m'(i) **n'(i))$$

possible outcomes with 1 < i < 1. If a questionnaire has n items, all with the same number m of possible outcomes, there are m**n possible outcomes for the entire questionnaire. For 10 questions allowing yes/no answers, i.e. having two outcomes, there are 2**10=1024 patterns of responses possible. If a third answer option like 'don't know' is allowed, the possible outcomes of this test would amount to 59049.

On the other hand, a general medical history questionnaire designed for a broad range of relevance will for reasons of practicability contain only a few items for each decision in the frame of reference.

Determination of the 'U' values for each item of the questionnaire and each decision in the range of relevance then constitutes a selection of appropriate subsets on the basis of the actual performance of the questionnaire under given conditions in a given population. The selection of the subset is therefore no longer based on conjecture but on actual data and will be representative for further application of the questionnaire, to such an extent as the population and the conditions of application are representative.

The composite test made up of a questionnaire subset may again be represented by a single 'U' value. The qualities of such a subset may also be illustrated by a sensitivity - specificity graph, as suggested by COLLEN (18, 19).

This procedure requires to determine the likelihood ratio for each outcome of the composite test. Ranking of the observed test outcomes in the order of increasing likelihood ratio (the ratio of the probability of this particular test outcome in a population with positive decision outcome to its probability in a population with negative decision outcome), makes it possible to discern two classes of outcomes. The one with likelihood ratios below a given threshold level will be regarded as corresponding to negative decision outcomes, the others, with likelihood ratios exceeding the threshold value, will be considered as corresponding to positive decision outcomes.

In this manner, the sensitivity and specificity values for each threshold level in the ranked list of test outcomes can be chosen for characterizing the performance of the composite test. The obtained values represent estimates for the probabilities of correctly positive decisions and correctly negative decisions for each threshold level, given the conditions of test application. This means that the essential prerequisites for second and third level standardization are given, because it becomes possible to estimate the probabilities of type 1 and type 2 errors (probabilities of false negative and false positive decisions) and to adapt the test instrument so as to meet medical requirements.

Although the basic assumption is not strictly justified that the tests, which contribute singly to a maximum reduction in uncertainty, also are the optimal subset of the questionnaire, if used in combination, practical application of the principle shows that the obtained results are not misleading (38).

5.4 VALIDATION OF THE MSH AUTOMATED HISTORY - A MODEL APPROACH

The principles outlined above were applied to the data acquired using the third version of the MSH Automated History, in order to give an example of the principle. Since the questionnaire had not been designed in accordance with the principles outlined for questionnaire design in section 5.2, we were not able to validate the data acquired against a true range of relevance. Instead we used the diagnoses that happened to have been observed and documented for the patients answering the questionnaire as substitute for such a frame of relevance. Still, the results are interesting in a number of respects.

5.4.1 FRAME OF REFERENCE

The diagnoses established for the patients of the Department of Internal Medicine of the Medical School Hannover are recorded in a standard documentation procedure, which is currently extended to include therapies and complications in order to be used more effectively by other medical specialties (54). The procedure in use during the trial application of our automated history form, required that the physician treating the patient, marked the diagnoses on the cover sheet of the medical record when the patient was discharged from the hospital. These diagnoses were then converted into a five digit code based on the KDS (Klinischer Diagnosen Schluessel) developed by IMMICH (55) which is continuously adapted in our institution (54).

For 525 patients, on who's data this model evaluation was based, these diagnoses were retrieved from the patient data bank (113, 114), or, if they had not reached the data bank yet, collected from the original patient records. A total of 510 different diagnostic codes had been used to record a total of 1472 diagnoses for the 525 patients. Since only very small patient samples were available for each diagnostic entity, the diagnoses were regrouped under a small number of headings and subheadings. A total of 13 headings resulted having up to four subheadings. Together they formed a total of 37 diagnostic classes. Even though the number of discerned classes was reduced in this fashion to 7.3 percent, the number of total recorded diagnoses was reduced only to 70 percent (from 1472 to 1016).

Table 5.4.1-1 lists the diagnostic classes, a short description of their medical meaning and the sample sizes observed for each. The diagnostic classes were arrived at with two goals in mind:

    1 to combine pathophysiologically and/or symptomatically
      related diagnostic classes
    2 to arrive at classes with large enough sample size.

Although classification was often possible in accordance with pathophysiological similarity, distinctly different symptomatology made it sometimes necessary to distinguish small groups (e.g. eyes, ears). For analogous reasons some pathophysiologically rather unrelated groups were sometimes combined into a single class because of similarities in symptomatology. This was in particular done, if each of the classes as such were represented by small sample sizes only. The classification was therefore not made, irrespective of symptomatology.

In the following we will discuss our results as if this arbitrary collection of diagnostic classes, in the manner they were defined, really constituted a medically valid frame of reference, and as if the population had been selected according to it and in consideration of other characteristics of the desired application of the questionnaire.

5.4.2 VALIDITY DETERMINATION

'I' values and 'U' values were determined for all items of the systems review section of the third questionnaire version and all 37 diagnostic categories.

All three possible answer options (yes, no, missing answer) were taken into consideration. For questions which could be skipped by branching instructions, the answer given to the branching question was assumed, if no other answer had been marked by the respondent. The results are exemplified in the following by a subsection of the questionnaire , comprising 72 questions related to 19 diagnostic classes D13 (diseases of the heart) through D31 (other G.I. disorders). Fig. 5.4.2-1 gives a semiquantitative illustration of the 'I' values obtained for each of the 72 questions and each of the 19 diagnostic classes. A look at table 5.4.1-1 shows that sample sizes for the diagnostic subclasses (D14, D15, D16, D17, D19, D20, D21, D22, D24, D25, D26, D28, D29, D30, D31)

Table 5.4.1-1

Diagnostic Classes   in the
Validation Experiment

Code	Designation	No. of cases
D01	other diseases	54
D02	malignant neoplasm, leukemia	102
D03	nutrition, metabolism, hormonal defects	35
D04	thyroid diseases, malnutrition	31
D05	hyperlipidemia, adiposity	4
D06	diabetes mellitus	96
D07	diseases of the blood system	58
D08	psychic disorders	33
D09	nervous system, sensory apparatus	39
D10	central and peripheral nervous system	25
D11	ears	9
D12	eyes	8
D13	heart	104
D14	insufficiency of the heart	39
D15	arrhythmias	27
D16	myocardial infarction	58
D17	valvular disease	14
D18	vessels and circulatory system	123
D19	hypertonia	48
D20	hypotonia	15
D21	arterial disease	55
D22	veinous disease	24
D23	respiratory tract disease	82
D24	spastic bronchitis, emphysema	36
D25	pneumonia, pleuritis, tuberculosis	17
D26	tonsillitis, sinusitis, other resp. dis.	44
D27	digestive tract	170
D28	diseases of the liver	63
D29	acute abdomen	39
D30	disorders of the stomach/intestines	61
D31	other G.I. disorders	54
D32	diseases of the urogenital tract	132
D33	kidney diseases	94
D34	other diseases of the urinary tract	53
D35	skelettal disease, muscular disease	109
D36	accidents, trauma	8
D37	musculo-skelettal system	64

Main groups are underlined, subgroups follow main groups of diseases.

ranged from 14 to 63. For the main groups (D13, D18, D23, D27) they
ranged from 82 to 170. The corresponding prevalence rates are then in
the range of .027 to .12 for the subclasses and in the range of .156 to
.323 for the main groups. It is evident from Fig. 5.4.2-1 that for each
diagnostic class there are relatively few items that contribute to a
reduction in uncertainty concerning this particular diagnostic class.
Among the first 36 questions (node number 818 to 949), which were aimed
at diagnoses involving the cardiothoracic and circulatory systems,

there are a fair number that contribute information to the decisions concerning the corresponding diagnostic classes D13 to D26. Some of these questions even contribute to some extent to the digestive tract diseases (D27). The questions aiming at disorders involving the abdominal organs (questions 37 through 72, node number 959 to 1074, diagnostic classes D27 to D31), on the other hand, contribute only moderately to the reduction in uncertainty concerning the corresponding diagnoses. With few exceptions (node number 1040 concerning diarrhea for D23 (respiratory tract disease), and node number 1042 (concerning incontinence of feces) for D26 (tonsillitis sinusitis)), none of the items contributes to the diagnoses of the cardio thoracic regions. The two exceptions are certainly surprising. They may be due to chance, although the probability is low (< 0.05), or to association of the registered disease conditions with other disease conditions.

Furthermore, it becomes evident that some items contribute a little to a number of different diagnostic categories. Examples are node number 4232 concerning heart palpitation, node number 862, concerning heart pain, angina pectoris and nodes number 959 (change of appetite) as well as 1040 (diarrhea). It is evident that these, in fact, are all symptoms which may be caused by a number of different organic conditions, but which also are a common feature of psychosomatic response patterns.

A different type of items contributes considerably to certain diagnostic categories and somewhat less to others. Examples are nodes number 4447 and 954 pertaining to the fact that elevated blood pressure had been recorded by a physician at an earlier time and to antihypertensive treatment respectively. These questions contribute considerably to D19 (hypertension), but also somewhat to D18, (diseases of the vessels and circulatory system), the heading under which D19 falls, and to D16 (myocardial infarction) and D13, (diseases of the heart), the heading under which myocardial infarction was placed. The associations are medically plausible. Another example is node number 896, concerning earlier diagnosis of myocardial infarction which loads highly on D16 (myocardial infarction) and D13 (diseases of the heart) but also on D15, (arrhythmia) D18, (diseases of the vessels and circulatory system), D21 (arterial disease) and D27 (gastrointestinal disease). Apart from the last category, for which the association might again be due to chance or to an association of disease categories, all associations are medically plausible.

Also it becomes easily possible to identify the items which contribute to none of the disease categories on the basis of the matrix - e.g. node number 4230, (heart pains precipitated by swallowing), 888, (prior diagnosis of rheumatic fever), 911 and 948, (tachycardia and pallor of fingers (digiti mortui) respectively), 4235, (heart burn caused by certain foods), 1046 and 1051 (obstipation and obstipation of short duration respectively). This group of items clearly contains some, which are either extremely rare (911, 948), unpopular (888) or extremely common (4235, 1022, 1046, 1051). In the same manner the diagnostic categories that are not picked up with sufficient certainty by any of the items, are identifiable. Examples are D20, (hypotension), and D25, (pneumonia, pleuritis). If one is sure that such categories belong justly in the list making up the frame of reference, and that the catalogue of available items in the questionnaire has been exhausted (which is not the case in our example), one would have to try to find new items which differentiate these categories better from the others. On the other hand, if one is sure that the range of relevance is complete, one might at least eliminate those items that do not contribute information because or in spite of high prevalence. For those items for which no association with any of the target decisions is found because of low prevalence, one would have to weigh what would be missed if the item was present in an individual but not picked up by the questionnaire, against its useless presentation in most cases.

Figures 5.4.2-2 and 5.4.2-3 give a quantitative illustration of 'U' values, which are better comparable between various disease categories, since they account for differences in disease prevalence. All 72 questions are represented by numbers on the abscissa (1 through 72). The ordinate gives a scale for the observed values of 'U'. The values observed for a given disease category are represented by specific symbols and interconnected by lines. It becomes evident from the graphs that these relative measures, which may vary between 0 and 1 attain rather high values for some combinations of questions and diagnoses.

Thus a maximal value of U = .44 is observed for question number 5 (node number 4191) with respect to D24 (spastic bronchitis and emphysema). The question asks whether the patient suffers from asthma attacks.

The graphs also show that the 'U' values for the more generally defined categories are lower than for the subcategories, which are more stringently defined. Thus the questions number 5, node number 4191 asking for asthma attacks loads also quite high for general respiratory diseases. The value approximates, however, only one third of the value for the spastic bronchitis and emphysema group. This demonstrates how the definition of disease categories among other factors influence the validity measures. The fuzzier the definition of a disease category, the lower the validity measures of a test item.

On the basis of the observed 'U' values, it is now possible to select the best test items for any given target decision. The questions selected in this way form a close to optimal subset, the composite validity of which may be determined in the manner outlined above.

The procedure will be exemplified for three diagnostic categories:

        D21   diseases of arteries
        D22   diseases of veins
        D24   spastic bronchitis, emphysema

These categories were selected, since only a few questions apply for each, which makes the process transparent, and because there were rather high 'U' values observed for categories D22 and D24 but low ones for D21. These differences should emphasize the principle.

Since our questionnaire accepts three kinds of questions:

  - no
  - yes
  - missing answer,

each individual test item will have m=3 possible outcomes. The answer pattern may be considered a ternary number system. A response pattern for n questions could be considered a n digit ternary number. A total of $3^{**}n$ distinct response patterns are possible.

In the following examples the questions will be characterized by numbers 0 through n-1 in correspondence with their positions as a digit of such a ternary number. Question 0 will be represented by the right most digit. In this way it becomes possible to characterize the response patterns by decimal numbers ranging from 0 to $(3^{**}n - 1)$ and to derive the corresponding response pattern.

KN.NR.	TEXT	D13	D14	D15	D16	D17	D18	D19	D20	D21	D22	D23	D24	D25	D26	D27	D28	D29	D30	D31
818	Husten		○									◉	◉	○						
819	Husten - seit länger als 4 Wochen		○											○						
825	Husten assoziiert mit Auswurf											◉	◉	○						
837	Husten verbunden mit Pfeiffen und Brummen											◉	◉							
4191	Asthma-Anfälle		○									●	●	○						
849	Luftnot - oft	◉	○	○	○							◉	●			○				
850	Luftnot beim schnellen Gehen oder Treppe	○	○	○								○	○							
854	Luftnot beim Gehen mit norm.Geschwindigkeit	○	○									○	○			○				
857	Luftnot beim langsamen Gehen	○	○									○	◉			○	○			
3231	Luftnot beim flachen Liegen	○	○	○																
3229	Luftnot - nachts	○	○										◉			○				
3230	Luftnot nachts verbunden mit Engeg.	◉	○		○							○	◉			○				
867	Herzschmerzen, Angina pectoris	○		○	○		○	○												
4229	Herzschmerzen, Auftreten nur in Ruhe	○		○	○															
4230	Herzschmerzen, Auftreten durch Schlucken																			
869	Herzschmerzen, Auftreten bei emotion.	○																		
870	Herzschmerzen, Auftreten bei schwerer kö.	○		○																
871	Herzschmerzen, Auftreten bei leichter kö.	◉	○	○																
887	Herzerkrankungen	◉	○	○																
3959	Herzerkrankungen: angeb. Herzfehler		○																	
896	Herzerkrankungen: Herzinfarkt	●		○	●		○			○						○				
4535	Herzerkrankungen: Klappenfehler	○	○	○		○														
888	Herzerkrankungen: rheumat. Fieber																			
3960	Herzerkrankungen: andere als abgefr.	◉	○	○	○	○							○							
4447	Erhöhter Blutdruck früher v.Arzt festg.	○			○		○	●												
952	Überwachung d. Blutdrucks wurde bei fr.	○		○			○	◉												
953	Behandlung gegen zu niedrigen Blutdruck							○												
954	Behandlung gegen zu hohen Blutdruck	○			○		◉	●					○							
4231	Für Pat. beunruhigende Herzfrequenzen	○	○		○		○									○				
4232	Für Pat. beängstigende Unregelmäßigk.	○	○	○	○								○			○				
911	Gelegentlich Anfälle sehr raschen Herzs.																			
948	Finger o. Zehen werden in Kälte wachsb.																			
924	Ödeme der Beine und Füße	◎	○				○													
941	Thrombophlebitis Venenthrombose						○			○	●									
943	Arterieller Thrombus od. Embolie früh.						◉			○	◉									
949	Claudicatio intermittens						○			○										
959	Appetitsveränderungen							○								○		○	○	
962	Gewichtsveränd. von mehr als 5 Pfund																		○	
4233	Bestimmte Speisen verurs. Magenschmerz															○			○	
4234	Bestimmte Speisen verurs. Völlegefühl															○		○	○	
4235	Bestimmte Speisen verurs. Sodbrennen																			
4236	Bestimmte Speisen verurs. Schmerzen															○		○	○	
4237	Pat. muß wegen Magenschm.nachts essen																		○	
4239	Häufiges Aufstoßen von Luft																		○	
4240	Häufiges Aufstoßen von Magensäure																		○	
4241	Häufiges Aufstoßen von Speiseresten																		○	
1032	Blähungsbeschwerden															○			○	
1010	Ulcus Magengeschwür v.Arzt diagnostiziert															○			○	○
3528	Gallenkolik															○	○			
1021	Gallensteine od. Gallenblasenerkrankung																○			
1022	Anorektale Erkrankungen																			
1030	Pat. hat nach d. Stuhlgang das Gefühl.																		○	
1031	Pat. hat das Gefühl, daß die Darmwand																		○	
3535	Ziehende Schmerzen beim Stuhlgang															○				
1040	Episoden v. Diarrhoe innerh.d.Vergangenh.											○			○	○		○		
1042	Stuhlinkontinenz innerh. d. Vergangenheit														◉					
1046	Obstipation																			
1051	Obstipation akute																			
1052	Veränderungen des Stuhls - Konsistenz															◉		○	○	
1055	Stuhl wie Oel - od. Fetteilchen im Wasser															○			○	
1056	Stuhl faul stinkend															○				
1057	Stuhl selbst im Wasser schwimmend																			
1058	Stuhl v. abnehmenden Durchmesser - Bleis.															○·		○	○	
3206	Stuhl bestehend aus lauter kleinen Kugel.																			
1059	Stuhl breiig, schleimig oder flockig															○		○		
3533	Stuhl unverdaute Speiseartikel enthaltend															○		○		
3534	Stuhl Würmer enthaltend																			
1061	Blutbeimengungen im Stuhl															○		○		
1067	Teerstuhl innerh. der verg. 6 Monate															○			○	○

Figure 5.4.2-1

Matrix of 72 questions and 19 diagnostic categories illustrating I values obtained in 525 patients semiquantively. Symbols used:

solid dots : $I > .1$
encircled dots: $.1 > I > .05$
circles: $.05 > I > .01$
empty fields: $I < .01$

For abbreviations of symbols for diagnostic categories refer to table 5.4.1-1.

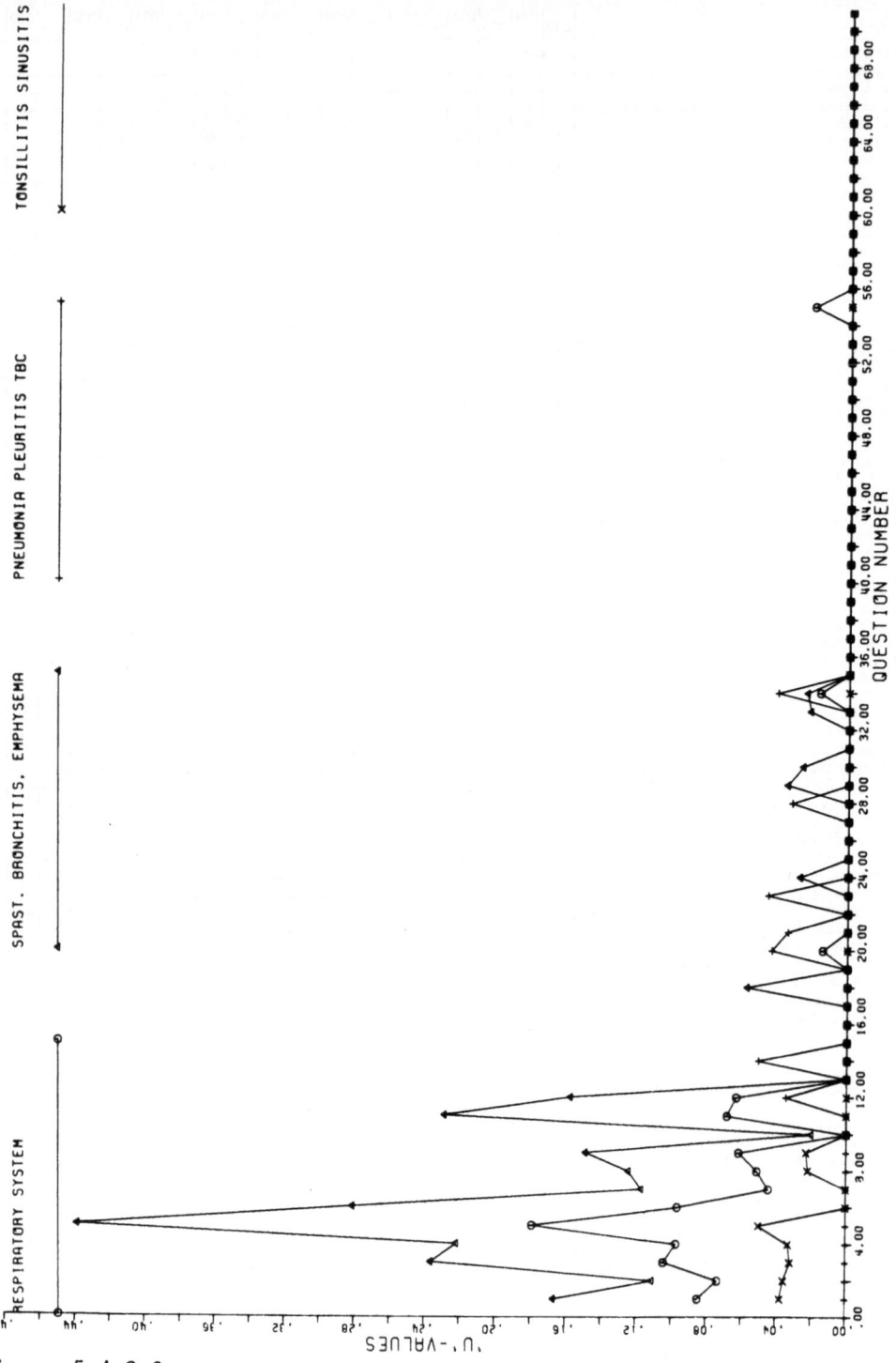

Figure 5.4.2-2

'U' values for respiratory tract diseases.
The numbers on the abscissa correspond to the top down sequence of
questions in figure 5.4.2-1 numbered consecutively 1 through 72.

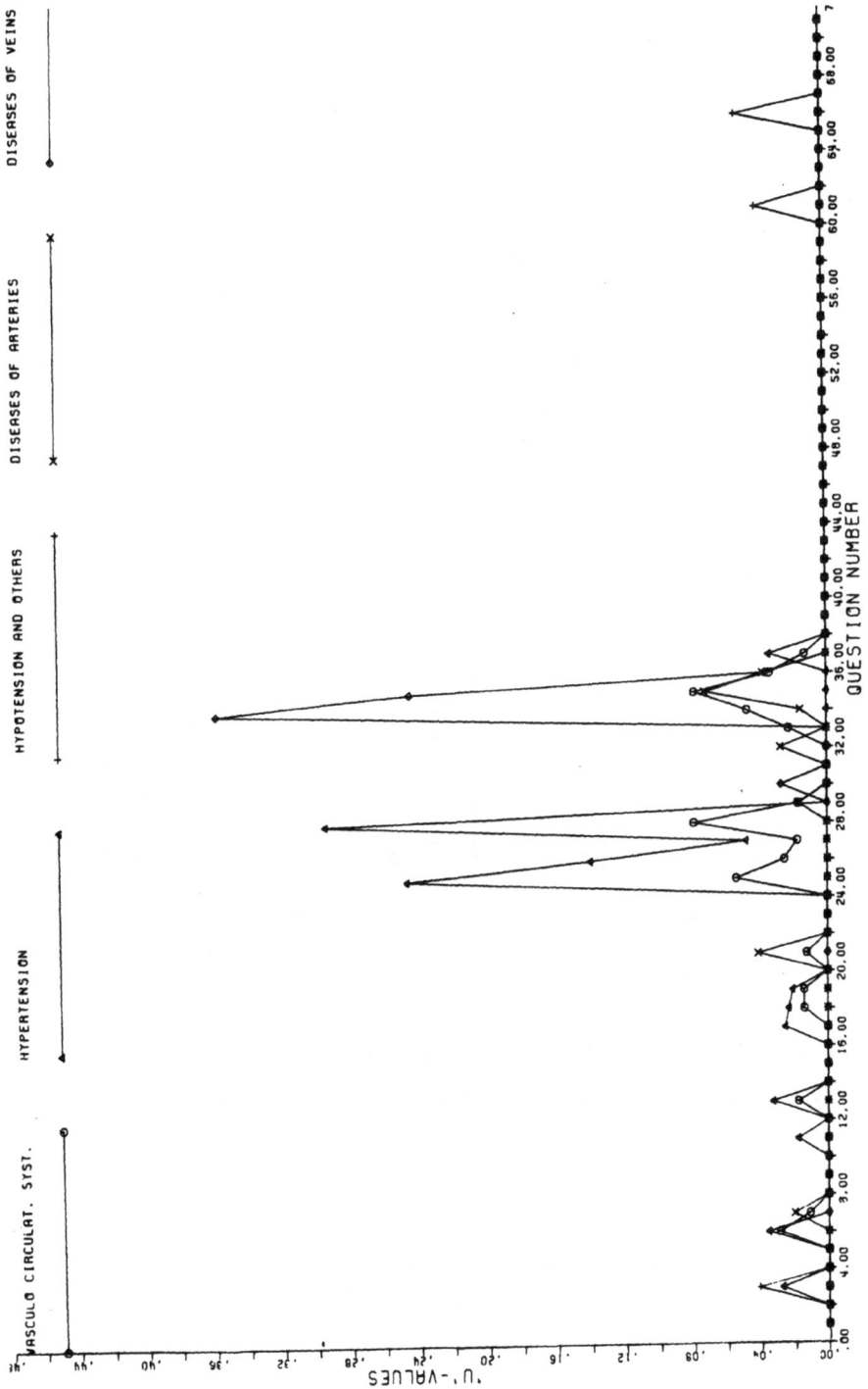

Figure 5.4.2-3

'U'-values for diseases fo the circulatory system. Analogue
representation to figure 5.4.2-2.

Pattern number 15 means that the observed response pattern was:

120

If we define '0' as code for 'no', '1' as code for 'yes', and '2' as code for 'missing answers', this means that a no answer was obtained for question 0, a missing answer for question 1 and a yes answer for question 2 (the third question, counting from the right).

Since our examples have a maximum of three questions, a table will be given for referencing numbers and patterns:

Table 5.4.2-1
Table of cross references between response patterns and pattern numbers.

Response codes :   0 = no
                   1 = yes
                   2 = no answer

Pattern number	Question number 2 1 0	Pattern number	Question number 2 1 0	Pattern number	Question number 2 1 0
0	0 0 0	9	1 0 0	18	2 0 0
1	0 0 1	10	1 0 1	19	2 0 1
2	0 0 2	11	1 0 2	20	2 0 2
3	0 1 0	12	1 1 0	21	2 1 0
4	0 1 1	13	1 1 1	22	2 1 1
5	0 1 2	14	1 1 2	23	2 1 2
6	0 2 0	15	1 2 0	24	2 2 0
7	0 2 1	16	1 2 1	25	2 2 1
8	0 2 2	17	1 2 2	26	2 2 2

For a subquestionnaire consisting of 2 questions, patterns 0 through 8 will apply, omitting the leading zero. For a subquestionnaire consisting of 3 questions, all 27 patterns will apply.

Example 1: Diseases of arteries.

For this category the following questions were selected

digit number	node number	text	'U'
0	943	Has a physician detected an occlusion of an artery (thrombosis or embolism)?	.072
1	869	Has a physician diagnosed myo-cardial infarction?	.041

These are questions number 35 and 21 respectively in the list of 72 questions for which 'U' values are illustrated in Fig. 5.4.2-2 and 5.4.2-3. It is apparent that both questions require considerable medical knowledge for correct answering. Especially the question pertaining to arterial occlusion seems to have been misunderstood, since it loads higher for venous disease than for arterial disease (figure 5.4.2-2). The 'U' value for the composite test consisting of these two questions for deciding on a classification as 'arterial disease' amounts to .117.

Example 2: Diseases of veins.
The selected questions comprise:

digit number	node number	text	'U'
0	943	Has a physician detected an occlusion of an artery (thrombosis or embolism)	.244
1	941	Has a physician diagnosed venous inflammation (thrombophlebitis)	.357

Even though the questions again would demand a high degree of medical knowledge, their 'U' values are high for the disease category taken into consideration. (In the case of the question aiming at arterial occlusion, this is obviously due to a misinterpretation of the question by the patients). The 'U' value of the composite test of .430 is relatively high.

Example 3: Spastic bronchitis, emphysema.
For this disease category, the selected questions comprised

digit number	node number	text	'U'
0	849	Do you suffer frequently from shortness of breath?	.221
1	4191	Do you suffer from attacks of asthma?	.439
2	837	Do you suffer from cough with wheezing and rales?	.281

In this case symptoms are asked that are commonly known and specific for a diseased state. The composite test gave a 'U' value of .620.

In tables 5.4.2-2 to 5.4.2-4 the response patterns are listed in the order of increasing likelihood ratio and the sensitivity and specificity values with concommitant standard deviations are given for each level of the likelihood ratio.

Fig. 5.4.2-4 illustrates the same numbers for all three diagnoses in the form of a sensitivity / specificity plot.

The figure demonstrates that for identifying 'spastic bronchitis and emphysema' on the basis of the three indicated questions under the conditions of the test, one would have a choice of setting a likelihood threshold so that sensitivity values approach 1. In this case a threshold value of .05 would be adopted. The specificity values would then be in the range of .75. In this case, reponse patterns 2, 5, 6, 9, 15, 18, 19 20, 23, 26 and 0 would have to be considered to indicate absence of disease, while patterns 1, 10, 8, 7, 4, 13, 14, 16, 22 would be handled as indicating disease (of table 5.3.2-4).

64

Table 5.4.2-2

Diseases of arteries

Pattern.

number	L	a	b	c	d	Se	s(Se)	Sp	s(Sp)
8	.33	54	444	1	26	.98	.02	.06	.01
2	.41	53	423	2	47	.96	.03	.10	.01
6	.60	49	366	6	104	.89	.04	.22	.02
0	.61	28	73	17	397	.51	.07	.84	.02
3	1.85	20	36	35	434	.36	.06	.92	.01
7	2.44	18	29	37	441	.33	.06	.94	.01
1	4.07	8	8	47	462	.15	.05	.98	.01
5	4.26	5	2	50	468	.09	.04	1.00	0
4	21.14	0	0	55	470	0	0	1.00	0

L = Likelihood   Se= Sensitivity
a = no. of true positives   s(Se) = standard deviation of Se
b = no. of false positives   Sp= specificity
c = no. of false negatives   s(Sp) = standard deviation of Sp
d = no. of true negatives

Table 5.4.2-3

Diseases of veins

Pattern

number	L	a	b	c	d	Se	s(Se)	Sp	s(Sp)
6,7,4	0	24	484	0	17	1	0	.03	.01
1	.12	23	106	1	395	.96	.04	.79	.02
9	.55	22	67	2	434	.92	.06	.87	.01
3	3.48	21	55	3	446	.88	.07	.89	.04
5	6.96	19	43	5	458	.79	.08	.91	.01
2	8.35	13	14	11	487	.54	.10	.97	.01
8	13.89	0	0	24	501	0	0	1	0

L = Likelihood   Se= Sensitivity
a = no. of true positives   s(Se) = standard deviation of Se
b = no. of false positives   Sp= specificity
c = no. of false negatives   s(Sp) = standard deviation of Sp
d = no. of true negatives

An extreme alternative would be to adopt a threshold value of 5. In
this case specificity of the test would be close to 1 while sensitivity
values would be in the range of .85.   The response patterns 2, 5, 6, 9,
15, 18, 19,   20, 23, 26, 0, 1, 10,   8 and 7 would all be considered to
indicate absence of disease and only patterns 9, 13,   14, 16   and 22
would be considered to indicate disease.

It is evident from table 5.4.2-4 that the response patterns 11, 12, 17,
21, 24 and 25 had not been observed in the   test population. A program
of automatic test interpretation should be able to handle them, if they
occur.   This property is the advantage of the algorithms used by
HENDERSON for automatic interpretation of test results (see below,
section 5.5.1).

The curve for 'diseases of veins' differs from the one discussed just
now, in that it is an example of a curve, where high sensitivity values

Table 5.4.2-4

Spastic bronchitis, emphysema

Pattern number	L	a	b	c	d	Se	s(Se)	Sp	s(Sp)
2,3,6,9, 15,18, 19,20 23,26	0	36	404	0	85	1	0	.17	.02
0	.05	35	125	1	364	.97	.03	.74	.02
1	.66	31	43	5	446	.86	.06	.91	.01
10	.76	30	25	6	464	.83	.06	.95	.02
8	1.36	29	15	7	474	.81	.07	.97	.01
7	4.52	27	9	9	480	.75	.07	.98	.01
9	9.03	23	3	13	486	.64	.08	.99	0
13	81.97	5	0	31	489	.14	.06	1	0
14,16 22		0	0	36	489	0	0	1	0

L = Likelihood
a = no. of true positives
b = no. of false positives
c = no. of false negatives
d = no. of true negatives

Se= Sensitivity
s(Se) = standard deviation of Se
Sp= specificity
s(Sp) = standard deviation of Sp

may be attained without a possibility of attaining also comparable specificity without appreciable loss in sensitivity. A sensitivity of close to .95 may be reached by adopting a likelihood value of .55 as threshold. Specifity in this case is in the order of .85. In order to attain a specificity level in the same range, a likelihood ratio of 8 should be exceeded. Sensitivity in this case would drop down to values in the range of .5.

The curve for diseases of arteries finally is an example of a curve which at no point reaches satisfactory levels. If one were sure that the target category was adequately defined and that it should be a member of the set of decisions defined as frame of reference, and if on the other hand, the possibilities of the available questionnaire had been exhausted - which in our example was not the case - one would have to modify the questionnaire by adding or replacing questions.

Questionnaire adaption to a device of third level standardization would therefore consist of two steps

1. Modification of the questionnaire, until desired levels of validity are obtained for each target decision
2. Selection of a decision threshold in consideration of the medical requirements of sensitivity and specificity.

5.5 CONSEQUENCES AND FUTURE PROSPECTS

Following the principles outlined for construction and standardization of history questionnaires, it should be possible

1 to arrive initially at a close to optimal questionnaire for a given application
2 to measure the validity of this instrument for the spectrum of desicions characteristic for a particular application

QUESTIONNAIRE VALIDITY

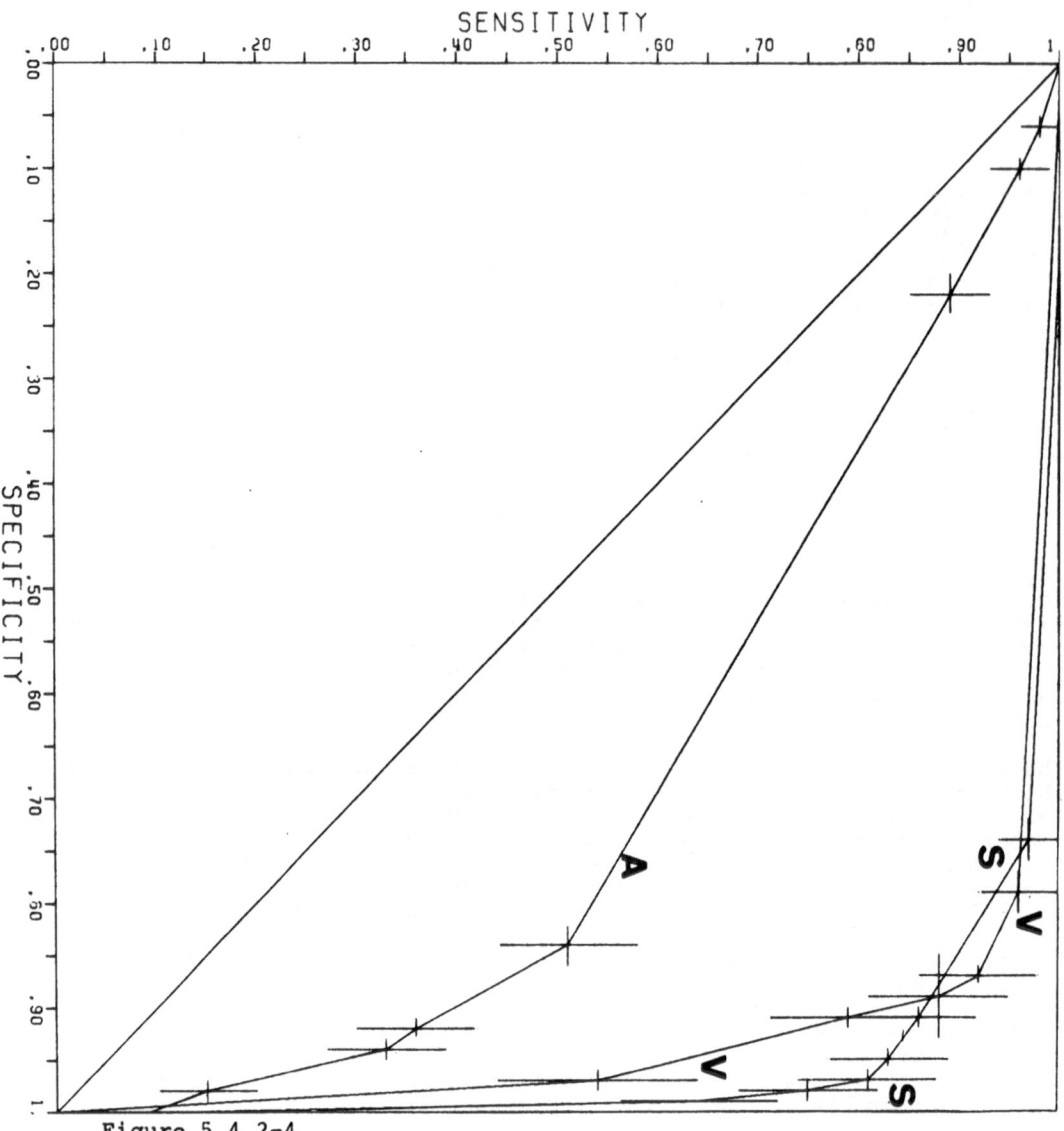

Figure 5.4.2-4

Questionnaire validity.
Questions selected on the basis of the 'U' values obtained for specific diseases are combined into composite tests, the validity of which is represented in a sensitivity specificity graph. Satisfactory values are obtained for 'spastic bronchitis, emphysema' (S) and 'veinous diseases' (V), whereas results for 'diseases of arteries' (A) are unsatisfactory. Standard deviations are given for each discrete point of measurement.

3 to progressively adapt it to desired levels of validity
4 to base question sequencing during interactive data
  acquisition on statistics
  reflecting the actual performance of a sample population using the
  questionnaire
5 to achieve compact, problem oriented and intelligible
  presentation of results.
6 to increase transparency of the instrument.

Two approaches realizing some of these principles will be reviewed in
the following.

5.5.1 NEW APPROACHES TO BRANCHING LOGIC AND PRESENTATION

WARNER described a system integrated into routine patient care
activities (131, 132, 133, 134), which seems to be the first one
realizing third stage features.

This automated history system comprises 320 questions screening for 134
disease categories. At least 50 questions are presented to a patient, 5
at a time, on a CRT- terminal. The patient may respond with 'yes'
answers only. This is accomplished by way of the patient's entering a
single digit index number which is displayed with each question. The
average time needed for completing the questionnaire is said to lie in
the order of less than 10 minutes. The program uses statistical data
contained in a matrix relating each question with each diagnosis. This
matrix is used for question selection on the basis of differential
diagnostic considerations carried out by the system. The matrix is also
referred to for the presentation of the results.

Each cell of the matrix which corresponds to one each of the questions
and diagnoses, contains a subjective estimate for the conditional
probability, that a patient with that disease will respond with 'yes'
to the particular question. After each question answered affirmatively
the probabilities for all diagnoses are determined using BAYES'
formula. The program starts by presenting a set of five of the fifty
key questions that are presented to all patients, each set pertaining
to a particular system, body area or body function. Depending on the
answers a number of modifying questions may be presented. These have to
be answered before the program proceeds to a different set of key
questions. After all modifying questions have been answered,
probabilities for disease are calculated and the program proceeds by
selecting the two most likely diagnoses. For each of these, one
question likely to confirm the respective diagnoses is selected from
among the unanswered. The criterion for selection is the ratio of the
probability that a patient with the particular disease would answer
'yes' to the question and the probabilities that a member randomly
selected from the entire population would respond by 'yes'. The latter
probabilities are calculated for every question from the probability
matrix. For this purpose, the probabilities given for each diagnosis to
the particular question are weighted according to the prevalence of the
disease and averaged over all diseases.

Another three questions are selected on the basis of their power for
discriminating between the two diseases. In this case the ratio of the
probabilities of a patient answering 'yes', if he has the disease, is
calculated for the two diseases under considerations for all remaining
questions. Questions having a probability of 0 for one or the other of

the diseases considered are preferred over any other question, since they would rule out one of the diseases.

The five selected questions are then presented and answered by the patient and the process is continued until one of two stopping rules are met:

1) the probability for a particular diagnosis exceeds .9.
2) the ratio of the probabilities of a patient answering 'yes' to the two diagnoses currently under consideration (or their reciprocals) is below 1.2.

If the last criterion applies, the most probable diagnosis will be marked for inclusion in the printout, if the sum of the probabilities for both diagnoses exceeds .5. If the probability of one diagnosis exceeds .2 it will also be presented.

The algorithm proceeds then to present the next set of five key questions. In this case all disease probabilities will be reset to a common value. This avoids that pertinent information is not picked up due to bias produced by questions previously asked and diagnoses previously arrived at. A system of flags and pointers provides that questions already answered are not presented again to the patient. The answers previously obtained are used, however, in calculating the disease probabilities. If all sets of key questions have been answered, the program concludes the session.

The history presented to the physician consists of a differential diagnostic part and a systematic part. In the differential diagnostic section, each diagnosis that the system marked for inclusion in the printout, is listed together with statements reflecting the answers that were obtained from the patient. The answer statements are printed only once in the order of decreasing probability of diseases to which they pertain. Their inclusion in a list of answers corresponding to a particular diagnosis depends on whether the ratio of the probability of a patient having the diagnosis to the corresponding average probability exceeds a value of 1.3.

In the systems review section, the positive answers not included in the previous section are reported.

The system is adaptable by using the answers obtained from patients with confirmed diagnoses for updating the probability matrices.

A different possibility has been suggested by HENDERSON (52, 53). This system concept aims at classifying a fixed set of input data with the aid of trainable pattern dichotomizers. The system requires a set of correctly classified cases as medical experience during a training phase.

The algorithm used by HENDERSON has its roots in the early approaches to artificial intelligence which resulted in the perception model of ROSENBLATT (109), and a hardware device called adaline (ADAptive LINEar device) (137). NILSSON treated this concept of pattern dichotomizers comprehensively (93), calling them 'threshold logic units' (TLU). In our experiments concerning the decision module concepts promoted by MOORE (80, 81, 86) we found that a decision module as realized in the CDSS system is also related to these 'threshold logic units'. As realized in the Clinical Decision Support System, the system that we used as supporting system for our automated history. The decision module turned out to have certain disadvantages, the most important being (75, 86, 97, 98):

1) Insufficient adaptivity since it required the programmer to programmer to explicitly specify any modifications to the decision logic and in this process to control complex decision networks.

2) Restriction to the realization of strictly boolean logic only. For this reason the system is unable to handle any condition that the programmer did not explicitly provide for.

In the form proposed by the workers in the field of artifial intelligence and neuron models, the threshold logic unit adapts automatically during a training procedure and is also able to handle patterns not previously encountered in a training set. These qualities are highly desirable in systems for history acquisition support. If there are 10 questions answered by yes-no alternatives relevant to a disease, $2**10$ response combinations are possible. If there are only a few hundred cases of this disease in the training sample, many of these combinations will not be encountered in the training set. Also the uncertainty about the real value of a question may make it necessary to delete questions from and add others to those contained in the questionnaire. In the case of addition of a new question, all previously classified cases will differ from subsequent training sets with respect to this question. The evidence available so far suggests, that threshold logic units will be able to adapt to the new situation and classify most of the new patterns correctly.

The concept has been challenged by MINSKY (74), who prooved that TLUs could not be trained to solve certain problems, and that with increasing complexity of the training task, the training process becomes computationally unfeasible. The work of HENDERSON suggests, that classification problems such as presented in the context of automated medical histories may do not belong to the unfeasible tasks.

Essentially , a threshold logic unit (TLU) is a linear discriminant function, which assigns pattern vectors to one of two classes by generating the sum of the scalar product of the pattern vector and a weight vector. Depending on whether this value is positive or negative one of the other classification (decision) outcome is assumed. Training consists essentially in generating a weight vector that produces correct classification of all offered patterns of a training set.

The process converges to a nonunique solution. The result is influenced by

- the starting weights
- the orientation of the hyperplanes corresponding to the pattern vectors
- the size of the increment
- the order in which the pattern vectors are included in the in the training process.

The weighting vector resulting from the training may therefore be suboptimal. Heuristic rules for obtaining close to optimal weighting vectors comprise

- starting with the pattern vectors that have the best discriminating power.
- expanding the training set stepwise until optimal classification of all patterns in the testing set is obtained
- including further patterns in the training set in the order of decreasing frequency, with which they have been observed.

It is conceivable that subsets of questions contained in a questionnaire are selected according to their validity for each decision represented in the set which has been defined as the range of relevance for a history taking device. The training process will then result in a weight vector for each of these decisions. This vector may be employed in the classification process and for presenting test results which may be grouped according to the categories the classification resulted in.

In a strict sense, the approach applies only to patterns that are linearly separable. The fact that this condition is rarely satisfied in medical applications makes it necessary to classify the observed patterns of responses according to their likelihood ratio, as suggested by COLLEN (18, 19) on the basis of the proposals of NEYMAN (91, 92). Practical application of this approach in clinical routine has not been described yet.

5.5.2 FURTHER PROSPECTS

Currently the compilation of an item collection according to the principles outlined above has been initiated. For this purpose, 68 problem categories were selected from the 'Verdener Problemliste' (Verden Problem List, named after a North German town, where it was developed), a diagnostic index tailored to the needs and means of the general practitioner (22, 23). They were selected according to two criteria: whether it appeared both useful and feasible to collect information concerning these target categories on the basis of anamnestic data. Seven general practitioners formulated a total of 1676 questions for this so defined range of relevance. These were grouped according to common semantic content into 476 groups of questions. These are currently further reduced in order to arrive at a manageable questionnaire size of less than 300 questions. For this, purpose an algorithm was applied in the first step, which scanned the questions and eliminated those which were considered of little use according to such criteria as

- quality of question phrasing,
- quality of target category
- number of questions available for a given target category
- number of physicians suggesting a given question
- number of target categories a question was estimated to apply for
- a threshold of a minimum number of questions per target category that should not be exceeded.

Setting the threshold value to 9, a list of 290 questions was arrived at by application of this algorithm. These are currently reevaluated by the group of physicians and edited in order to yield a practicable questionnaire.

This questionnaire is intended as a screening instrument for backup in special problem management in private offices or specialized acute care environments. It is expected to be completed by the patient himself, either at home, in his family environment, in the waiting room or on the ward. It will therefore be subdivided in at least two sections, one containing items touching the private sphere, the other items of greater general acceptability. Depending on the size of the final instrument, further subdivision or the development of parallel versions for use in different settings is contemplated. It will be realized as a portable paper and pencil device that may be read by the physician either through scanning the answers or through presentation of a problem oriented summary presentation.

Although the final form is not yet available, it becomes already evident that the spectrum and quality of questions are considerably different from those of most existing questionnaires. About 1/3 of the questions refer to social conditions. The bulk would have to be categorized under systems review. Questions pertaining to family history are practically nonexistent, those regarding past diseases are rare. Since these differences are in accordance with what was to be expected from the evaluation of the medical utility of data acquired by our experimental questionnaire, it seems not unrealistic that the instrument will prove in general to be of greater utility than instruments based on a more or less subjective compilation of questionnaire items. Further improvements of practical utility are expected from better practicability for patients and physicians and especially from progressive adaptation towards an optimized standardized instrument.

Design of an adaptive system for acquisition and evaluation based upon HENDERSON's suggestions has been initiated.

6. CONCLUDING SUMMARY

Technical aids to medical history acquisiton, frequently referred to as self-administered or impersonal medical histories have come into widespread use. The main reason for employment of such aids stems from perceived and documented shortcomings of conventional procedures of acquisition and documentation of medical histories in a variety of medical care situations. The most important shortcomings have been characterized as errors of omission and commission.

Technical aids may serve primarily to reduce the error of omission. The error of commission is likely to be only indirectly influenced in as much as provision of a more complete data base improves the result of interpretation of these data.

Apart from the realization of the need for support, the availability of the computer as potential tool for solution has stimulated research in this respect. Computer applications were at first directed at reducing the effort of acquisition and presentation of detailed histories through deterministic modeling of a physician's conduct of a medical interview. This was achieved by incorporation of branching logic into questionnaire sequences and presentation techniques. Shortcomings of this approach were due to differences in the interpretation of questions between questionnaire designer and respondent, which rendered the execution of branching instructions unreliable. Also a difference between the information needed by the physician and that provided by the history acquisition system was often perceived.

The proposed solutions are based on a review of purpose and characteristics of history taking and of basic concepts of information in medicine as well as on practical experience with an experimental history acquisition system.

The experimental basis was provided by a system developed on the basis of existing collections of questions for medical history questionnaires. The questionnaire was completed by the patient himself. Computer processing of the completed mark sense forms generated a summary which was forwarded to the physician and evaluated in several respects by testing three versions of this questionnaire on over 900 patients in internal medicine and private practices.

Prominent features of the results were that the device was well received by the patients who were also able to handle it satisfactorily despite of crude appearance and considerable volume. Detailed analysis of the medical utility of the acquired data showed that they were for the most part correct, but not always considered necessary. Also analysis of patient responses with respect to reliability and validity indicated that patients were not in every instance able to provide the required data.

In order to achieve a match between the physician's need of information, the patient's ability to provide it, a modified procedure for construction and implementation of history systems and an extension of computer application beyond the support of acquisition and presentation of data to their validation has been developed.

This proposal includes an adaptive strategy of optimization towards the identified information need of a physician. The strategy takes into account the characteristics of performance of tests and questions designed to provide this information. Instead of considering the spectrum of possible symptoms of a patient, an appropriately defined set of decisions the physician has to face is suggested as basis for definition of the contents of a questionnaire device.

In connection with adaptive techniques for acquisition and presentation of the data the history acquisition systems may become reliable and valid test instruments standardized to the extent of matching defined requirements under given circumstances.

In this respect, the proposed solutions seem relevant for the field of computer assistance in the medical decision process. In the proposed manner, the computer assisted history becomes a test which may be applied under defined conditions.

Rather than backing up the decision process in the manner of a consultant with detailed interpretation of selectively acquired data, the computer acts as an assistant preparing available data to assist in an ongoing decision process. Because the medical decision process is initiated under a variety of conditions and leads to a similar variety of outcomes its complexity is difficult to control. Computer assistance intended as an aid in the solution of problems presented by certain problem data has therefore nowhere reached the stage of routine application. The cascade of decisions unleashed by a leading symptom or symptom constellation is often so vast that the ensuing problem of data acquisition tends to render the system impracticable. Still the resulting decision networks tend to be incomplete.

The proposed approach to select the data to be acquired according to a defined spectrum of needed information enables to control the scope of a system intended as an aid in medical care decisions. Automated support of the acquisition of medical histories may in this mannner add an additional tool comparable in reliability and validity to other laboratory tests, but less costly in terms of danger to health, inconvenience and money. In this fashion it may contribute to the welfare of the patient.

LITERATURE

1 BEISSERT, A.: Die Trennung klinischer Gruppen im Fragebogenversuch, Dissertation, Heidelberg (1967)

2 BERNER, W.: Erfahrungen bei der Anwendung des Anamnesefragebogens der MHH in der Allgemeinpraxis Arbeitstagung ARO und Arbeitskreis Praktische Medizin der GMDS, Koeln (3.-5.12.1973)

3 BERNER, W.: Untersuchungen zur Automatisation der Erhebung einer Basisanamnese II. Experimentelle Anwendung des MHH-Fragebogens in der Allgemeinpraxis, Vortrag, Seminar "Systemanalyse II", Abt. Medizinische Informatik der Med. Hochschule Hannover vom 13.2.1974

4 BLOCK, H.: The Perceptron: A Model for Brain Functioning, Reviews of Modern Physics 34 (1962) 123-135

5 BLOHMKE, M.: Reproduzierbarkeit und Gueltigkeit von Fragebogen, Meth.Inf.Med., Suppl. 5, (1971) 195-205

6 BRAUN, R.N.: Die Allgemeinpraxis und der Zeitfaktor, Deutsch.Med.Wschr. 88 (1963) 2084-2092

7 BRAUN, R.N.: Lehrbuch der aerztlichen Allgemeinpraxis. (Muenchen - Berlin - Wien: Urban & Schwarzenberg 1970)

8 BRODMAN, K., ERDMANN, A.J., LORGE, I., WOLFF, H.G.: Cornell Medical Index. An Adjunct to Medical Interview, JAMA 140 (1949) 530-534

9 BRODMAN, K., ERDMANN, A.J., LORGE, I., WOLFF, H.G.: The Cornell Medical Index Health Questionnaire II as a Diagnostic Instrument, JAMA 145 (1951) 152-157

10 BRODMAN, K., ERDMAN, A.J., jr., LORGE, I., GERSHEMON, C., WOLFF, H.G.: The Cornell Medical Index Health Questionnaire III, The Evaluation of Emotional Disturbances, J.clin.Psychol. 8 (1952) 119-124

11 BRODMAN, K., ERDMANN, A.J., jr., LORGE, I., GERSHEMON, C., WOLFF, H.G.: The Cornell Medical Index Health Questionnaire IV. The Recognition of Emotional Disturbances in a General Hospital, J.clin.Psychol. 8 (1952) 289-293

12 BRODMAN, K., ERDMANN, A.J. jr., LORGE. I., WOLFF, H.G.: The Cornell Medical Index Health Questionnaire VI. The Relation of Patient's Complaints to Age, Sex, Race and Education. J. Gerontology 8 (1953) 339-342

13 BRODMAN, K., ERDMANN, A.J. jr., LORGE. I., DEUTSCHBERGER, J., WOLFF, H.G.: The Cornell Medical Index Health Questionnaire VII. The Prediction of Psychosomatic and Psychatiatric Disabilities in Army Training. Amer.J.Psychiatry III, (1954) 37-40

14 BRODMAN, K., DEUTSCHBERGER, J., ERDMANN, A.J. jr., LORGE, I., WOLFF, H.G.: Prediction of Adequacy for Military Service, U.S. Armed Forces Med.J. 5 (1954) 1802-1808

15 BUDD, M.A., BLEICH, H., BOYD, G.E., REIFFEN, B., SHERMAN, H., STRONG, R.M.: The Acquisition of Medical Histories by Questionnaires Dept. of Health, Education and Welfare HSRD 70-37 National Center of Health Service and Research Development, Report Contract HSM 69-294, Rockville, Md., (1970)

16 CEDERLOEF, R., JONSSON, E., LUNDMAN, T.: On the Validity of Mailed Questionnaires in Diagnosing "Angina Pectoris" and "Bronchitis". Arch.Env.Health 13 (1966) 738-742

17 COCHRANE, A.L., CHAPMAN, P.J., OLDHAM, P.D.: Observer's Errors in Taking Medical Histories, Lancet I, (1951) 1007-1009

18 COLLEN, M.F.: Machine Diagnosis from Multiphasic Screening Program, Proc. 5th IBM Symposium, (1963) pp. 129-153

19 COLLEN, M.F.: Automated Multiphasic Screening and Diagnosis, Am.J.Publ.Health 54 (1964) 741-750

20 COLLEN, M.F., CUTLER, J.L., SIEGELAUB, A.B., CELLA, R.L.: Reliability of a Self-Administered Medical Questionnaire, Arch.Int.Med. 123 (1969) 664-681

21 DAHMER, J.: Die aerztliche Untersuchung. (Muenchen - Berlin - Wien:

Thieme 1967)
22 DREIBHOLZ, K.J., ROHDE, P.A.: Die Verdener Diagnosenliste. Prakt.Arzt 12 (1973)
23 DREIBHOLZ, K.J., ROHDE, P.A.: Eine Diagnosenliste fuer die Allgemeinpraxis. Allg.Med.Int. 2 (1973) 94-96
24 ELSHTAIN, E.L., HAESSLER, H.A., HARDEN, C.M., HOLLAND, T.: Field Study of an Automated Pediatric Data Base History, Manuscript, (1973)
25 ENCARNACAO, J., GILOI, W., NEGRETE, J., SEYFARTH, A.: Anamnesis Dialog Assistant, Vortrag, Methoden der Informatik in der Medizinischen Datenverarbeitung, (12. - 14. Oct. 1972), Hannover
26 ERDAMNN, A.J. jr.: Experiences in the Use of Selfadministered Health Questionnaire, AMA Archives of Industrial Medicine 19 (1959) 339-343
27 ERDMANN, A.J. jr., BRODMAN, K., DEUTSCHBERGER, J., WOLFF, H.G.: Health Questionnaire Use in an Industrial Department, Indus.Med. and Surg. 22 (1953) 355-357
28 ERDMANN, A.J. jr., BRODMAN, K., LORGE, I., WOLFF, H.G.: The Cornell Medical Index Health Questionnaire V. The outpatient admitting Department of a General Hospital. JAMA (1952) 550-551
29 FAHRENBERG, J.: Methodenprobleme bei der Fragebogenkonstruktion, Meth.Inf.Med.Suppl. 5 (1971) 165-182
30 FAIRBIRN, A.S., WOOD, C.H., FLETCHER, C.M.: Variability in Answers to a Questionnaire on Respiratory Symptoms, Brit.J.Prev.Soc.Med. 13 (1959) 175-193
31 FASSL, H.E.: Die Anamnese als Informationsgewinnungsprozess, Habilitationsschrift, Mainz (1970)
32 V. FERBER, C.: Die Rolle des Arztes in der modernen Gesellschaft. Prakt.Arzt 8 (1971) 1146-1163
33 V. FERBER, L.: Verstehen und Verstaendigung zwischen Arzt und Patient, Fortschr.Med. 91, 8 (1973) 311-312, 345
34 FIELD, M.G.: Doctor and Patient in Soviet Russia, Cambridge Mass. (1965)
35 FORKNER, C.L.: Delivering the Essentials of Medical Care to all Segments of the Population, The Contribution of Systems of Computerized Medical Histories and Computerized Automated Medical Technology, Amer.J.Med.Sc. 226 (1971) 194-203
36 FRICKE, R.: Testguete - Kriterien bei lehrzielorientierten Tests (Ein Mass zur Bestimmung von Objektivitaet, Zuverlaessigkeit, Gueltigkeit und Trennschaerfe bei lehrzielorientierten Tests) Zeitschr. Erziehungswiss. Forsch. 6 (1972) 150-175
37 FRITZE, E.: Oekonomische und zugleich forschungsgerechte Krankenblattdokumentation, Verh.Dtsch.Ges.Inn.Med. 66 (1960) 1103-1105
38 GLESER, M.A., COLLEN, M.F.: Towards Automated Medical Decisions, Comp.Biomed.Res. 5 (1972) 180-189
39 GOEPEL, H.: Screeninguntersuchungen in der Allgemeinpraxis, Allg. Med. Int. 1 (1972) 54-57
40 GOLDSTEIN, S.: Assisted Recording of the Medical History (ARM): A Method of Recording the Medical History during the Interview, Comp.Biol.Med. 4 (1974) 215-222
41 GROSS, R.: Medizinische Diagnostik, Grundlagen und Praxis. (Berlin - Heidelberg - New York: Springer 1969)
42 GROSSMANN, J.H., BARNETT, G.O., MCGUIRE, M.T., SWEDLOW, D.B.: Evaluation of Computer Acquired Patient Histories, JAMA 215 (1971) 1286-1291
43 GRUENTZING, A., BLOHMKE, M.: Pruefung der Zuverlaessigkeit medizinischer Fragen in der epidemiologischen Forschung, Meth.Inf.Med. 9 (1970) 159-165
44 GRUETZIG, A., GALLA, J.: Die Ergebnisse eines Fragebogens im Vergleich mit der aerztlichen Diagnose, Meth.Inf.Med. 9 (1970) 21-26
45 GRUND-KREHL, K.: Untersuchungen zur Systematisierung der Anamnese - dargestellt am Beispiel einer chirurgischen Klinik. Dissertation, Tuebingen (1973)
46 HAESSLER, H.A., HOLLAND, T., ELSHTAIN, E.L.: Evolution of an

Automated Database History, Arch. Int. Med. 143 (1974) 586-591

47 HAESSLER, S.: Allgemeinmedizin Gegenwart und Zukunft, Stuttgart (1969)

48 HALL, P., MELLNER, CH., DANIELSSON, C.: J5 - A Dataprocessing System for Medical Information, Meth.Inf.Med. 6 (1967) 1-6

49 HARTMANN, F.: Die Anamnese (Teil 1), Klinik der Gegenwart 19 (1965) 691-718

50 HARTMANN, F.: Anamnese, Fischer Lexikon Band 1

51 HARTUNG, J., VALLEE, I.: Ueber die Reproduzierbarkeit der Anamnese, Meth.Inf.Med. Suppl.5, 81-94 (1971)

52 HENDERSON, C.: A Trainable Pattern Classifier for Medical Questionnaires, Ann.Biomed.Engin. 1 (1972) 115-133

53 HENDESRON, C.: System Design Considerations for Automated Health Screening, Meth.Inf.Med. 13 (1974) 23-29

54 HOLTHOFF, G., MOEHR. J.R.: Zur Bedetung der klinischen Basisdokumentation fuer Information und Kommunikation im Krankenhaus, Krankenhausarzt 48 (1975) 276-282

55 IMMICH, H.: Klinischer Diagnosenschluessel. (Stuttgart: Schattauer 1966)

56 JAMBON, J.R.: Interactive Medical Report System, Master Thesis, University of Minnesota, Minneapolis (1972)

57 KANNER, J.F.: Programmed Medical Historytaking with or without Computer, JAMA 207 (1969) 317-321

58 KANZLER, G., GIERE, W., MICHELS, B.: Computer Anamnese - Erfahrungen und Perspektiven, Diagnostik 6 (1973) 644-648

59 KEELE, K.D.: Uses and Abuses of Medical History, Brit.Med.J. II (1966) 1251-1254

60 KEREKJATO, M. v., MEYER, A.E., ZERSSEN, D.V.: Die HHM-Beschwerdenliste bei Patienten einer internistischen Ambulanz, Zeitschrift fuer psychosomatische Medizin und Psychoanalyse 18 (1972) 1-16

61 LANGEN, D.: Anamnese und Untersuchungen in ihrer Wechselwirkung, Meth.Inf.Med.Suppl. 5 (1971) 133-139

62 LIENERT, G.A.: Testaufbau und Testanalyse. (Weinheim - Berlin: Beltz 1961)

63 LUETH, P.: Sprechende und stumme Medizin. Ueber das Arzt-Patienten-Verhaeltnis. (Frankfurt - New York: Harder & Herder 1974)

64 MARTIN, M.J., MAYNE, J.G., TAYLOR, W.F., SWENSON, M.N.: A Health Questionnaire Based on Paper and Pencil Medium Individualized and Produced by Computer, II Testing and Evaluation, JAMA 208 (1969) 2064-2068

65 MAULTSBY. , M.C., SLACK, W.V.: A Computer Based Psychiatry History System, Arch.Gen.Psychiat. 25 (1971) 570-572

66 MAYNE, J.G., WEKSEL, W., SCHOLTZ, P.N.: Toward Automating the Medical History, Mayo Clinic Proc. 43 (1968) 1-25

67 MAYNE, J.G., MARTIN, M.J., MORROW, G.W., TURNER, R.M., HISEY, B.L.: A Health Questionnaire Based on Paper and Pencil medium Individualized and Produzeced by Computer. I Technique, JAMA 208 (1969) 2060-2063

68 MAYNE, J.G.: Experiences with the Use of Automation for Collection and Recording Medical History Data, Meth.Inf.Med. 8 (1969) 53-59

69 MAYNE, J.G., MARTIN, M.J.: Computer Aided History Acquisition, Med.Clin.North America 54 (1970) 825-833

70 MAYNE, J.G., MARTIN, M.J., TAYLOR, W.F., O'BRIEN, P.C., FLEMING, P.J.: A Health Questionnaire Based on Paper and Pencil Medium, Individualized and Produced by Computer, II Usefulness and Accepatbility to Physicians, Ann.Int.Med 76 (1972) 923-930

71 MELLNER, CH.: The Selfadministered Medical History, Acta.chir.scand.Suppl. 406 (1970)

72 MELLNER, CH., GARDMARK, S., PARKHOLM, S.: Medical Questionnaires in Clinical Practice, in Anderson, J., Forsythe, J.M., (ed.): Information Processing of Medical Records, Amsterdam - London (1970) pp 106-115

73 MEYERINGH, H.: Diskussionsbemerkung, Tagung des "Aerztlichen Sachverstaendigenbeirates fuer Fragen der Kriegsopferversorgung der BMA", Oktober 1958, Cited according to (116)

74 MINSKY, M., PAPERT, S.: Perceptrons, (Cambridge - Mass. 1969)

75 MOEHR, J.R., ODRIOZOLA, J., RIES, P.: Einsatz und Erfahrungen mit einem System fuer Klinische Entscheidungshilfe (Clinical Decision Support System) Meth.Inf.Med.Suppl. 6 (1972) 347-357

76 MOEHR, J.R., HARTMANN, W., FABEL, H.: Computerunterstuetzung fuer klinische Entscheidungen: Automatische Interpretation von Ergebnissen der Blutgasanalyse, Meth.Inf.Med.Suppl. 7 (1973) 317-323

77 MOEHR, J.R.: Prinzipien der Konstruktion und Bewertung von Anamnesefrageboegen Arbeitstagung ARO und Arbeitskreis Praktische Medizin der GMDS, Koeln (3.-5.12.73)

78 MOEHR, J.R.: Methoden zur Konstruktion und Bewertung von Frageboegen zur Erfassung einer Basisanamnese, Verh.Dtsch.Ges.Inn.Med. 80 (1974) 930-932

79 MOEHR, J.R., HAEHN, K.D.: Wer zu frueh kommt, wartet laenger - Zeitanalyse in einer Allgemeinmedizinischen Bestellparxis , Prakt. Arzt 12 (1975) 454-470

80 MOORE, F.J.: Concept of a Clinical Decision Support System, IBM Technical Report 17-209 9/66 Yorktown Heights, New York (1966)

81 MOORE, F.J.: Development of a Clinical Decision Support System, IBM Yorktown Heights, New York (1968)

82 MOORE, F.J.: Information Technologies & Health Care I. Medical Care as a system, Arch.Int.Med. 125 (1970) 157-161

83 MOORE, F.J.: Information Technologies & Health Care II. The Need for New Technologies to Offset the Shortage of Physicians, Arch.Int.Med. 125 (1970) 351-355

84 MOORE, F.J.: Information Technologies & Health Care III. The Need for New Technologies to Support the Conveyence & Use of Knowledge, Arch.Int.Med. 125 (1970) 503-508

85 MOORE. F.J.: Information Technologies & Health Care IV. The Need for New Technologies to support Planning and Management, Arch.Int.Med. 125 (9170) 711-715

86 MOORE, F.J.: Implementation of an Experimental Clinical Decision Support system, IBM Yorktown Heights, New York (1971)

87 MUIC, V., PETRES, J.J., TELISMAN, J.J.: Validity of a Diagnostic Test Designated by a Single Function, Meth.Inf.Med. 12 (1973) 244-248

88 MORCUZ, J.: Zur Beurteilung serologischer Reaktionsergebnisse, Z.Immun.Forsch. 130 (1966) 339-353

89 NEGRETE, J.: Report on the automatic Coding of Answers to the Medical Question. Where? Interner Bericht, Heinrich Hertz Institut, Berlin (1970)

90 NEGRETE, J., GILOI, W., ENCARNACAO, J.: The Application of Computer Graphics to Automate Medical Interviews, IEEE Mexico 1971, Conferencia sobre sistemas, redes y computadoras

91 NEYMAN, J.: Outline of the Statistical Treatment of the Problem of Diagnosis, Pub.Health Rep. 62 (1974) 1449-1456

92 NEYMANN, J.: First Course in Parobability and Statistics, Chapter V, New York (1950)

93 NIE, N. et al: SPSS Statistical Package for Social Sciences. (New York: Mc Graw Hill 1970

94 NILLSON, N.J.: Learning machines, New York (1965)

95 NUESSEL, E.: Das aerztliche Gespraech und die Anamnese, Dtsch.Med.Journ. 19 (1968) 45-51

96 OSHER, W.J.: Physician Evaluation of a Computer Based Automated Medical History System, Oklahoma State Med.Ass.Journ. 66 (1973) 100-104

97 PAPE, H., ODRIOZOLA, J., MOEHR, J.R.: Automatisierte Diagnostik von Knochenmarkausstrichen im Onlineverfahren mit einem Netz von Schwellenlogikelementen, Meth.Inf.Med.Suppl. 7 (1973) 311-316

98 PAPE, H.: Entwicklung und Anwendung eines Programmsystems zur Teilautomatisation der Befundung von Knochenmarkausstrichen,

Dissertation, Medizinische Hochschule Hannover (1974)

99 PEARLMAN, M.H., HAMMOND, W.E., THOMPSON, H.K.: An Automated "Well Baby" Questionnaire, Pediatrics 51 (1973) 972-979

100 PIPBERGER, H.V., KLINGEMAN, J.D., COSMA, J.: Computer Evaluation of Statistical Properties of Chest Pain, Meth.Inf.Med. 7 (1968) 79-92

101 POCKLINGTON, P.: AMAP - A General Optimal Mark Reader Form Evaluation Program, Meth.Inf.Med. 12 (1973) 211-222

102 PONDOEV, G.G.: Notes of a Soviet Doctor, London (1959)

103 REICHERTZ, P.L.: Moderne Computertechniken zur Anamneseerhebung, Meth.Inf.Med.Suppl. 5, Stuttgart/New York (1971)

104 REICHERTZ, P.L.: Medical School of Hannover Hospital Computer System (Hannover), in Collen, M.F. (ed.): Hospital Computer Systems, pp 598-661, New York (1974)

105 REICHERTZ, P.L.: Informationssysteme in der Medizin, (Bonn/Bad Godesberg: IBM, 1975)

106 REISNER, I.: Die Bedeutung von Screening-Fragen im Prozess der Anamneseerhebung, Meth.Inf.Med.Suppl. 5 (1971) 321-325

107 ROSE, G.A.: The Diagnosis of Ischaemic Heart Pain and Intermittent Claudication in Field Surveys, Bull. W.H.O. 27 (1962) 645-658

108 ROSE, G.A.: 2. Chest Pain Questionnaire, Milbank Mem.Fun.Quart. 43 (1965) 32-39

109 ROSENBLATT, F.: Principles of Neurodynamics Perceptrons and the Theory of Brain Mechanism, Washington (1962)

110 ROSENTHAL, I., HARTMANN, F.: Theophraste Renaudot, Idee und Form seiner Taetigkeit als Polikliniker

111 RUBIN, T., et al.: The Use of Interview Data for Detection of Association in Field Studies, J.Chron.Dis. 4 (1956) 253-266

112 RUBIN, L., COLLEN, M.F., GOLDMAN, G.E.: Frequency Decision Theoretical Approach to Automated Medical Diagnosis, LeCam, L.M., Neyman, J. (ed.): Proc. 5th Berkeley Symposium, Los Angeles (1967) 867-886

113 SAUTER, K.: Integrierte Datenbank und Patienteninformationssystem im Medizinischen System Hannover, Habilitationsschrift, Medizinische Hochschule Hannover, Hannover (1972)

114 SAUTER, K., REICHERTZ, P.L., ZOWE, W.: Die zentrale Patientendatenbank in einem integrierten Hospital Informationssystem, Meth.Inf.Med. 11 (1972) 91-96

115 SCHAEFER, M.: Faktorenanalytische Ueberpruefung klinischer Frageboegen , Dissertation, Heidelberg (1968)

116 SCHENK, E.G.: Kunstfehler und mangelndes Verstaendnis bei der Aufnahme der Anamnese, Med. Welt 50 (1960) 2631-2638

117 SCHWARZROCK, R.: Untersuchungen zur Automatisation der Erhebung einer Basisanamnese, I Experimentelle Anwendung des MHH-Fragebogens in der Medizinischen Klinik, Vortrag, Seminar "Systemanalyse II", Abt.Medizinische Informatik der Medizinischen Hochschule Hannover vom 13.2.1974

118 SEYFARTH, A., ENCARNACAO, J., NEGRETE, J.: AMANDA - Automatized Medical Anamnesis Dialog Assistant, Technischer Bericht Nr. 147, Heinrich Hertz Institut, Berlin (1971)

119 SIMMONS, Jr., E.M. MILLER, O.W.: A New Concept in Automated Patient Histories in Anderson, J., Forsythe, J.M. (ed.): Information Processing of Medical Records, Amsterdam - London (1970) 116-132

120 SIMMONS, E.M., MILLER, O.W.: Automated Patient History Taking - Automated Patient History Acquisition System (APHAS) Provides Valid Information and Conserves Physician's Time and Energies, Hospitals JAHA 45 (1971) 56-59

121 SLACK, W.V., HICKS, G.P., REED, C.E., VAN CURA, L.J.: A Computer Based Medical History System, New Eng.J.Med. 274 (1966) 194-198

122 SLACK, W.V., VAN CURA, L.J.: Patient Reaction to Computer Based Medical Interviewing, Comp.Biomed.Res. 1 (1968) 527-531

123 SLACK, W.V., VAN CURA, L.J.: Computer Based Patient Interviewing, Postgraduate Medicine, 68-74, 115-120 (1968)

124 SLACK, W.V., SLACK, C.W.: Good Questions and Bad in Anderson, J., Forsythe, J.M. (ed.): Information Processing of Medical Records, Amsterdam - London (1970) pp 133-143

125 SLACK, W.V.: Computer Based Interviewing System Dealing with Nonverbial Behaviour as well as Keyboard Responses, Science 171 (1971) 84-87

126 SLACK, W.V., SLACK, C.W.: Patient Computer Dialogue, New Eng.J.Med. 286 (1972) 1304-1309

127 STERLING, T.D., GLESER, M., HABERMAN, S., POLLACK, S.: Robot Data Screening: A Solution to Multivariate Type Problems in the Biological and Social Sciences, Comm.A.C.M. 9 (1966) 529-532

128 STERLING, T.D., HABERMAN, S., POLLACK, S.: Robot Data Screening, an Automated Search Technique, Biomed.Comp. 1 (1970) 61-73

129 VECCHIO, T.J.: Predictive Value of a Single Diagnostic Test in Unselected Populations, New Eng.J.Med. 274 (1966) 1171-1173

130 WAITZKIN, H., STOECKLE, H.: The Communication of Information About Illness - Clinical, Sociological and Methodological Considerations, Adv. Psychosom.Med. 8 (1972) 180-215

131 WARNER, H.R., OLMSTED, C.M., RUTHERFORD, B.D.: HELP - A Program for Medical Decision Making, Comp.Biomed.Res. 5 (1972) 65-74

132 WARNER, H.R., RUTHERFORD, B.D., HOUTCHENS, B.: A Sequential Bayesiaen Approach to History Taking and Diagnosis, Computers Biomed.Res. 5 (1972) 256-262

133 WARNER, H.R..: Health Evaluation Through Logical Processing - HELP Kansai Institute of Information Systems, Proc. Medis'73, Osaka (1973) pp 197-303

134 WARNER, H.R., MORGAN, J.D., PRYOR, T.A., CLARK, S., MILLER, W.: HELP - A Self-Improving System for Medical Decision Making, in Anderson, J., Forsythe, J.M. (ed.): Medinfo'74, Amsterdam: North Holland (1974) pp 989-993

135 WEED, L.L.: Medical Records, Medical Education and Patient Care. (Cleveland: Press of the Case Western Reserve University 1969)

136 WESTRIN, C.G.: The Reliability of Auto-Anamnesis - A Study of Statements Regarding Low Back Trouble, Scand.J.Med. 2 (1974) 23-25

137 WIDROW, B.: Generalization of Information Storage in Networks of Adaline "Neurons", Marshall et al. (ed.): Washington, (1962) pp 453-461

138 YOUDEN, J.: Index for Rating Diagnostic Tests, Cancer 3 (1950) 32-35

139 YARNALL, S.R., SAMUELSON, P., WAKEFIELD, B.S.: Clinical Evaluation of Automated Screening History, North West Medicine (1972) 186-191

140 YOUNG, D.W.: Assessment of Questions and Questionnaires, Meth.Infor.Med. 10 (1971) 222-228

141 YOUNG, D.W.: Comparison of Information Collected by a Questionary with that in the Patient's Hospital Record, Meth.Inf.Med. 11 (1972) 20-22

142 YOUNG, D.W.: Evaluation of Questionnaire, Meth.Inf.Med. 11 (1972) 11-19

143 ZEINER-HENRIKSON, T.: The Repeatability at Interview of Symptoms of Angina and possible Infarction, J.Chron.Dis. 25 (1972) 407-414

144 ZERSSEN, D.V.: Die Beschwerdenliste als Test, Therapiewoche 21 (1971) 1908-1920.

MEDICAL LANGUAGE DATA PROCESSING

Friedrich Wingert, Münster

1   Need and Application Areas for Formal Representation of Language Data

The present form of the medical record has been developed when patient care was primarily a single physician-patient relation. It has been used by the physician to record his observations and orders. Thus the medical record has been, in the legal sense,
the rationale of clinical decisions and actions. It is most important that the data
have been written down by a physician to be read again by himself, if necessary. This
fact has led to an extremely physician-related document with subjective associations,
omissions, ordering, nomenclature, style etc.. The largest part of the medical record
contains free text, often handwritten and illegible to other people.

In modern medicine the environment has changed, but document has not. Several physicians, nurses and technical personnel take care of a patient in a hospital and several medical specialities are engaged in the process of diagnostics, therapy and surveillance [1]. All these people may add data to the medical record which suffer from
the same weaknesses. The result is a fairly unstructured document, unreliable with
respect to completeness and correctness and in general useless for research. Hundreds
of medical students each year and not only students extract data from these documents
for "research".

In this situation it is not sufficient to argue that the system is running. It is unknown, how many important data have not been captured, how many data have been captured several times, how often relevant data in the medical record are not recognized
or are misunderstood by an attending physician, especially when he is short in time,
and how many hours medical students waste their time in generating tables and false
hypotheses or even "proofs" from medical records.

The goal is the generation of documents which really support health care delivery in
every day routine and in research, i. e., communication, justification and analysis.
Tasks that have to be done to reach this goal are

- *standardization* of the medical terminology, procedures and
  data structures,
- explicit *rules* for data aggregation and communication.

It seems to be reasonable to investigate, how far qualitative characteristics for computer programs, like portability, adaptability and reliability [10] can be applied to the medical record.

Basically there is only one alternative to natural language-based systems in the documentation of medical language data: Language data have to be coded by men into a highly formalized artificial language. Experience shows, that physicians are in general neither willing to learn such an artificial language and work as a code clerk, nor are they well performing this job. In other words, special personnel has to be used to translate natural language statements into artificial language statements. Despite the fact that such personnel is expensive and is available in a limited number only, the results are loaded with a high error rate due to errors in interpretation and transcription and due to inconsistency of interpretation.

Because most of the data in medicine are in language form, use of computers in medical data processing directly leads to the problems connected with the processing of language data. If computers are accepted as a powerful tool for the improvement of communication of data and information, than the problems of processing of language data have to be solved.

Communication in general is the application area which can be subdivided according to the links of communication chains:

Physician A ⟷ file ⟷ Physician A, B: Report, consultation, document, medical record.

Patient ⟷ Physician: Diagnostic chain (Speech analysis: drug influence, psychoses); medical history taking; orders.

Another scheme can be derived from clinical routine:

- Initiating and performing the diagnostic and therapeutic procedures,

- timely collecting, summarizing and reporting data,

- storage and retrieval of medical records for retrospective studies.

In the broader sense, language used in medicine is natural language, which becomes more specific when only physicians or paramedical personnel are linked in the communication chain.

2   Goals of Automated Processing of Medical Language Data

Let me first give a rough scheme of the decision process in clinical medicine:

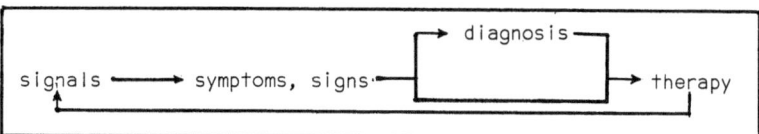

The signals are perceived by physicians and are interpreted as *symptoms* or *signs*.
Symptoms and signs are collected and can be abstracted and classified as a *diagnosis*.
Symptoms and signs either lead directly or via diagnosis to a *therapy* which may generate new signals. These processes include comprehensing and generating language-based
informations and indexing of these informations due to accepted classification schemes.

Computer-based processing of medical language data involves

- *recognition* resp. *analysis* (morphological, syntactical, semantical)
  of a language string,

- *representation* of the content using a data structure.

2.1   FUNCTIONAL GOALS

Functional goals are derived from the mental processes involved in extracting, collecting, ordering and retrieving informations in medicine. They are:

- Automated *indexing* of medical utterances due to a given classification
  scheme.

- Automated *abstracting* of medical documents.

- Automated *retrieval* and counting of medical facts and documents.

There is a significant gap between theoretical terminology and language which is
used in practice. This gap may lead to contradictions between several goals such as
serving of local needs versus international compatibility.

2.2   DERIVED GOALS

Derived goals are combined functional goals and/or are combined with functional goals
of areas of interest other than medical language data processing. Examples are:

- Support for medical decision making,

- support for medical education,
- generation of medical reports,
- machine translation,
- health cost estimation,
- linking of different classification schemes,
- generation of hypotheses about syndromes that have to be verified
  genetically, etiologically or pathogenetically,
- language-based question-answering systems.

3 Components of Language Data Processing

3.1 DEFINITIONS

Natural language: This is not the place and I do not have the competence to evaluate the extensive literature on natural language. So far, there seems to be no definition of natural language which is fundamentally different from: *General-purpose tool of communication within a speech community*. That means, language is used by a transmitter to encode informations out of a human information store and has to be decoded by a receiver. Language elements are words, signs and rules for combination of words in such a way, that a message can be understood by human beings in a special domaine of discourse.

Natural language in medicine: Fuzzy subset of natural language which is used by competent speekers in medicine speaking about medicine.

Artificial language: Designed for a restrictive purpose by and for specialists for use in a limited domaine of knowledge and application [25].

An artificial language consists of words and rules for combining words. Mapping of an utterance formulated in natural language into an utterance formulated in an artificial language has to be done in such a way that the information content of both formulations is approximately identical.

Medical language: Artificial language for the communication of medical informations.

Medical language is not just natural language in medicine. As we will see later, there are additional rules and there is dominance of semantics over syntax which is different from natural language. On the other hand, medical language lacks of most of the advantages present in highly formalized artificial languages, like (1) precision, (2) axiomatic characterization, (3) suitability for computer processing, (4) lack of ambiguities, (5) inferential power, (6) explicit specification of rules for determination of language structure and content, (7) formal rule notation [25].

Medical Document: Collection of data representing medical informations with concern to a special patient. The types of data in a medical document are:

- Identification data (patient identification, hospital identification, etc.),
- content data (lab results,(medical) language data, pictures, etc.).

Term: Word or phrase used for denotation of a semantic concept.

Descriptor: Term which can be used in an artificial language for denotation of a semantic concept. Descriptors can be *simple* descriptors or *compound* descriptors (denotation of compound semantic concepts).

Synonyms: Different terms denoting the same semantic concept.

Quasi-synonyms: Different terms denoting different semantic concepts which are not differentiated in the respective system.

Homonym: Term denoting context-dependent different semantic concepts.

Equivalence class: Set of all synonyms and quasi-synonyms.

Preferred term: Selected descriptor representing an equivalence class, i. e., representing a semantic concept. Sometimes the terms "descriptor" and "preferred term" are used as synonyms.

Nomenclature: List of terms for denotation of semantic concepts.

Terminology: List of terms related to semantic concepts.

Classification: Set of all preferred terms and of their (hierarchical) relations.

Thesaurus: List of descriptors and relations between descriptors:

- Used for *terminologic control,* i. e., translation from natural language utterances into artificial language utterances and vice versa.
- *Controlled* and *dynamic vocabulary* containing all terms, which are used to describe a specific domaine of discourse.

A thesaurus contains implicitly a classification, but is restricted to those terms and relations which are used. Additional weights of descriptors may be defined to identify the relevance of a descriptor for information retrieval.

Equivalence relation: Establishing of an equivalence class.

Hierarchical relation: Logical subordination, expecially

>   Generic relation: The semantic concept denoted by the more specific
>   term is fully contained in the semantic concept denoted by the more
>   general term and differs from the more general semantic concept with
>   concern to at least one characteristic (e. g., inflammation - acute
>   inflammation).
>
>   Partitive relation: The more specific term denotes a part of a whole,
>   the latter being denoted by a more general term (e. g., kidney-urogenital
>   system).

Associative relation: Each important relation which is neither an equivalence relation nor a hierarchical relation, e. g., marking of terms with the same generic general term (e. g., urogenital system - kidney, ureter, urinary bladder, ...) (see section 7.1).

3.2   TYPES OF MEDICAL UTTERANCES

The most important types of utterances with respect to medical language data processing are symptoms, signs, diagnoses, orders and descriptions.

The data collected in the usual medical history taking are subsumed here under
"descriptions". In general, these descriptions lack in precision and standardization
and they are on a low level of objectivity and abstraction. In pathology, for example,
where the data seem to be more reproducable than in other medical areas, the descriptive part of a report serves several objectives:

- *Justification* of a diagnosis by verbalizing a picture and listing
  the criteria related to the diagnosis.
- *Modification* of a diagnosis when the diagnostic term available does
  not meet fully the findings.
- *Compensation* for a missing unique diagnosis.

Experience leads to the conclusion, that a diagnosis usually cannot be derived from
descriptions alone, which is even true for that pathologist who formulated the description. In general, he prefers to look at the specimen. That means, a diagnosis
contains more or other informations than the related description does. Therefore, and
because descriptions are formulated in natural language in medicine, processing of
pure descriptions will be excluded from the discussion for the present. But because
there is no sharp distinction between medical language (e. g. diagnoses) and natural
language in medicine, the problems may nevertheless occur and will have to be handled.

4   Morphology

Morphology is the theory of minimal meaningful units or morphemes and their arrangements in forming words. Morphemes are also called *basic productive constituents*. Morphemes are strings of characters of minimal length, carrying grammatical and/or semantic information which is relevant in automatic language data processing. It is important to mention that morphemes are not only defined by a *sequence* of characters
but also by their *position* in a sequence of morphemes forming a word. This can be demonstrated by the following examples (e. g., VERBINDUNG - UNGEBUNDEN, PERFORATING -
INGENIOUS). The order of morphemes forming a word is usually much more rigid than the
order of words forming an utterance. This fact has been used to justify a contrast
between *morphology* and *syntax*. On the other hand, it can be argued that the inflectional morphemes in inflectional languages are markers not only of *morphological* relationships but also of *morphosyntactic* and *morphosemantic* relationships or values
and indicate the boundaries of syntactic structures. For this reason, it does not seem
to be useful to draw a sharp distinction between morphology and syntax.

For conveniance the following formal notation for case and number will be adopted:
S denotes singular, P denotes plural and the digits 1, 2, 3 and 4 denote the different cases, e. g., S1 (nominativ singular), P14 (nominativ and accusative plural).

In morphosyntactical analysis a word w can be split into a *stem form* t and an *inflectional morpheme* s:

$$w = t * s.$$

In general, the stem form t carries the semantical information and the inflectional
morpheme carries syntactical information:

$$w = MAGENS \longrightarrow t = MAGEN, \quad s = S.$$

The syntactical information of the morpheme s is not one-valued but is a function
of both components of a word. This issue can be formulated by a bivariate function,
where the same inflectional morpheme s may have different values:

$$
\begin{aligned}
f(MAGENS) &= f(MAGENS*S) &= S2 \\
f(TESTS) &= f(TEST*S) &= S2\ P1234
\end{aligned}
$$

Because stems can be connected to different inflectional morphemes and the same inflectional morpheme can be connected to different stems, the number of different words
is by far greater than the sum of the numbers of stems and inflectional morphemes. If

the number of stems is n_+ and the number of inflectional morphemes is n_s, than the total number of components is $n = n_+ + n_s$, whereas the product $n_+ \cdot n_s$ is an upper limit for the total number of words. In natural languages the number of different words is much less then this upper limit, because most of the theoretical combinations of stems and inflectional morphemes are not used. But this number is still by far greater than the sum of the numbers of the components. For this reason, most projects in machine translation use morpheme dictionaries instead of dictionaries of full forms. Following this *segmentation* approach [27, 30, 41] we have several advantages:

- The dictionaries are relatively small, leading to substantial savings in *storage space* and *access time*.

- New words can be segmented, even if they have not been considered when the dictionary has been constructed. Therefore, necessary *dictionary update* is significantly reduced.

- About 2/3 of medical terms are based on Greek and Latin. Therefore, a dictionary of morphemes may serve as a basis for *multilingual dictionaries*.

These advantages are partly compensated by the need for the development of rules for the combination and disambiguation of morphemes. Especially a *discovery procedure* for the segmentation of words and a *synthesizer* for the construction of words or even phrases from morphemes have to be developed.

4.1   FORMAL REPRESENTATION OF RESULTS

There are several formal representations of the results of a morphosyntactical ana-lysis in computable form, such as

- Tree representation (Fig. 1),
- Formation rules (Fig. 2),
- Matrix representation (Fig. 3),
- Decision table (Fig. 4).

4.2   MORPHOSYNTACTIC ALGORITHMS

So far, the notion of stems and inflectional morphemes has been introduced. German language and medical language make extensive use of compound word forms which may even paraphrase whole sentences. In medical language the reason for this behaviour is quite clear: utterances are shorter, simpler and therefore less ambiguous:

LARYNGOTRACHEOBRONCHITIS = Inflammation of the larynx, trachea and bronchus

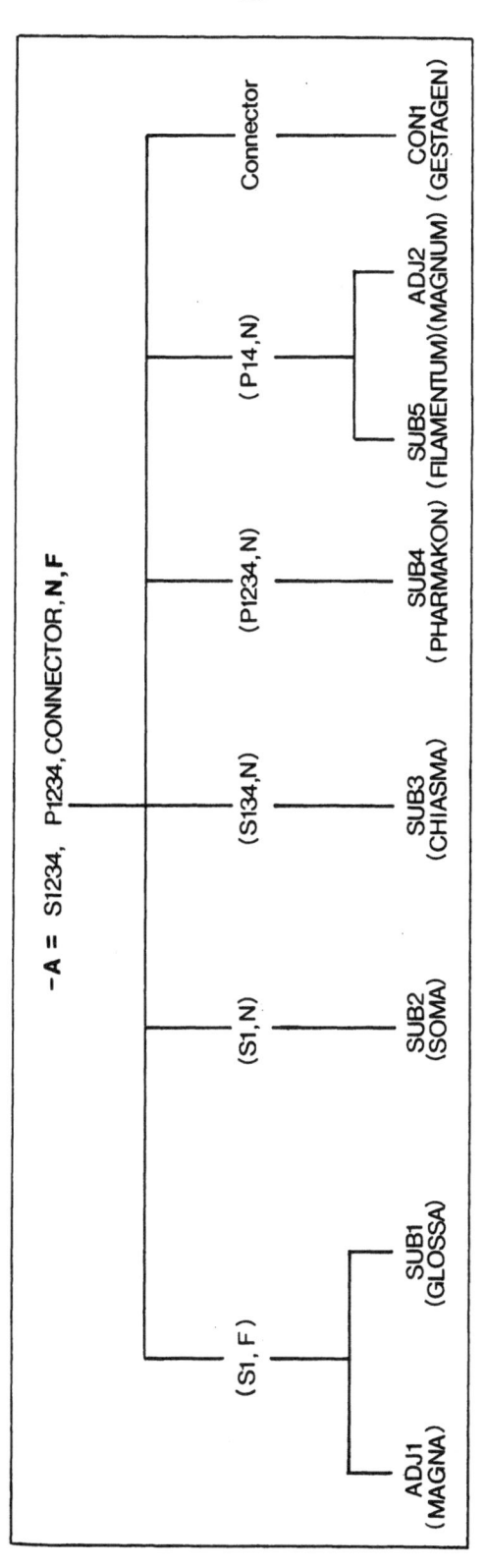

Fig. 1: Tree representation of the results of the morphosyntactical analysis of suffix -A in German medical language data. There are 2 adjectival classes (ADJ) and 5 noun classes (SUB). For each class an example is given. The genders are denoted as N for neutrum and F for feminine.

$$- A \cdot (SUB1 \cup ADJ1) \subset (S1, F)$$
$$- A \cdot (SUB2) \qquad \subset (S1, N)$$
$$- A \cdot (SUB3) \qquad \subset (S134, N)$$
$$\cdots\cdots\cdots\cdots$$

Fig. 2: Formation rules for the results of the morphosyntactic analysis of suffix -A in German medical language data.

	SUB1	SUB2	SUB3	SUB4	SUB5	ADJ1	ADJ2	CON1
S1	F	N	N			F		
S2								
S3			N					
S4			N					
P1				N	N		N	
P2				N				
P3				N				
P4				N	N		N	
Con-nector								*

Fig. 3: Matrix representation for the results of the morpho-syntactic analysis of suffix -A in German medical language data.

	SUB1	SUB2	SUB3	SUB4	SUB5	ADJ1	ADJ2	CON1
−A	(S1, F)	(S1,M)	(S134,N)	(P1234,N)	(P14,N)	(S1,F)	(P14,N)	*
−AE	. . .							
.								
.								
.								

Fig. 4: Decision table for the results of the morphosyntactic analysis of suffix -A in German medical language data.

The paraphrase uses 7 words, a comma and 41 characters other than blank, whereas the compound word form uses only 24 characters. The compound word form carries additional information, because the sequence of the site markers follows a logical path. It may therefore be more efficient to segment stems into morphemes.

Two models may be presented here. In one model terminal morphemes are identified, in the other one there is a full segmentation of words.

4.2.1   Identification of Terminal Morphemes

Suffixes are analyzed from right to left and are compared with a tree-structured set of "productive" suffixes [30]. The longest entry found in the tree, matching the analyzed suffix, is taken. The length of suffixes is restricted to 4 characters. Productive suffixes are connected to a set of rules, identifying parts of speech, as well as

- adjective to noun transformations,
- noun to noun transformations,
- noun plural to noun singular transformations.

Parts of a rule are <type> and <remainder>. <type> identifies a suffix as adjective (A) or noun (N). The remainder consists of permissible morphological transformations (Fig. 5). If necessary, the transformations are applied and are verified using a reference dictionary. A permissible transformation consists of a target parts of speech symbol, an integer, denoting the number of characters which have to be deleted and a

```
L

AL        A N2A N2E N2UM N2US

NAL

INAL      A N4EN

EAL       A N3US N3ES

GEAL      A N4X

CEAL      A N4X

IAL       A N3US

CAL       A N4IX N4EX N4ERY

ICAL      A N4IX N4EX N4ERY

RAL

ORAL      A N4UR
```

Fig. 5: **L-tree of productive suffixes [30].**

string, which has to be appended to the right of the remaining string. The model will be discussed in more detail in section 8.4.1.

4.2.2   Segmentation Approach

The second model uses a segment dictionary [41] and will be discussed in more detail because it seems to be more efficient for medical language.

Ultimate goal is the segmentation of every word used in medical language into pieces (*segments*) carrying syntactical and/or semantical information which cannot be broken down into smaller pieces. The linguistic entity "morpheme" often imposes problems, which may be avoided. Therefore, an approach is taken, which is slightly different from the usual linguistic approach.

The principles underlying the model are:

- There are different types of segments, listed in dictionaries; the dictionaries are linked by a set of rules.

- There is an explicit structure of words as a repetitive sequence of elements, where each element consists of segments of different types in fixed order.

- Segmentation of words is done from left to right and follows a principle of longest valid match.

4.2.2.1 Words and Segments

For further description there have to be definitions of different types of *segments*.

A *root* is a string of characters carrying semantical information which cannot be decomposed into meaningful parts by splitting the root. Note, that not every string, which carries semantical information has to be a root. In practice, the definition is done by enumeration.

A *secondary string* is every string which is not part of a root and which is used for building a word. The empty string is a secondary string. In general, a secondary string consists of two parts:

(1) *derivational* suffix,
(2) *terminal* suffix.

The terminal suffix can be an *inflectional* suffix or it can be a *connector* (Fig. 6).

$$w = R_1 s_1 t_1 R_2 s_2 t_2 \ldots R_n s_n t_n \quad (n \geq 1)$$

Fig. 6: Canonical form of a word w in terms of roots (R), derivational suffixes (s) and terminal suffixes (t).

For simplicity, I will not differentiate between the two parts of a secondary string in the following discussion.

With some language specific exceptions there is:

- The derivational suffix determines the connector(s) and the inflectional suffixes.

- In many noun-adjective transformations only the exchange of the secondary string is necessary.

- Many roots are derived from Latin or Greek roots, sometimes used in their original form, sometimes adapted to the English or German language. In the latter case, mostly the replacement of language specific parts of the secondary string is necessary for translation from English to German and vice versa.

Sometimes suffixes carry semantic informations. This has been analyzed for the suffixes *-osis* and *-iasis* in English and French [27]. Other examples are: *-itis* (inflammation), *-oma* (tumors), *-ase* (enzymes), *-one* (ketones), *-ite*, *-ide* (salts). In these cases the decision is arbitrary whether the segment belongs to the set of roots, or to the set of secondary strings carrying semantic information. So far, these segments are used as secondary strings due to a more or less technical reason: These segments are always preceded by roots. If they would be defined as roots, than the number of roots, which can be connected by the empty string would increase and the degree of ambiguity would be raised.

A *morphosyntactical class* number n contains a set (family) S_n of secondary strings

$$S_n = \{s_{n1}, s_{n2}, \ldots\}, \quad 0 \leq n \leq 255,$$

where each member s_{ni} is associated with a specific syntactical and/or semantical information.

For a root R associated with class number n all the constructions

$$R * S_n = \{Rs_{n1}, Rs_{n2}, \ldots\}$$

are *valid*, that is, the sequence Rs_{ni} is correct in a word. Each construction Rs_{ni} carries the syntactical information associated with s_{ni}.

If a secondary string s_j is associated with class number n, than s_j is a member of family S_n.

There are about 250 classes with morphosyntactical (Fig. 7) and semantical information. Each root is assigned to at least one class. The maximum number of classes a root belongs to is 14.

Morphosyntactical and semantical values are assigned to constructions and are not related to secondary strings alone. Thus there is no problem to distinguish between suffix -om marking a tumor and suffix -om in Coelom (Fig. 16).

	Case	Number	Gender	Degree of comparison	Person	Tense	Voice
Nominals	*	*	*				
Pronominals (excl. personal pronouns)	*	*					
Adjectivals Participles	*	*	*	*			
Verbals	*	*			*	*	*
Personal pronouns	*	*			*		

Fig. 7: Syntactical informations for different parts of speech.

The purpose is the same information PRATT [30] gets by the identification of terminal morphemes. The advantage is the handling of smaller pieces of information and the knowledge of the root and secondary string usable with the respective root, i. e., there is a direct relation between the various possible forms derived from a root, thus reducing the number of noise words generated significantly and establishing a direct relation between the original Latin or Greek form and the equivalent English or German form in about 2/3 of all cases. This is a basis for the translation of diagnostic statements. The disadvantage is the need for a larger dictionary.

Detailed class descriptions go beyond the purpose of this paper, but a few examples may show the principles (Fig. 8 - 12).

A construction $d_i d_{i+1}$ is a *valid pair*, if d_i is a root and d_{i+1} is a secondary string and d_i and d_{i+1} are associated with the same class number (there may be more than one).

A sequence $d_1 d_2 \ldots d_j$ is a *sequence of valid pairs*, if each pair $d_i d_{i+1}$ (i being an odd number) is a valid pair and if - for an odd number j - d_j is a root.

The *canonical form* of a word w is a sequence of valid pairs (Fig. 6)

$$w = R_1 s_1 R_2 s_2 \ldots R_n s_n .$$

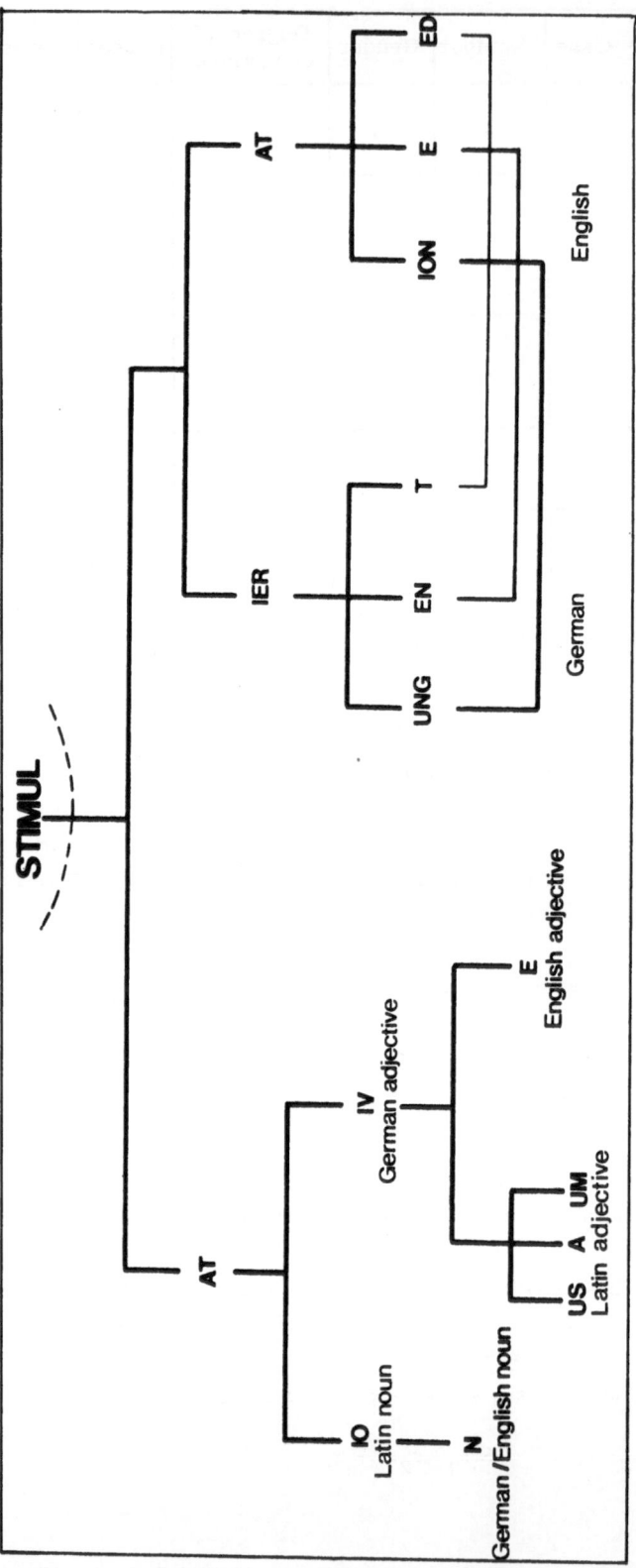

Fig. 9: Suffix families S_{31} and S_{86}[41].

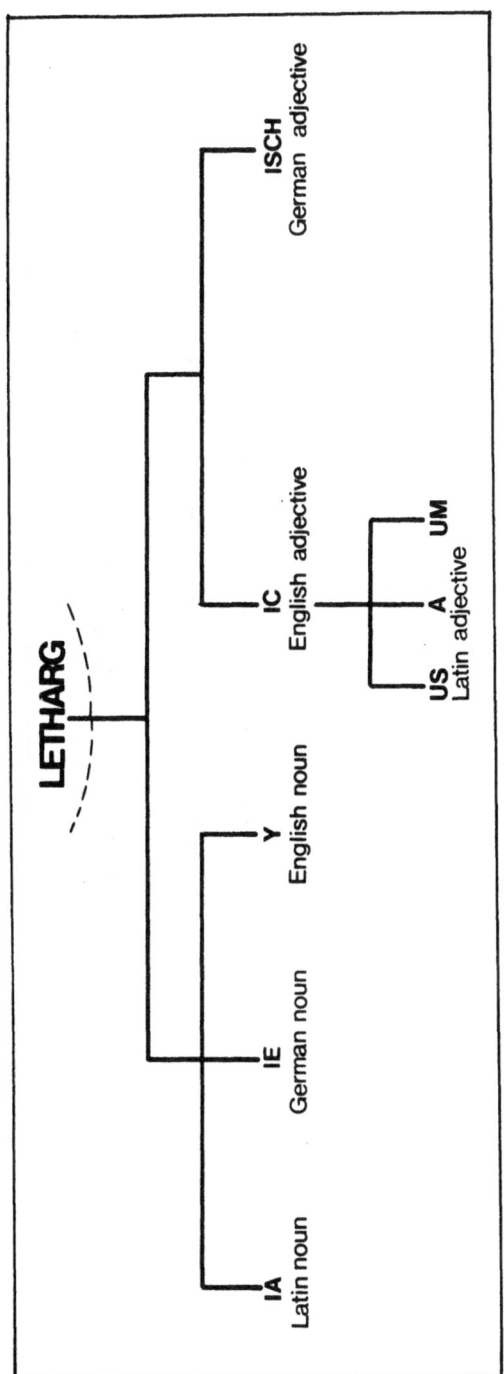

Fig. 10: Suffix families S_{33} and S_{66}[41].

596

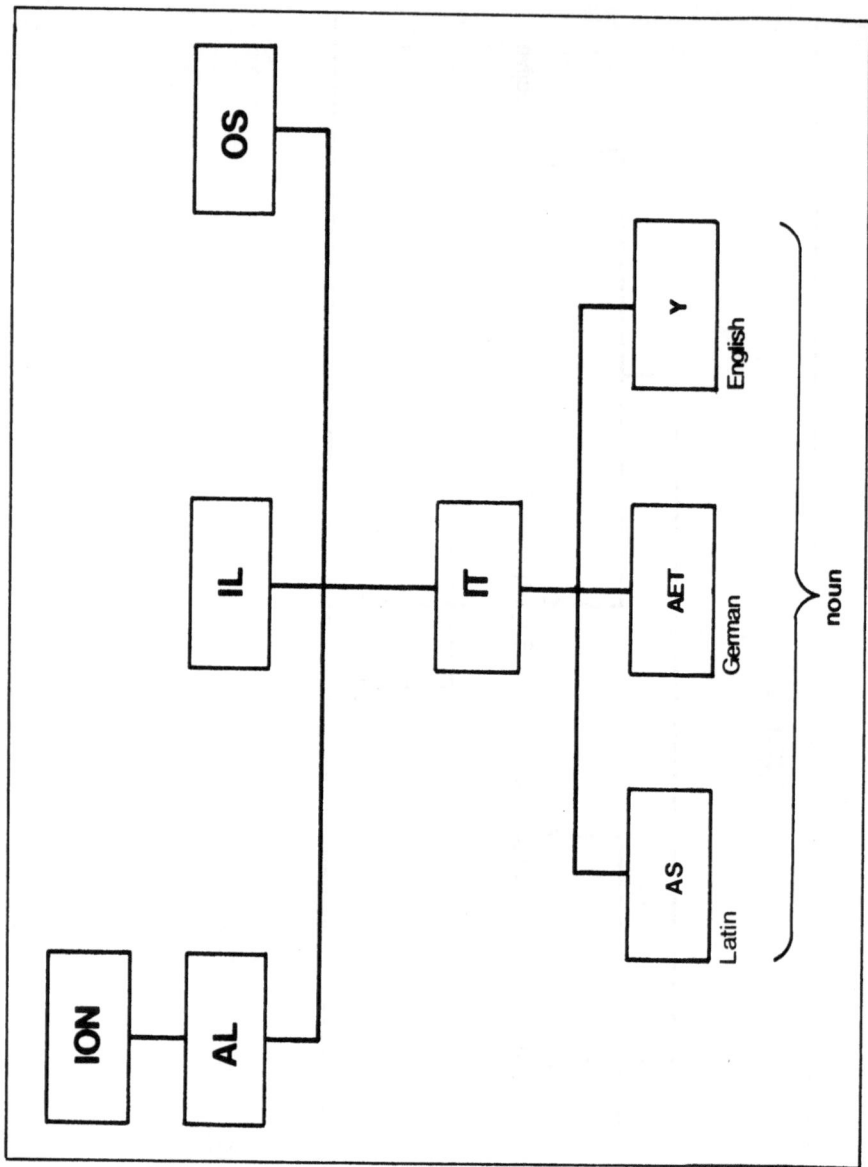

Fig. 11: Part of a suffix tree. Each box belongs to another family [41].

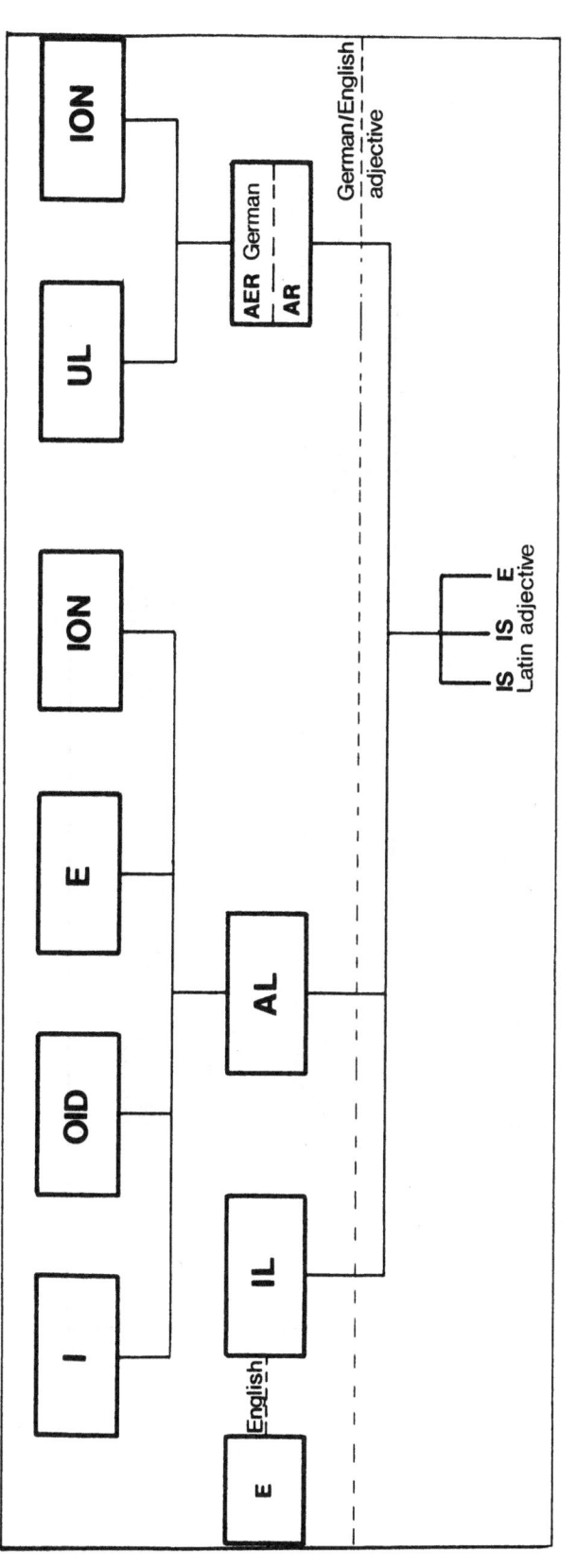

Fig. 12: Part of a suffix tree. Each box belongs to another family [4].

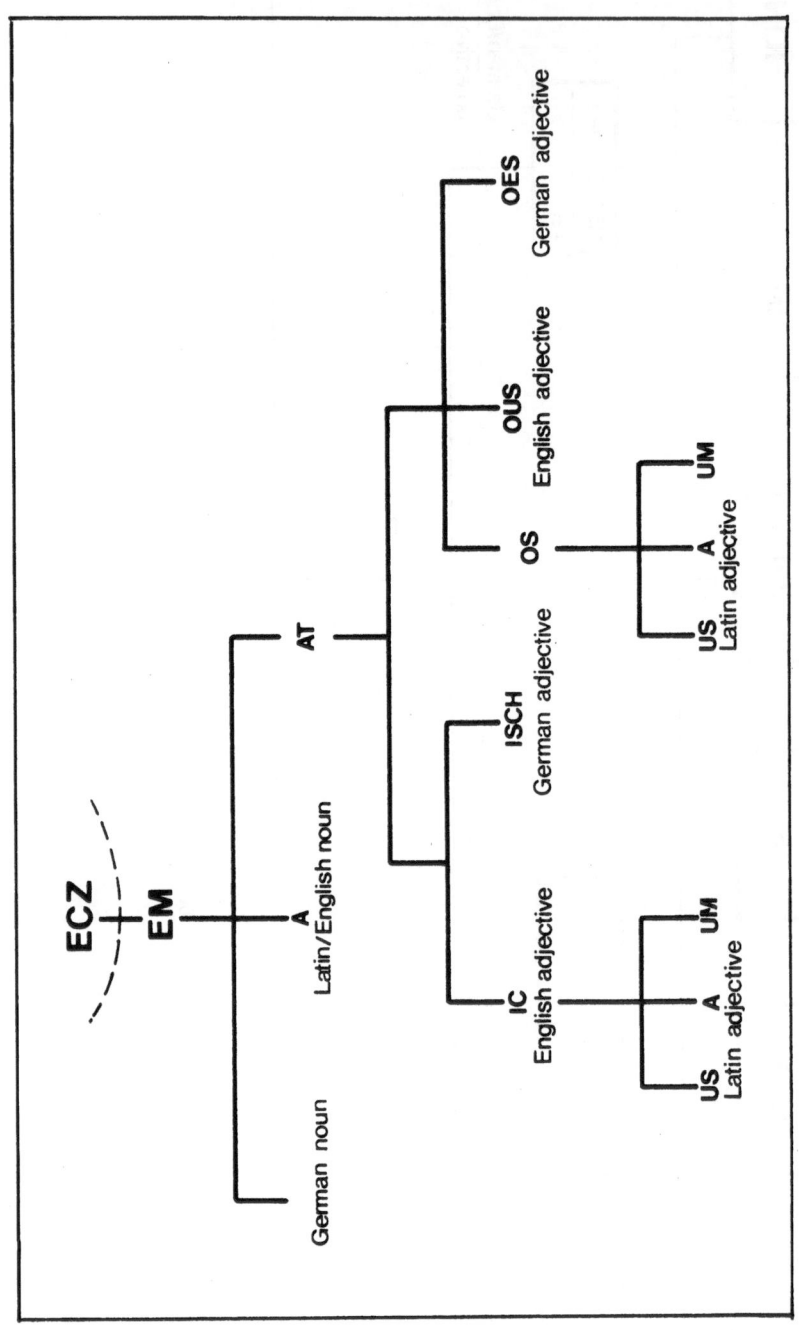

Fig. 8: Suffix family $S_{80}[41]$.

There are a few additional rules, e. g., segments which must not be terminal segments
or segments which have to be terminal segments.

Preliminary analyses showed, that the similarities proven for English and French in
special examples hold also for German in the majority of cases. Therefore a German
segment dictionary has been constructed semi-automatically by use of the segmentation
algorithm (see section 4.2.2.3) and starting from a word-oriented German thesaurus [32]
containing about 28,000 different words from autopsy and biopsy reports. To this about
12,000 different words from a German SNOP translation [42] have been added. Then the
resulting German segment dictionary has been used for the segmentation of about 8,000
different words from the English SNOP version [38], not considering chemicals and drugs.
Without any addition to the dictionary about 70 % of the English words could be segmented automatically. This number increased to more than 80 % after addition of about 20
specific English suffixes. The rest consisting of specific English roots and secondary
strings has been added manually (Table 1).

Number of	Roots	Secondary strings		Segments	%
		Derivational suffixes	Terminal suffixes		
German	1583	122	7	1712	21
English	814	111	1	926	12
German and English	5139	179	52	5370	67
Total	7536	412	60	8008	100

Table 1: Statistics for a segment dictionary for medical language data processing.

4.2.2.2 Organization of the Segment Dictionary

Because of the extensive intersection, English and German segment dictionaries are
merged and each segment is assigned a *language marker* L, which identifies, whether it
belongs to the German, to the English or to both versions of the dictionaries.

The general form of an element of the dictionary is

$$\left\{{R \atop s}\right\} L\ i_1 \ldots i_j \ldots i_k, \quad 0 \le i_j \le 255,\ j = 1,2,\ldots,k, \quad k \le 14\ ,$$

where R and s are strings of characters (root, resp. secondary string), L is the language marker and i is a class number. Every construction of $R * S_n$ is possible ($n = i_1$,
$\ldots, i_k$), that is, every construction Rs is valid, where s belongs to the union of all
sets S_n (Fig. 13).

4.2.2.3   The Segmentation Algorithm

The segmentation algorithm is searching *alternatively* for roots and secondary strings
in a word. The principles of the algorithm are: There are two dictionaries, a dictionary D_r of roots and a dictionary D_s of secondary strings. The segments are assigned
class numbers. Both dictionaries are in lexicographical order. Thus the relation $d_1 < d_2$
means, d_1 stands before d_2 in lexicographical order. The empty string belongs to D_s.
Segments are searched from left to right. Given a sequence

$$w = d_1 d_2 \ldots d_i X ,$$

$d_1 \ldots d_i$ being a sequence of valid pairs and X the remainder of word w, the algorithm
is searching for the *longest* segment d_{i+1}, such that

$$w = d_1 d_2 \ldots d_i d_{i+1} Y ,$$

and $d_1 \ldots d_{i+1}$ is a sequence of valid pairs (**principle of longest valid match**). If such
a segment is found the algorithm proceeds for Y. Otherwise, a mistake is assumed in
the preceding sequence. First d_i is assumed to be wrong, the correct sequence then
being

$$w = d_1 \ldots d_{i-1} t_i Z ,$$

where $t_i < d_i$ and $d_1 \ldots d_{i-1} t_i$ being a sequence of valid pairs. If such a segment t_i is
found, the algorithm proceeds to the right. Otherwise d_{i-1} is assumed to be wrong, etc..

The algorithm terminates when either the whole word has been segmented, i. e.,
$w = d_1 \ldots d_n$ is in canonical form, or there is no root as first root.

The basic assumptions underlying this model are:

> (1) The semantic content of a word is the logical sum of the semantic
> contents of its roots. This is the most simplistic assumption, which
> can be made to reduce the size of any semantic structured reference
> dictionary. A much more complicated set of rules has to be developed
> for the prediction of the value of compound words, where this sim-
> plistic model is insufficient (Examples [26] may demonstrate some as-
> pects (Fig. 14)). In many cases, the semantic category of the compound
> descriptor is identical to the semantic category of the last segment.

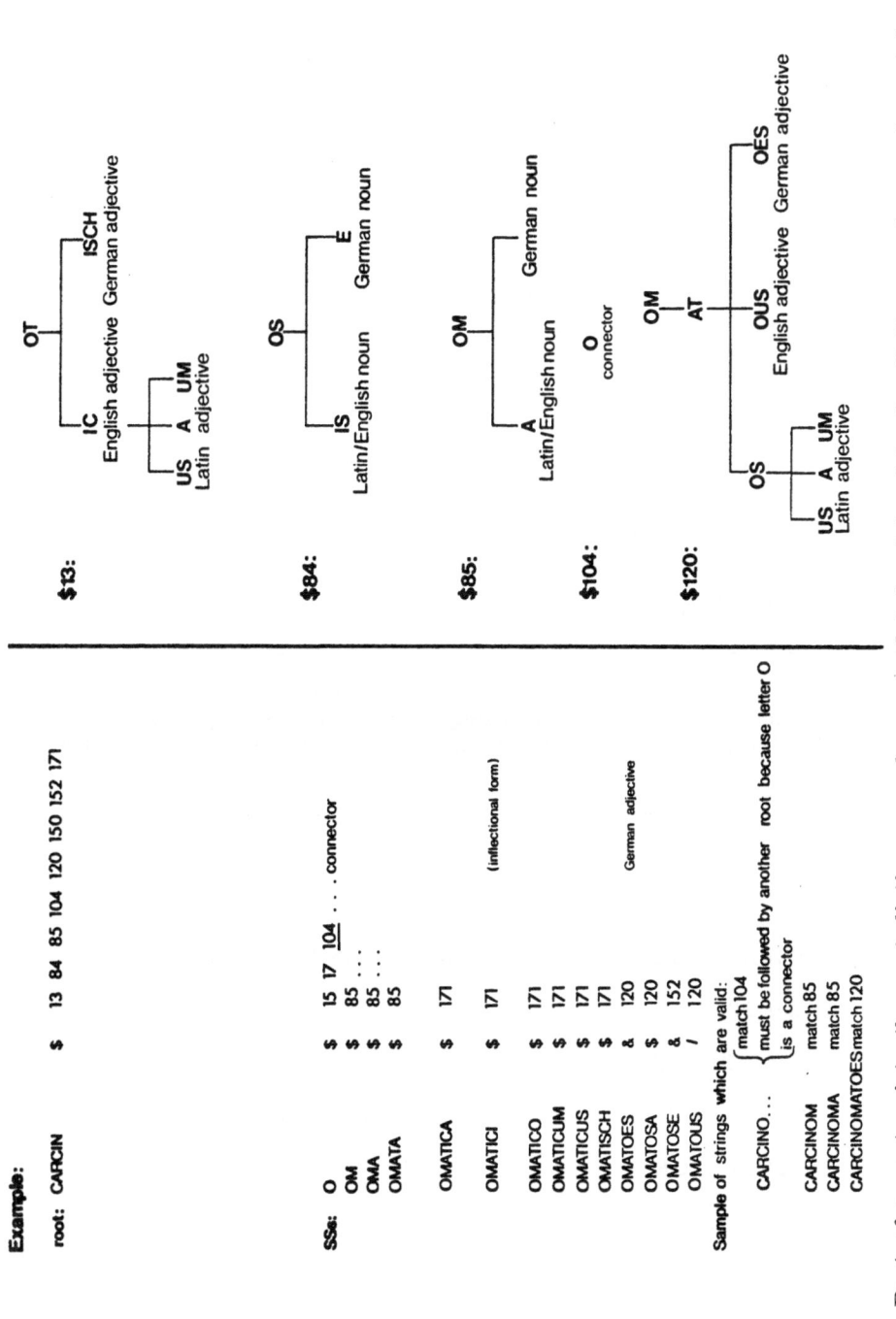

Fig. 13: Part of an entry into the root dictionary and some related entries into the dictionary of secondary strings (SS_S) on the left side. Some suffix families related to the root on the right side [41].

Semantic Category of Constituents	Graphemic Segmentation of Word Form	Semantic Category of Word Form
T T	MYO, CARDIUM	T
T M	BRONCH, ITIS	M
T E	MENINGO, COCCUS	E
T F	VASO, SPASM	F
M T	VARICO, BLEPHARON	M
E F	AMEB, IASIS	F
E E	BACTERIO, TOXIN	E
F F	ALGO, SPASM	F
T T M	GLOMERULO, NEPHR, ITIS	M
F T F	HYPER, TRICH, OSIS	M
T E F	THYRO, TOXIC, OSIS	F
F T M	MENO, METRO, RRHAGIA	F
T T T T M M	PERINEO, COLPO, RECTO, MY, OM, ECTOMY	M

Fig. 14: Semantic patterns of compound words and resulting semantic values [26]. The semantic categories due to SNOP [38] are: T = topography, M = morphology, E = etiology, F = function.

SCHLÜSSELBEIN

LANDKARTENZUNGE   -   GEOGRAPHIC TONGUE

SANDUHRMAGEN   -   HOURGLAS STOMACH

KEIMEPITHEL

NARBENHERNIE

SCHUSTERBRUST   -   COBBLER'S CHEST

CYSTENLUNGE   -   HONEYCOMB LUNG

{NIERENBECKEN   -   RENAL PELVIS }
{BECKENNIERE   -   PELVIC KIDNEY}

Fig. 15: Examples where decomposition of compound descriptors lead to changes in the semantic concepts.

(2) The parts of speech can be derived from the bivariate function
$f(R_n, d_n)$ using last root R_n and *derivational* suffix s_n.

(3) Case, gender, etc. can be derived from the three-variate function
$g(R_n, s_n, t_n)$ using last root R_n, derivational suffix s_n and terminal
suffix t_n. There is a substantial number of derivational suffixes,
where this information can be derived from a bivariate function using
only the secondary string.

There are several exceptions to these basic rules, which have to be handled separately.
Types of exceptions to rule (1) are:

- Words with a semantic meaning differing from the sum of the semantic
  meanings of the constituents (Fig. 15).

- Ambiguous semantic meaning of components (MYEL - referring to "bone
  marrow" or to "spinal cord", SCLER - referring to SCLERA or SCLEROSIS).

- Secondary strings carrying a specific semantic meaning, like -OM,
  -OMA (tumor) (Fig. 16), -IASIS (diseases), -ITIS (inflammation)
  except capitis, linitis plastica, rhachitis.

SYNDROM	FIBROM
SKOTOM	SPIDER ANGIOM
COLOBOM	OSTEOM
HAEMATOM	TRACHOM
GRANULOM	GLAUKOM
TUBERCULOM	MYCETOM
STAPHYLOM	RHINOSKLEROM
LEUCOM	PARAFFINOM
NEUROM	CONDYLOM
ATHEROM	KERATOACANTHOM
XANTHOM	FIBROMA PENDULUM
PSAMMOM	ANGIOMA SERPIGNOSUM
CHOLESTEATOM	OSTEOFIBROM
PAPILLOM	COELOM

Fig. 16: Exceptions to the $\left\{\begin{matrix} \text{-OM} \\ \text{-OMA} \end{matrix}\right\}$ rule with respect
to SNOP [38].

The semantic meaning of suffixes often is not connected to the suffix alone but is a bivariate class function. For example, the suffixes -IA (Latin), -IE (German) and -Y (English) constitute two classes with the same morphosyntactical but with different semantical information:

$$f(FAMIL* \begin{Bmatrix} IA \\ IE \\ Y \end{Bmatrix}) = \text{noun, singular}$$

$$f(ANODONT* \begin{Bmatrix} IA \\ IE \\ Y \end{Bmatrix}) = \text{noun, singular, disease}$$

4.2.2.4 Synthesis rules

Insofar, we have used the classes and analysis rules for the segmentation of compound word forms. The same rules can, however, be used for synthesis and for transformation. This has been made possible by two different features:

- combinatorial classes consisting of subclasses for noun form, adjectival form and so on (Fig. 8),

- membership of a root in several classes, e. g.

$$\text{ENTZUEND} < \{UNG\} \cup \{-EN\} \cup \{-ET\} \cup \{-LICH\}.$$

The following transformations are possible:

- Noun singular ⟷ noun plural,

- noun ⟷ adjectival,

- noun ⟷ verbal,

- German noun ⟷ English noun ⟷ Latin noun, if possible using class functions.

- German adjectival ⟷ English adjectival ⟷ Latin adjectival, if possible using class functions.

4.2.2.5 Eponyms

Eponyms are used extensively in medicine and have to be treated specially. Eponyms mostly are

- names of people (e. g., HODGKIN'S DISEASE, MORBUS LITTLE),

- names of geographical regions (e. g.,CHRISTMAS DISEASE, COXSACKIE VIRUS),

- names of professions (e. g.,WOOLSORTER'S DISEASE, COBBLER'S CHEST).

The eponyms have to be listed in their full forms in the root dictionary and they make up a good portion of it. Additionally some of these eponyms are inflected like Latin roots (e. g.,FALLOPIAN TUBE, TUBA EUSTACHII, ANGINA LUDOVICI).

4.2.2.6 Problems

Some of the problems arising from the fact that there are only a few principles under-lying the model have already been mentioned. Therefore, I will concentrate on some spe-cial failures, which are of practical interest.

Ambiguities have to be handled, e. g., the word ECTOPIA can be segmented formally in-to the segments

$$\underbrace{EC}_{R_1} \quad \underbrace{\emptyset}_{s_1} \quad \underbrace{TOP}_{R_2} \quad \underbrace{IA}_{s_2} \quad \text{and} \quad \underbrace{ECT}_{R_1} \quad \underbrace{O}_{s_1} \quad \underbrace{P}_{R_2} \quad \underbrace{IA}_{s_2} \, .$$

The first sequence is the correct one, but the second sequence is the canonical form due to the principle of longest valid match (the root dictionary contains the longer prefix ECT, which may be connected by letter O, e. g. ECTODERM). This problem arises from the unsymmetrical segmentation algorithm and it is not detected automatically. It may occur whenever roots are combined with some "reactions" in the combination area, e. g.,

(1) elision of vowels (MYOPIA instead of MYOOPIA),

(2) "smoothing" of combinations (ECTOPIA instead of ECTOTOPIA),

(3) dropping of one consonant in case the preceding root ends with the same (double-)consonant the following root starts with (FLUSS-STAUUNG ⟶ FLUSSTAUUNG),

(4) gemination (TAR ⟶ TARRING).

Errors like the example given occur in a surprisingly small number of less than 3 % in a large sample of more than 50,000 different words. In most of these cases the am-biguities are caused by short prefixes, like A-, E-, and so on. There are different types of failures, which can be arranged into classes.

Practically all ambiguities could be detected, if the same principle of longest match would be applied not only in a left to right scan, but also in a right to left scan. But because it is intended to develop a segmentation algorithm, which can be used fully automatically, there is no advantage in the knowledge of more than one possible formal segmentation, as long as there are no explicit rules for the decision, which of the different versions should be taken.

The ambiguities can be handled by special rules or by addition of pseudo-roots to the dictionary. Where the number of cases is small the latter has been done.

5   Syntax

Syntax deals with the order or structure of word strings with respect to the parts of speech. I will not go into the discussion about the usefulness of special types of grammars, which is much more up to a linguist. It has often been argued, that linguistics has not yet delivered powerful tools for practical retrieval systems. I do not know, whether this is because of the insufficiency of formal grammars for natural languages or because of the insufficiency of people working with practical retrieval systems with a very limited knowledge of linguistic theories.

Therefore I will mention some types of formal grammars very briefly to introduce just the notions. *Formal grammars* intend to develop a formal model of a language and are therefore most relevant to automatic language data processing. The definition of language is by generation, using *rewrite rules:* "Rewrite a string X as a string Y". Such a grammar is adequate , if it generates just all sentences of the language. If more sentences are produced, than rules have to be more restrictive. Formal grammars are totally restricted to formal relationships and disregard semantic content.

A *phrase-structure* grammar consists of a finite *vocabulary,* V, and a finite set, $\{P\}$, of *rewrite rules.* The vocabulary, V, consists of two disjoint parts, a *terminal* vocabulary, V_T, and a *non-terminal* vocabulary, V_N. The terminal vocabulary is a lexicon of the language, the non-terminal vocabulary contains symbols, such as S = sentence, NP = noun phrase, VP = verb phrase, etc..

Each rewrite rule has the form

$$\alpha \ A \ \beta \longrightarrow \alpha \ \gamma \ \beta \ ,$$

where A is a member of V_N and α, β and γ are members of V. α and β may be null, A may be not. This general form of a phrase-structure grammar is called *context-sensitive.* If the rewrite rules have the special form

$$A \longrightarrow \gamma$$

then the grammar is called *context-free.* A special context-free grammar is a *finite-state* grammar, with rewrite rules

$$A \longrightarrow cB$$
$$A \longrightarrow c$$

where A and B are members of V_N and c is a member of V_T.

A finite state grammar is the most restricted phrase-structure grammar, which can generate an infinite number of sentences with a finite set of rewrite rules.

Another more restricted grammar may have only rewrite rules of the second type

$$A \longrightarrow c,$$

A grammar like this one is essentially a finite list of phrases, which constitute the language (Fig. 17).

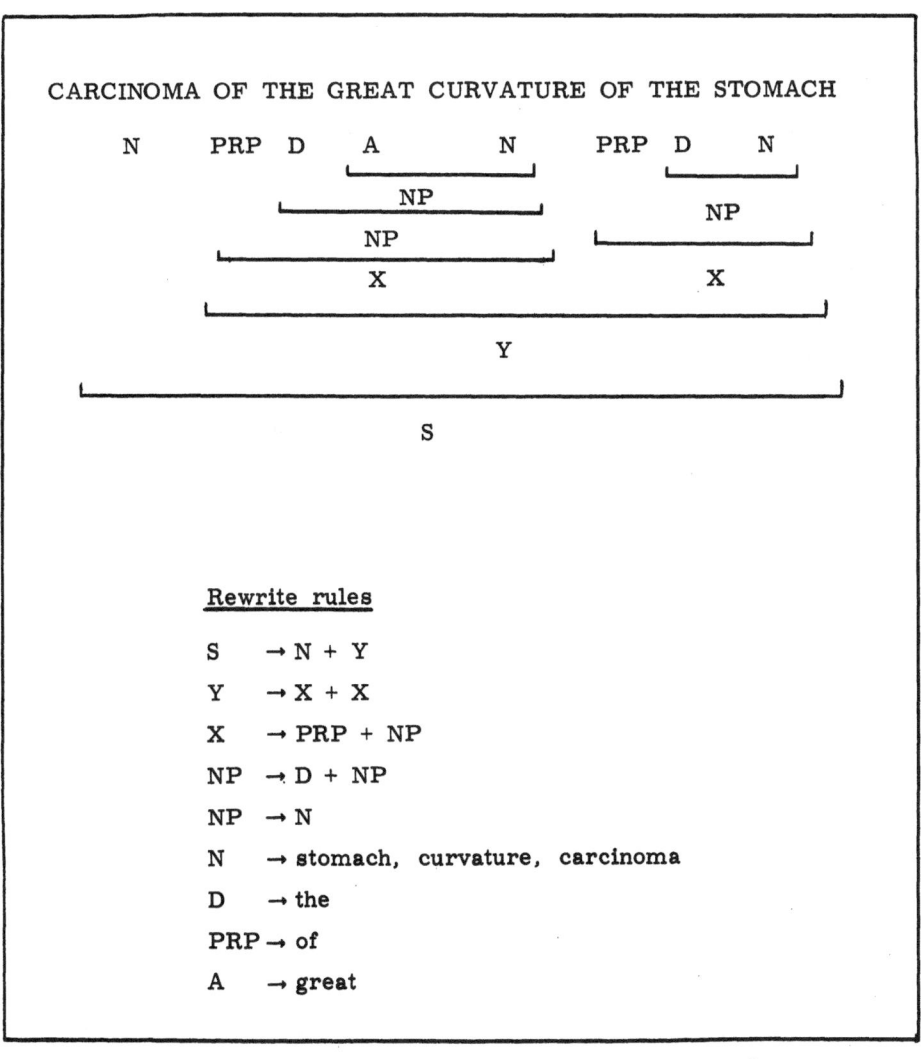

Fig. 17: Example of the syntactical analysis of a medical utterance.

Another type of grammars is called *transformational* grammar [4]. Two structures are
assigned to each sentence: A *surface* structure and a *deep* structure. The latter one
determines the semantic interpretation.

6   Semantics

The different types of medical utterances have to be seen in the light of the semantic structure of informations in medicine. This semantic structure is always preliminary due to the limited knowledge about the universe. Formal representation of informations requires a model of the universe, which contains a finite number of elements:

- *Characteristics* and their respective *values* (semantic concepts),

- *relations* between different characteristics and values,

- a *terminology* containing the terms denoting the characteristics
  and their respective values,

- a *classification* to make explicit the relations between characteristics and values.

That is, modelling the universe leads directly to the problems of classification and
terminology. Because models are used for a special purpose and depend on diagnostic
and therapeutic possibilities, classification and terminology are a valuable resource
but they cannot be the goal. The classification used depends on the goals and there
is a variety of such classifications in medicine, a fact, which often leads to serious problems in communication instead of solving these problems.

There are efforts to *standardize* terms with respect to their meaning, which is an important requirement for every kind of language processing. For example, the terms
"breathlessness" and "dyspnea" are often used synonymously to describe shortness of
breath of normal individuals as well as of individuals suffering from pulmonary disease. Agreements in the medical community have to be made, which are the basis for
unambiguous usage of terms.

The *Current Medical Information Terminology* (CMIT) [11] contains about 3,500 diseases
and their definitions in terms of etiology, symptomatology, and X-ray and laboratory
findings. In another system developed in Germany [20] data about rare or newly described syndromes are collected. There are efforts for the standardization of syndrome
and symptom nomenclature. Further efforts are mainly in the area of tumor nomenclature [35, 36, 37].

Diagnostic terms are a good example to demonstrate the difficulties. In a common sense
the diagnosis serves for different purposes, e. g., unambiguous and short denotation
of a disease, explanation of disturbances, classification due to a given scheme. Be-

cause most of the diseases are complex in nature with respect to etiology, pathogenesis, combination of signs and symptoms and with respect to their time dependance and individual reaction, simplification has to be done. The classification therefore has to be - at least in principle - *polyhierarchical,* it has to be an *open system* to allow for additions, deletions and update. The necessary degree of *completeness* depends on:

- data,
- structure of search questions,
- handling by computer or by man.

The semantic categories, which are used to categorize medical informations can be explained, at least in part, by the history of medical systematization. I will not go into the interesting, but sometimes philosophical discussions about the value of a diagnosis. This has been done and this discussion is carried out by experts in the field [14]. From a pragmatic point of view, the semantic categories should meet - at least approximately - the following objectives:

- *Decomposition* of information, i. e., the elements should be disjoint and complete in the sense of set theory.

- Orientation towards the *diagnostic* and *therapeutic possibilities.*

- Differentiation between different *prognostic entities.*

- Reflection of known important *relations* and *pathogenetic processes.*

Some of the categories used in different systems are:

- Topography (location of a disease),

- nosology (disease entities),

- morphology (what can be seen, for example using tissue specimens and a microscope),

- etiologic agents (causes of alterations),

- functional disturbances,

- pathogenetic processes,

- histochemical alterations,

- medical procedures (diagnostic procedures, therapeutic procedures).

This list is far from being complete and it contains categories, which are not mutually exclusive. For example, the category "nosology" is based on the assumption that diseases are well definable states, which can be arranged in some type of a natural system in analogy to the natural system of elements [14]. In the light of the discussion whether this is right or wrong, terms like "disease" or "syndrome" already reveal different points of view. Without sticking to the assumption of the existence of a natural system of diseases, one can say that morphology, etiology, function etc. are semantic subdivisions of the category "nosology".

Diseases usually have projections into several semantic categories, e. g., *acute appendicitis* as a patho-anatomical diagnosis is made up from acute inflammation (morphology) + appendix (topography), whereas the same term as a clinical diagnosis is made up from abdomen (topography) + pain, nausea, emesis, fever (function).

In a consequent classification – if ever one such classification exists – one has to consider

- *multiple causes* of a disease or state,
- projections into *several semantic categories,* depending on the point of view and on the available facilities and knowledge,
- *inconstancy* of the projections depending on time and patient characteristics.

Taking into account these considerations, available systems are rather poor. Nevertheless there are developments, which are an important step forward.

The semantic categories, which have to be used, depend on the special demands in information retrieval and on the available resources with respect to dictionaries, classifications, thesauri, data and software.

It is agreed that more sophisticated language processing requires semantically ordered *lexicons*. These lexicons list the morphemes, words or phrases, which have some value of meaning in the respective domain of discourse. This value is identified by *semantic markers*, which reveal the meaning-defined use of these elements in terms of syntax, denotation, connotation, etc. [29]. In addition, thesaurus functions should be preserved, like:

- Entry by letter strings to yield concepts, and
- entry by concepts (semantic markers) to yield lists of words and phrases related to the concepts.

There are three general approaches to the construction of a semantic lexicon.

The *scaling* method uses judgements along semantic dimensions from language users about the meaning.

The *statistical derivation* method examines the contextual distribution of two words or phrases to determine their similarity of meaning.

The *componential analysis* decomposes the sense of each word or phrase into a number of components. This is done by assigning to each word-sense in the dictionary:

    (1) A set of semantic markers, which are *overall* semantic features, occuring in more than one word sense.

    (2) A *specific* marker, which represents the semantic features unique to the given word sense.

    (3) *Combinatorial rules,* that are the conditions under which the given word-sense may be combined with other word senses.

Additionally there are *projection rules* describing the methods of combining the readings of a pair of words or phrases to obtain a reading for the longer string.

The above listed requirements are best met by *thesauri,* possibly completed by a set of special dictionaries (*microglossaries*). It has already been mentioned, that a thesaurus is a list of *descriptors* and *relations* between descriptors, containing all the terms, which are necessary to formulate the semantic concepts in a domain of discourse. The descriptors can be divided into a set of simple descriptors and a set of compound descriptors. A *simple descriptor* denotes a semantic concept, which cannot (or should not) be divided into subconcepts. A *compound descriptor* denotes a compound semantic concept, that is a semantic concept, which should be divided into its elements.

The approach of taking compound descriptors into the thesaurus is called *precoordination* in contrast to *postcoordination,* where a compound semantic concept is denoted by combination of simple descriptors during information retrieval. The distinction between precoordination and postcoordination is related to the decision whether descriptors are only single-word terms or, in general, compound words and multi-word phrases. Usually, a thesaurus is a compromise between both methods. There is a general rule for the decision where each one of the two methods should be used:

    - *Postcoordination* should be used, when the morphological decomposition of a compound descriptor is identical with the semantic decomposition (*semantic factoring*). In other words, the logical sum of the semantic values of the components is equal to the semantic value of the compound descriptor. Otherwise the precision (see section 9) of information retrieval is decreased.

The advantages of postcoordination are in principle the advantages that have been mentioned in the discussion of the segmentation approach (see section 4).

Technical considerations may lead to variations of the given rule. For example, if there are two morphemes m_1 and m_2, which are used (nearly) always in the aggregate m_1m_2, than the compound descriptor may be taken into the thesaurus to save time, decrease ambiguity etc..

To some extent, *relations* can substitute precoordination. These relations can be fixed in the thesaurus and belong to the type of associative relations (see section 3.1 and 7.1). Or they can be payed regard to in the data structure (see section 7.2). It may be sufficient here to mention that a sophisticated data structure may replace a lot of precoordinated descriptors in medical language.

On the other hand, there is an important relation between *dictionary size* and the use of *rewrite rules* in the analysis of medical language data. This may become clear when considering a sample of synonymous phrases:

HERZINFARKT
CORONARINFARKT
INFARKT, CORONARGEFAESS
INFARKT, CORONARARTERIE
INFARKT, HERZKRANZGEFAESS
INFARKT EINER CORONARARTERIE

There are numerous ways of paraphrasing a given sentence without alteration of its meaning. The rewrite rules have to be handled with care, as an example may show, where each phrase represents another complex concept, constructed from the same two single concepts (CYST, INFLAMMATION):

CYSTITIS   - CYSTITIS
INFLAMMED CYST   - ENTZÜNDETE CYSTE
CYSTIC INFLAMMATION - CYSTISCHE ENTZÜNDUNG
INFLAMMATORY CYST   - ENTZÜNDLICHE CYSTE

7   Relations and Data Structure

7.1   RELATIONS

Relations have to be defined on every level of data representation. There are relations on the level of simple descriptors and segments as well as on the level of data aggregates. Some relations have already been mentioned and they are well known when classification and thesauri are discussed. Additional relations exist due to medical logic, for example,

- Antonyms (e. g., malignancy - benignancy),

- <u>disease-symptoms</u> (e. g.,meningitis - rigidity of the neck),

- <u>cause-effect</u> (e. g.,cytomegalic inclusion disease - cytomegalic inclusion disease virus; secondary effects of drugs),

- <u>pathogenesis</u> (e. g.,obstruction *due to* tumor, paleness *due to* anemia, pneumonia *complicating* paralysis transverse),

- <u>differential diagnosis - diagnostic procedure</u> (e. g.,meningitis - sub-occipital puncture),

- <u>location and location - specific alterations</u> (e. g., limbus corneae - arcus senilis),

- <u>influence of time</u> with respect to the age of the patient and the age of the disease.

7.2   DATA STRUCTURE

A data structure is the physical basis for the formal representation of language data. It is not only a technical tool, but reflects also the selected semantic categories and additional features like time, origin of data, security, relations, sureness.

Data atoms contain informations related to a single semantic category. *Data aggregates* can be built with varying levels and degrees of complexity: Signs, symptoms, syndromes, "simple" diseases, "complex" diseases.

There are some systems where the idea of the data structure is related to the concept of the *Kernel sentence* [13], which is a non-decomposible entity and carries the information of a sentence. It can be used to generate new sentences carrying the same information by application of well defined rules. Therefore the data structure cannot be seen separate from the structure of the thesaurus resp. classification underlying the thesaurus. In theory, the data structure has to reflect additional information like relations between Kernel sentences (*semantic operators*).

Besides logical problems, technical problems have to be considered to define a good data structure, which can be handled by man and/or by computer.

There are three systems for computer-based retrieval of medical language data utilizing the concept of the Kernel sentence for precise representation of information in a language data string. ACORN (Automatic Coding of Report Narrative) [3] is an automated natural language question-answering system for surgical reports. A Kernel extractor mappes the language data into the structure "$F(x) = y$", where x and y are "words or short phrases" and F is a function corresponding to phrases like "size of", "state of", "location" and so on. For example, a sentence like "the tumor is small" will be mapped into

SIZE (TUMOR) = SMALL .

The same will happen to all paraphrases of this sentence.

The authors point out, that natural language-based question-answering systems may
even be simpler than systems based on artificial languages, which have to be learned
by the human user. If we restrict relations between Kernel sentences to boolean relations, than answering a question formulated in natural language is nothing else than
extracting the Kernel sentences out of the question and matching these sentences with
the data base consisting of Kernel sentences.

Another system for automatic analysis of natural language pathology reports is based
on the semantic categories: site, diagnosis and modifier [43]. The data are processed
by a parsing routine, mapping into one out of five possible major data formats:

Data format:	Example:
(1) DIAGNOSIS of SITE	Carcinoma of urinary bladder
(2) DIAGNOSIS-ive SITE (adjectival diagnosis)	normal vermiform appendix
(3) SITE-al DIAGNOSIS (adjectival site)	renal amyloidosis
(4) DIAGNOSIS = SITE-itis	Appendicitis
(5) SITE with DIAGNOSIS	uterus with leiomyoma

The algorithm extracts delimiters out of the language string. These delimiters belong
to a list of 62 morphemes, words or phrases, grouped into 13 groups, like conjunctions,
diagnostic suffixes (-ITIS, -OSIS, ...), garbage words, diagnostic adjectival delimiters (-ating, -ed). After this, a preliminary assignment to one of the formats is done
and tested for consistency. Inconsistency means, for example, that a diagnostic delimiter is found in a place, where the format expects a site delimiter. A limited set
of rewrite rules is used (e. g., site adjectivals ⟶ site nouns, diagnostic nouns ⟶
⟶ site nouns). The authors report low error rates of about 10 % in 2 samples of
diagnostic statements.

The third system will be explained in section 8.4.1 .

8   Systems for Management of Medical Language Data

8.1   SECTIONING OF REPORTS

In pure sectioning of reports there is no analysis of language data. Reports are formalized by a rigid scheme of sections and subsections and data input is done in natu-

ral language [40].

The pay-offs of this approach are:

- Higher degree of completeness of reports in a restricted domain of discourse, mostly connected to higher expenses in generating these reports,

- lower degree of ambiguity compared with the scanning of unformatted reports,

- increase in precision and improvement of communication,

- automated generation of reports and journals, automated monitoring of report generation if combined with man/machine systems (see section 8.3).

8.2   TECHNICAL SYSTEMS

In technical systems language data are handled mechanically. There is no data analysis except plausibility checking in terms of completeness and formal relations (e. g., mutually exclusive values of characteristics). Reports are generated by aggregation of selected items from various lists. Usually the items in a special list denote mutually exclusive informations. Some systems offer additional support by implementation of branches in the otherwise rigid sequence, dependant on simplistic text structure like "yes", "no", "male", "female" and so on [7, 22, 23, 28]. Sometimes supplementary remarks in free text are also possible.

There is a widespread use of technical systems in medicine with a great variety of data catching methods (mark sense forms, punched cards, CRT's) and flexibility. Some developments are combinations between purely technical systems and formulation of the input data in highly formalized artificial language [9, 12].

Technical systems offer possibilities, which may be extremely useful for further developments of medical information systems. The more specific the domain of discourse is, the more helpful these systems are. The main *advantages* are:

- *Sectioning* of reports,
- *standardization* of the "skeleton" of a report,
- combination between *documentation* and *report generation,* which ensures documentation.

The main *disadvantages* are:

- Need for usage of a special artificial language by physicians,
- high degree of formalization of input data resulting in a more time-consuming generation of reports.

8.3   MAN/MACHINE SYSTEMS

Man/machine systems are exclusively computer-based and require time-sharing and teleprocessing facilities. Human intelligence is combined with the advantages of computers with respect to large storage capacity, fast access to data and fast processing
of explicit procedures. Man/machine systems are in use for report generation [2, 17,
18, 21, 31], access to lexicons [8, 39], and augmenting the use of structured questionnaires.

8.4   DESCRIPTOR SYSTEMS

The replacement of a document by a set of descriptors is common to all these systems.
It is intended, that the set of descriptors reflects the informational content of the
document:

$$D \simeq \{d_1, d_2, \ldots, d_n\} \quad .$$

In *descriptor-out-of-context* systems descriptors are added to the document, usually
by human indexers after reading the document. In *descriptor-in-context* systems the
descriptors have to be part of the language string from the document. Descriptor
systems always depend on the existence of thesauri and dictionaries. The best known
descriptor systems have been introduced in the documentation of literature (e. g.,
Universal Decimal Classification) and they are widely used in medicine.

The *International Classification of Diseases* (ICD) [33, 44] has emerged from a classification of causes of death presented in 1893. During a conference in 1900 delegates from 26 countries accepted the updated version of this classification of diseases
and traumata. The current, 8th, revision has been published in 1967. There is an obligatory version encoded with 3 digits and an extended official version encoded with
4 digits. Based on the official ICD there are national adaptations like the American
version ICDA and probably thousands of hospital- or even physician-based adaptations.

ICD is a logically ordered list of diseases, where each entry is denoted by a rigid
numeric code. The numeric codes are running numbers. The main structure is by *topography* and on the second level by *nosology*.

The sections "malignant tumors" and "congenital malformations" have an inverted structure, e. g., the nosological main class "malignant tumors" is topographically structured on the second level.

In the dictionary sense the characteristics are:

- One-dimensional structure, mixed between nosology and topography,

- complete list of descriptors for the domain of discourse by definition,

- primitive semantic marker in the form of the numeric code,

- terminologic control of synonyms and quasi-synonyms.

To give better support for retrieval in the two dimensions topography and nosology, IMMICH [16] has developed the *Klinischer Diagnosenschlüssel* and a cross reference table to ICD. There is a 5 digit code equivalent with 2 digits for topography and 3 digits for nosology. The last nosological digit can be subdivided further for special needs.

The *Standard Nomenclature of Diseases and Operations* (SNDO) [34] is no longer maintained by its sponsors but some of the ideas have been absorbed in later developments.

The *Medical Subject Headings* (MeSH) [24] are used by human indexers in the MEDLARS-system to index the content of published medical literature.

Word oriented descriptor-in-context-systems are in widespread use. There are two better known systems following almost the same principles. One system is called the Lamson-IBM-Thesaurus [6, 19], the other one is the AGK-Thesaurus [32]. Both thesauri have been developed for pathology data processing and contain only single word descriptors (Fig. 18). The elements of the original text are called *input words*. In the first step these input words are replaced by *standard words*. The transformations performed during this step are:

- Replacement of *derivational forms* by their underived forms,

- replacement of *adjectival forms* by their noun forms,

- replacement of *synonyms* by their preferred terms,

- deletion of *insignificant* words (e. g., articles).

The second step contains:

- *Classification* of a standard word according to site, finding, and modifier,

- *subclassification* of site words and findings (one more level),

- *supply* of simple descriptors for compound descriptors, i. e., explicit notation of some hierarchical, partitive and associative relations (Fig. 19).

The AGK-thesaurus now contains about 50,000 input words and 12,000 standard words.

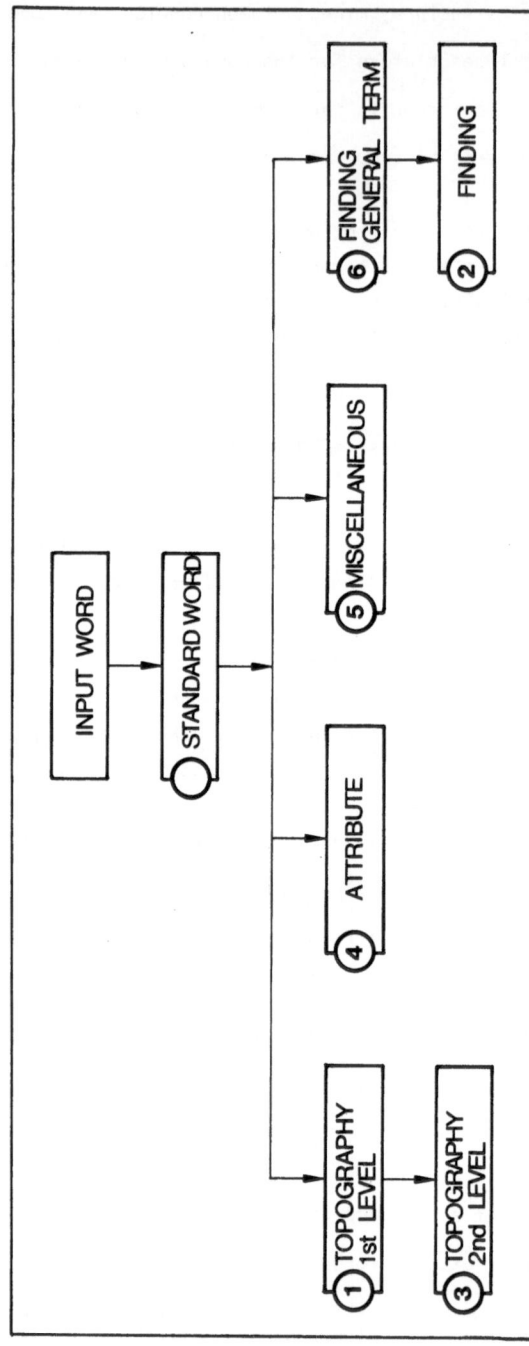

Fig. 18: Structure of the AGK-thesaurus [32].

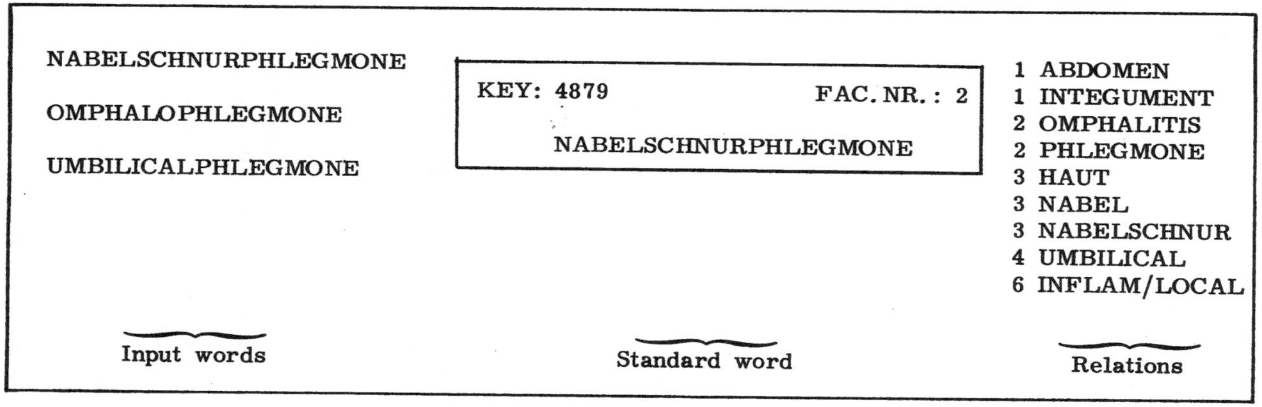

619

NABELSCHNURPHLEGMONE

OMPHALOPHLEGMONE

UMBILICALPHLEGMONE

Input words

KEY: 4879   FAC. NR. : 2

NABELSCHNURPHLEGMONE

Standard word

1 ABDOMEN
1 INTEGUMENT
2 OMPHALITIS
2 PHLEGMONE
3 HAUT
3 NABEL
3 NABELSCHNUR
4 UMBILICAL
6 INFLAM/LOCAL

Relations

Fig. 19: Example taken from the AGK-thesaurus [32].

Language processing is done by replacing every nonsignificant input word from a pathology report by its standard word and its explicit relations. Query is done by "stan-
dardizing" the search question in the same way and comparing the descriptor sets of
the search question and of the documents. Some primitive syntactical informations can
be used, like

- restriction of the data fields to single sentences,
- neighbourhood-relationships.

The main advantage of such a system is, that mainly the language practically used has
to be considered and that there are almost no constraints on the pathologist. The
main disadvantage is the amount of postcoordination that has to be done by the user
during search phase if he wants to increase precision and recall (see section 9).
Syntactical information is almost totally lost. Another disadvantage is the primitive
data structure, which cannot serve as a basis for logical deduction.

In 1965 the College of American Pathologists published the *Systematized Nomenclature
of Pathology* (SNOP) [38], which has been an important step forward. It provides the
necessary thesaurus functions to describe diseases by a pathologist and it introduces
an explicit data structure based on the semantic informations underlying the terms.
SNOP contains about 15,000 single word- or multi-word-descriptors, which are categorized into 4 lists (Fig. 20). SNOP has been translated into German [42].

Topography - a list of the names of the body sites

Morphology - a list of the names of structural changes that occur in
tissues as a result of disease

Etiology - a list of the names of causative agents of disease such as
microorganisms, drugs and chemicals

Function - a list of the names of the physiological manifestations
associated with disease plus a limited number of specific
infectious diseases

Fig. 20: Semantic categories of SNOP [38].

There is a high degree of precoordination. Related terms are listed together, (quasi-)
synonyms belong to the same equivalence class. Each list is highly structured, the
depth of the structure varying between 2 and 3 levels. Each entry has a code-equiva-

lent consisting of 5 characters. The first character, T, M, E, F, denotes list membership, the following 4 characters are markers for the position of the descriptor in the respective list. Hierarchical relations, both generic relations and partitive relations are represented in the code structure (Fig. 21, 22). Code numbers on the same level are markers for the associative relation "parallel classes".

Another important step into the direction of a poly-dimensional approach is done by introduction of *cross references*. For example, the term APPENDICITIS is listed under M4001 and carries an additional semantic marker T66 for the site (APPENDIX). The cross references are only in the 2-digit form as pointers to topography.

The basic philosophy underlying the data structure is, that a diagnosis may be formulated by a pathologist as:

> There are *morphological* alterations in a *topographic* site due
> to an *etiologic* agent combined with a *functional* disorder.

Therefore, in general, all 4 lists have to be used in combination for full description of a pathology finding.

Handling of *modifiers* is done in SNOP in different ways. If a modifier is part of a concept, the compound descriptor is listed in the dictionary, either explicitly or implicitly. For example, in the inflammation section the modifier "acute" is used as a concept modifier and is encoded in the 2nd digit as number 1:

M4000	INFLAMMATION, NOS	→	M4100	ACUTE INFLAMMATION, NNB
M4000	CERVICITIS (T83)	→	M4100	ACUTE CERVICITIS (T83)

The same principle is used for "acute" when combined with leukemia, where it is encoded in the 4th digit as number 5:

M9803	LEUKEMIA, NOS	→	M9805	ACUTE LEUKEMIA

If the modifier "acute" appears in other concepts, it may be handled otherwise:

M3812   ACUTE CONGESTION, NOS

M5472   ACUTE INFARCT

The same modifier is not only used in concepts but also as a general modifier in me-

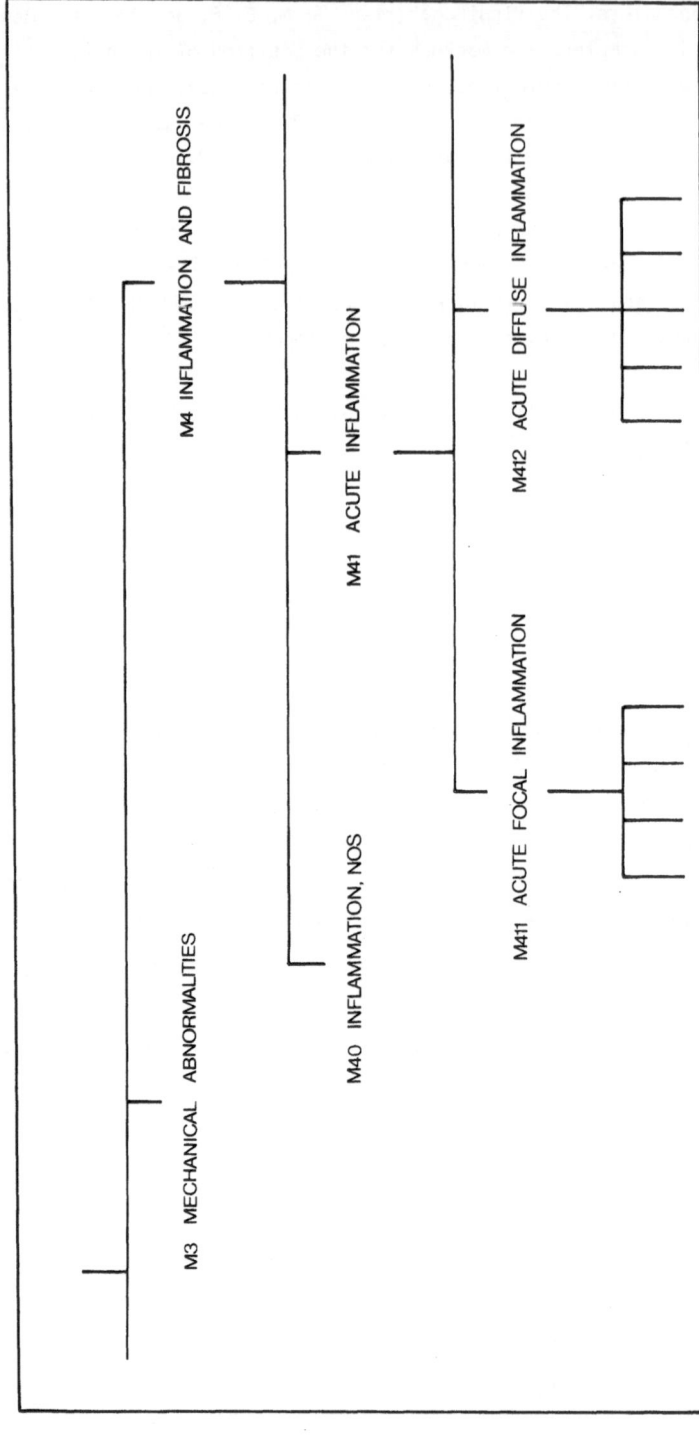

Fig. 21: Example of structure of SNOP (MORPHOLOGY) with generic hierarchical relations [38].

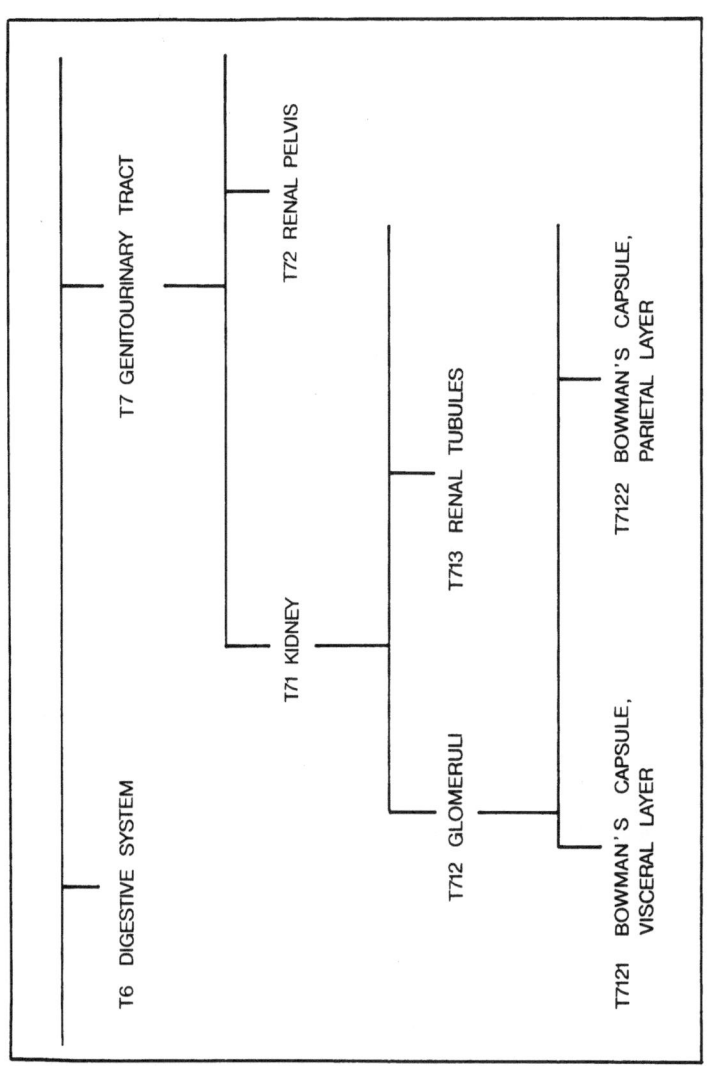

Fig. 22: Example of structure of SNOP (TOPOGRAPHY) with partitive hierarchical relations [38].

dicine, e. g., ACUTE ABDOMEN, ACUTE BLEEDING, and so on. Modifications like the latter ones cannot be coded, and they are lost if no special features are prepared for
"general modifiers".

The success of SNOP led to the development of an expansion, called *Systematized
Nomenclature of Medicine* (SNOMED) [5], which shall provide a dictionary for all of
medicine. The major expansions are:

- Additional categories *procedures* and *complex diseases*.

- Increase in the number of descriptors (total number is about 40,000).

- Reclassification of several sections according to the development
  of medical knowledge (e. g., malignant tumors, leukemias, lymphomas).
  There is an important sign for convergence: the section "malignant tumors"
  of SNOMED will be identical to the analague section of the 9th revision
  of ICD (ICD-O).

- Expansion of the code to 6 digits in some sections.

- More specific cross references to topography.

- Expansion of cross references to other categories than topography.

The underlying assumption is, that a general utterance in medical language may be
formulated as:

> There is a *procedure* for a *complex disease* or for *morphological*
> alterations in a *topographic* site due to an *etiologic* agent com-
> bined with a *functional* disorder.

There is one system for medical language data processing on the basis of SNOP developed by PRATT and his group [29, 30]. Each pathology finding is mapped onto the
TMEF data structure and retrieval is done against this structure. All pathology data
are stored in artificial language form and in their original form:

> Txxxx   Mxxxx   Exxxx   Fxxxx   <Language string>.

The complete medical record therefore is a sequence of such TMEF statements
(Fig. 23) (see section 8.4.1).

Another data structure is introduced in the REMAID-system, which can be arranged
between technical systems and descriptor systems [15]. The physician has to use a
special syntax and semantic categories: *symptoms, topography, etiology, treatment,
results*. Descriptors have to be used according to dictionaries, which are different
for different specialities. It is intended to implement the system for rheumatology
and orthopedics first.

T2600	M8103	E0000	F0000	Bronchus, Carcinoma
T0000	M0000	E6927	F0000	Tobacco (Cigarettes)
T0000	M0000	E0000	F7103	Paroxysmal Nocturnal Dyspnea
T5600	M8106	E0000	F0000	Liver, Metastatic Carcinoma
T5600	M3850	E0000	F0000	Liver, Hemorrhage
T0000	M7051	E0000	F0000	Cachexia
T0000	M0000	E8816	F0000	Fluorouracil Therapy
.	.	.	.	
.	.	.	.	
.	.	.	.	
Txxxx	Mxxxx	Exxxx	Fxxxx	<Language String>

Fig. 23: Example of a part of a medical record encoded
due to SNOP [29, 30, 38].

8.4.1 A System for Pathology Data Processing

The most advanced system for automatic processing of medical language data has been developed by PRATT and his group [29].

For the explanation of the algorithm some definitions are necessary.

The formal structure of a dictionary entry of SNOP is represented in Fig. 24. SNOP is organized in indexed sequential manner, with the dictionary English $<k \; w_1 ... \; w_m>$ as key. Access by the encoder program is done by specifying a character string v corresponding to a first word (k) of the dictionary English. By using the generic key feature, all entries having the string v as first word k are then available.

The encoding process is divided into 3 major steps:

(1) *Organization* of the original utterance into a special data structure, access to several dictionaries and associating of their contents with the utterance for processing in the following steps.

(2) Access to SNOP to obtain those dictionary entries relevant to encoding (*look-up matching* phase).

$$\{k, W\} = <k \ w_1 \ldots w_m \quad CR \quad CODE >$$

k = first word of english language part (key)

w_i = ith word of english language part, except key $(i = 1, 2, \ldots, m)$

CR = cross reference SNOP-code

CODE = SNOP-code

Examples:

<k w_1 .... w_m	CR	CODE >
UTERUS LOWER SEGMENT	∅	T8230
PHARYNX	∅	T6010
PHARYNGITIS	T6010	M4000
INFLAMMATION BLENORRHAGIC	∅	M4040

Fig. 24: Formal structure of SNOP due to PRATT [29, 38].

(3) Use of dictionary entries obtained in step (2) and utterance structure obtained in step (1) to generate SNOP-statements (Fig. 23).

8.4.1.1 Preparation of an Utterance

From the original utterance an *item array* and an *item symbol array* are generated. *Items* are words or punctuation symbols. Abbreviations are regarded as words, for example, L4, meaning "4th lumbar vertebra".

Hyphens and quotation marks are deleted from the utterance. Abbreviations are expanded to their full form or to an abbreviation without a period. Some fixed phrases are transformed into single items ("consistent with" → CW).

Several dictionaries are accessed during this step. They are organized either as binary prefix trees in main storage or in indexed sequential manner on disc, depending on the frequencies of access and on available main storage space. Otherwise the dictionaries are equivalent. The dictionaries are accessed using as key the items or affixes obtained from the item array and deliver the elements of the item symbol array. One element of the item symbol array consists in general of different parts:

<item symbol> : = <mode> <type> <remainder>.

<mode> : identifies informations about the conditions under which the item symbol will be used. The values of <mode> may be:

- '0': obligatory transformation, exceptions to general rules, e. g., a word is used as key in nominal <u>and</u> in adjectival form,

- '/': item symbol is to be ignored,

- '-': the item has to be concatenated with its right neighbour,

- null: normal use of an item symbol.

<type> : indicates special functions to the encoder (Fig. 5), such as

- phrase delimiter,

- parts of speech (noun, adjective, ...),

- transformation from plural form to singular form for English, Latin and Greek words,

- transformation from adjectival to noun,

- transformation from noun to noun,

- deletion of some prefixes (MIDBACK ⟶ BACK),

- transformation of synonyms,

- replacement of plural forms of bilateral organs by their singular forms plus the words "LEFT" and "RIGHT",

- degree of relevance of a word with respect to SNOP,

- direct association of SNOP-codes (MUSCLE: T1300),

- specification of SNOP-code modifiers (ACUTE: CN21 CN45),

- exceptions to general rules.

The output of this step is an item array u_i $(i=1,2,...,n)$ and an item symbol array, which is a list of elements t_{ij} denoting for every item u_i possible transformations (<mode> = null in this example):

u_i:	t_{i1}	t_{i2}	t_{i3}
MALIGNANT	A	N1CY	
LYMPHOMA	N		
TESTIS	N	A1CULAR	
BOWEL	NINTESTINE		
ATYPICAL	A	N3X	N3A

For explanation of the symbols used in the item array see section 4.2.1.

8.4.1.2 Look-up Matching Phase

There are two general parts in this step:

- *Selection* of text structures from the original utterance,
- *transformation* of these text structures and *look-up* in the
  dictionary.

Words from the utterance may be used with two different functions. They may be used
either as a *key* or as a member of a set of words related to another key (*match list*).
The possible transformations t_{ij} in the item symbol array are divided into two sets.
One set of transformations is applied, if the word is used as key, and the other set
of transformations is applied, if the word is a member of a match list.

A *minimal noun phrase* is a non-empty set of words in the context of a special word
between words of type L (phrase delimiters including beginning and ending of the
utterance).

From the item list a variable number of *syntactic potential noun phrases* is generated. A syntactic potential noun phrase consists of a key and of a match list:

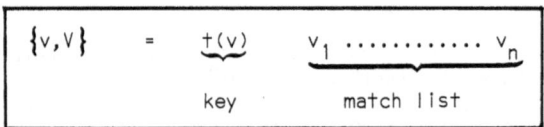

$$\{v,V\} \quad = \quad \underbrace{t(v)}_{\text{key}} \quad \underbrace{v_1 \dots\dots\dots v_n}_{\text{match list}}$$

All v's are words form the item array and t is a key-transformation of v. t may be
the identity transformation. The elements $\{v,V\}$ are directly related to the SNOP-
entries $\{k,W\}$. It is assumed, that the meaningful parts of the language, defined by
the dictionary, may be paraphrased in the utterance in a way, that the semantic elements are contained in the syntactic potential noun phrases. Therefore, for look-up,
the syntactic potential noun phrases have to be compared with the dictionary entries.

Selection of a Key

The item array is scanned and each word is marked as a possible key, if it has a
letter N(noun) or A(adjective) as the first symbol in its item symbol list. Keys are
selected from right to left. Within a minimal noun phrase first all nouns and then
all adjectivals are selected.

Selection of a Match List

To every selected key v a match list V is generated. Members of the match list are
items surrounding the key in the item list. Selection is done using two different
algorithms.

The first algorithm is used in case of *compound acjective phrases* such as "GASTRIC,
PYLORIC, CELIAC, RIGHT COLIC AND AXILLARY LYMPH-NODES". For the noun-noun structure,
"LYMPH-NODES", as key item, the match list will be in turn, each of the adjectivals
or adjectival phrases to the left.

In all other cases each word to the left of the selected key and to the right of the
next delimiter is selected. If there are less than 6 words, than each word to the
right of the selected key and to the left of the next delimiter is selected. This
process is repeated as long as there are less than 6 words in the match list and
there are words left:

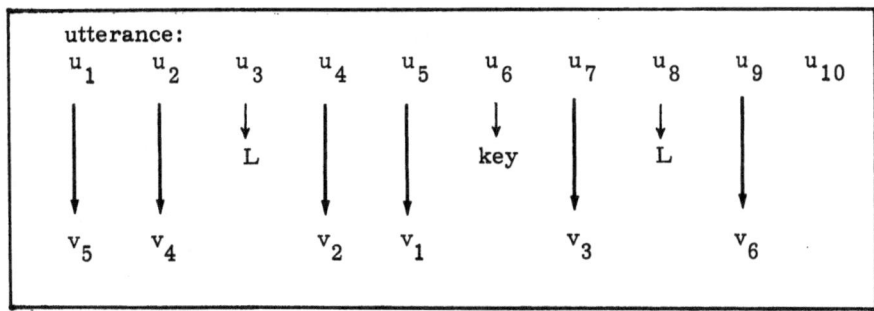

Key and match list represent, in general, a minimal noun phrase and fragments of
other minimal noun phrases.

Look-up Phase

An element $\{k,W\}$ of SNOP is said to be __matched__ with an element $\{v,V\}$ of the original
utterance if the following conditions are met:

$$k = t(v)$$

$$\{w_1,\ldots,w_m\} \subset \{t_{ij}(v_i), \quad j = 1,2,\ldots,n_i; \ i = 1,2,\ldots,n\}$$

That means:

- SNOP contains an element, whose key k is identical to a transformation t(v) of the selected key.

- Every additional word $w_1, \ldots, w_m$ is identical to a transformation of a member of the match list.

- Different words w have to be matched with different elements of the match list.

A selected key v is transformed for access to SNOP as long as there has been no match and there are possible key-transformations left.

After the successful use of a key item, the rightward extent of match lists for later key items may be restricted on the grounds that distinct dictionary entries from the same category are most likely parts of distinct noun phrases, and should not appear in the same match list. That is, inference about the syntactic structure is made from the semantic context. Autopsy summaries often contain long lists of topographic sites, separated by commas or semicolons. This technique limits the inclusion on match lists of significant words from distinct topographic sites occurring to the right of the key item in the utterance.

After a successful look-up on a key item, the SNOP-categories of the resulting dictionary entries are checked for consistency. If there is more than one SNOP-category represented, the restriction is not applied. A search to the right for the previous key item is made. If the results for this key item are also of the same consistent SNOP-category, and the first, or high order, digit of SNOP-code number of the last dictionary entries of each set of results do not match, it is assumed that the two key items belong to separate noun phrases of the same category:

```
MALIGNANT            A N1CY
LYMPHOMA             N
,                    L
TESTIS               N OA1CULAR
,                    L
CERVICAL             A * G
LYMPH-NODE           NLYMPH*$SNODE&LYMPH ANODE*
,AND                 L
TONSIL               N *
.                    LB


T6110      TONSIL
T0820      LYMPH NODE CERVICAL
```

After matching LYMPH NODE CERVICAL and comparing the results with those of the previous key, TONSIL, it is assumed that their respective noun phrases are unrelated. A
"block" to halt the filling of match lists is placed at the previous key item. Under
this modified condition, the program now selects a new key item and its match list.
This simple conclusion on such general evidence is sometimes wrong. It does not appear
to be possible to make accurate deductions about noun phrase structure in medical
language on the basis of the semantic structure of the present SNOP-dictionary.

There are some more additional rules or exception rules, which will not be explained
in detail.

For each selected key, pointers are generated to the items of the item list, which
have been part of a match.

Possible Improvements of Look-up Matching Phase

There is need for optimization of this step due to pragmatic and technical reasons.
Minimal syntactical informations are involved in the generation of the syntactic potential noun phrases. After selecting the elements of a match list, no more syntactical information is used. This approach has two effects:

- Entirely different Kernel sentences will become undistinguishable:

$$
\left\{ \begin{array}{l} \text{NIERENBECKEN} \\ \text{KIDNEY PELVIS} \\ \text{T7200} \end{array} \right\} - \left\{ \begin{array}{l} \text{BECKENNIERE} \\ \text{PELVIC KIDNEY} \\ \text{T7100 M3315} \end{array} \right\}
$$

- The step becomes very expensive. For each key-transformation $t(v)$,
  up to πn_i transformations in the match list have to be performed
  and compared with the set W. This product depends on the number
  of words in set V and it depends on the numbers n_i of possible
  transformations for a word v_i. Another factor is the number of
  possible key transformations, which influences the number of disc
  accesses.

Because the whole algorithm is a match of a language string against a dictionary,
improvements may be

- by identifying syntactic potential noun phrases with less "noise",

- applying only those transformations, which are highly productive.

Weaknesses of the dictionary result in longer lists of exceptions to general rules.
In other words, weaknesses of the dictionary result in longer lists of possible
transformations.

(1) <u>Minimizing the Number of Syntactic Potential Noun Phrases</u>

The number of syntactic potential noun phrases is determined by the number of keys. The number and types of keys are dependent on the structure of initial words of the dictionary. If the structure of the initial words can be described by symbols, which can be derived from an analysis of an utterance, than keys can be recognized and must not be guessed. (For example: keys may be only noun singular words).

(2) <u>Reduction of the Number of Key-transformations</u>

Other formal descriptions of the initial words may be developed, which reduce the number of key transformations to those, which are productive with respect to the dictionary. These transformations may be kept, for example, in a special dictionary based on morphemes or stems. Again, changes to the dictionary SNOP are alternatives to changes of the algorithm.

(3) <u>Minimizing the Length of the Match List</u>

An optimal solution would be a syntactic parser identifying the noun phrases. Experience shows, that general syntactic parsers are of no great value. In medical language some important features of natural language are rarely used, such as verbs, verb phrases, prepositions and so on. Words composing a noun phrase are frequently found in discontinuous sequences of the sentence.

The syntax of natural language may be violated while preserving the content carrying functions of the language (CORTICAL CYST OF THE KIDNEY).

(4) <u>Minimizing the Number $\pi_i n_i$ of Transformations</u>

This is done by minimizing the length of the match list (see (3)) and by minimizing the numbers n_i (see (2)).

8.4.1.3 <u>Mapping Onto the Data Structure</u>

The procedures in this step serve the following purposes:

- Removal of dictionary entries carrying redundant or unwanted SNOP codes.

- Generation of the SNOP-statements combinatorially from the 4 categories represented in the dictionary entry array.

- Application of the SNOP-code number modifications for the inflammation, neoplasm, and leukemia code groups.

- Application of semantic consistency rules embodied in the code structure and cross-references of SNOP.

- Retentions or deletions for improving the readability of the encoder's output.

The respective algorithms are:

(1) <u>Principle of longest match</u>

This principle has already been mentioned. A SNOP-entry is deleted if his English language part is a subset of the English language part of another SNOP-entry, which has been matched. This principle is based on two contradictory assumptions:

- A SNOP-entry implicates every entry containing a subset of his English language part (hierarchical relations):

```
┌─────────────────────────────────┐
│ T0800 LYMPH NODE, NOS            │
│                                  │
│ T0820 CERVICAL LYMPH NODE, NOS   │
└─────────────────────────────────┘
```

```
┌─────────────────────────────────┐
│ M3850 HEMORRHAGE, NOS            │
│                                  │
│ M3851 HEMORRHAGE, PETECHIAL      │
└─────────────────────────────────┘
```

- A matched SNOP-entry consisting of an English language part, which is a subset of the English language part of another SNOP-entry, is an artefact:

```
┌─────────────────────────────────┐
│ [T0X40 PLASMA, NOS]              │
│                                  │
│ M9733 PLASMA CELL MYELOMA        │
└─────────────────────────────────┘
```

(2) SNOP-entries with 4 or more adjacent items dominate other SNOP-entries matching or overlapping on exactly one of these items and having at least 2 fewer matched items:

```
┌────────────────────────────────────────────────────┐
│ FOREIGN BODY GIANT CELL REACTION, KNEE JOINT         │
│                                                      │
│       M4414 FOREIGN BODY GIANT CELL REACTION         │
│       T1272 KNEE JOINT                               │
│       [M3911 JOINT BODY (T1200)]                     │
└────────────────────────────────────────────────────┘
```

An exception is made when the overlapping item is a topography modifier such as LEFT.

(3) Expansion of the entry array by inclusion of the cross-references.

(4) Expansion of the entry array to include new entries generated from those unmatched items carrying a default SNOP-code in their item symbol list:

```
┌─────────────────────────────────────────────┐
│  SMALL              G                         │
│  ARTERIES           XT4100 ⌀SARTERY           │
│  OF                 L                         │
│  LEFT               GTL                       │
│  ARM                N                         │
│                                               │
│  TY802   ARM LEFT                             │
│  T4100   ARTERIES                             │
└─────────────────────────────────────────────┘
```

(5) The dictionary entry array is reduced to include only one entry having any given SNOP-code. Duplicate codes are removed.

(6) SNOP topographic region codes (TY000 to TY999) are deleted, when the matched items overlap the matched items of a dictionary entry having a non-region topography code:

```
┌──────────────────────────────────┐
│   T1111    FRONTAL BONE           │
│  [TY011    FRONTAL REGION]        │
└──────────────────────────────────┘
```

(7) The dictionary entry M9593 MALIGNANT LYMPHOMA is deleted, as redundant, if any of the malignant lymphoma class morphologies (SNOP codes M9603 to M9703, and M9750 to M9799) are present in the dictionary entry array:

```
┌──────────────────────────────────────────────────┐
│  MALIGNANT LYMPHOMA, HODGKIN'S GRANULOMA           │
│                                                    │
│  [M9593  MALIGNANT LYMPHOMA, NOS]                  │
│   M9673  HODGKIN'S GRANULOMA                        │
└──────────────────────────────────────────────────┘
```

(8) Dictionary entries carrying the general neoplasm class codes (M8000 to M8009) are deleted, as redundant, from the dictionary entry array when a more specific neoplasm class code (M8010 to M9799) is present.

(9) SNOP-code modifications (see section 8.4) are applied to appropriate codes, if and only if there is exactly one dictionary entry in the particular code modification class. The item array is scanned from left to right for items, such as ACUTE, which indicate code modifications but which are unmatched. Modifications to a SNOP-code number digit are not made if the digit already has been modified.

(10) SNOP-statements are now generated combinatorially from the remaining dictionary entries. Some of these are deleted because of inconsistency of SNOP-codes in the generated statement with the cross-reference SNOP-codes carried by the dictionary entry of another category of the statement.

To generate a SNOP-statement, each topography code in the dictionary entry array is paired with each morphology code and each of these pairs with each etiology code, then each of these triples with each function code.

Those SNOP-statements are not retained if a cross-reference SNOP code carried by one of the dictionary entries is inconsistent in the first two digits of SNOP-number with the SNOP-code of the same category in the generated SNOP-statement:

```
CERVICITIS, CHRONIC CYSTIC AND ATROPHIC ENDOMETRIUM

-------------------------------------------------------------

M4384   CERVICITIS, CHRONIC CYSTIC (T83)  ⎫
M7837   ATROPHIC ENDOMETRIUM (T84)        ⎪
                                          ⎬ matched entries
T8400   ENDOMETRIUM                       ⎪
T8300   CERVIX UTERI                      ⎭

-------------------------------------------------------------

T8300   M4384   E0000   F0000             ⎫
                                          ⎪
T8300   M7837   E0000   F0000             ⎪
                                          ⎬ SNOP-statements
T8400   M4384   E0000   F0000             ⎪
                                          ⎪
T8400   M7837   E0000   F0000             ⎭
```

The combinatorial generation of SNOP-statements from an array of dictionary entries assumes, that the utterance for which the statements are generated, states that all members of each SNOP-category are present with each member of the other SNOP-categories. This is frequently true. For example, in surgical pathology an examination of a single specimen is fairly common, or a single diagnosis from the morphology category may be stated for several specimens from the same case. It is also frequently untrue, for example, "necrosis of spleen, hyperemia of liver". The algorithm uses the semantic rules implied by the cross-reference SNOP-codes, where available, to purge some of the possible erroneous combinations. However, the errors arising from this method cannot be generally eliminated without the use of medical language syntax to help establish the proper semantic combinations to be generated from dictionary entries matched on noun phrases.

In this final phase a sequence of individually simple algorithms, some of them semantically contentless, has been used for a kind of semantic processing. When a dictionary is developed with a more complete representational structure for its domain of medicine the linguistic processes operating on a well-developed semantic dictionary should become both simpler and more interesting academically.

The viability of the current techniques against the current dictionary may be summed up as follows. A single simple algorithm can often make multiple changes to a data structure. These changes may cut across the boundaries of quite diverse portions of a conventional, intuitively satisfying linguistic or semantic theory. The "meaning" of these contentless algorithms is partly to be found in their sequential relationships. In constructing them, one considers what structure the data have before and after their application, which algorithm follows, and if the effect produced at this point in the sequence is desirable. This kind of system is relatively easy to program but the interdependencies among its components make certain kinds of modifications difficult or impossible.

Modifications, which do fit easily into this framework are treatment of high frequency problems, which can be recognized from SNOP-codes, such as the treatment of the malignant lymphomas and topographic regions.

8.4.1.4 Adaptability of the Algorithms to German Medical Language

So far, there is no reason why the algorithms could not be applied to German medical language too. Our experience is, that there are neither serious semantical nor structural problems. Nevertheless, the direct implementation would be inefficient because of the widely used possibility of generating compound words in German language.

Listing all the possible paraphrases in SNOP, would probably lead to an enlargement by a factor of about 4. Furthermore,most compound words denote compound concepts from several semantic categories. This would result in a much more complex cross-reference structure. For this reason a modification using the segmentation approach should be done. If the basic entity "word" is replaced by "segment", than SNOP can even be reduced.

Therefore, semantic markers have been associated with segments. Each segment, which appears only in a single SNOP-entry, is marked by the respective SNOP-code. Each entry in SNOP, whose semantic content can be generated from the semantic contents of its segments can be deleted from SNOP. In other words, if the segmentation of SNOP-entries delivers the same result as the semantic factoring does, then the SNOP-entry can be generated both by language and by meaning.

8.4.1.5 Expansion of the Data Structure

SNOMED [5] is the basis for expansion of the above described methods to medicine. It imposes a fundamental data structure, which has to be proved in practical use.

Depending on the accurateness of encoding, provision has to be made to encode modifiers, which are not part of the concepts listed in SNOMED (e. g., size, degree, time, number, quality, extent, and so on). Furthermore relations have to be established between the fundamental SNOMED-statements (Fig. 25).

The language tokens and the grammatical functions for representation of these relationships have to be defined. This is a medical and a linguistic problem. After this has been done, it seems to be possible to develop algorithms for the recognition of

- pathogenesis

  TUMOR OBSTRUCTING SMALL INTESTINE

  EPIDURAL HEMATOMA COMPRESSING TEMPORAL LOBE

- logical relationships

  BLINDNESS DUE TO ACCIDENT

- qualifications

  CARCINOMA OF THE ADRENAL GLAND WITH EXTENSION INTO THE RENAL CORTEX

  CARCINOMA OF THE STOMACH INFILTRATING INTO THE PANCREAS

- relations between elements of PTMEF-statements

$$B\left(A\left\{I\left[L(t_i, m_j), e_k\right], f_\ell\right\}, P_n\right)$$

A statement like this one would be read as:

a procedure p_n "B" ("as therapy for") a lesion m_j L

("in", "contained in", "of") site t_i I ("due to")

e_k A ("associated with") f_ℓ.

Fig. 25: Examples for relations which have to be considered in medical language data processing using SNOMED [5].

the full semantic content of language data and for data structures, which allow for formal representation and retrieval of the semantic content.

9   Automated Retrieval of Language Data

Automated retrieval of language data is done by

- document identification (patient identification),

- content.

Retrieval by document identification shall not be discussed here because it offers
no special problems in medical language data processing. Retrieval by content means,
that there is a search question, asking for all documents whose semantic content mat-
ches the semantic content of the question.

If there is only a *sectioning of reports* (see section 8.1), then information retrieval is accomplished in one of two ways:

   (1) Retrieval of the content of (sub-)sections,

   (2) scanning of specified (sub-)sections for the appearance of
       user-defined descriptors.

In *technical systems* (see section 8.2) data search may be done by explicit data field
and value. In computer-based systems boolean expressions are used for query across
data fields. Additional specification of strings for free text supplements may be
possible. The same remarks can be done for *man/machine systems* (see section 8.3).

In *descriptor systems* (see section 8.4) data search is done by explicit or implicit
specification of descriptors. This is most easily be understood in descriptor-in-
-context-systems, using word-oriented thesauri. For every descriptor asked for, all
its synonyms and all the descriptors in a downward hierarchical relation are additionally supplied. This has to be done either by man or by computer.

In systems using the idea of Kernel sentences, search questions are manipulated in
the same way as language data. The Kernel sentences are extracted from the search
question and these Kernels are compared with the data base of Kernel sentences from
the original data, if there is no cross-referencing between different Kernel sentences.

Measures for the quality of retrieval systems

The best known measures for the quality of retrieval systems are

$$recall = \frac{\text{number of relevant elements retrieved}}{\text{number of relevant elements in the collection}} \quad ,$$

$$precision = \frac{\text{number of relevant elements retrieved}}{\text{number of elements retrieved}} \quad .$$

The value of the two measures ranges between 0 and 1. Ideally, both values are equal
to 1. The computation of the two measures requires a knowledge not only of what is
retrieved, but also of what is relevant to a given query. For the *recall*-computation,

furthermore, information must be available concerning the number of relevant items in the collection. This information is available only for small test queries because it requires additional indexing by experts. In general, the two measures are dependant, and improvement of one measure results in deterioriation of the other one.

Another problem is the definition of *relevance*. If we use descriptor systems, than we can represent the documents D_i in the collection in a first level approach by a set of descriptors

$$D_i \simeq \{d_{i1}, d_{i2}, \ldots, d_{im_i}\} \quad , \quad i = 1, 2, \ldots, m \; ,$$

and the query q by another set of descriptors

$$q = \{q_1, q_2, \ldots, q_n\} \text{ with the notion of length of } q = n \; .$$

It is fair to say, that a document D_i is relevant, if q is a subset of $\{d_{ij}\}$. Looking at normal communication, a well defined boundary between relevant documents and irrelevant documents is unnatural. Medical informations build an information continuum and discrete dots are enforced only when people communicate. It may be possible to find a fuzzy definition of "relevance" in terms of:

> a document is *relevant,* if *some* or *most* of the descriptors q_i are members of the set $\{d_{ij}\}$.

Then we may give the following definition of

$$\textit{degree of relevance} = \frac{\text{number of descriptors } q_i \text{ matched with set } \{d_{ij}\}}{n} .$$

In this case it may be up to the user to define his own boundary of relevance.

Using this approach, every descriptor has the same weight. This may be changed for descriptor systems with different information "load". For example, in a medical descriptor system, there is not much information in descriptors like "lobe", "disease", "morbus", "disturbance", and so on. More information is contained in descriptors like "heart", "carcinoma", "right upper lobe", and so on. Therefore, a weight may be introduced for each descriptor in the system. This may be done by experts, or it may be done by a formal algorithm. A better known formal algorithm is a definition of the weight of every descriptor proportional to a number 1/p, where p is the relative frequency of the descriptor in the data base. This introduces the notion of a *rank number* R for every document with respect to a given query:

$$R \sim \sum_{k=1}^{n} \delta_k / p_k \; , \qquad \delta_k = \begin{cases} 0, & q_k \notin \{d_{ij}\} \\ 1, & q_k \in \{d_{ij}\} \end{cases}$$

If a thesaurus is used, another approach may be taken to define some sort of neighbourhood to a special dot defined by a query. *Associative relations* may be used to define for each pair of descriptors the degree S of similarity between the semantic concepts denoted by the descriptors. If this is the case, the query may be extended from each descriptor q_i to a set of descriptors r_j with $S(q_i, r_j) \geq p$ where p has to be selected by the user. This type of similarity is defined implicitly in a nomenclature like SNOP or SNOMED by the neighbourhood in the respective lists and it has become explicit in the similarity of the SNOP-codes. Due to the hierarchical structure of the SNOP-code, a "distance" between two semantic concepts may be defined in terms of the difference of the respective SNOP-codes. It is quite clear, that the code-equivalent of a descriptor is not a value of a quantitative variable called T or M. Nevertheless the hierarchical organization introduces some properties of mathematical variables. It is possible to define in the M-category a subspace by the limits M4 and M4999(inflammation), or M41 and M4199 (acute inflammation) or M411 and M4119 (acute focal inflammation). Using this notion of a variable, reflecting the similarity of medical concepts, queries like the following one seem to be naturally formalizable:

All documents with inflammatory diseases of bones, caused
by bacteria and associated with pain:

T11**   M4***   E1***   F753*

This query defines not only a set of dots but also a 4-dimensional subspace of the total information space defined by SNOP. These features have been used for the development of a retrieval language [29]:

All records of "primary choriocarcinoma of the uterus
with metastases to the liver and with no metastases to
the lung":

IF SNOP   EQ T8300 M8823 /

AND SNOP EQ T5600 M8826 /

AND NOT SNOP EQ T2800 M8826.

9.1   DATA PRESENTATION

There are other improvements that are enabled in data presentation using a semantically structured lexicon that may only be demonstrated shortly. If we look at an autopsy
report represented as a set of dots in the 4-dimensional discrete information space
defined by SNOP, it is possible to give formalized projections of this report using
2 dimensions:

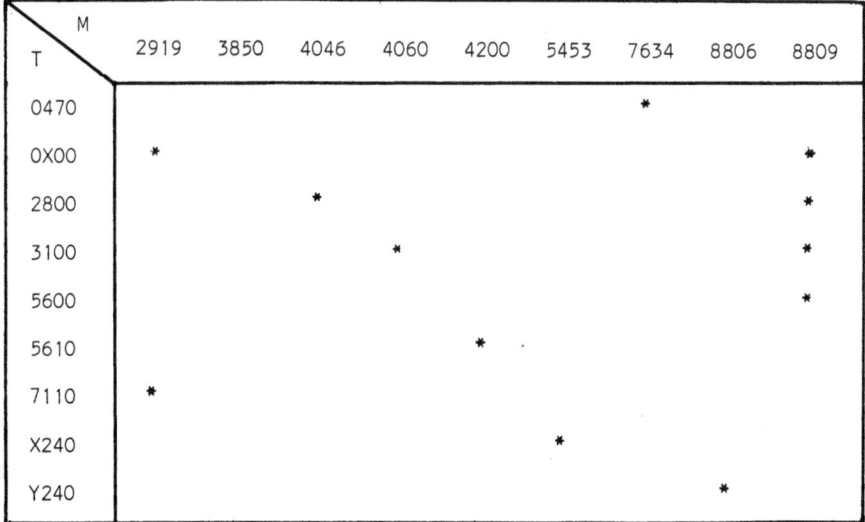

T \ M	2919	3850	4046	4060	4200	5453	7634	8806	8809
0470							*		
0X00	*								*
2800			*						*
3100				*					*
5600									*
5610					*				
7110	*								
X240						*			
Y240								*	

It is quite clear that a data presentation like this one provides some capabilities
of pictures. A whole set of informations can be seen at "one glance". The same type
of data presentation may be used for the projection of a 3rd dimension (write the
3rd "coordinate" in the matrix element) or for a statistical analysis (write the
frequency in the matrix element). Matrixes like the one demonstrated may be further
input to statistical analysis for classification algorithms.

10   Literature

[1]   ANDERSON, J.: Information System in the Hospital
        Lecture Notes

[2]   BARNETT, G.O., GREENES, R.A., GROSSMAN, J.H.: Computer Processing of
        Medical Text Information
        Meth. Inform. Med. 8 (1969) 177 - 182

[3]   BROSS, I.D.J., PRIORE, R.L., SHAPIRO, P.A., STERMOLE, D.E., ANDERSON, B.B.:
        Feasibility of Automated Information Systems in the Users' Natural Languages
        Americ. Scientist 57 (1969) 193 - 205

[4]   CHOMSKY, N.: Aspects of the Theory of Syntax
        Cambridge, Mass.: MIT-Press 1965

[5]   COLLEGE OF AMERICAN PATHOLOGISTS: Systematized Nomenclature of Medicine.
        Trial Version
        Chicago: College of American Pathologists 1975

[6]   DIMSDALE, B.: A Thesaurus Processor
        IBM Form 320 - 2628 (1969)

[7]   VAN EGMONT, J., WIEME, R.J.: Systematized Codification of Medical
        Diagnostic Statements
        In: ANDERSON, J., FORSYTHE, J.M. (eds.): Proceedings of the MEDINFO 74
        Amsterdam: North-Holland Publ. Comp. 1974

[8]   ENGELBRECHT, R., SCHERTLEIN, G., REICHERTZ, P.L.: AKOS - Allgemeines Codie-
        rungssystem
        In: REICHERTZ, P.L. (Hrsg.): Das medizinische System Hannover (MSH)
        IBM Form G 12 - 1166 (1972)

[9]   GIERE, W., BAUMANN, H.: Zur Erfassung und Verarbeitung medizinischer Daten
        mittels Computer. 1. Mitteilung: Ein Datenerfassungs- und Speicherprogramm
        (DUSP) zur Dokumentation von Krankengeschichten
        Meth. Inform. Med. 8 (1969) 11 - 18

[10]   GOOS, G.: Basic Notions of Informatics
        Lecture Notes

[11]   GORDON, B.L. (ed.): Current Medical Information and Terminology (CMIT)
        Chicago, Ill.: Americ. Medic. Ass. 1971

[12]   HALL, P., MEILNER, CH., DANIELSON, T.: J5 - A Data Processing System
        for Medical Information
        Meth. Inform. Med. 6 (1967) 1 - 6

[13]   HARRIS, Z.S.: Mathematical Structure of Language
        New York: Wiley 1968

[14]   HARTMANN, F.: What Could and Should Doctors Learn From Their Experiences
        With Computers in Medicine
        In: ANDERSON, J., FORSYTHE, J.M. (eds.): Proceedings of the MEDINFO 74
        Amsterdam: North-Holland Publ. Comp. 1974

[15]   DE HEAULME, M., MERY, C.: REMAID: An Artificial Language for Medical
        Reports on Computer
        In: ANDERSON, J., FORSYTHE, J.M. (eds.): Proceedings of the MEDINFO 74
        Amsterdam: North-Holland Publ. Comp. 1974

[16]   IMMICH, H.: Klinischer Diagnosenschlüssel (KDS)
        Stuttgart: Schattauer 1969

[17]   KOEPPE, P.: Zum Problem der EDV-gerechten Erfassung medizinischer Befunde
        Meth. Inform. Med. 10 (1971) 25 - 29

[18]   KOEPPE, P., SCHAEFER, P., GUTENMORGEN, W., SCHWOERE, I.: Das System ORVID,
        ein Beitrag zur programmierten Dokumentation in der Röntgendiagnostik
        Fortschr. Röntgenstr. Nukl. Med. 112 (1970) 103 - 110

[19]   LAMSON, B.G.: Natural Language Retrieval System, Pathology Thesaurus
        UCLA 1970

[20]   LEIBER, B.: The German Syndrome Identification and Information
        System (DOFONOS)
        Meth. Inform. Med. 14 (1975) 69 - 72

[21]   LODWICK, G.S., REICHERTZ, P.L., PAQUET, E., HALL, D.L.: "ODARS", A Computer
        Aided System for Diagnosing and Reporting
        Part I: Clinical Problems
        In: DE HAENE, R., WAMBERSIE, A. (eds.): Computers in Radiology

(Proceedings of the International Meeting on the Use of Computers in
Radiology, Brussels, Sept. 1969)
Basel (1970)

[22]   MAYNE, J.G., WEKSEL, W.: Toward Automating the Medical History
        Mayo Clin. Proc. 43 (1968) 1 - 25

[23]   MAYNE, J.G., MARTIN, M.J., MORROW, G.W., TURNER, R.M., HISEY, B.L.:
        A Health Questionnaire Based on Paper-and-pencil Medium Individualized
        and Produced by Computer
        J. Amer. Med. Ass. 208 (1969) 2060 - 2068

[24]   NATIONAL INSTITUTES OF HEALTH: Medical Subject Headings, Index Medicus
        NIH Publ. No. 72 - 265, Vol. 13, part 2
        Nat. Libr. of Med. U.S. Gov. Printing Office, Washington, D.C.

[25]   PACAK, M.: Computational Linguistics and Information Handling
        In: HOWERTON, P.W. (ed.): Management of Information Handling Systems
        Rochelle Park, New Jersey: Hayden Book Comp. Inc. 1974, 19 - 47

[26]   PACAK, M.: Automated Morphosemantic Analysis of Compound Word Forms in
        Medical Language
        Personal note

[27]   PACAK, M., COUSINEAU, L., WHITE, W.: The Segmentation Approach to Dic-
        tionary Construction
        National Institutes of Health: NIH-Publ. 32801

[28]   POCKLINGTON, P.L.: AMAP - A General Optical Mark Reader Form Evaluation
        Program
        Meth. Inform. Med. 12 (1973) 211 - 222

[29]   PRATT, A.W.: Medicine, Computers and Linguistics
        Adv. Biomed. Engineering 3 (1973) 97 - 140

[30]   PRATT, A.W., PACAK, M.: Identification and Transformation of Terminal
        Morphemes in Medical English
        Meth. Inform. Med. 8 (1969) 84 - 90

[31]   REICHERTZ, P.L., LODWICK, G.S., PAQUET, E., HALL, D.L.: "ODARS", A Computer
        Aided System For Diagnosing and Reporting.
        Part II: Technical Problems

In: DE HAENE, R., WAMBERSIE, A. (eds.): Computers in Radiology
(Proceedings of the International Meeting on the Use of Computers in
Radiology, Brussels, Sept. 1969)
Basel (1970)

[32] RÖTTGER, P., WINGERT, F., FEIGL, W., GRAEPEL, P., GROSS, W.M., RIES, P.,
MATAKAS, F.: Structure and Development of a Thesaurus for Accomodation of
Autopsy and Biopsy Records to Automatic Free Text Evaluation
4th Congress of the "Europäische Gesellschaft für Pathologie",
Budapest 21. 9. 1973

[33] STATISTISCHES BUNDESAMT: Internationale Klassifikation der Krankheiten (ICD),
8. Revision
Stuttgart, Mainz: Kohlhammer 1968

[34] THOMPSON, E.T., HAYDEN, A.D. (eds.): Standard Nomenclature of Diseases and
Operations
New York: McGraw-Hill 1961

[35] UICC (International Union Against Cancer): Illustrated Tumor Nomenclature
Berlin, Heidelberg, New York: Springer 1969

[36] UICC (International Union Against Cancer): TNM Classification of Malignant
Tumors
Geneva 1974

[37] UICC (International Union Against Cancer): TNM General Rules
Geneva 1974

[38] WELLS, A.H. (chm.): Systematized Nomenclature of Pathology
Committee on Nomenclature and Classification of Disease
Chicago, Ill.: College of American Pathologists 1965

[39] WINGERT, F.: Klartextverarbeitung in der Pathologie
In: REICHERTZ, P.L. (Hrsg.): Das medizinische System Hannover (MSH)
IBM Form G12-1166 (1972)

[40] WINGERT, F.: Pathologie-Befund-System
Meth. Inform. Med. 12 (1973) 150 - 155

[41]   WINGERT, F.: Word Segmentation and Morpheme Dictionary for Pathology
        Data Processing
        In: ANDERSON, J., FORSYTHE, J.M. (eds.): Proceedings of the MEDINFO 74
        Amsterdam: North-Holland Publ. Comp. 1974

[42]   WINGERT, F.; GRAEPEL, P.: Systematized Nomenclature of Pathology,
        Deutsche Übersetzung
        Schriftenreihe des Instituts f. Mediz. Informatik und Biomathematik
        der Univ. Münster 1975

[43]   WONG, R.L., GAYNON, P.: An Automated Parsing Routine for Diagnostic
        Statements of Surgical Pathology Reports
        Meth. Inform. Med. 10 (1971) 168 - 175

[44]   WORLD HEALTH ORGANIZATION: International Classification of Diseases,
        8th Revision (ICD/VIII)
        Geneva 1967

The computer utility in a health enviroment

W. Schneider

1. Introduction

A health information system (HIS)must be arranged so as to be useful for
widely different circumstances of care. These include information processing where requirements have different timing requirements, levels of detail, need for readiness of access, etc.

a. For anticipatory screening to prevent illness and disability and to
   achieve improved personal health as well as to recognize and control
   early disease resk factors.
b. For periodic and episodic acute or short term care designed to reme-
   dy or cure illnesses and injuries. This may involve management of
   life threatening situations. Data access is almost unpredictable in
   respect to whom and when.
c. For comprehensive, continuing, or extended care (often called "long
   term"), where the purpose is to restore healthful status or to achieve rehabilitation or restoration of function. Predictability of usage
   is high and repetitive. Extended life maintaining services may have to
   be aided when the original medical condition is incurable or unavoid-
   able as can occur with advanced age, etc. In this circumstance it is
   crucial that the system assist in achieving comprehensiveness and
   continuity.
d. For population health educational purpose largely directed toward
   better personal health practices preserving the capacity to cope with
   illness and disability. Here, generality of data usage and elective
   usage of data is common.

It also becomes evident that the most promising strategy for further
development of computer usage in health care is to create a common data
base (CDB) as a core around which the various - step-by-step developed
- application systems are grouped. Together with the common data base
these application systems form the HIS. They can be considered as subsystems of HIS, and it is this notion which is used in this report.

There are mainly two types of such HIS-subsystems. One type, which
may be called CDB independent or dedicated, is used to improve information handling and communication within a structural element of a health

care system such as a clinical laboratory, a pharmacy, a payroll office, a laundry or a kitchen. This type also applies for special care units as e.g. intensive care. These subsystems can be essentially independent of the common data base in their function and can, therefore, preferably be developed, installed, and run autonomously. In many cases they will even use special hardware. It is, of course, an important requirement that these subsystems are designed in such a way as to permit coupling to the hardware and software of the CDB, both for entering data into it and for acquiring data from it. These subsystems are, as a matter of fact, generally used for information processing and communication within such elements of a health service system or a hospital which are responsible for the execution of the above mentioned medical and, to some extent, managerial acts.

The question whether data emanating from these subsystems should be included in the common data base or not depends on whether the introduction of such data are necessary for a subsystem of the second type, i.e. an application system working directly on the information aggregated in the CDB. It is important to note that this second type of subsystem may well require data from subsystems of the first independent dedicated type which are irrelevant to the specific function of the independent subsystem. Subsystems which work directly on the common data base are those where data processing applications assist decision making in the medical care process, or provide analyses for epidemiological follow up and for financial management. The concept of a common data base and two types of subsystems provides a strategy of controlled stepwise progression in developing and establishing a health information system. It is compatible with the general requirements associated with successful computer applications in hospital operation which have been set by Lamson et al. [13] . The principles of setting goals with realistic timetables and selecting departments for initial and subsequent applications are inherent in this concept as well as the principle of modular approach. It is very important at this point to establish clearly the difference between the modular approach in the strategic meaning and the modular hardware approach.

A subsystem as described above is, in the strategic meaning, a module which, from the hardware point of view, may be implemented on a hardware module specific for this subsystem. In the total, single systems hardware approach, it would be installed on the same computer hardware as all the other modules.

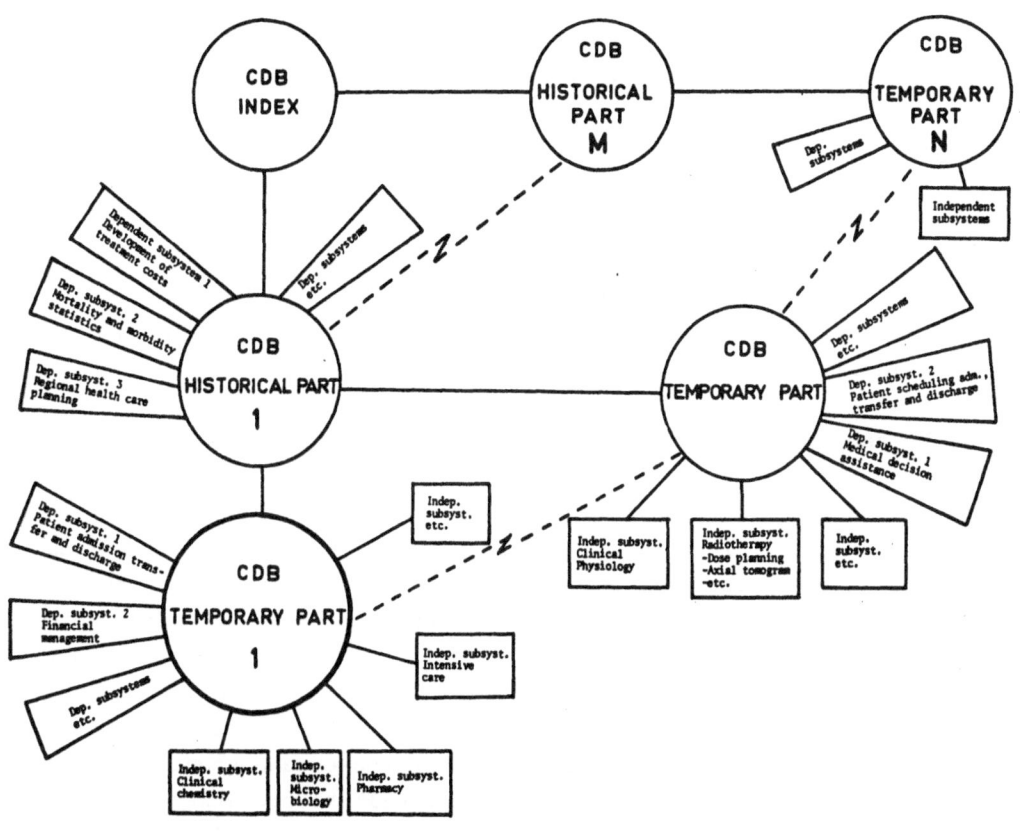

Fig. 1. Basic structure of the health information system.

2. Software

The software for any computer-based handling system must be viewed from two related but significantly different aspects of computer science, namely, systems software and applications software. The systems software comprises a large number of complex computer programs that organize the computer hardware modules into a functioning machine that will process a given job or application. Application programs define the job, that is, the application programs define the form of the data to be processed and the logical constructs of the processing. The analogy of an ambulance may be helpful to the hospital administrator in understanding the relation between systems programs and application programs. Consider that an ambulance cen be driven from point A to B carrying a patient receiving emergency treatment if the driver is competent to drive the vehicle, avoids traffic accidents and knows the route between points A and B.

For practical reasons, it is advantageous to divide the common data base into two parts. The first part consists of data aggregated during a patient's continuing treatment, and the second part consists of historical data. As already stated, only those data should be aggregated in the historical part that are required by existing application programs subsystems, or those under development. In the temporary part - in addition to those data which are necessitated by the historical part - data are aggregated for medical and managerial acts for which subsystems exist, operating shortly before or during a patient's disease or immediately after discharge.

The temporary part of the common data base is favorably located and controlled by the setting of the health service system (e.g. a hospital) responsible for the patient during a specific interval in the course of disease. If a patient is transferred from one organizational entity to another, the data available in the temporary part of the master file can be copied to the temporary part of the second unit, which may or may not use the same computing facility. In many cases, a copy of the reduced data set for the historical part of the common data base will be sufficient. The problem of reduction is significant and yet unsolved. Except for research facilities only those data should be transferred to the historical part of CDB which will be processed by an application subsystem and is motivated by cost reasons. Obviously, the historical part of the CDB will become a huge data base.

This implies that hardware and software resources necessarily have to be shared between a number of organizational activities in the health service system. For many different reasons, in many cases, it will not be possible to have one central implementation of the historical part; instead, shared units will be established, probably on a regional base. This implies, however, that a special index file has to be created, through which any authorized decision maker will get access to the data stored in this regionally distributed common data base, consisting of the historical part of the CDB. This CDB-index file may either be implemented on a central facility at the location of supervising of the health service system, or it may be distributed in accordance with some optimization criteria within such a system or through circular polling of multipel data locations. A further possibility could be to distribute the index file on patient cards with a magnetic strip storage capacity of at least 800 characters [14]. The basic structure of HIS is visualized in fig. 1 (see also [5]).

This aspect of the ambulance is analogous to the applications aspect of the computer - the task to be performed. But consider that an ambulance is a complex mechanical object in its own right. It consists, in addition to a cargo space and a driver's seat, an engine described in terms of parts and horsepower, a transmission which is a complex gear box that transmits the power of the engine to a drive shaft which delivers the force or power of the engine to the drive wheels. In addition, the vehicle has a frame, a steering system, a braking system, a heat exchange system to name some of its complex structure. It is this integrated structure of functional parts of the vehicle that is analogous to the systems programs and the integrated hardware components that we recognize as a functional computer.

There is a purpose to this analogy. The hospital administrator and his supporting staff should not and probably cannot be involved in writing computer systems except for the most trivial of computers. The competence to create de novo, competent computer systems stands totally apart from any hosptial function and involves staff competence and costs that no hospital or consortium of hospitals can afford. It should be expected that the hospital administrator can rent or buy a competent computer (equivalent to a functional ambulance) that as well-defined hardware components and competent systems programs to integrate these hardware modules in the functional sense. However, the hospital administrator's staff should have some systems programming competence but only at the level necessary to evaluate the computer vendor's product or interface application programs efficiently.

Providing suitable applications software for the efficient storage and processing of medical and administrative data is the responsibility of the administrators and their staff. Irrespective of their common functions, most hospitals tend to have unique operations requirements. Thus, no complete general purpose software for hospital functions has been invented the hospital administrator cannot purchase applications software in the same sense that he can purchase systems software. Thus, the design, implementation and utilization of the applications software is the responsibility of the hospital administrator and his staff. This responsibility of the hospital administrator cannot be put aside; only the hospital administrator can provide the managerial and scientific leadership for the difficult task of defining and designing the applications software.

Clearly, the design task for the applications software represents

a challenging task. There is a basic requirement on the one hand to
establish dedicated files which support the activity of the several services of the hospital, e.g., the registration of patients, the operation of the clinical laboratory, the operation of the blood bank, etc.
These data files and their interlocked computer applications programs
sustain the operation of the individual services. There is on the other
hand a different basic requirement, namely, the creation of an integrated, computer-based medical record for every patient which includes the
pertinent medical data for every hospitalization and out-patient visit
and which is current or medically up-to-date for any current medical
episode. The integrated, medical data file, the common data base CDB
supports the medical decision-making process that sustains the clinical
management of a patient.

For the dedicated applications, it is clearly the case that existing software technology can provide the hospital with efficient systems for data storage and processing. The systems requirements for such
applications tend to be straightforward since typically, the dedicated
files are designed with their own data storage space such as magnetic
tape or a direct access storage device. Definition of the data and data
formats is easily controlled since the dedicated application supports
a homogeneous user population. Thus, the tasks of data editing, file
entry and data retrieval are greatly simplified. In addition, the standard compilers have proven quite satisfactory for writing the data dependent computer programs required to process the data involved in the
execution of a dedicated application.

Creating applications software for the efficient management of an
integrated common data base such as that required to represent the complete medical record constitutes a more difficult problem. In fact, the
creation and efficient management of an integrated data base may well
represent the key or primary problem to be solved in the developing
of a computer-based hospital medical information handling system.

It is convenient and highly arbitrary to speak of three approaches
to this problem. Two of these approaches are quite traditional and both
involve the use of dedicated data files. The first of these two traditional approaches calls for redundant storage of multiple-use data in
the several dedicated data files. This approach has proven to be unsatisfactory. It is usually the case that new data do not get added to all
the files on a regular and carefully monitored basis and thus files be-

come incomplete and often out of date. It is also the case, that the redundant data stored in the different files are of different formats and are incorporated in specific data organizations and structures which are matched to specific storage devices. Thus, any change in data format, data value and structure or storage devices can lead to a chaotic state of the data files. The second of the two traditional files calls for the normal up-to-data maintenance of the individual dedicated data files. From these files pertinent data necessary for an integrated data file are gathered by a set of multiple job steps. In this action data are extracted from each of the dedicated data files for entry into the integrated data base. This organization of applications software is in widespread use and has proven to be reliable. However, the multiple job step organization of software tends to be costly and usually involves a large amount of reformating of data for construction of an integrated data file.

The third approach to the creation and management of an integrated common data base represents a newer dimension in computer science and is often referred to in terms of "data base concepts" and "data base management". Current data base concepts presume that these undesirable attributes of data files can be eliminated by the concept of "a data base". A data base is defined as a non-redundant collection of interrelated data elements that can be processed by one or many application programs. The data base concept is founded on the notion that the physical storage of data is achieved independent of any direct association with the application program. Thus, the data base provides for flexibility of data organization and allows addition, deletion, update and change of data without requiring modifications in existing programs.

In summary, the advantages of the data base concept are: (1) Elimination of redundant data from the data file and elimination of redundant data maintenance procedures. (2) Reduction in storage costs and applications processing costs. (3) Independence of physical storage of data and data organization from application programs. (4) Greater reliability of data and a more consistent use of data.

The software used for data base management consists of at least two major components: (a) the data base manager component and (b) the data communications component.

The data base manager component must provide data organization methods that are suitable for creation, interrelation and maintenance of large common data bases that can be expeditiously used by multiple application programs.

The data base communications component must provide for data base processing in the batch mode but more importantly must provide the ability to do data base processing in the teleprocessing environment and finally provide an efficient telecommunications sub-system to support large volume - useful time response for an applications area.

Much progress has been made in the design and implementation of data base managers. Increasingly, such software systems are coming on the market. None of these new products have proven their worth for integrated data handling on the scale that is required by a large general hospital. However, progress is rapid and the existing progress that has been made in generating these complex software systems for data base management has already made the development of a computer-based medical data handling system a far more tractable problem (see e.g. [15,16]).

3. Hardware

It is now traditional to speak of two different "approaches" to the development of medical information systems; the "modular" approach and the "total system" approach. There is in fact a third concept which can be called for want of a better name, the "utility" concept. All have much in common and have the same long-term goal, namely that of providing integrated medical data processing and data communication services.

The modular approach places primary emphasis on identifying and, in fact, isolating functional units of medical activity which have clearly articulated information processing requirements. These functional units of medical activity are called modules and may comprise a hospital function such as "admission and discharge" or may represent a hospital department such as X-ray or the pharmacy. In the modular approach, the primary concern is to provide a data processing capability which will sustain the operational integrity of each of the identified modules. Since each of the hospital modules is usually implemented on highly standardized, limited capacity, hardware/software systems, the presumption is that ultimately, the several modules in a hospital can be linked together as a distributed capacity computer network to form a total medical information system for a hospital. A detailed discussion of the advantages and disadvantages of the modular approach to medical information systems is in the literature [1]. The total systems approach initially takes a more holistic view of a medical information system as contrasted with the more atomistic view of the modular approach for a hospital [2,3,4,12]. The design effort is oriented from the outset to integrate the units of medical activity (the modules) into an integrated total system designed to accomodate total data flow both within a module and among modules. This approach presumes that by a detailed, systematic study of some sample of existing data flow patterns, it is possible to specify and develop for a relatively large computer configuration, the components of a highly reliable operating system that can accommodate existing and future requirements for total data flow without forcing major systems changes.

The hardware and systems software utility concept is fully compatible with either the modular or total system approaches. The utility concept also places primary emphasis on the careful definition of the information tasks of the medical units and recognizes the need to isolate (make "stand-alone") or integrated the individual functional information tasks. In most other aspects, the utility concept differs significantly. The utility concept is basically conceived as a hierarchically organized hardware/software configuration comprised of small, medium and large capacity machines. The hierarchy has a minimum of two levels; additional levels are easily accommodated and are in fact, encouraged. Human-dependent interaction by terminal is possible at all levels in the hierarchy. At the lowest level of hierarchy are the indispensible minicomputers, the new microprocessors and special-task hardware that perform the on-line functions of the clinics and laboratories. These machines comprise a variety of types and can be used in the stand-alone mode or can be intermittently or continuously linked to computers of larger capacity that are in the hierarchy. At the highest level in the hierarchy is a large, centralized computer capacity shared by many users. The centralized computer facility has multiple operating systems and provides a variety of user services in both the batch and interactive mode. The utility concept for medical information systems attempts to take advantage of the current trends in the evolution of computer technology. In addition, this approach attempts to match computer capacity and power to the information handling tasks of the clinical and laboratory applications.

The evolution of computer technology has emphasized in recent years two highly contrasting trends in an effort to (1) improve equipment reliability and flexibility and (2) reduce costs of computer services. One trend has resulted in the introduction of minicomputers, microprocessors and inexpensive, increasingly standardized, digital interfacing equipment. Minicomputers have become common instruments throughout the world. Very innovative use has been made of these instruments by scientific professionals who have no computer science competence because these machines are free of any complex operating system and are relatively easily interfaced to transducers (measuring devices) and other computers. The advent of this kind of digital equipment has provided highly reliable, flexible computer equipment at the local level and has placed control of a computer-based task in the hands of those responsible for the application. The other trend in the evolution of computer technology has emphasized the development of highly centralized computer facilities. The effort has focused on the attachment of various kinds of input/output terminals to large central computer facilities and in turn, these large central computer facilities are being linked together in the form of computer networks. Via these centralized facilities, it becomes possible to share costly program libraries and data bases at greatly reduced costs. The cost of communicating data to a remote site for processing is far less than the cost of establishing a redundant and usually limited autonomous data processing and computation facility. Clearly, the progress in computer technology is at the two ends of the computer technology spectrum - the small and the large. These trends in the evolution of computer technology will continue since the areas of great opportunity lie at the two ends of the computer technology spectrum.

It is rational and correct to argue that the current evolution of computer technology is in the best interests of biomedicine. Experience has shown that the conduct of the work in the clinics and laboratories requires, at a minimum, varying degrees of two different levels or modes of digital equipment support. It is convenient and arbitrary to refer to these levels as (1) the process level and (2) the analysis level. At the analysis level, digital equipment support is equipment support for data gathering, on-line control and real-time event monitoring with respect to the execution of the procedures and protocols of the clinics and laboratories. This mode of operation is well served by minicomputers acting as flexible, reliable, inexpensive, process level control devices. The minicomputers and the newer microprocessors readily provide the computer support environment for on-line processes involving real-time instrumentation applications and human-dependent interactions.

At the analysis level, digital equipment support is required for extensive transformation, analysis, integration and reporting of clinical, laboratory and administrative data and their derivative information. There is a universal and rapidly increasing demand for medical documentation in support of cost accounting and financing of health activities, quality assurance of health care, continuing medical education and research and the planning and rationalization of health oriented functions. The increasingly large data handling tasks which characterize the analysis level are well served and probably can only be served by large, well integrated centralized computer facilities.

It is generally agreed that modern computer equipment can provide all the technological capability required for medical information systems. Translating this technological capability into a useful medical data handling capability requires that a well defined information system design be superimposed on the hardware/software configuration. As noted above, the utility approach to computer-based information systems is based on a hierarchical design. This design presumes that any set of information processing tasks can be represented as a well defined hierarchy comprising levels which will range from highly localized data gathering tasks - the medical process level, to the complex tasks involving transformation, translocation, analysis and integration, and reporting of data and their derivative information - the medical analysis level. By assignment of the individual tasks to a given level in the hierarchy, the task is identified and the relation among tasks is explicitly expressed.

In the hierarchical design, the levels in the hierarchy are defined by the functional requirements of the specific information processing task to be performed and the equipment employed is matched to the task. It is expected in the hierarchical design that a variety of equipment will be employed in the hierarchy, particularly at the level or levels where minicomputers and microprocessors are employed. It is also expected that new equipment can be added or substituted in the hierarchy thus enabling the information system to benefit from technological progress. The hierarchical design is an effective design. It preserves the integrity of both localized and centralized information processing operations and places control of these operations at the responsible level. The hierarchical design combines the outstanding advantages of localized,

dedicated processing facilities and minimizes the disadvantages of such
facilities when either is used in the independent mode. Maximum advantages is taken (1) of the flexibility and power of small capacity equipment and (2) of the multiprocessing, multiple services capability of
large capacity equipment.

The utility concept has a firm basis in reality. This concept with
strong emphasis placed on the hierarchical design, has been successfully
used in military applications, industrial process control applications
and commercial applications - particularly banking. In recent years, as
more funds have become available, the utility approach has been increasingly applied in the biomedical and physical science research laboratories. In this environment, the technology underlying the utility concept has evolved rapidly because of (1) the sheer complexity of the subject matter to be processed, (2) the broader task spectrum that is inherent in the processing and analyzing of scientific data and (3) access
to large cost-shared, central facilities such as those existing in the
university. The rapid evolution of the technology underlying the utility
concept plus the acquisition of productive experience has encouraged
the medical computer scientist to attempt adapting this concept approach
to computer-based medical information systems for specific clinical activities and support of the delivery of health care. For example: the
"Multi-Satellite System" (MSS) at Uppsala University, Uppsala (Sweden)
which has been in operation since 1966 is an excellent example of the
utility concept [5]. This system, which is used for processing administrative data and some clinical care support data, comprises a network
for a large geographic area and links together local, regional and centralized computer resources. The University Hospital at the University
of California, Los Angeles, California (USA) has a central computer facility for hospital administration, financial management, medical record search and retrieval that is linked with the extensively computerized clinical laboratories [6]. The Medical System Hannover (MSH) at the
Hannover University Hochschule for Medicine, Hannover (West Germany)
includes plans for the linkage of special purpose computer hardware to
the central computer facility [4]. The National Institutes of Health
(NIH) computer facility, Bethesda, Maryland (USA) also represents a pio-
neering effort in developing the computer utility concept for medical
data handling [7].

References

1 G.O. Barnett, The Modular Hospital Information System. Comp. & Biomed. Res., Fourth Vol., B. Waxman and R.W. Stacy, eds., Academic
   Press (in press).
2 M.F. Collen, Implementing hospital computer systems: general requirements, in: Hospital Computer Systems, M.F. Collen, ed. (John Wiley
   & Sons, New York, 1974).
3 P.F.L. Hall, Implementing hospital computer systems: current status
   of the Karolinska hospital computer system (Stockholm), in: Hospital
   Computer Systems, M.F. Collen, ed. (John Wiley & Sons, 1974).
4 P.L. Reichertz, Implementing hospital computer systems: Medical
   School of Hannover Hospital Computer System (Hannover), in: Hospital
   Computer Systems, M.F. Collen, ed. (John Wiley & Sons, New York,
   1974).
5 W. Schneider, Integrattion of data from a computer automated laboratory into a generalized hospital information system, in: Automati-
   sierung des klinischen Laboratoriums (F.K. Schattauer Verlag, Stutt-
   gart-New York, 1968) pp. 301-305;
   W. Schneider, MSS, a centrally planned decentralized medical information system in Sweden, Proc. of MEDIS 1972, Osaka International
   Symposium on Medical Information Systems, Kansai Institute of Information Systems, Japan.
6 B.G. Lamson, personal communication. Director, Center for Health
   Sciences, School of Medicine, UCLA, Calif.
7 A.W. Pratt, NIH computer hardware complex. Federation Proceedings
   of the Federation of American Societies for Experimental Biology
   Computer Conference, Vol. 33, No. 12 (1974).
8 R. Fajman and J. Borgelt, Communications of ACM, V. 16, N5 (1973).
9 R. Sproull, Omnigraph Decsystem-10 Display Systems. Technical Report, DCRT, NIH, DHEW, Bethesda, MD.
10 G. Knott, MLAB" An On-line Modeling Laboratory. Technical Report,
   DCRT, NIH, DHEW, Bethesda, MD.
11 R. Shrager, MODELAIDE: A computer graphics program for the evaluation of mathematical models. Technical Report DCRT, NIH, DHEW,
   Bethesda, MD.
12 W. Spencer, R. Baker and C. Moffet, Hospital computer system, Adv.
   Biomed. Engin. 2 (1972) 61.
13 B.G. Lamson, W.S. Russel, J. Fullmore and W.E. Nix, The first decade of effort: Progress towards a hospital information system at
   the UCLA hospital, Los Angeles, California, Meth. Inform. Med. 9
   (1970) pp. 73-80.
14 U. Ericsson, W. Schneider and K. Vogel, The problem of privacy in
   a computer based integrated health care information system, Proc.
   of MEDINFO 74, Vol. 2 (North-Holland, Amsterdam, 1975) p 694.
15 K. Sauter, (Ed.): A Data Structure Model for a Health Information
   System, Computer Programs in Biomedicine 6 (1976) issue 3.
16 M. Jainz, and T. Risch, ed.: A Data-Manager for a Health Information System. Computer Programs in Biomedicine 6 (1976) issue 3.

LABORATORY

W. Schneider

1. General considerations

1.1. The hospital-laboratory function

A clinical laboratory can be defined as one of the basic structural elements in a health service system, especially designed to perform
observations on the patient.

The main task of the laboratory is to perform the different investigations required by the request stations, i.e. the consumers of laboratory service, (e.g. the wards of a hospital). The result of the investigations performed in the laboratory, the operative station, is a
report, which is transferred to the request station.

Operationally this laboratory function can be considered as consisting of a number of modules, each defining a restricted part of the
laboratory. Structurally a module consists of (i) a input, i.e. that

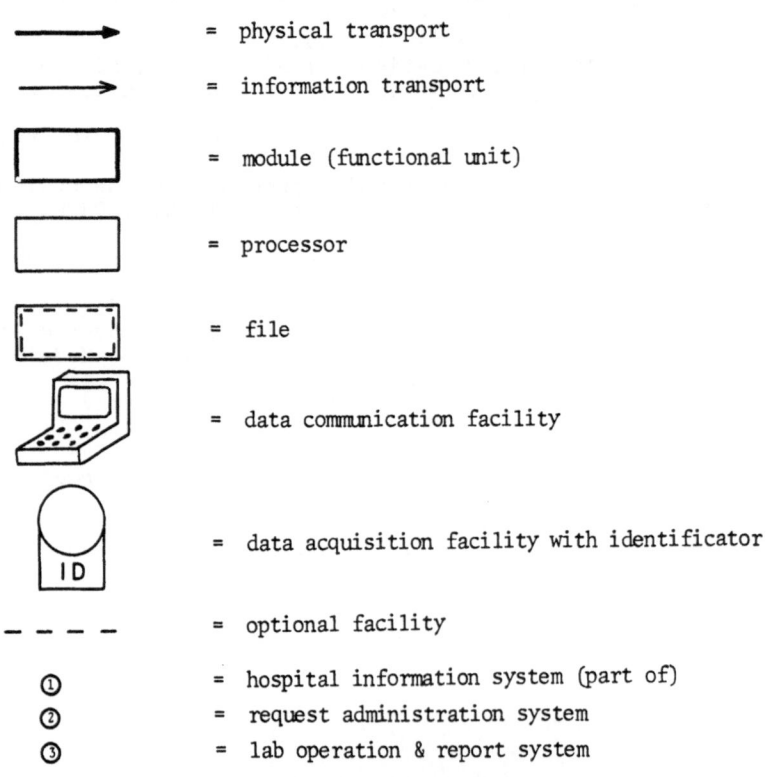

→	= physical transport
→	= information transport
▭	= module (functional unit)
▭	= processor
⬚	= file
	= data communication facility
◯ ID	= data acquisition facility with identificator
- - - -	= optional facility
①	= hospital information system (part of)
②	= request administration system
③	= lab operation & report system

Fig. 3 Explanation of symbols used in Fig. 2

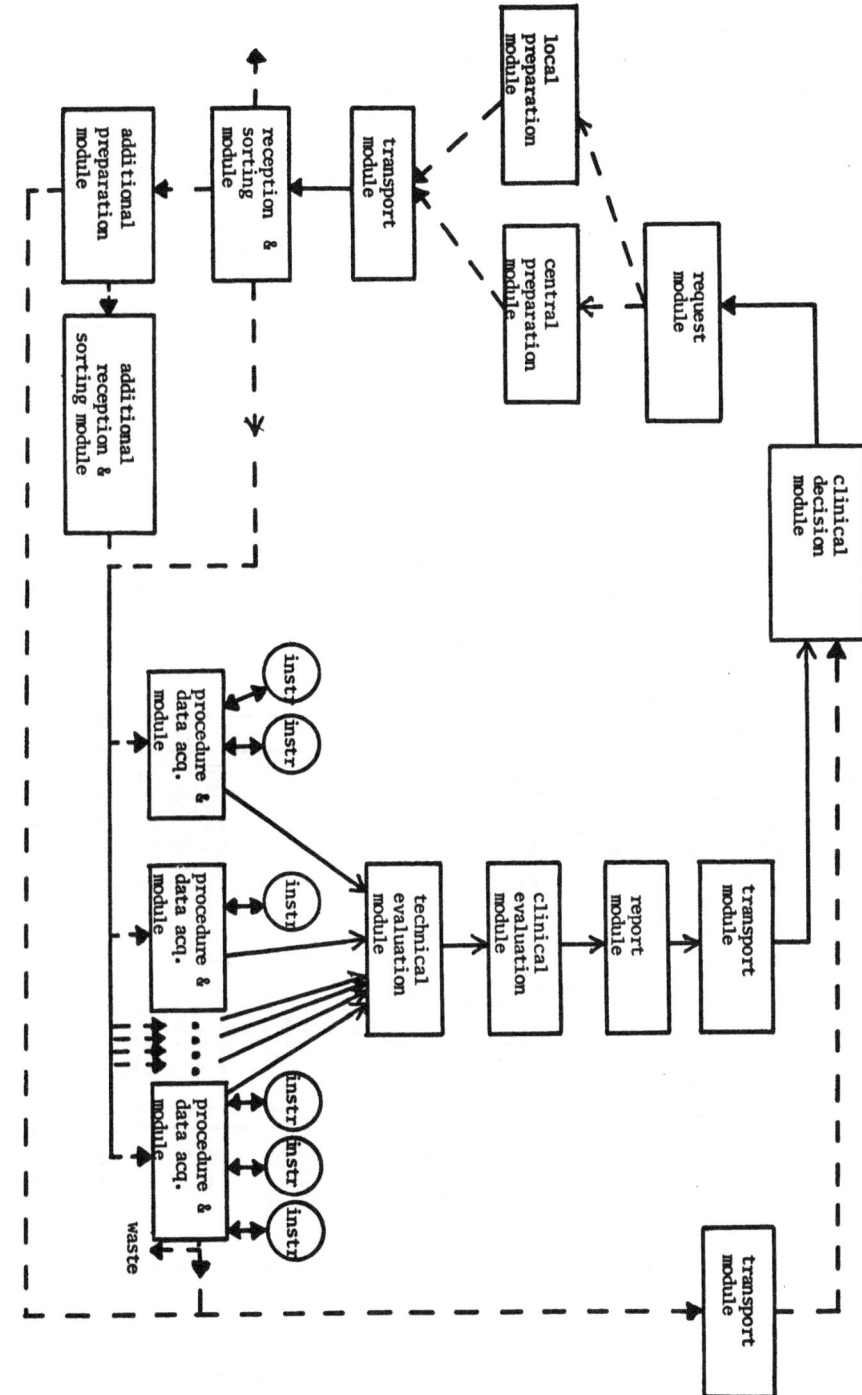

Fig. 1 The laboratory function.

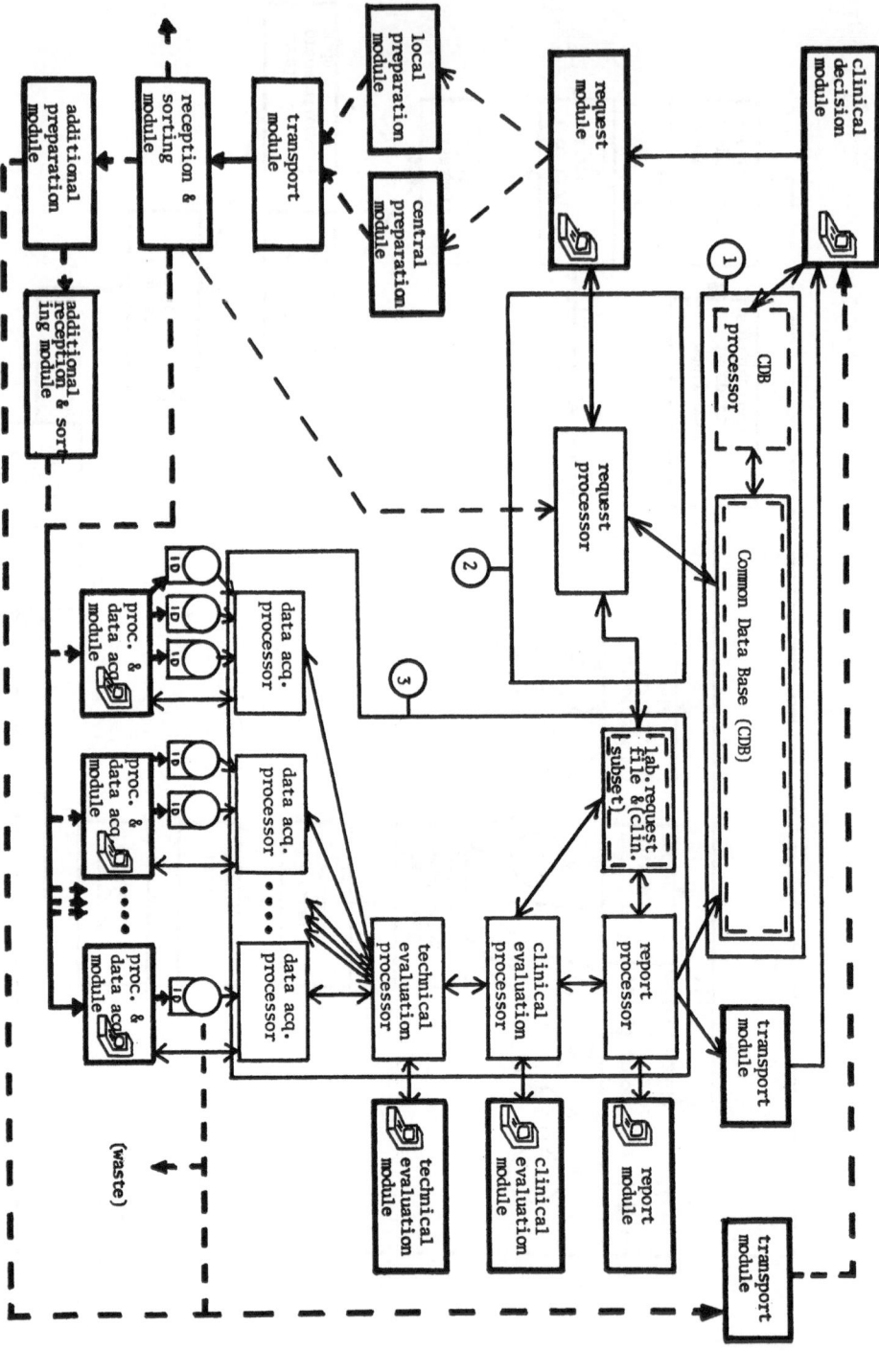

Fig. 2 The laboratory information system.

set of physical entities and information on which the module is operating, (ii) a number of activities that defines the algorithms according
to which the module is operating, and (iii) an output, i.e. the result
of the operations of the module.

The concept could be used to define very large blocks of actions,
each describing a large part of the laboratory function. This results
in a laboratory model consisting of a few modules only, corresponding
to a rather high level of abstraction. On the other hand, the separation into a great number of modules leads to a description of the laboratory in much more detail, involving much less abstraction.

' In the following we have chosen a degree of abstraction which is
consistent with our objectives, i.e. to define a model of the laboratory function appropriate for the description of the structure of the
laboratory information system (fig. 1-3). The ordering of laboratory
service is an integrated part of the clinical decision process. Therefore the first module in the sequence is the clinical decision module,
the output of which is the ordering of a specific laboratory investigation. The clinical decision module can also be considered to be the last
module in the sequence, and it's input is among other things the laboratory report concerning the ordered investigation, which is used in
future decisions. A request is handled by the request module, which is
designed in different ways, depending on what sort of investigation that
is requested, the actual laboratory organization etc. The request process is e.g. influenced by how (i) request registration takes place if
(ii) a booking-procedure of the laboratory resources is necessary and
if (iii) the preparation procedure (e.g. blood sample taking) is going
to be effectuated by a "central" laboratory staff, or by a "local" one,
i.e. by the ward staff.

Request registration may take place after the preparation and transport procedures, if no booking or actual preparation has to be performed. In many cases requests are registered in connection with reception
procedures or during data acquisition. Such a restricted request module
may therefore be placed elsewhere in the model of a specific laboratory.
If booking or central preparation is performed, request registration is
done before the preparation and transport procedures. It is directly
followed by the booking or central preparation procedures which are performed by the administrative part of the request module.

The preparation is effectuated by the <u>local preparation module</u> or the <u>central preparation module</u>. After the preparation the physical entity (e.g. a patient or a sample) is transported to the laboratory in question (<u>transport module</u>).

On arrival to the operative station - the laboratory - the physical entity and possibly the request form are taken care of by the <u>reception and sorting module</u>. Its main activities are to notify the reception of the entity and to send it to one of the succeeding modules, the choice depending on the nature of the entity, the investigation requested and the laboratory structure.

The entity can (i) be transported to another laboratory designed to perform the investigation; (ii) or be transferred to an <u>additional preparation module</u>. In this module it can either be treated in some way and then passed on to the succeeding module, or be transformed into a new physical entity. After the additional preparation, the entity is transported to an <u>additional reception and sorting module</u> with activities analogous to the reception and sorting module above. In the case of additional preparation the original physical entity might have to be sent back to the request station.

The actual investigation takes place in the <u>procedure and data acquisition module</u>. Each laboratory can consist of several such modules, corresponding to different types of investigations. Each of these modules may comprise one or several instruments. Examples of such modules are, in the clinical chemical laboratory, the manipulation and analysing of the samples; in the radiology laboratory, the preparation and adjustment of patient and apparatus, as well as the film registration. In the clinical physiological laboratory it comprises e.g. the application of electrodes and the ECG-registration.

The output from the module are the raw or derived data required by a specific investigation. The physical entity can, at this point if necessary, be transported back to its origin, the request station. The data acquired by the procedure and data acquisition module may not serve as a final result from the investigation. They may have to be further evaluated in different ways. The first phase of this process takes place in the <u>technical evaluation module</u>, where the data are treated with respect to technical and statistical criteria. This evaluation is strictly technical, and no consideration is taken to the clinical parameters such as patient data, the medical relevance and so on. It includes immediate quality control procedures, one of the most important and successful application areas of computers in laboratories.

Input to the next module, the <u>clinical evaluation module</u> is a technically corrected value, and the output is a result which has been corrected, evaluated and commented on, on the basis of the clinical situation of the patient, on which the investigation has been made. The final
step in the result evaluation process is the construction of the final
laboratory investigation report. This is done by the <u>report module</u>. The
laboratory function circle is closed, when the report has been transported back to the decision module (<u>transport module</u>). The information can
be used in the clinical decision process for diagnosis, therapeutical
considerations and as a data base for future requests for complementary
laboratory investigations. It may also result in a decision to initiate
complementary investigations within the laboratory which performed the
original analysis.

1.2 <u>The laboratory information system</u>
The description above deals with the laboratory <u>function</u>, and is
valid for a small manual laboratory as well as for a large, highly automated and computerized central laboratory. Information handling is an
integrated part of almost all activities in each module, independent of
the special character of a laboratory. There is therefore a potential
use of computing power in all modules, because basically information
handling always is intended to be improved. Whether computing power already has or ever may be applied meaningfully within a specific module
of a specific laboratory, depends primarily on the actual need and the
possibilities to adapt technology to the information handling process
of the module and secondarily on the state of the art of computer technology, and on pricing of computing equipment. The structure of such an
information system, within the frame work of the description above, is
shown in fig. 2, and described below.

1.2.1. <u>The health information system</u>.* The part of the <u>health information system</u> which is relevant to consider, as far the laboratory func

---
* For definitions as e.g. "common data base" see chapter "Computer Unility in a Medical Environment".

tion is concerned, consists mainly of the temporary part of the common data base. This part contains demographic information on the patient, his clinical situation and results from previous investigations. It is continuously updated.

1.2.2 The request administration system. The request administration system is the part of the laboratory information system which deals with the requests for laboratory investigations and is implemented on the request processor. In our model, it can be considered to consist of two parts. The first communicates with the clinical decision module and registers all the information given in the order for a laboratory investigation. If necessary it can also update the temporary part of the common data base with data concerning the request. Later in the laboratory process there is a great need for information about the nature of the investigations, and therefore a special file is created inside the laboratory information system, the laboratory request file. Secondly we have the part, which in the case of booked procedure and/or a central preparation procedure takes care of the scheduling of the laboratory resources.

1.2.3. The laboratory operation and report system. The laboratory operation and report system is the part of the laboratory information system which handles the technical part of the laboratory process, and the evaluation of data into a final laboratory report.

Local to each of the procedure and data acquisition modules, and to their respective group of instruments, is a data acquisition processor which performs and controls the data acquisition process. As appropriate it also takes care of direct instrument control. In cases where the instruments are equipped with an identificator, it also executes the reading and transmission of identification codes.

The technical and statistical processing of the acquired data is effectuated by the technical evaluation processor, communicating with the technical evaluation module. Here, the data are treated and corrected in a way specific to each of the different types of laboratories, as described in the following sections. A common function is the possibility to sort out data which are not approved from the technical point of view, resulting in a direct feed-back to the procedure and data acquisition module for repeated action. When the result is technically processed, it must be checked and evaluated from the clinical point of view. This is done in the <u>clinical evaluation processor</u>, which works in communication with the clinical evaluation module. Here the result from the observation must be coupled to the request, i.e. the clinical evaluation processor must have access to the laboratory request file, described above. If a more advanced clinical evaluation is wanted more data is needed, and the laboratory request file must be complemented from the common data base by some sort of a <u>clinical subset</u> containing relevant data describing the patient's clinical situation.

The final information processor necessary to complete the information system is the <u>report processor</u>, which in communication with and under control of the report module prepares the final laboratory investigation report. This has to be done according to what actually was requested, and therefore this processor must have access to the lab. request file.

The report is transported to the request station as described above, but also used for updating the temporary part of the common data base, in order to create the clinical data base for the decision process.

1.3 <u>Hardware and software implementation</u>
Regardless of the type of clinical laboratory, some basic requirements have to be fulfilled independently of the specific hardware and software solution chosen. These are that the system must be highly reliable, rapidly responsive, and provide user-oriented, interactive programming.

It is difficult to exactly define system reliability needs. Most clinical laboratories in medical centers function twenty-four hours a day, seven days a week, and it is desirable that the data processing system be continuously operational. An occasional short duration failure may be tolerable, but frequent brief or lengthy failures or infrequent lengthy failures are not. It is important to note that, in addition to the computer system itself, consideration must be given to the reliability of the power source, air conditioning, communication lines, remotely located terminal or instrument interfaces, and the supporting personnel.

It is not possible to approach continuous operation without some system redundancy. The throughput and response time requirements are such that, even at the present state of the art, a computer system which has sufficient capacity will also be moderately expensive. A single system of this type may be beyond the reach of many clinical laboratories or hospitals, and a completely duplicated system beyond that of most.

There are several possible solutions to the cost versus reliability dilemma. One is to carry out the clinical laboratory data processing operations using a redundant computer facility which is shared with other application areas. The facility may be composed of two or more processors at a single center or multiple computers which are physically separated but are connected together through a network. The two key advantages of this approach are that the shared system typically has better capacity for handling peak loads, and the cost of the redundancy is minimized. In the case of a network, a third potential benefit is the ability to easily communicate data between the various computer centers.

When using a computer system which is dedicated to clinical laboratory data processing, some redundancy can be provided by distributing the total computing between two or more processors which are configured so that if one fails there is still sufficient capacity to continue the critical functions. It is also possible to duplicate those components of the system which are most prone to failure. Finally, provision can be made for using an alternate computer facility for back-up only at times of catastrophic failure of the local system. This latter approach suffers from the practical difficulties of quickly establishing the required data and program files.

Throughput capability is equally difficult to describe in quantitative terms, and, unfortunately, there are no mathematical methods for accurately simulating the time-sharing load. Twenty to thirty interactive terminals and instrument groups are typical for a medium-sized laboratory. The number of interactive terminals may increase substantially if it is necessary to provide data communication for satellite laboratories or patient care areas. Whatever the hardware configuration, the principal throughput requirement is that the system must be able to support the required number of terminals with a "question and answer" interactive response time of one hundred to two hundred milliseconds and a retrieval time of two to five seconds for a request not requiring sophisticated searches.

Minimum peripheral equipment includes mass storage and a communications multiplexor. The amount of mass storage required varies with the clinical laboratory and the extent to which data files may be distributed if a computer network is employed. Ten million characters should be provided as a minimum in the case of a "stand-alone" system coupled to a common data base. The laboratory data base is frequently accessed and in the case of moving head disk systems, it is essential to distribute the access load over multiple separate drives, connected to separate controllers and channels, in order to reduce the disk seek and data transfer times. Critical components of the data base should be duplicated on different storage devices in order to meet system reliability requirements.

The "ideal" time-sharing operating system is one which is flexible, highly reliable, user oriented, multilingual, and contains a good data base manager. An interpretive language with either a hardware implemented interpreter or a compiler is highly desirable.

A problem area in any system is the interface between instruments and the computer. Medicine now faces the complex decision whether to use (a) standardized interfaces or (b) a standardized computer input/ output bus or (c) microprocessors and microcomputers adapted to process individual signals [*]. The first alternative is supported by the fact that a large number of products already exist. The second is supported by the efforts, already made by computer manufacturers, to standardize the in/out bus.

The third alternative seems to be the design adopted by the medical equipment manufacturers. Also, for many other reasons e.g. flexibility, this approach seems to be the most promising.

The incorporation of a small computer within an instrument has mixed benefits. The replacement of complex hardwired logic with a microprocessor has definite advantages, as have been discussed. A microprocessor can also assist materially with the monitoring of instrument performance, initial data reduction, and the formatting of information for output.

---

[*] Bulletin No. 1 of IFIP Working Group 4.2, in Computer Programs in Biomedicine 5 (1975) 84-90.

There are two potential disadvantages. First, the instrument manufacturer does not always implement the optimum performance monitoring or data reduction procedures and, depending on the system, the microprocessor may make it either easier or much more difficult for a user to modify these operations. Second, the functions of some instrument computer systems have been expended to include data files, the printing of complex reports, and other operations of a more general clinical laboratory data processing system. These features may have some benefit to the clinical laboratory which does not have a general data processing system, but for the one which does, they are unneccessary, add significantly to instrument cost, and may increase the difficulty of communicating instrument data.

It is necessary to use an external interface with instruments which do not contain serial communication circuitry. Such an interface contains level converters (if required) for handling digital signals and analog to digital converters which transform incoming analog signals to a standard digital format; a buffer memory with sufficient capacity for storing five to ten seconds of data; asynchronous or bisynchronous data transceivers; a command decoder, and circuitry for connecting one or more interactive terminals.

In typical operation, information is transferred from the instrument to the interface as soon as it is available. Any necessary data conversions are carried out and the digital information is stored in the buffer memory. At some point in time, a command is transmitted from the time-sharing computer system, requesting that data be sent from the buffer memory when available. The transmission then occurs automatically after the buffer has been filled to a predetermined value. The computer system is also able to transmit information directly to the instrument for control purposes, to retransmit data in case of a transmission error, to control the pattern of analog to digital conversions, and to carry out other control functions. In addition to the instrument/computer data transfers, the interface controls the communication of information between the computer system, the buffer memory, and one or more interactive terminals.

With the availability in 1972 of medium- to large-scale integrated circuits capable of handling the parallel to serial conversions and other complex logic functions, for the first time it was feasible to fabricate this type of interface with a reasonable component package count and cost. A typical interface using this technology approaches that of the older parallel interfaces used for connecting instruments to real time computing systems.

In 1974 there was a further advance in the technology with the availability of the "second generation" microprocessors. This approach results in a 70 percent to 80 percent reduction in the package count in comparison with units which are fabricated using medium- or large-scale integrated circuit components. The principle of operation of the micro-processor-based system is identical to that described above. The difference is that a microprocessor program and a larger memory replace many of the hard wired functions. The flexibility and system capability are greatly enhanced, fabrication cost is reduced, and, at least in theory, reliability is improved.

The "second generation" microprocessors such as the Intel 8080, and Motorola 6800,have processing capabilities comparable to those of many minicomputers. If desired, complex arithmetic computations can be carried out in the interface; for example, the raw instrument data can be reduced prior to transmission or instrument performance monitored. Local computing within the interface has the advantage of reducing the load on the central facility. The disadvantage is that the complexity of programming the overall system may be slightly increased. This is not, however, a significant problem if the microprocessor programs are written in the same high level language utilized by the time-shared computer system and then automatically converted to microprocessor ma-chine language for storage in either read only or random access memory. The latter can be loaded directly from the time-shared system using the serial communication link, thus this is a simple and rapid process.

A number of interfaces based on both microprocessors and more dis-creet technology are now commercially available. The microprocessor-based version is easily fabricated, a minimum system requiring less than fifteen circuit modules.

Microprocessor technology is advancing at a very rapid rate. It is estimated that, by the end of 1975, high capability N and P channel, metallic oxide semiconductor-based micro-processor elements will be available for a cost of less than $50, that the use of integrated in-jection technology will result in a tenfold of better increase in pro-cessor speed, that the capacity of semiconductor memory chips will be

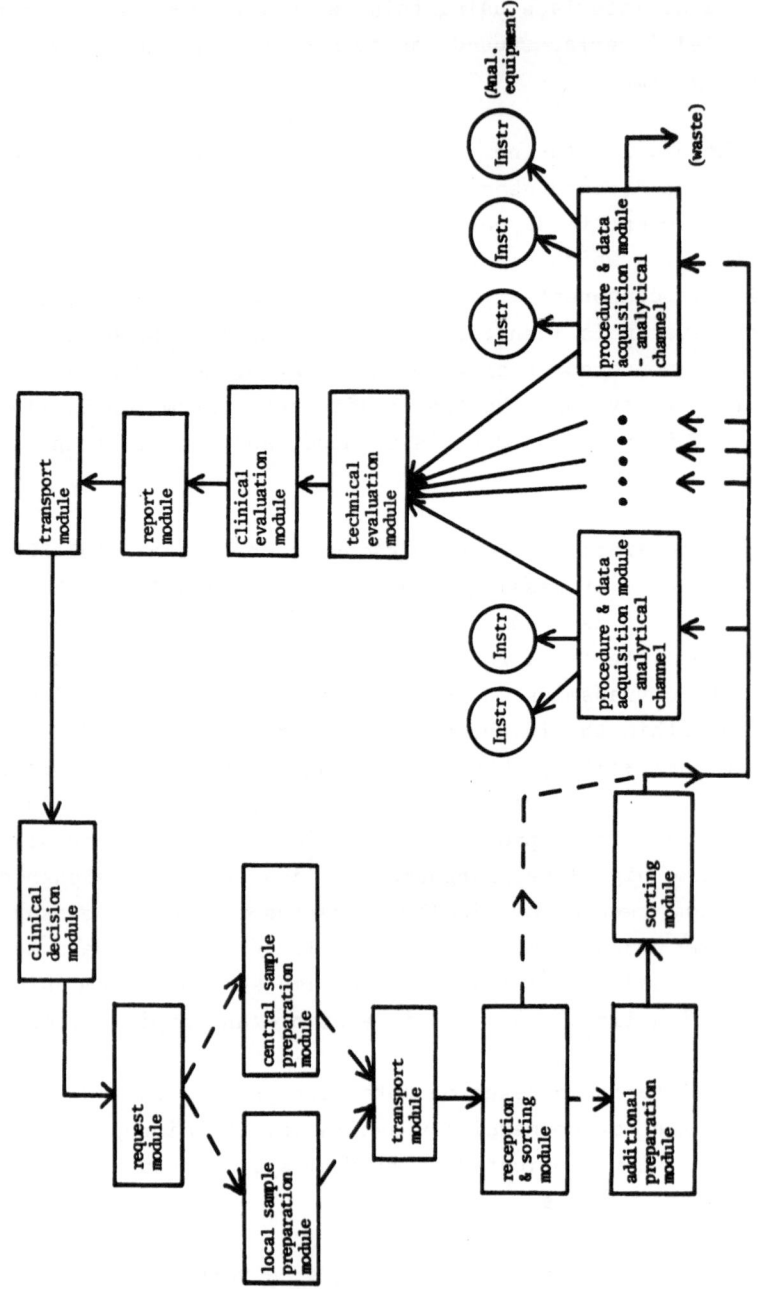

Fig. 4 The clinical chemical laboratory function.

673

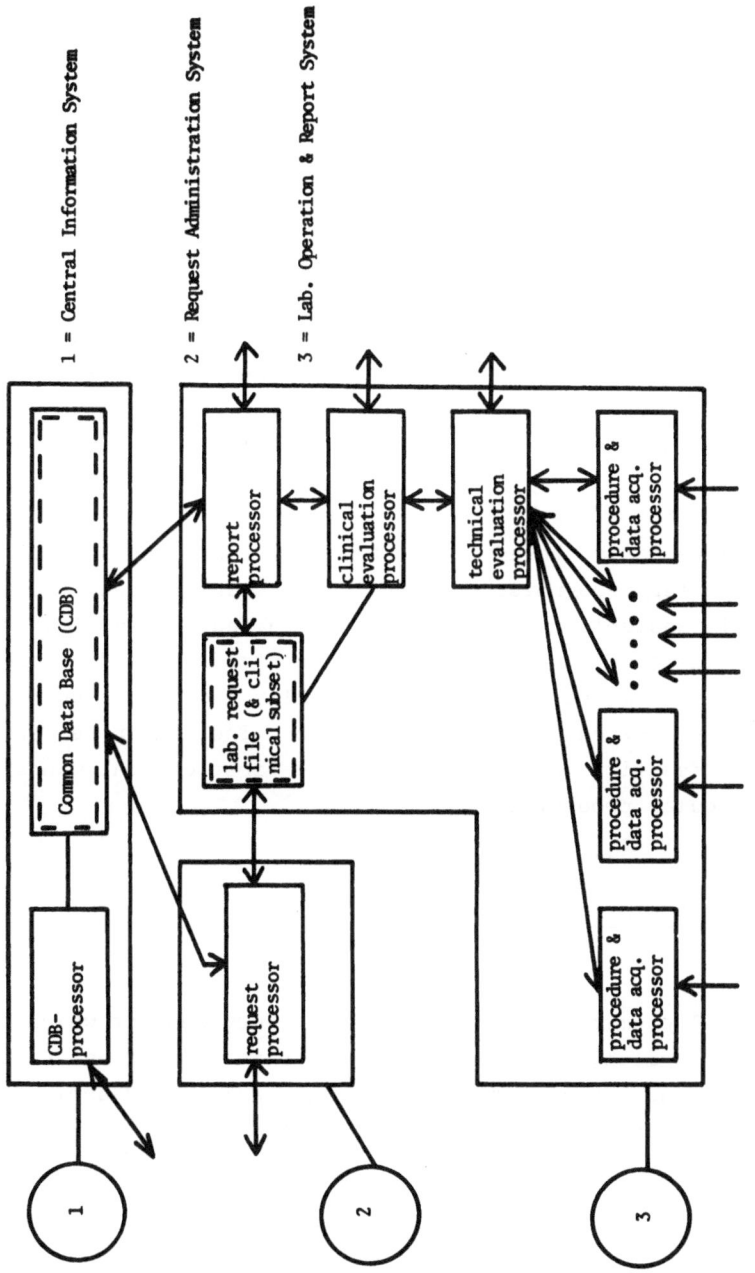

Fig. 5 The laboratory information system (Clin. Chem.).

expanded from 4K to 16K, and that single chips incorporating both the
microprocessor and memory elements will be available. All of these developments will have a significant impact on microprocessor-based systems.

Another problem, which is common to any hardware and software solution is <u>specimen identification</u>. The clinical laboratory data processing operations are dependent on knowledge about the patient, including
his or her identification, location, medical problems, medications, physician , and other information. The best hope for sample identification
lies in the technology being developed for the retail point-of-sale
systems. The ideal system is one in which machine-readable information
can be imprinted inexpensively and read by hand-held and instrument-
mounted sensors.

The best alternative based on the present technology appears to
be optical character recognition, which is the standard recently adopted by the Retail Dealer's Association in the United States. Its advantages are that the code may be imprinted with standard credit card im-
printers, it is both machine and human readable, and it can be read
with a relatively inexpensive hand-held sensor. The sensor research
and development is still in progress, and the first optical wands have
just entered regular production.

2. <u>The clinical chemical laboratory</u>

The clinical chemical laboratory is that service unit which performs the hematological, chemical, and similar investigations (analyses)
requested by the care units. Its function can easily be described in
terms of the different modules defined in Section 1.1.

2.1 <u>The function</u>
The ordering of a clinical chemical laboratory investigation is a
result of the considerations taken inside the clinical decision module.
The order itself contains a request both for the investigation as
such, as well as for the preparation of the sample. This request is
transported to the request administration module at the operative station in question. In general no patient transports from request to op-

THE LABORATORY INFORMATION SYSTEM (CLIN.CHEM)

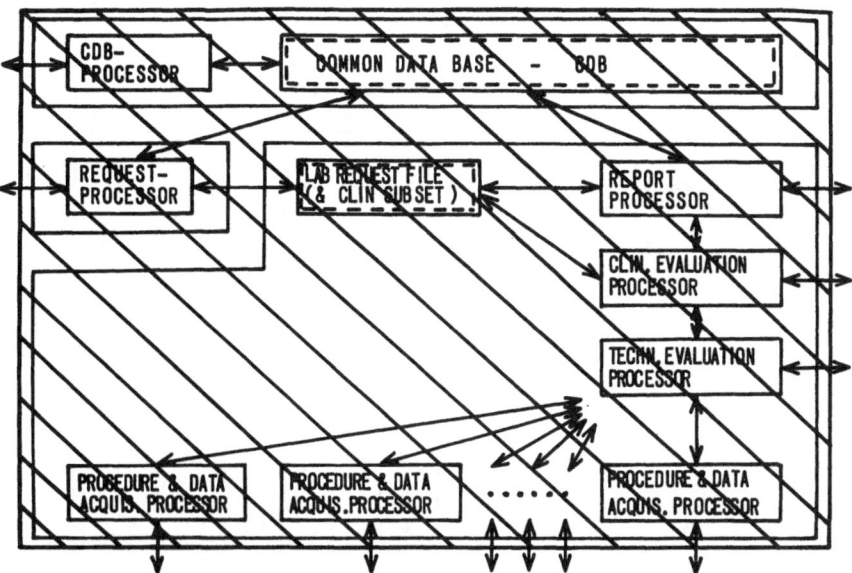

Fig. 6   Single hardware-unit implementation. This approach can now be considered obsolete.

THE LABORATORY INFORMATION SYSTEM (CLIN.CHEM)

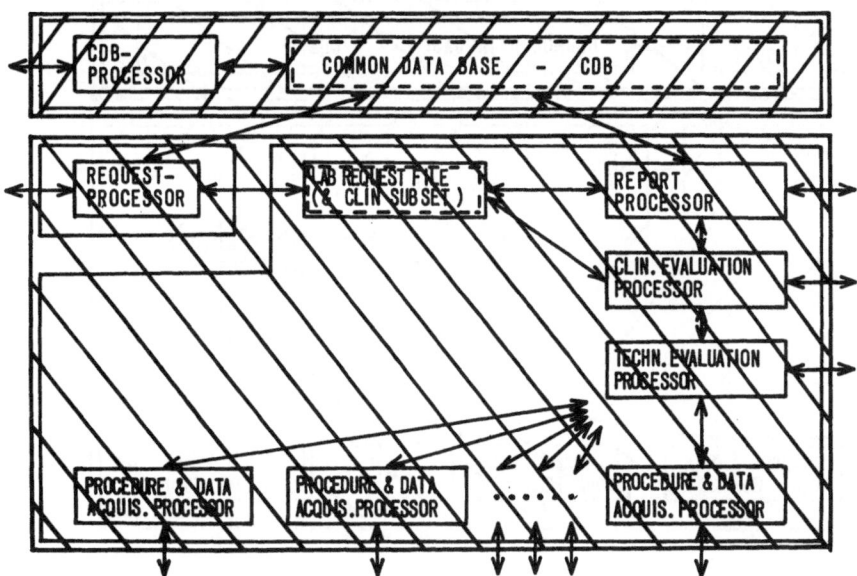

Fig. 7 Comprehensive chemical laboratory system implementation separate from the common data base (e.g. CLS-IBM 1800, University Hospital Umeå, Sweden)

THE LABORATORY INFORMATION SYSTEM (CLIN.CHEM)

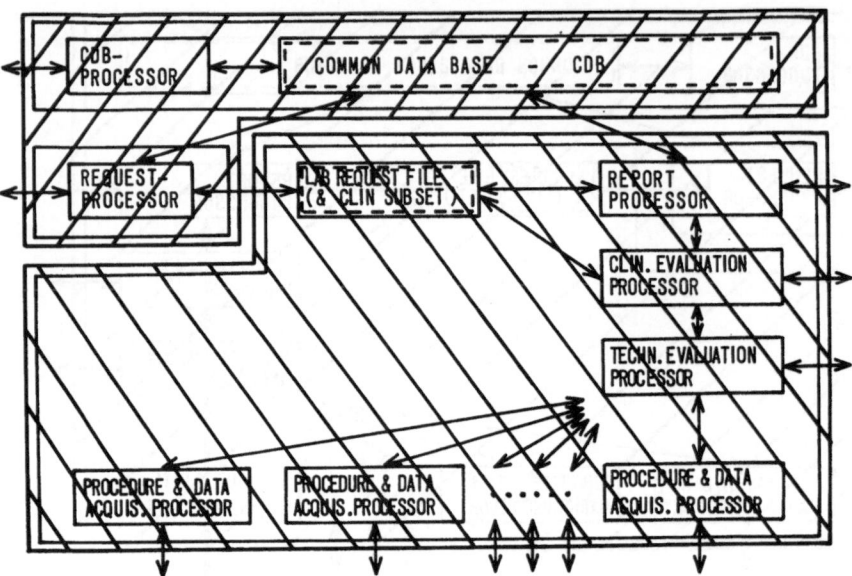

Fig. 8 Same as Fig. 7, but request processing implemented in the same hardware as the common data base.

THE LABORATORY INFORMATION SYSTEM (CLIN.CHEM)

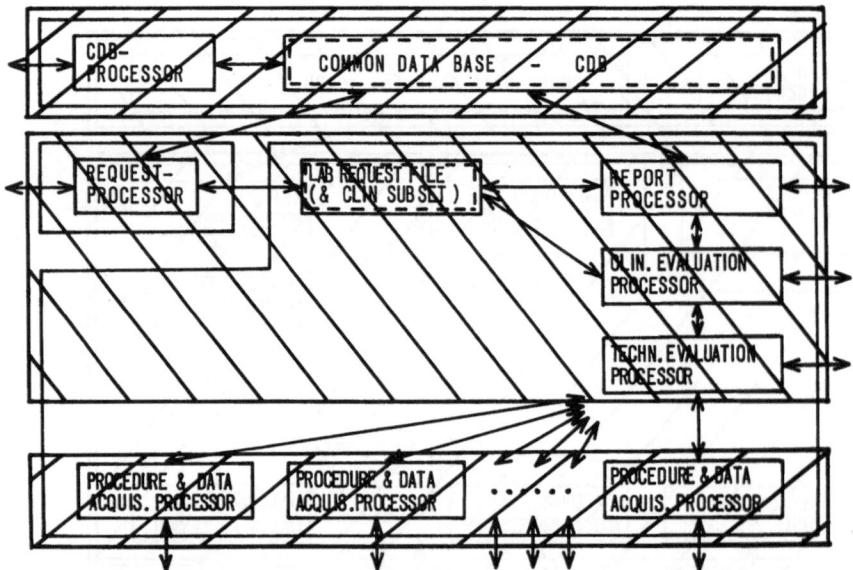

Fig. 9 Same as Fig. 7 but procedure- and data acquisition processing implemented on separate single hardware unit. (e.g. CLS on IBM 1130-S/7 or KLS on IBM S/3-S/7 in a number of European Hospitals. See also Aronsson et al, in Proc of MEDINFO'74, Vol 2, p. 959. North-Holland Publ. Co. 1974.

THE LABORATORY INFORMATION SYSTEM (CLIN.CHEM)

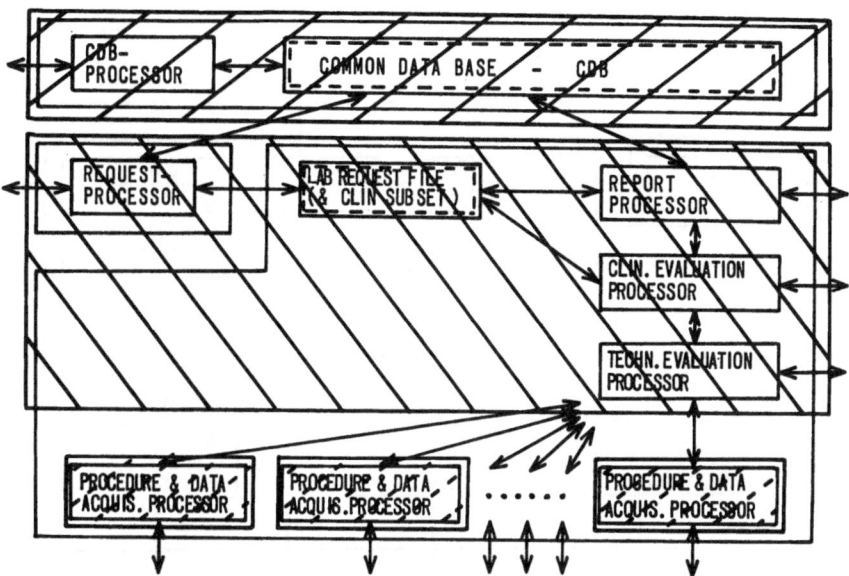

Fig. 10 Same as Fig. 9, but procedure- and data acquisition processing
implemented on different hardware components, ranging from a
number of microprocessors to minicomputers (e.g. Olli System
400 KLS, Uppsala)

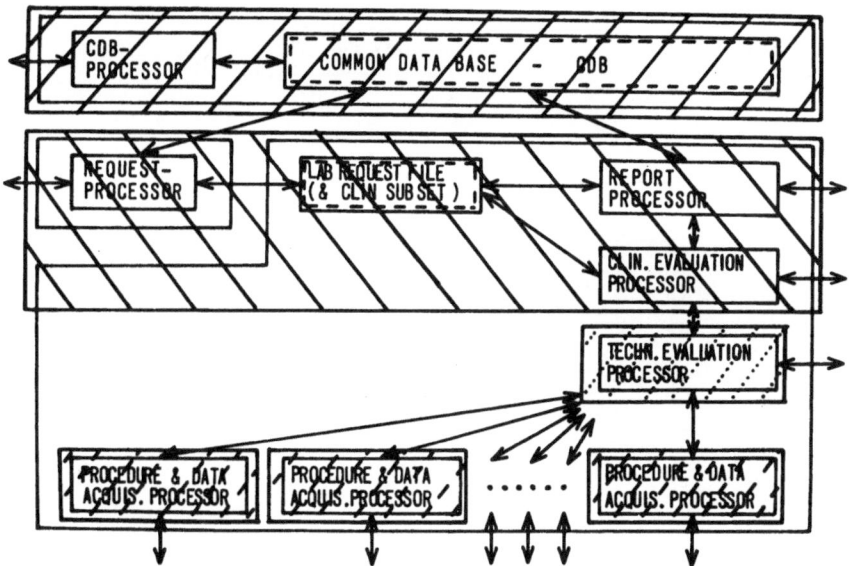

Fig. 11 Same as Fig. 10, but technical evaluation processing implemented
on a separate hardware unit(s). (E.g. Philips Labosys).

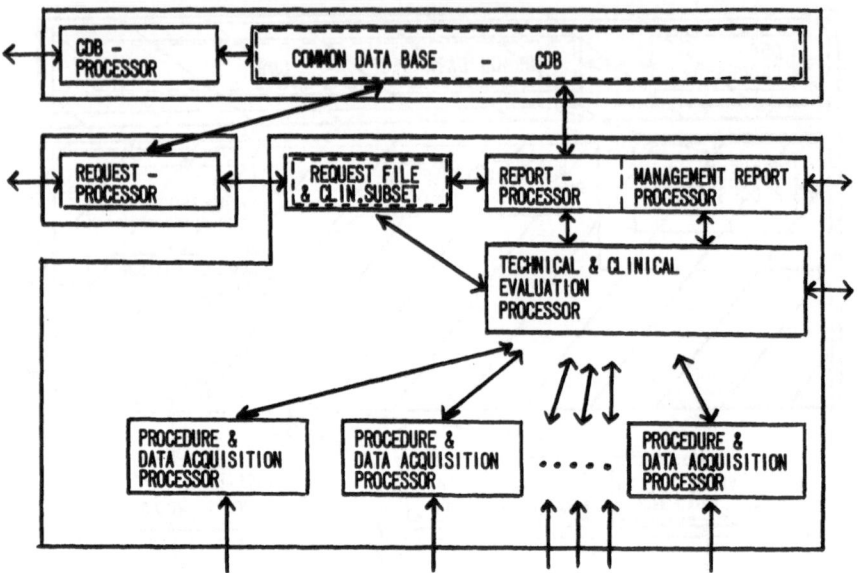

Fig. 12 Laboratory information system - radiology.

erative stations are necessary. There is no general need for booking
procedures at the chemical laboratory, so the activities of the request
module are restricted to the scheduling of sample preparation. The result of this scheduling is often a "walking list", according to which
the sample preparation staff execute their duties. After preparation,
local or central, the sample is transported to the operative station
together with relevant information, such as patient identification, address of request station, requested investigation, special demands concerning report time, or layout of report.

At the operative station the sample is taken care of by the reception and sorting module. If no computerized request system is implemented, the relevant request information is entered to the lab. information
system via the request processor. The further treatment of the sample
is a function of the nature of the sample and of the requested investigation. The sample may be given some additional preparation in the module designed to do this.

This can e.g. be centrifugation of blood samples, or if several
different determinations are requested, the parting of the original sample into several secondary samples.

The samples are then delivered, each one to an observation module
corresponding to the type of determination requested and capable of performing the determination under the stated circumstances, concerning
e.g. the time factor (emergency samples). Actions of this observation
module are the analytical procedures, and the output are the raw values
from the analysis. As described in Section 1.1, these values are evaluated both technically and clinically in the succeeding two modules, in
the last of them with respect to the clinical situation of the patient.

In the report module various reports are produced, outgoing from
routine formates and from special demands defined in the request.

2.2. The laboratory information system
The clinical chemical information system interacts with the temporary part of the common data base in the same way as other clinical laboratory systems. Still, the question to what extent the analytical data
are needed in the common data base for future use, e.g. in the decision
process and for billing purposes, has not been answered.

2.2.1. <u>The request administration system</u>. The request processor is an important part of the clinical chemistry information system. Its main functions are to update the lab. request file and to schedule any central sample preparation, e.g. procedure "walking-lists" for the preparation staff.

2.2.2. <u>The laboratory operation and reporting system</u>. The data acquisition processors in a chemical laboratory work mainly as process controllers of the analytical equipment, but can also handle the sample identification, execute alarm functions, etc.

From the data acquisition processors the information is transferred to the technical evaluation processor. Common qualities of this processor are automatic calibration, corrections for different kinds of analytical errors e.g. base line drift, statistical evaluation of results, printing of results from quality control etc. All this is done without access to patient identification.

Much less developed is clinical evaluation processing which often is restricted to a check against normal values. One function can also be the check of result vs request, i.e. the check that all requests have been effectuated. The future possibilities of this evaluation, if an access to a clinical subset was possible, must be pointed out. This subset could contain information on diet, pharmacological therapy etc. of the patient.

The last part of the clinical chemical information system is report processing. Its main duty is to present the results of the investigations, the analyses, in a way as well adapted to its purpose as possible.

2.3. <u>The hardware and software implementation</u>
The description above, of the clinical chemical laboratory function, and of the connected information processing possibilities are strictly formal, and nothing has been said about the implementation of the information systems. This is of course very natural, because the implementation must always be adapted to the real needs, at a specific laboratory.

From the structure of the Clinical Chemical Laboratory information

system in fig. 4 and 5 it is obvious that the implementation can be made
in many different ways, and therefore just a few examples will be discussed. On one extreme it is possible to implement all laboratory information system processors and files in one single computer, and this
has often been done. This can, however, be a less suitable approach,
among other things for break-down reasons. The request administration
system can be common to all laboratories inside a hospital, and therefore best be placed in the same hardware as the temporary part of the
common data base (CDB). It can be exclusive to each laboratory, and
implemented in the same computer as all or parts of the laboratory operation and report system.

A hardware structure for this latter system which will probably
dominate the future is based on a hierarchical approach. On the lowest
level, the observation processor will preferably be implemented on microcomputers. The higher levels can be implemented in one or several minicomputers, depending on the needs of the higher modules and on whether
and how the CDB is realised and implemented. The latter influences highly the layout and implementation of the request processing modules and
the lab request file. If no CDB is available and no information processing is done before the sample and a handwritten request arrives at the
laboratory, all information needed in the lab request and clinical subset file has to be entered directly at the laboratory by terminal or
punching. This input routine has anyway to be available in the system
for emergency reasons as e.g. if the connection with the CDB is down.

In fig. 6-11 some examples of alternative implementation, as realized at different places throughout the world, are presented. It should
be mentioned here that several fairly complete laboratory systems can
be obtained from commercial sources, and that these products have already shown themselves able to fulfill the requirements of a cost-benefit analysis.

3. Microbiological laboratory

Microbiological laboratories for diagnostic work in clinical bac-
teriology, clinical virology, immunology and parasitology etc. usually
exist in larger hospitals, but they may also be selfdependent laboratory
service units independent of the organizational structure of the regio-

nal hospitals. Regardless of the manner in which they are connected to
the health administration system they share the common problems of all
clinical laboratories, i.e. a steadily increasing workload due to the
increased demands from doctors, health centers and hospitals. It is thus
only natural that many laboratories have tried to work out various types
of computer systems in order to facilitate at least some parts of the
process of producing an intelligent answer to a sometimes not too intelligent request. In addition the problem of hospital-acquired infections has made the need for some kind of system capable of registering
the infections occurring within a hospital more and more pressing.

Using the structural outline introduced earlier the function of a
microbiological laboratory may be described in the following manner.

A request for a microbiological examination usually reaches the
laboratory together with the sample; most examinations are acute and the
resources of the laboratory elastic, which means that advance booking is
not necessary. Any preparation for collecting the specimen, e.g. venepun-
cture,. is generally carried out locally without help from the laboratory.
In a laboratory where the requests are handled manually, work lists may
be prepared at this stage. The specimens are usually given a unique laboratory registration number before processing. After the necessary preparations the samples are transferred to the various stations within the
laboratory for further processing and analysis as culturing, titration,
microscopy etc. The results of the examinations are checked in technical
and clinical evaluation modules and reports are prepared for the request
stations and, if necessary, for the administration as material for billing.

The supervising of hospital infections is usually the responsibility of an infection control officer or nurse and it is done both by a
day-to-day control or reports and by recording the findings over longer
periods of time.

If one looks at the general outline of the clinical laboratory as
discussed in section 1 it is obvious that at the present time only few
modules in the microbiological laboratory are ripe for computerizing.

Thus only two procedure and data acquisition modules in the routine
laboratory may at present be automated: some serologic tests (mainly for
syphilis) and antibiotic sensitivity determinations. The first of these

requires such a large number of tests to be carried out in order to be economical, that few laboratories can use it and the second is yet too expensive and poor in performance for routine work. If and when these and other processes are available at reasonable costs they will, like the chemical analyses, be suitable for computer handling with the advantages concerning method control etc. that this makes possible.

At the present time the possibilities to introduce a computer in the microbiological laboratory are in the reporting of answers and the preparing of epidemiological surveys for the infection control. This means, using the nomenclature adapted above, that the report module is linked to a report processor. It also means that, unless an information processor has been established in connection with the common data base, all preparation of surveys must be carried out by analyzing the locally stored information, i.e. a subsystem dedicated data base must be set up for this purpose.

The simplest, but not most efficient and economic way, to reach this goal is to transfer all reports to a data register via punch cards or punched tape. This can either be done in coded form, which is error prone, or as free text, which necessitates the use of a large computer. A more efficient way is to record the findings of the analysis at the bench and then leave the work of preparing the request report to the computer. This will mean that, since all data needed for a correct report including patient data from the request form are already stored in the computer, the preparation of surveys etc. will be a question of programming according to the desires of the infection control officer and/ or the hospital management.

The recording of patient data is usually by punching, but the recording of laboratory data may be performed by several methods. One is by the use of ferrite pencil and subsequent punching of cards after magnetizing the ferrite marks but this hardware is no longer on the market.

The second is by using so-called Port-a-Punch cards, 40 column preperforated punch cards, where the punching is done by punching out holes with e.g. a pencil. This means that codes must be used and this may lead to errors if many, varied results have to be reported.

The third way is to use optical mark recognition; many optical mark readers are on the market. Here one is free to design the form according to the wishes of the customer and there is usually enough space to permit the use of ordinary, though abbreviated, text instead of code designations.

The laboratory data may also be entered as the results of all fermentation tests etc. performed, leaving to the computer to make the species diagnosis, but since the majority of organisms encountered are easily identified such a system will hardly be rational.

The above mentioned systems all work batchwise off-line and one may, of course, also design systems working on-line. This is more costly and so far, no on-line system has been designed using either typewriter terminals or display systems with lightpens, which has been able to meet the demands of the laboratory customer for speed and practical usefulness.

Regardless of the manner in which the patient and laboratory data are acquired the output of the microbiology system may vary according to local needs. Generally speaking all systems produce standard nomenclature reports to the customers and some kind of list is also produced daily for the laboratory to keep as copy of the results, and also for the use of the infection control officer who wants to keep an eye on the bacteriological findings in the hospital. If desired, the necessary lists for internal cost allocation and/or external billing should also be produced, depending on the structural framework of the health service system.

Of more interest from the purely medical point of view is the preparation of epidemiological and other surveys e.g. changes in sensitivity of various bacteria to commonly used antibiotics, the results of which may affect the antibiotic policy in the hospital. The recording of infections occurring in the hospital is the most important of the epidemiological surveys and the resulting cumulative lists should be prepared often and the results communicated to the responsible department heads etc.

The reports and surveys mentioned above may be prepared on a sub-system dedicated data base. If further analysis requires clinical or other data not contained in this data base, communication must be set up with a central common data base, or alternatively, a special program designed to introduce these data.

Though it may seem as if the microbiological laboratory's use of information processing is still in its rather unsophisticated youth, the laboratories using computers have found it very difficult to be without them once the initial troubles (it would be silly to deny that these exist) have been overcome, the main advantages being the production of uniformly worded answers from all the responsible persons, the production of invoice material as a spin-off process and perhaps as the greatest help: the preparation of cumulative reports of hospital infections for the infection control.

4. Radiology

4.1 Introduction

Radiology departments for carrying out standard X-ray procedures and many other dynamic investigations using radioopaque substances now exist in most hospitals or hospital groups, in health care centres and other health care facilities in the community. The systems for handling patient investigation are still largely based on paper and voice communication to speed the flow of work and so far few automatic controls are used to try to improve the efficiency of the operation.

Often some quite considerable improvement has been achieved by standard work study methods and the design of appropriate documentation, job definition and communication routines. Nevertheless the area for error and problem situations is still quite large and this throws a burden on those who expect and give a high performance in their demanding technical duties. Safety because of ionising radiation is very important and personnel cannot afford to be tired and slipshod.

4.2 The information system as related to the laboratory function

In the following the functions of the radiology laboratory are analyzed according to the general principles described for the hospital laboratory, cf. fig. 12. It is obvious that computer techniques may be used for many purposes but, so far, very few actual working solutions exist and those mentioned here may be regarded as a sample catalogue.

4.2.1. Request module - laboratory administrative system   The task of

the clinical decision module to initialize the request for an investiga-
tional procedure, can be performed in many ways, some of which depend
on the use of computer systems. For example input can be by paper from
a doctor arriving at a central area and be entered into the radiological department information system by a clerk. The data that are entered
must include patient identification data and other necessary data. Other
systems can include doctors using peripheral computer terminals and some
health care screening systems can use patient questionnaires to generate
the appropriate data either on-line or off-line. In a developed health
information system it would be possible to retrieve all pertinent patient data for identification as well as clinical data from the common
data base described.

Once requests reach the radiology department some type of appointment system is essential. It can be based on the principle of first in
first out and related to the arrival of routine patients or be a little
more sophisticated and indicate to wards and outpatients the possible
routine waiting time. Provision must be made for emergency investigations at every level. This applies also to longer time scale appointments where facilities have to be booked in advance (especially difficult standard procedures or special dynamic studies). Different approaches to patient appointment systems have varied from simple descriptions offering only long term appointments to those that deal with all
requests whether urgent or routine or for long term arrangements.

Usually such appointment systems are linked to machine and staff
booking systems so that resources are allocated correctly. Here facilities may be provided not only for producing booking lists but also to
allow for immediate updating if the users wish to use computer techniques to assist them in their every day work. Using such a system a
radiographer can keep up-to-date with the work load and decide what steps
can be taken to deal with queues etc. without moving from her station.
The request module should also issue instructions to the requesting unit
regarding the correct way of preparing the patient for the diagnostic
procedure, i.e. whether he should be fasting, receive an enema etc.

It is clear that more and further sophisticated computer applications can be thought of. The ensemble of all applications defines the
request administrative system as described in section 1. One of its
main functions is also here to create the request and clinical subset
file for the laboratory operating and reporting system.

4.2.2. <u>Local preparation module</u>.   The object here is to present to the
transport module a patient prepared according to the instructions mentioned above.

4.2.3. <u>Transport module</u>.   Links through an appointment system and machine booking system can be made to porters and other means of transport
to ensure that patients reach the department at the appropriate times.
For example, the booking system for a routine machine can generate lists
for individual patients ordering transport facilities within the hospital
and also ambulances for patients who are not fit to make the journey from
their homes. Such computer applications form - of course - another part
of the laboratory administrative system.

4.2.4. <u>Reception and sorting module</u>.   There are problems dealing with
patients at reception, ensuring they have proper identification, understand what type of investigation is to be undertaken, showing them where
to go, and getting them into the appropriate clothing for the investigation. It is often here that much time is spent, and accordingly may be
saved. In a local study of patients, waiting time around the X-ray department took about forty minutes and the X-ray itself and quality check
and reporting back took twenty minutes.

     It is thus useful if patients arrive with identification and the
information about the investigation that is required as well as the
computer system already transferring this data to the radiological department. This provides not only a useful check of identification and
procedure and so reduces patient waiting time, but also provides a fail
safe system in case of computer failure.

4.2.5. <u>Procedure and data acquisition module.</u>   This module produces
the films by the use of man and machine. Some procedures are simple
standard ones whereas others are highly sophisticated using machinery
directed by intelligent computer-like devices. In contrast to therapeutic radiology little has been done to introduce computers into this
field, but it should be fairly easy to automatize the setting of the
machines through presenting the necessary data on the patient and his
examination in a suitable manner.

4.2.6. <u>Technical and clinical evaluation module</u>.   Here the films are
checked for technical quality - correct exposure etc. - and clinical
quality - so that the requests may be answered through studies of them.
Also at this stage there must be a means of indicating that X-ray films
have been approved for quality and that the patient can return to the
ward. On the other hand it may be necessary for them to wait until the
radiologist has reported. Image analysis may, theoretically, be performed through pattern recognition computer programs. These are still, however, in their infancy and will not be practically available for many
years. The raw values, i.e. the films must thus be processed by humans.
A different kind of image analysis, axial tomography, has, however, recently proven to be highly successful.

Concerning dose registration all departments keep records of operator actions if only for medico-legal purposes and usually record important machine settings so that the radiation dose can be determined.
This dose depends on a number of factors including the type of machine,
the distance of the patient from the machine and the field of radiation.
It is important that this type of data should be transferred to the patient's record, but few systems have reached this degree of sophistication. It is also important that the radiation exposure of radiographers
be recorded and some centres do hold records about this. X-ray films
have also to be labelled and it is possible to provide this service automatically by using printing devices to produce the appropriate markers
from the patient's record via the request module. Document control is
another important application area and one which is now easily implemented using point-of-sale technology.

4.2.7. <u>Report module and medical reports</u>.   The reporting system input
requires adequate films for reporting and old films and reports where
appropriate. An adequate film library system must have the appropriate
communications with the reporting module. In some systems reports can
be made by the radiologist direct to a typist using a teletype or video
terminal, and either entering the report in a fairly fixed overall format or as free text. In other systems it is possible to use multiple
choice text descriptors displayed on a visual display unit to create
inputs into the record system. However, the creation of such display
systems is not easy and requires a considerable effort on the part of
the user to ensure that these are correct and useful.

4.2.8. <u>Report module and managerial reporting</u>.   Data from requests,
appointments or machine booking systems or reports on machine usage and
radiologists reports can be used for administrative and accounting purposes. Billing data can be derived form requests or appointment data or
radiologists reports. Indeed perhaps it is best derived from at least
two different files of data for the sake of accuracy and reliability.
Of course, records can be created solely to operate a billing system
and in many hospitals this is true. In any case these reports are in
general best produced directly from the active part of the common data
base of the health information system, located in the care unit to which
the radiological laboratory is belonging.

4.2.9. <u>Report transport module</u>.   Reporting often stops at the door of
the radiology department and the medical report is despatched over the
ordinary hospital communication system or by post. Films may also be
dispatched to the wards along with the report or the report and the film
sent separately or the report may take another route. In this way gross
errors may be stopped from affecting care. Often in hand driven systems
such communications are slow and can be much more timely if proper automated communication systems are used. Urgent reports are often telephon-
ed but as they are transferred from person to person this may produce
errors and it certainly requires extra people to man the telephone terminal.

The reports should also be transferred to the active part of the
common data base in order to update the patient's records.

4.3. <u>Review of existing systems</u>
In general few systems have been implemented and are used and only
a few manufacturers have produced sub-systems which can perform some of
the functions already outlined. Hall and his colleagues at the Karolinska Hospital and Peterson et.al. at Huddinge Hospital both in Stockholm
have introduced a sophisticated booking system. Systems for reporting
have been developed by Reichertz and his colleagues in Hannover, at the
Uppsala University Hospital and elsewhere in Europe. Other reporting
systems have been developed in the United States, e.g. by Robinson et.
al.

Brolin has worked on the development of display systems for radiological reporting. However, these require some sophistication on the

part of users and many radiologists feel that they are better dictating
their reports, either structured or unstructured, than trying to use
display systems. However, opinions do alter as experience grows. The
more a radiologist wants from his reports in the way of analysis, the
more likely is he to demand a sophisticated system.

Image processing has a future but it is complex to develop such
automated analysis systems at present. Very few systems have been described and most deal with one type of X-ray, for example a chest X-ray.
So far only elementary rules of processing have been extablished and
much more work needs to be done in this area.

On the whole there is a need for a lot of work to be done to apply
information processing in departments of radiology. To some extent the
systems implemented depend not only on the department itself, but other
users of such information systems in the hospital or other organization.
However, given certain basic facilities and equipment there are benefits to be obtained from automation and the use of computer techniques.

Bernhard, H.J. and Dockray, K.T., Computerized operations in the diag-
nostic radiology department, Amer. J. Roentgenol. 109 (1970) 628.
Brolin, I., Medela: An electronic data-processing system for radiologi-
cal reporting, Radiology 103 (1972) 249-255.
Háll, P., Medical Information Processing, the KS Project, (IBM Corp.
Stockholm, 1969).
Källström, S., Lund, G. and Peterson, H., A Planning and Scheduling
System for Patient Admission to Srugical Departments. Medinfo 74 (North
Holland Publishing Company 1974) pp. 509-511.
Riedler, L., Possibility of documentation of static X-ray pictures with
the aid of electronic data processing, Method. Inform. Med. 13 (1974)
38.
Robinson, R.E. III and Mescahn, I. Computerized radiological reporting
with word retrieval using MT/ST, Radiology 101 (1971) 323-329.
Stein, M.A. and Winter, J. System desing of a computer based library
circulation system for a radiology file room. Method. Inform. Med. 12
(1973) 207.
Templeton, A.N., Reichertz, P.L. and Paquet, E., Radiate-up-dated and
redesigned for multiple cathode ray terminals, Radiology 92 (1969) 30.

5. Clinical physiology and neurophysiology

Within the field of clinical physiology and neurophysiology information processing techniques have been successfully used for treating
the results of blood gas analyses, lung function tests, ECG, EEG, EMG,

heart catheterization etc. Here, as with radiotherapy and clinical chemistry, most progress has lately been made in instrument automation through the application of microprocessor technology. Several of these applications are at present available from commercial sources. In principle the conclusions regarding laboratory function and the related information system made in previous sections of this chapter are also applicable here.

It is considered to be beyond the scope of this report to iterate the detailed description of laboratory functions etc. and to present different applications in detail. In the following the discussion will therefore focus on the existing differences between clinical physiology and other laboratory disciplines.

In clinical physiology and neurophysiology the technical evaluation is much more extensive and complicated than, for instance, in clinical chemistry (cf. fig. 2). This may lead to technical evaluation processing being preferably implemented on separate hardware units (cf. fig. 11).

A prerequisite for the successful application of computers in this field is the development of suitable clinical evaluation modules (cf. fig. 2). Accordingly much more work has been devoted to this problem here than in other laboratory specialties. The fact that most examinations in this field use the patient as "specimen" instead of a patient-derived sample explains why only through application of suitable microprocessors for instrument automation may significant advances be made. In many cases use of this technique will eliminate the need for transporting the patient to and from the laboratory and will thus lead to substantial saving of staff time. Also the use of microcomputerized instruments enables distant health care units to have access to centrally placed interpretation expertise through data communication.

Acknowledgement

The chapters "The computer utility in a health environment" and "Laboratory" are slightly revised and reedited versions of the corresponding sections of the report "The application of computer techniques in health care", prepared by a special study group of the International Hospital Federation (IHF). The group, which was chaired by Prof. W. Schneider, Uppsala, consisted of the following members:

J. Anderson, King's College Hosp. Med. School. London, UK

S. Bengtsson, University of Uppsala, Uppsala, Sweden

V. Kästner, Sen. f. Ges. u. Umweltschutz, Berlin, FRG

B. Lamson. Univ. of Calif., Hospitals and Clinics, Los Angeles, USA

A. Pratt, Div. of Comp. Res. and Techn., NIH, Bethesda, USA

P. Reichertz, Med. Hochschule, Hannover, FRG

R. Robinson, Univ. of Calif., Hospital and Clinics, Los Angeles, USA

B. Sandblad, Uppsala University, Uppsala, Sweden

W. Schneider, Uppsala University, Uppsala, Sweden

W. Spencer,Texas Inst. for Rehab. and Research, Houston, USA

The report was financially supported by a grant of IBM Sweden and published by North-Holland Publishing Company in "Computer Programs in Biomedicine" Vol 5 (1976 pp. 169-250. The permission of North Holland Publ. Co. for reprinting parts of the report in the present volume is highly appreciated.

FOUR TECHNOLOGIC APPLICATIONS OF MEDICAL
INFORMATICS TO RADIOLOGY

Gwilym S. Lodwick, M.D.
University of Missouri - Columbia

Columbia, MO. 65201/USA

While this excellent conference has been concerned with the application of computers to informatics and medical informatics in particular, the subjects discussed so far have been concerned largely with theoretical considerations of the content of information. In the field of radiology, which is a branch of medicine dealing very largely with images, one is confronted with not only optimum speed and quality presentation of image information, but also with the problem of determining whether one kind of image contains more information than another, and also with the problem of how best to extract information from an image which is of ultimate value to the patient and to the physician. Perhaps the most stunning recent advance in imaging, the CAT scanner, combines radiological physics and imaging, computer technology, image reconstruction algorithms, and image display systems to provide images which offer the interpreter the greatest accuracy that is known to date.

The presentation which follows is necessarily brief, because the volume and complexity of the material presented do not permit a comprehensive review. However, the bibliography which accompanies this presentation offers those sufficiently interested an excellent insight into the subject of medical informatics in radiology. Four subjects are covered: 1) MARS (Missouri Automated Radiology System), a medical information management system; 2) CAD (computer-aided diagnosis), with respect to lesions of bone; 3) automated image analysis where the computer uses shape and texture measurements to assist in the evaluation of radiant images, and 4) direct measurement of image information content, as an evaluation experiment, where a manipulated image system is compared with the original system to determine the loss of information which would degrade the accuracy of the radiologist's interpretation. While the evaluation experiment was presented first in order of the spoken presentations for the purpose of introducing a multi-disciplinary audience to the problems of radiologic practice, in a written presentation it logically follows last because of the tremendous importance of measuring cost effectiveness and medical efficacy in determining the true value of any change in a costly health care system. In the United States today, evaluation, cost effectiveness, and efficacy are potential key words for almost any major research presentation.

MARS

A Computer Mediated System for Information Management in a Functioning
Radiology Department

Radiology is a major clinical discipline in any hospital, clinic, or health care
system. Because of its highly technological nature, costly instrumentation ($500,000
for a CAT scanner), high overhead costs, and the complexity of the chain of events
leading from examination of the patient to the delivery of the diagnostic report
(figure 1), it is extremely important that radiology departments be managed effective-

INFORMATION MANAGEMENT IN DIAGNOSTIC RADIOLOGY

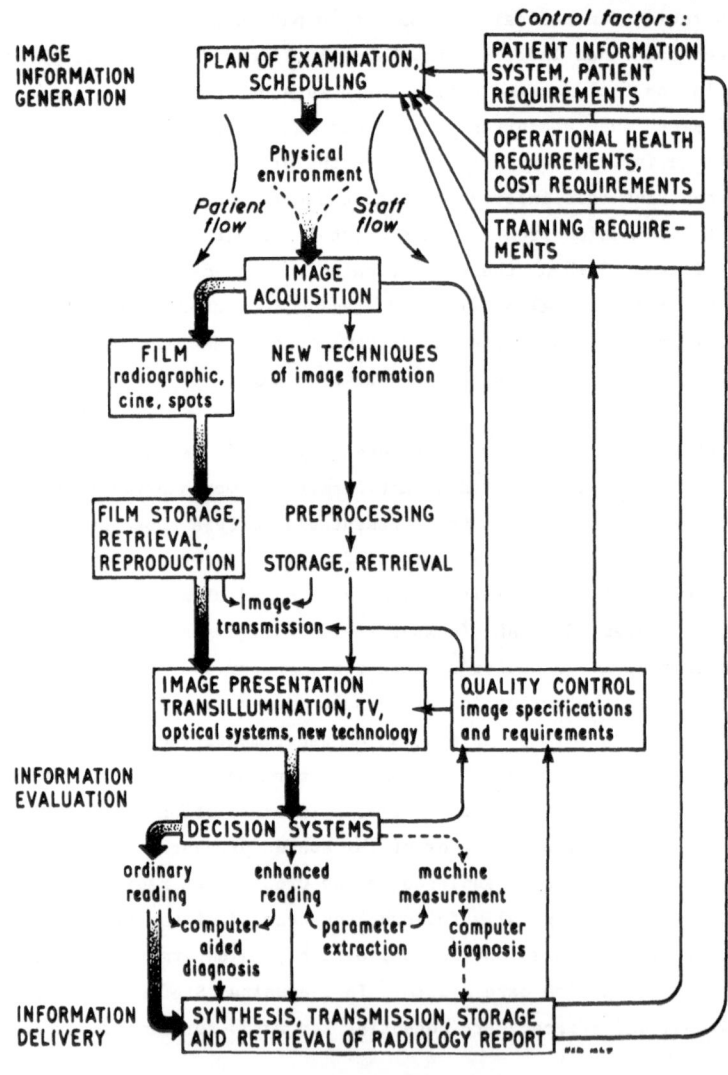

ly. There must be a speedy turnaround of information from the beginning to the end of the examining process. There are a number of key areas where efficient management is difficult: 1) patient reception and waiting areas where the length of time that a patient remains in the department must be reduced to an absolute minimum; 2) the examining process itself where time, quality control, and cost are extremely important; 3) the film filing and management area, where new examinations are assembled together with existing films and interpretations. Here film library control must be extremely tight and effective; 4) film interpretation area, where the radiologist examines and reports films or sends them back for further studies, the final product being a hard copy of the radiologist's opinion; 5) for management purposes, billing, collection of statistical information, retrieval capability, and feedback information for the examining and waiting areas. Each of these five areas is of great sensitivity to the effectiveness of a radiology department. The scope of the radiology examination includes diagnostic x-rays, fluoroscopic examinations, vascular procedures, special neurological procedures, CAT scans, nuclear medicine procedures, in vitro and immunoassay studies, and radiation oncology. With so many variables, management has become exceedingly complex, volumes of procedures running to more than 1000 per day, and each element of every procedure bearing requirements of accuracy and speed, plus specialized requirements. Accuracy and speed are ever-increasingly important in order to reduce per diem hospital costs, and to meet the extremely high expectations of the medical public.

Effective management coordinating all elements of radiology diagnostic and therapeutic services is heavily dependent upon information feedback. A department with considerable excess capacity is capable of easily managing periods of peak load. However, the typical department of radiology, because of the growth of demand and expectation of services, is likely to be marginal in size and capacity, with periods of excessive loads throughout the day. To meet this situation, efficient systems management and adequate feedback are essential. During the past ten years, at the Department of Radiology at the University of Missouri-Columbia, the staff has evolved an efficient computerized management system which is capable of scheduling patients, maintaining an excellent data base, providing feedback from admissions to file control, providing a time-tested and proved reporting interface between the radiologist and the computer, and offering speedy turnaround time from the admission of the patient to the completion of the report. Billing is automatic. The radiologist has the choice of direct computer interface or dictation for reporting. In an entirely voluntary choice setting, approximately 85% of all reports are managed through direct radiologist computer interface rather than by dictation. Rapid turnaround time makes it possible for the patient to be admitted, examined, and return to the out-clinic with film, bill and interpretation in reasonable time.

A system is no better than its weakest functional link. Further implementation of MARS has required that the traffic control manager be made aware of each sequential step in the link from admission to interpretation. This is provided by a scope monitor which shows the stage of the examination and the total elapsed time each patient has been in the department. This new feedback mechanism has proved effective in eliminating or at least minimizing the number of patients with prolonged stay due to some unperceived breakdown in the examination sequence. The MARS system is now being extended to the Department of Radiology at the Harry Truman Veterans' Administration Hospital nearby, and to the nuclear medicine division with sections in both hospitals. MARS is now regarded as an unusually well-designed, effective, and accepted example of a radiology information system. Elsewhere many other systems are under design or are in use, reflecting principally efforts to improve the radiologist-computer interface. At least one system is now focusing on reporting through direct computer recognition of voice.

Finally, a few remarks about the hardware and software systems. Most effective radiology information systems have been designed to operate with small computers under direct control of department management. It is extremely important that control of a system so vital to department operation be under the control of professional management. A factor of great importance in the evolution of such stand-alone systems as MARS is the interactive language MUMPS, specially designed for medical data management. Evaluation of MARS is the subject of a doctorate thesis in economics available in microfilm form from Dr. Reichertz.

Evolution of the system has continued since this 1974 evaluation. Another added refinement is the physician and resident scheduling algorithm, which offers optimal professional coverage of all services of the department, interfaces vacation and leave requests with daily professional work schedules.

REFERENCES
RADIOLOGY INFORMATION SYSTEMS

Brolin, I.: Automatic typing and transmitting of radiological reports, Proc. Conference on the Use of Computers in Radiology, University of Chicago, October 20-23,1966.

Kricheff, I. I., and Korein, J.: Computer processing of narrative data: Progress and problems, Proc. Conference on the Use of Computers in Radiology, University of Chicago, October 20-23, 1966.

Templeton, A. W., Lodwick, G. S., and Turner, A. H.: RADIATE: A new concept for computer coding, transmitting, storing, and retrieving radiological data, Radiology 85:811, 1965.

Lodwick, G. S., Reichertz, P. L., Paquet, E., and Hall, D.L.: ODARS: A computer aided system for diagnosing and reporting, presented by Eleonore Paquet at 32nd Annual Meeting of the Canadian Association of Radiologists, Vancouver, British Columbia, Canada, March 10-14, 1969.

Lehr, J. L., Lodwick, G. S., Garrotto, L. J., Manson, D. J., and Nicholson, B. F. : MARS - Missouri automated radiology system, AFIPS-Conference Proc., Vol. 40.

Barnhard, H. J.: Automatic coding and manipulating of radiology diagnostic reports, Proc. Conference on the Use of Computers in Radiology, University of Chicago, October 20-23, 1966.

Barnhard, H. J., Jacobson, H., and Nance, J. W.: Diagnostic radiology information system (DRIS), Proc. of Conference on Computer Applications in Radiology University of Missouri-Columbia, Sept. 23-26, 1970.

Koeppe, P., and Schaefer, P.: ORVID - An on-line roentgen diagnosis using video display and including documentation, Computer in Radiology, Proc. Int. Meeting Bussels 1969, (Basel: S. Karger, 1970), pp. 328-332.

Covert, R. P., Lodwick, G. S., and Wilkinson, E. W.: Simulation modeling of a diagnostic radiology department, Proc. Conference on Use of Computers in Radiology, University of Chicago, October 20-23, 1966.

Hsieh, R. K. C.: Scheduling of patients, technologists, and facilities in a hospital radiology department, Proc. Conference on Use of Computers in Radiology, University of Chicago, October 20-23, 1966.

Lodwick, G. S.: Computer simulation and information system in radiologic departmental operations, EDV in Medizin und Biologie, April 1971.

Lodwick, G. S.: Recommendations for obtaining the maximum benefit of radiation exposure in diagnostic radiology through improved production and utilization of image information, Report to National Center of Radiological Health on a Study of X-Ray Image Analysis and Systems Development, July 1968.

Kundel, H. L., and Revesz, G.: Effects on non-linearities on the television display of x-ray images, Invest. Radiol. 6:315, 1971.

Zimmerman, J.(ed): Proceedings of the 1974 MUMPS Users' Group Meeting, Biomedical Computer Laboratory, St. Louis, November 1974.

Brolin, I.: Radiologic reporting, Acta Radiol. [Suppl](Stockh) 323:1, 1973.

Koeppe, P., Schaefer, P., and Treichel, J.: ORVID - A report on termination of routine application of the system. Lecture given at 18th annual meeting of Deutsch Gesellschaft fur Medizinische Dokumentation und Statistik, Bielefeld, Sept. 30 - October 3, 1973.

Lang, G.: Review of the State-of-the-Art: Diagnostic Radiology Reporting/Information Systems (Washington, D.C.: Veterans Administration, June 1973).

Dickhaus, E. A.: Economic evaluation of Missouri automated radiology system, MARS- A case study. Dissertation presented to Faculty of Graduate School, University of Missouri, May 1974.

Lodwick, G. S.: The applications of computers in diagnostic radiology, Current Problems in Radiology, Vol 5, No.1, Jan-Feb, 1975.

Computer-aided Diagnosis

The average diagnostic accuracy of a radiologist, estimated from the literature and from the experience of the evaluative program reported later, is of an order of 68%. While the detection of abnormality rate is higher, it is quite clear that of the chain of events which leads from x-ray examination to discover disease to the correct diagnosis, detection and diagnostic classification are the weakest links.

Computerized axial tomographic images through better representation of gray levels in digital displays of specialized areas have led to an increase in detection rate reportedly to as high as 94%. However, in standard diagnostic situations which represent 99% of the total, there has been little improvement in diagnostic accuracy. Clearly there is a task yet to be accomplished.

Beyond improvement of the image itself, which has been accomplished with a CAT scan in a very specialized situation, the effort which should lead to the greatest chance of improvement lies in the area of improving radiologist perception and diagnostic competence. At Missouri, an effort to accomplish better diagnoses through computer assistance in the evaluation of images has been funded by the National Cancer Institute since 1962. In this approach, the radiologist acts as the perceiver of information in the image, and the computer compares the perceived information with known information about frequency of signs in the various disease processes, and classifies the new information to match best with diagnostic possibilities. Since 1970, another effort parallel to the computer-aided diagnostic effort has been to allow the computer to directly examine complex images, with the goal of extracting measurements of size, shape, and texture, which are similarly treated as problems in computer-assisted diagnosis. Both efforts have demonstrated areas of success, and in the instance of computer-assisted diagnosis, practical application.

A basic part of analyzing any image system is the modeling of the image itself. Most of the basic work in image modeling has been accomplished with bone tumors and other kinds of bone disease which must be distinguished from bone tumors. Our first modeling attempts were initiated in 1951 at the Armed Forces Institute of Pathology in Washington, D.C. Throughout the sixties the models of bone disease were refined to their present status. In the context of bone tumors, modeling means that one examines the images of a large number of lesions carefully, dissecting patterns of disease and determining basic variables. One attempts to identify all variables that are present, and to describe and illustrate them to the point where they are understandable by others. With variables clearly identified, their rate of occurence can be studied in different disease states and a probability matrix built from this information. Some modification of Bayes' Rule has been our basic decision rule, and because of the large number of variables involved, a very substantial data base has been necessary. Much of our work throughout the years of dealing with bone tumors has been the collection and organization of an adequate data base.

Once we had established an approximation of a valid probability matrix, an on line interactive and interogative program was developed to ask the radiologist user to identify each variable, which one after another is compared by the computer with the probability matrix to determine the best classification. This kind of approach to diagnosis, with nine disease classes, can yield an accuracy of the order of 90%. However, to be practical, a program must recognize all common diagnoses, which is a problem of an order of magnitude greater than nine classes. In recognition of this basic problem of numbers of classes, limited Bayes concept was evolved to break statistical data into smaller probability sets through the use of decision trees. This narrows the range of possibilities to a number which can be more effectively managed by Bayesian analysis of images.

Using a difficult test set characterized by overlapping patterns, the limited Bayes program has yielded an accuracy rate of approximately 75%. Where the first three choices of the computer were considered, one of the first three choices was the correct diagnosis 95% of the time.

Today, the most important impact of computer-aided diagnosis of bone disease has been 1) identification and illustration of the variables necessary to accurate diagnosis by humans, and 2) establishment of the concept of rate in evaluation of radiant images of bone disease. These have become powerful tools in the human recognition and classification of bone disease and are now widely used. Future efforts are now underway to improve accuracy, speed, and acceptance of computer programs to classify bone disease and to improve data base acquisition processes. We see no reason why the acquisition of the data base needs to be an off line activity, and are developing mechanisms to make the process automatic in the routine work day.

These kinds of activities have renewed interest in bone diagnosis, and have encouraged the development of diagnostic centers where skilled specialists examine problem cases for physicians throughout the United States. One of these centers is the Mid-America Bone Diagnostic Center and Tumor Registry in Columbia. It is a source of constant new experience and knowledge, and a service to our profession.

Additional research of similar nature has been done in the differential diagnosis of gastric ulcers, congenital and acquired heart disease, and pulmonary neoplasms. These programs have been successful in identifying disease with satisfying accuracy, but need to be made available through on line programs to fully exploit their diagnostic usefulness. This remains a problem which we plan to resolve.

REFERENCES
COMPUTER AIDED PROGRAMS

Lodwick, G. S., Haun, C. L., Smith, W. D., Keller, R. F., and Robertson, E. D.: Computer diagnosis of primary bone tumors: A preliminary report, Radiology 80:273, 1963.

Bayes, T.: An essay towards solving a problem in the doctrine of changes, Philosophical Trans. of the Royal Society, Vol. LIII, London, 1763.

Ledley, R. S. and Lusted, L. B.: Reasoning foundations of medical diagnosis: Symbolic logic, probability and value therory aid our understanding of how physicians reason, Science 130:9, 1959.

Wilson, W. J., Templeton, A. W., Turner, A. H., and Lodwick, G. S.: The computer analysis and diagnosis of gastric ulcers, Radiology 85:1064, 1965.

Templeton, A. W., Lehr, J. L., and Simmons, G.: The computer evaluation and diagnosis of congenital heart disease using roentgenographic findings, Radiology 87:658,1966.

Templeton, A. W., Jansen, C., Lehr, J. L. and Hufft, R.: Solitary pulmonary lesions, Radiology 89:605, 1967.

Youker, J. E., Welin, S., and Main, G.: Computer analysis in the differentiation of malignant polypoid lesion of the colon, Radiology 90:794, 1967.

DuBoulay, G. H., and Price, V. E.: Selecting the next neuroradiological investigation with help of a computer, Br. J. Radiol. 44:416, 1971.

Dubost, E., and Bargy, P.: Diagnostic radiologique d'une dysplasie osseuse par un methode informatique, J. Radiol. Electrol. Med. Nucl. 52:181, 1971.

Jeans, W. D.: An evaluation of radiological signs in small bowel examinations in children, Clin. Radiol. 23:78, 1972.

Cover, T. M.: Geometrical and statistical properties of systems of linear inequalities with applications in pattern recognition, IEEE Trans. on Electronic Computers, EC-14:326, 1965.

Lodwick, G. S., and Reichertz, P.: Computer assisted diagnosis of tumors and tumorlike lesions of bone. The limited Bayes' concept, Proc. Symposium Osseum, London, April 1968.

Inamoto, K., Hyogo College of Medicine, Nishinomiya, Japan. Personal communication.

Lodwick, G. S.: Computer Diagnosis in Radiology. Journ. of the Michigan State Medical Society. 61:1239-1242, October, 1962.

Lodwick, G. S., Keats, R. E., and Dorst, J. P.: The coding of roentgen images for computer analysis to lung cancer. Radiology Vol. 81, No. 2, pp. 185-200, August,1963.

Lodwick, G. S.: Computer analysis of tumor roentgenograms. 5th IBM Medical Symposium, Endicott, New York, October, 1963.

Lodwick, G. S.: A systematic approach to the roentgen diagnosis of bone tumors. In Tumors of Bone and Soft Tissue, Year Book Medical Publishers, Inc., pp. 49-68, 1963.

Lodwick, G. S.: Reactive response to local injury in bone. Radiologic Clinics of North America. Vol. II, No. 2, pp. 209-219, August, 1964.

Lodwick, G. S.: Radiographic diagnosis and grading of bone tumors, with comments on computer evaluation. Proceedings of Fifth National Cancer Conference, Philadelphia, September 1964, pp. 369-380, J.B. Lippincott Co.

Lodwick, G. S.: A probabilistic approach to the diagnosis of bone tumors. Radiological Clinics of North America, Vol. III, No. 3, pp. 487-497, December 1965.

Lodwick, G. L.: Solitary malignant tumors of bone: the application predictor variables in diagnosis. Seminars in Roentgenology, Vol. 1, No. 3, pp. 293-313, July 1966.

Lodwick, G. S. and Reichertz, P. L.: Computerunterstutzte diagnostik von TUMOREN und
tumorahnlichen veranderungen des knochens: Das begrenzte Bayes-Konzept. Rontgen-
blatter Heft 4. April 1969, 22. Jahrgang F55935 E.

Lodwick, G. S.: A dynamic atlas of tumors of bones and joints. Published April 15,
1971. Year Book Medical Publishers, Inc.

Automated Image Analysis

The National Institute of General Medical Sciences in 1970 funded a program project entitled "Diagnostic Content and Redundancy in Radiant Images" which has supported work in automation of diagnosis from images, an extremely difficult technical problem. The magnitude of the task of teaching the computer to see and interpret is mind-boggling. However, since we see this technology as an important asset in improving human performance and providing better diagnosis, automated interpretation remains a worthwhile effort. However, we have found it necessary to reduce the scope of problems to be solved to certain specific structures visualized from specific projections. Examples are the heart and vascular structures as seen from the postero anterior position. Less complicated problems are attacked first. It is easier for the computer to see the long sharp lines or gross details than to describe textures. We have focused on solving two-dimensional problems before attempting much more difficult three-dimensional ones. Since the problems of describing the details of automated image analysis are beyond the scope of this manuscript, references made to the progress report of the grant, "Diagnostic Content and Redundancy in Radiant Images," for the period September, 1973, through May, 1975, available on microfilm from Dr. Peter Reichertz. Very extensive and significant bibliography is included at the conclusion of this progress report which covers the subject material well. Reference is also made to a publication concerned with our efforts in automated image analysis at Missouri, from a medical perspective. Our earlier work was to classify various kinds of heart disease according to cardiac size and silhouette. We now are taking a more interactive approach, where the physician outlines the cardiac silhouette with a graf pen, segmenting the silhouette into areas representing the aortic arch, the pulmonary conus and artery, and the left ventricle. Early results with this new approach are yielding sufficient improvement in accuracy of classification results that this approach is being intensively studied. Our program to recognize textures has progressed to the point where we are now able to recognize diminished vascularity, normal vascularity, and increased vascularity with accuracy substantially greater than that of radiologists. We are now interactively outlining disease areas in the pulmonary fields, and are training the computer to recognize differences between normal pulmonary texture, alveolar type infiltrations and interstitial type infiltrations. We plan to bring these technologies into the radiology department where they can be evaluated in the clinical setting.

By way of summary, it is clear that interactive analysis will probably be the major thrust for the immediate future. Total automation of chest film interpretation seems to be beyond the reasonable scope of our project, and we have found it necessary that the problems of automation be broken into manageable segments. The best mechanism for introducing a manageable segment into the clinical domain appears to be through the interactive approach, where the human perceives and asks the computer for help in analyzing a pattern or shape. We are carrying this same approach into a new effort to marry computerized axial tomography to radiation dosimetry and simulation.

REFERENCES

AUTOMATED IMAGE ANALYSIS

LEHR, J.L., PARKEY, R.W., HARLOW, C.A., GAROTTO, L.J., and LODWICK, G.S.: Computer Algorithms for the Detection of Brain Scintigram Abnormalities. Radiology 97, 269-276, (November, 1970).

HALL, E.L., KRUGER, R.P., DWYER, S.J., III., HALL, D.L., McLAREN, R.W., and LODWICK, G.S.: A Survey of Preprocessing and Feature Extraction Techniques for Radiographic Images. IEEE Transactions on Computers, (September, 1971).

HALL, D.L., LODWICK, G.S., KRUGER, R. P., and DWYER, S.J., III.: Computer Diagnosis of Heart Disease. Radiological Clinics of North America, Vol. IX, No. 3, 533-541, (December, 1971). Also Technical Report: Image Analysis Laboratory, Departments of Radiology and Electrical Engineering, University of Missouri-Columbia, Columbia, Missouri, (June, 1971).

HALL, D.L., LODWICK, G.S., KRUGER, R.P., DWYER, S.J., III., and TOWNES, J.R.: Direct Computer Diagnosis of Rheumatic Heart Disease. Radiology, 101, No. 3., 497-509, (December, 1971). Also, Technical Report: Image Analysis Laboratory, Departments of Radiology and Electrical Engineering, University of Missouri-Columbia, Columbia, Missouri, (June, 1971).

HALL, E.L., and KAHVECI, A.E.: High Resolution Image Enhancement Techniques. Proceedings, Two-Dimensional Digital Signal Processing Conference, University of Missouri-Columbia, Columbia, Missouri, pp. 1-5-1, 1-5-9, (October, 1971).

HENDERSON, S.E., HARLOW, C.A., and LODWICK, G.S.: Feature Extraction of Knee X-Rays. Technical Report. Special Issue of IEEE Computers Transactions on Feature Extraction and Selection in Pattern Recognition, (September, 1971).

AUSHERMAN, D.A., DWYER, S.J., III., and LODWICK, G.S.: Feature Extraction for Computer Diagnosis of Primary Bone Tumors. Proceedings, Two-Dimensional Digital Signal Processing Conference, University of Missouri-Columbia, Columbia, Missouri, (October, 1971).

DWYER, S.J., III., HARLOW, C.A., AUSHERMAN, D.A., and LODWICK, G.S.: Computer Diagnosis of Radiographic Images. Proceedings, AFIPS 1972 Spring Joint Computer Conference, Atlantic City, New Jersey, (May, 1972).

AUSHERMAN, D.A., DWYER, S.J., III., and LODWICK, G.S.: Extraction of Connected Edges from Knee Radiographs. IEEE Transactions on Computers, (July, 1972).

KRUGER, R.P., HALL, D.L., LODWICK, G.S., DWYER, S.J., III., and TOWNES, J.R.: Radiographic Diagnosis via Feature Extraction and Classification of Cardiac Size and Shape Descriptors. IEEE Biomedical Transactions, (July, 1972).

EISENBEIS, S.A., OTTO, J., HARLOW, C.A., and DWYER, S.J.,III.: The Analysis of Images in Nuclear Medicine. 18th Annual Meeting, American Nuclear Society, (June, 1972).

DEGROOT, J.M., HALL, E.L., SUTTON, R.N., DWYER, S.J., III., and LODWICK, G.S.: Perception of Computer Simulated Lesions in Chest Radiographs. Proceedings, ACM 1972 Conference.

HENDERSON, S.E., HARLOW, C.A., SCHRUNK, D.G., and LODWICK, G.S.: An Approach to Direct Computer Diagnosis of Knee Radiographs. 3rd Computer Conference, University of Missouri-Columbia, Columbia, Missouri, (September, 1972).

KAHVECI, A., and DWYER, S.J., III.: Automated Lesion Detecting in Lung Cancer. 1972 ACEMB, Bal Harbour, Florida, (October, 1972).

DWYER, S.J., III., HARLOW, C.A., LODWICK, G.S., AUSHERMAN, D.A., BROOKS, R.C., HU, R.T., JAMES, R.V., and McFARLAND, W.D.: Computer Analysis of Radiographic Images. Proceedings, Conference on Applications of Optical Instrumentation in Medicine, Chicago, Illinois, (November, 1972).

EISENBEIS, S.A., HARLOW, C.A., and TSIANG, P.K.: Automated Processing of Radioisotopic Scans. Proceedings, IEEE Conference on Decision and Control, New Orleans, Louisiana, (December, 1972).

HARLOW, C.A., DWYER, S.J., III., and CASTLEMAN, K.: Biomedical Image Processing. ACM Graphics Workshop, Anaheim, California, (December, 1972).

EISENBEIS, S.A., OTTO, J., HARLOW, C.A., and DWYER, S.J., III.: The Analysis of Images in Nuclear Medicine. 18th Annual Meeting, American Nuclear Society, (June, 1972).

HARLOW, C.A., and DWYER, S.J., III.: Medical Image Processing. Image Processing, Coding and Transmission Workshop, Purdue University, (June, 1972).

HENDERSON, S.E., HARLOW, C.A., and LODWICK, G.S.: Computer Analysis of Knee X-Rays. Computer Image Processing and Recognition Conference, University of Missouri-Columbia, Columbia, Missouri, (August, 1972).

HARLOW, C.A., HENDERSON, S.E., and SCHRUNK, D.G.: Direct Computer Diagnosis of Knee X-Rays. Proceedings, 3rd Conference on Computer Applications in Radiology, University of Missouri-Columbia, Columbia, Missouri, (September, 1972).

HARLOW, C.A., and CAUDILL, P.: Computer Software. Proceedings, 3rd Conference on Computer Applications in Radiology, University of Missouri-Columbia, Columbia, Missouri, (September, 1972).

FARRELL, C., LODWICK, G.S., BOURGEOIS, C.H., LEHR, J.L., and MEYER, A.P.: What the Mid-America Bone Diagnostic Center has to offer. University of Missouri-Columbia (August, 1973). Proceedings, XIII International Congress of Radiology, Madrid Spain, (October, 1973).

LODWICK, G.S.: Recent Advances in Computer-Assisted Diagnosis. Proceedings, XIII International Congress of Radiology, Madrid, Spain, (October, 1973).

OESTREICH, A.E., and LODWICK, G.S.: Current Directions in Computer-Enhanced Radiology. Australasian Radiology, Vol. XVIII, No. 4, (December, 1973).

LEHR, J.L.: Automated Image Analysis in the U.S.A.. Proceedings, XIII International Congress of Radiology, Madrid, Spain, (October, 1973). (Abstract published in Excerpta Medica 301:111).

McFARLAND, W.D., and DWYER, S.J., III.: An Interactive Digital Image Display. 1973 Annual Meeting, Missouri Academy on Sciences, Columbia, Missouri, (April, 1973).

McFARLAND, W.D., and DWYER, S.J., III.: An Image Analysis Interactive Display. Society for Information Display International Symposium, New York, (May, 1973).

McFARLAND, W.D., and DWYER, S.J., III.: An Interactive Image Analysis System. Proceedings, Society of Photo-Optical Instrumentation Engineers. Applications of Optical Instrumentation in Medicine II, (November, 1973).

CHANG, J.K., and DWYER, S.J., III.: Rate Distortion Theory and Image Transmission. 1973 Annual Meeting, Missouri Academy of Sciences, Columbia, Missouri, (April, 1973).

CHANG, J.K., and DWYER, S.J., III.: New Multiclass Classification Method: Modified Maximum Likelihood Decision Rule. First International Joint Conference on Pattern Recognition, Washington, D.C., (October 30 - November 1, 1973).

HARLOW, C.A., DWYER, S.J., III., EISENBEIS, S.A., and LODWICK, G.S.: Analysis of Medical Images of Computer. Proceedings, VII International Congress on Cybernetics, Namur, Belgium, (September, 1973).

HARLOW, C.A.: Scene Analysis Techniques and Applications. Joint Meeting Computer/Control Systems Societies Engineering in Medicine and Biology, Dallas, Texas, (April, 1973).

CHANG, J.K., and DWYER, S.J., III.: Error Criterion for Image Quality. Proceedings, Princeton Conference on Information Sciences and Systems, Princeton University, New Jersey, (March, 1973).

ROELLINGER, F.X., Jr., CHANG, J.K., KAHVECI, A.E., DWYER, S.J.,III., and HARLOW, C.A.: Automatic Recognition of Congential Heart Abnormalities via Chest Radiograms. Proceedings, Princeton Conference on Information Sciences and Systems, Princeton University, New Jersey, (March, 1973).

HARLOW, C.A., DWYER, S.J., III., EISENBEIS, S.A., and LODWICK, G.S.: Analysis of Medical Images by Computer. Proceedings, VIII International Congress on Cybernetics, Namur, Belgium, (September, 1973).

HARLOW, C.A., and PREWITT, J.: Medical Graphics. SHARE XL, Denver, Colorado, (March, 1973).

HARLOW, C.A., DWYER, S.J., III., EISENBEIS, S.A., and LODWICK, G.S.: Digital Processing of Radiograms Utilizing Graphical Models and Shape Descriptors. Proceedings, 1973 International Symposium on Circuit Theory, Toronto, Canada, (April, 1973).

HARLOW, C.A., and EISENBEIS, S.A.: The Analysis of Radiographic Images. IEEE Transactions on Computers, (June, 1973).

HARLOW C.A.,: Approaches to Medical and Industrial Image Analysis Problems. Proceedings, U.S.-Japan Seminar on Picture and Scene Analysis, Kyoto, Japan, (July, 1973).

HARLOW, C.A., and LEE, S.M.: Boundary Detection of Chest Radiographs. Proceedings, First International Symposium on Computers and Chinese I/O Systems, Taiwan, Formosa, (August, 1973).

HARLOW, C.A.: Image Analysis and Graphs. Computer Graphics and Image Processing, Vol. 2, No. 1, 60-72, (August, 1973).

BROOKS, R.C., DWYER, S.J., III., and LODWICK, G.S.: Computer Diagnosis of Congenital Heart Disease using Discriminant Functions. Technical Report IAL-TR 25-73. Image Analysis Laboratory, University of Missouri-Columbia, Columbia, Missouri, (December, 1973).

LODWICK, G.S.: Information Management in Radiology. In Hospital Computer Systems: How to use Computers in Medical Centers for Better Patient Care. (Morris F. Collen, ed.) New York: John Wiley and Sons, 1974, 206-240.

LODWICK, G.S.,: The L-Bayes Concept. Presented at the Association of European Radiologists, Proceedings, Symposium Computers in Diagnostic Radiology, The Hague, Netherlands, (June, 1974). LEHR, J.L.: Computer and Effectivity of Department. Presented at the Association of European Radiologists, Proceedings, Symposium Computers in Diagnostic Radiology. The Hague, Netherlands, (June, 1974).

LEHR, J.L.: How and Why of Computer Applications in Radiology. Proceedings, Forty-Seventh Annual Clinical Assembly of Osteopathic Specialists, Bal Harbour, Florida, (October, 1974).

CHANG, J.K., and DWYER, S.J., III.: New Approach to Measurement Selection in Pattern Recognition. Second International Joint Conference on Pattern Recognition, Lyngby-Copenhagen, Denmark, (August, 1974).

TSIANG, P.K., HARLOW, C.A., and LODWICK, G.S.: The Computer Analysis of Chest Radiographs. Proceedings, ACM 1972 Conference, San Diego, California, (November, 1974).

BROOKS, R.C., DWYER, S.J.,III., and LODWICK, G.S.: Computer Diagnosis of Congenital Heart Disease. Proceedings, Systems, Man and Cybernetics 1974, International Conference, IEEE, Dallas, Texas, (October, 1974).

TSIANG, P.K., HARLOW, C.A., and DWYER, S.J., III.: Computer Analysis of Chest Radiographs using Size and Shape Descriptors. IAL-TR 39-74 (December, 1974).

LODWICK, G.S., : The Application of Computers in Diagnostic Radiology. Current Problems in Radiology. Year Book Medical Publishers Inc., (January-February, 1975).

LODWICK, G.S., and OESTREICH, A.E.: Extended Application of L-Bayes to the Diagnosis of Bone Disease. Proceedings, Fourth Conference on Computer Applications in Radiology, Las Vegas, Nevada, (March, 1975).

LEHR, J.L., SCHRUNK, D.G., LODWICK, G.S., McFARLAND, W.D., MOORE, G., KAHVECI, A., DWYER, S.J., III., HARLOW, C.A., and CONNERS, R.: Automated Analysis of Plain Chest Roentgenograms in Congenital Heart Disease. Proceedings, San Diego Biomedical Symposium, San Diego, California, (February, 1975).

SCHRUNK, D.G., LEHR, J.L., LODWICK, G.S., McFARLAND, W.D., MOORE, G., KAHVECI, A., DWYER, S.J., III., HARLOW, C.A., and CONNERS, R.: Automated Diagnosis of Congenital Heart Disease from Chest Roentgenograms: Comparisons and Evaluation. Proceedings, Fourth Conference on Computer Applications in Radiology, Las Vegas, Nevada, (March, 1975).

McCRACKEN, T.E., DWYER, S.J., III., and SHERMAN, B.W.: An Economical Tonal Display for Interactive Graphics and Image Analysis. ACM Conference on Interactive Graphics, Denver, Colorado (July, 1974). British Journal of Graphics, (April, 1975).

GLENN, W.V., JOHNSTON, R.J., MORTON, P.E., and DWYER, S.J., III.: Image Generation and Display Techniques for CT Scan Data, Thin Transverse and Reconstructed Coronal and Sagittal Planes. CT International Conference, (March, 1975).

LUSTED, L.B.: Diagnostic Video Data Processing, IRE Trans. on Medical Electronics, ME-7:293, (1960).

MEYERS, P.H., BECKER, H.C., SWEENEY, J.W., NICE, C.M., and NETTLETON, W.J., Jr.: Evaluation of a Computer-Retrieved Radiographic Image, Radiology 81,201, (1963).

BECKER, H.C., NETTLETON, W.J., Jr., and MEYERS, P.H.: Digital Computer Determination of a Medical Diagnostic Index Directly from a Chest X-Ray Image. IEEE Trans. Bio.Med. Engin. 11,67, (1963).

WINSBERG, F., and MACY, J., Jr.: Detection of Radiographic Abnormalities in Mammograms by Means of Optical Scanning and Computer Analysis. Proceedings, Conference on the Use of Computers in Radiology, University of Chicago, (October, 1966).

SELZER, R.: Improving Biomedical Image Quality With Computers. Jet Propulsian Lab., California Institute of Technology. Pasadena, California, Technical Report.

TORIWAKI, J., SUENAGA, Y., NEGORO, T., and FUKUMURA, T.: Pattern Recognition of Chest X-Ray Images. Computer Graphics and Image Processing, 2,252, (1973).

IDSTROM, L.G., DODD, G.D., and O'DONNEL, E.H.,: Image Enhancement of Radiograph by Digital Computer. Work in Progress. Radiological Society of North America, Chicago, (November - December, 1974).

KIMME, C., O'LOUGHLIN, B.J., and SKLANSKY, J.: Finding Abnormalities in Breast Xerograms by Computer. University of California, (in preparation).

KRUGER, R.P., THOMPSON, W.B., and TURNER, A.F.: Computer Diagnosis of Pneumoconiosis, IEEE Trans. on Systems, Man and Cybernetics, 40-49, (1974).

Evaluation of Image Content

Modern technology offers a variety of methods by which radiographic images may
be manipulated in order to increase their value. These include photographic reduction
of ordinary films into one of several formats which may be more convenient to handle,
copy, or store, as well as digital and television techniques for enhancing storing
transmitting images. Although such systems may improve the availability of images
or even decrease the overall cost of maintaining film files, by altering the original
roentgenograms they also run the risk of reducing the diagnostic information contained
in the images. Physical measurements such as modulation transfer function have been
employed to compare the fidelity of imaging systems or to assist in the design of
such systems. However, the measurements do not provide an answer to the basic question
of how well radiologists will be able to interpret the altered image as compared with
the original.

At the University of Missouri, a major interdisciplinary effort has been directed
at developing a method of evaluating the effect of altering an image system on the
radiologist's diagnostic ability. We have completed this four year effort of 1)
establishing a 5000 case data base, 2) copying the data base on the test medium, in
this instance a high quality 35mm film and display system, 3) establishing a logical
and statistically valid double blind testing procedure where diagnostic accuracy of
radiologist terms is measured in both media, 4) carrying the testing procedure to
the point where the results are accepted as statistically valid. This work has now
been completed and published as a direct method of measuring the effect of image minia-
turization on diagnostic accuracy.

In order to develop this new technology, we chose to examine a miniature imaging
system of very high quality which was under experimental production. For this particular system, the double blind study demonstrated that the error resulting from interpreting miniature redisplayed images lies somewhere between zero and 4.6%. A total
of 4,290 readings comprised the data base.

Comparisons of accuracy rates, timing data, suggestions for future work, and a
presentation of the statistical logic are included in the study. It is recommended
that the interested reader review the original article and its references for the
detailed presentation.

By way of final comment, application of this double blind technology to determining intelligence content of similar image systems may require a large number of read-

ings, reaching to infinity in identical systems. Where one imaging system is much less effective than another, only a small number of readings may be required to measure the difference. On the other hand, some kinds of images are much less challenging to a display system than others, as for example, nuclear medicine images as compared with chest films. Future possible applications include evaluation of digital image transmission and storage systems, where possible loss of diagnostic information may need to be measured against the advantage of speed and convenience.

REFERENCES
EVALUATION OF IMAGE CONTENT

Montgomery, W. J.: Improved radiograph file management through minification. Presented at the Association of Hospital Radiology Administrators Convention, New Orleans,
LA., Sept. 11, 1973.

Proceedings of the Symposium on X-Ray Records with Speical Reference to Film Copies.
London, Royal College of Surgeons, May 16, 1974.

Nealon, J. V.: Kodak RETNAR Products for Minification of Radiographs. Proceedings
of the Society of Photo-Optical Instrumentation Engineers, Chicago, IL, 43:29-30,
November 1973.

Revesz, G., Kundel, H.: Transmission of radiographic images via closed circuit and
microwave television techniques. Invest. Radiol. 8:392-395, Nov-Dec, 1973.

Lester, R. G., O'Foghludha, F., Prter, F., et al: Transmission of radiologic information by satellite. Radiology 109:731, Dec 1973.

Lehr, J. L., Lodwick, G. S., Nicholson, B. F., et al: Experience with MARS (Missouri
Automated Radiology System). Radiology 106:289-294, Feb. 1973.

Smith, M. J.: Error and variation in diagnostic radiology. Springfield, IL. Thomas,
1967.

Herman, P. G., Hessel, S. J.: Accuracy and its relationship to experience in the
interpretation of chest radiographs, Invest. Radiol. 10:62-67, Jan-Feb, 1975.

De Palma, J. J., Lwerey, E. M.: Sine-wave response of the visual systems. 11. Sine-
wave and square-wave contrast sensitivity. J. Optic Soc. Am. 52:328-335, March 1962.

Lowrey, E. M., De Palma, J. J.: Sine-wave response of the visual system. I. The
mach phenomenon. J. Optic Soc. Am. 51:740-746. July 1961.

Lehr, J. L., Lodwick, G. S., et al.: Direct measurement of the effect of film mini-
atureization on diagnostic accuracy. Radiology 118:257-263, February 1976.